Chronic Illness

Impact and Intervention

Seventh Edition

Ilene Morof Lubkin, RN, MS, CGNP
Professor Emeritus
California State University
Hayward, California

and

Pamala D. Larsen, PhD, RN, CRRN, FNGNA
Associate Dean and Professor
Fay W. Whitney School of Nursing
University of Wyoming
Laramie, Wyoming

JONES AND BARTLETT PUBLISHERS
Sudbury, Massachusetts
BOSTON   TORONTO   LONDON   SINGAPORE

World Headquarters

Jones and Bartlett Publishers
40 Tall Pine Drive
Sudbury, MA 01776
978-443-5000
info@jbpub.com
www.jbpub.com

Jones and Bartlett Publishers
Canada
6339 Ormindale Way
Mississauga, Ontario
L5V IJ2
Canada

Jones and Bartlett Publishers
International
Barb House, Barb Mews
London W6 7PA
United Kingdom

Jones and Bartlett's books and products are available through most bookstores and online booksellers. To contact Jones and Bartlett Publishers directly, call 800-832-0034, fax 978-443-8000, or visit our website www.jbpub.com.

Substantial discounts on bulk quantities of Jones and Bartlett's publications are available to corporations, professional associations, and other qualified organizations. For details and specific discount information, contact the special sales department at Jones and Bartlett via the above contact information or send an email to specialsales@jbpub.com.

The authors, editor, and publisher have made every effort to provide accurate information. However, they are not responsible for errors, omissions, or for any outcomes related to the use of the contents of this book and take no responsibility for the use of the products and procedures described. Treatments and side effects described in this book may not be applicable to all people; likewise, some people may require a dose or experience a side effect that is not described herein. Drugs and medical devices are discussed that may have limited availability controlled by the Food and Drug Administration (FDA) for use only in a research study or clinical trial. Research, clinical practice, and government regulations often change the accepted standard in this field. When consideration is being given to use of any drug in the clinical setting, the health care provider or reader is responsible for determining FDA status of the drug, reading the package insert, and reviewing prescribing information for the most up-to-date recommendations on dose, precautions, and contraindications, and determining the appropriate usage for the product. This is especially important in the case of drugs that are new or seldom used.

Production Credits
Publisher: Kevin Sullivan
Aquisitions Editor: Emily Ekle
Aquisitions Editor: Amy Sibley
Associate Editor: Patricia Donnelly
Editorial Assistant: Rachel Shuster
Associate Production Editor: Amanda Clerkin
Associate Marketing Manager: Rebecca Wasley
V.P., Manufacturing and Inventory Control: Therese Connell
Composition and Content Management Services: Newgen North America
Cover Design: Kristin E. Ohlin
Cover Image Credit: © Jeffrey Clattenburg/Dreamstime.com.
Printing and Binding: Malloy, Inc.
Cover Printing: Malloy, Inc.

Library of Congress Cataloging-in-Publication Data
Chronic illness : impact and intervention / Pamala D. Larsen,
Ilene Lubkin.—7th ed.
    p. ; cm.
  Includes bibliographical references and index.
  ISBN-13: 978-0-7637-5126-5 (alk. paper)
  ISBN-10: 0-7637-5126-X (alk. paper)
  1. Chronic diseases–Psychological aspects. 2. Chronic diseases—
Nursing. 3. Chronically ill–Family relationships. 4. Nurse and patient.
I. Larsen, Pamala D., 1958– II. Lubkin, Ilene Morof, 1928–2005
  [DNLM: 1. Chronic Disease—psychology. 2. Professional-Family
Relations. 3. Professional-Patient Relations. WT 500 C5577 2009]
RC108.L83 2009
616·044—dc22
                                        2008042656
6048

Printed in the United States of America
13 12 11 10 09   10 9 8 7 6 5 4 3 2

To my grandchildren,

Cody and Kai Larsen,

Jonah and Landon Fanning,

and

Abby and Carter Larsen

This text was developed by and originated with Ilene Morof Lubkin in 1986 and was the first work of its kind to address the psychosocial concepts of chronic illness. Pamala Larsen joined the project in its 4th edition in 1998. It remains a landmark work in the health care field.

CONTENTS

Our country has achieved great things, but providing *access* to health care and *quality* care for all continues to be an issue. The United States leads the world in total health expenditures, with $5,711 spent per capita per year (2003 data) as compared to countries such as the United Kingdom, US $2,317; Japan, $2,249; Canada, $2,998; France, $3,048; and Switzerland, $3,847. Although some of the lower amounts spent in other countries can be attributed to socialized medicine, others cannot. Perhaps we could justify our high cost of health care if we had consistently positive health outcomes for our citizens; unfortunately, this is not the case. Two health outcomes of the population are particularly troubling. Currently, citizens of 41 other countries have a higher life expectancy than those in the United States, and 20 countries have a lower infant mortality rate than we do. So what does one get for $5,711?

Chronic disease accounts for 75–80% of our healthcare costs. The percentage of the aging population of the United States continues to grow faster than other population groups; the first baby boomers will be eligible for Medicare in 2011, and we need to be creative in our approaches to caring for those with chronic conditions. To date, few models have been developed to address the needs of individuals with chronic illness and their families; there are models that address the *disease* process, but not the *illness* experience. Those of us who are passionate about caring for such individuals and families want to improve the situation now, with our generation. But there are no easy solutions on the horizon. Can a new president and his administration effect change in our healthcare system to provide better access to care and quality care for those with chronic illness? I would like to believe that change can happen; however, the complexity of the healthcare system and its payment systems seems overwhelming. Caring for someone with chronic illness is *nursing*, not medicine. It is nursing's domain of practice. If only we could provide a nurse to every individual with chronic illness . . . What better care management could there be?

Pamala D. Larsen

CONTRIBUTORS

Susan J. Barnes, PhD, RN
Chair, Graduate and Continuing Education
Kramer School of Nursing
Oklahoma City University
Oklahoma City, Oklahoma

Jill Berg, PhD, RN
Associate Professor
Program in Nursing Science
University of California, Irvine
Irvine, California

Diana Luskin Biordi, PhD, RN, FAAN
Associate Dean for Nursing Research and
    Scholarship
College of Nursing
University of Akron
Akron, Ohio

Donna Carruthers, PhD, RN
Assistant Professor
School of Nursing
University of Pittsburgh
Pittsburgh, Pennsylvania

Jacqueline M. Dunbar-Jacob, PhD, RN, FAAN
Dean, School of Nursing
Professor, Nursing, Psychology, Epidemiology and
    Occupational Therapy
Director, Center for Research in Chronic Disorders
University of Pittsburgh
Pittsburgh, Pennsylvania

Lorraine S. Evangelista, PhD, RN
Assistant Professor
School of Nursing
University of California, Los Angeles
Los Angeles, California

Sonya R. Hardin, PhD, RN, CCRN, ACNS-BC
Associate Professor
School of Nursing
University of North Carolina at Charlotte
Charlotte, North Carolina

Judith E. Hertz, PhD, RN
Associate Professor
School of Nursing and Health Studies
Northern Illinois University
DeKalb, Illinois

Alicia Huckstadt, PhD, RN, ARNP, FNP-BC,
    GNP-BC
Professor and Graduate Program Director
School of Nursing
Wichita State University
Wichita, Kansas

Faye I. Hummel, PhD, RN, CTN
Professor
School of Nursing
University of Northern Colorado
Greeley, Colorado

Cynthia S. Jacelon, PhD, RN, CRRN-A
Associate Professor
School of Nursing
University of Massachusetts,
    Amherst
Amherst, Massachusetts

Pamala D. Larsen, PhD, RN, CRRN, FNGNA
Associate Dean and Professor
Fay W. Whitney School of Nursing
University of Wyoming
Laramie, Wyoming

Ilene Morof Lubkin, RN, MS, CGNP
Professor Emeritus
California State University
Hayward, California

Barbara J. Lutz, PhD, RN, CRRN
Assistant Professor
College of Nursing
University of Florida
Gainesville, Florida

Kristen L. Mauk, PhD, RN, CRRN-A,
    GCNS-BC
Professor of Nursing
Kreft Chair for the Advancement of Nursing
    Science
Valparaiso University
Valparaiso, Indiana

Elaine T. Miller, DNS, RN, FAAN
Professor of Nursing
Coordinator, Center for Aging with
    Dignity
College of Nursing
University of Cincinnati
Cincinnati, Ohio

Nicholas R. Nicholson, Jr., MS, RN, MPH,
    PHCNS-BC
Doctoral Student
Yale University
New Haven, Connecticut

Lisa L. Onega, PhD, RN, APN, CNS-BC,
    FNP-BC, GNP-BC
Professor
School of Nursing
Radford University
Radford, Virginia

Linda L. Pierce, PhD, RN, CNS, CRRN, FAHA
Professor
College of Nursing
The University of Toledo
Toledo, Ohio

Barbara M. Raudonis, PhD, RN
Associate Professor
School of Nursing
University of Texas at Arlington
Arlington, Texas

Victoria Schirm, PhD, RN
Director of Nursing Research
Department of Nursing
Penn State Milton S. Hershey Medical Center
Hershey, Pennsylvania

Betty Smith-Campbell, PhD, RN
Associate Professor
School of Nursing
Wichita State University
Wichita, Kansas

James R. Steele, MSN, RN, ANP-C
Clinical Associate Professor
College of Nursing
East Carolina University
Greenville, North Carolina

Linda L. Steele, PhD, RN, APRN, ANP, BC
Associate Professor
Director, FNP/ANP Programs
College of Nursing
East Carolina University
Greenville, North Carolina

Diane L. Stuenkel, EdD, RN
Professor
School of Nursing
San José State University
San José, California

Margaret Chamberlain Wilmoth, PhD,
   RN, MSS, FAAN
Professor
School of Nursing
University of North Carolina at Charlotte
Charlotte, North Carolina

Vivian K. Wong, PhD, RN
Associate Professor
School of Nursing
San José State University
San José, California

I

Impact of the Disease

1

Chronicity

Pamala D. Larsen

INTRODUCTION

In 2005 it was estimated that there were 133 million individuals living with at least one chronic disease [Centers for Disease Control and Prevention (CDC), 2008a], and that 7 of every 10 Americans who die each year, or more than 1.7 million people, die of a chronic disease. Chronic disease accounts for one third of the years of potential life lost before age 65. However, perhaps more sobering are the CDC's (2008a) data that have quantified the costs from chronic disease.

- The direct and indirect costs of diabetes is $174 billion per year
- In 2008, the cost of heart disease and stroke is projected to be $448 billion
- Cancer costs the United States $89 billion annually in direct medical costs; and finally
- The medical costs of people with chronic disease account for more than 75% of the nation's $2 trillion medical care costs each year (CDC, 2008a)

These facts indicate that chronic disease is the nation's greatest healthcare problem and the number one driver of health care today. With our aging population and our advanced technologies that assist clients in living longer lives, the costs will only increase.

The prevalence of chronic disease worldwide is similar if not greater than that of chronic disease in the United States. Chronic diseases are the leading cause of death in the world (World Health Organization [WHO], 2005a; Yach, Hawkes, Gould, & Hofman, 2004). Twenty percent of chronic disease deaths occur in high-income countries, whereas the remaining 80% occur in low- and middle-income countries, where most of the world's population resides (WHO, 2005, p. 18–20).

There is a wide variety of conditions that are considered chronic, and with each condition a diverse array of services is needed to care for these individuals. For example, consider clients with Alzheimer's disease, cerebral palsy, heart disease, acquired immunodeficiency syndrome (AIDS), or spinal cord injury; each of these clients has unique physical needs, and each would need different types of services from a healthcare system that is currently attuned to delivering acute care.

The first baby boomer turns 65 in 2011, and this anticipated event has focused increased attention on the capabilities of the healthcare system. The Baby Boomer generation, in particular, has been vocal about the inability of the healthcare system to meet current needs, let alone future needs.

The influx of baby boomers into organizations such as AARP has distinctly flavored the activities of that organization. In addition, this new group of seniors will be the most ethnically and racially diverse of any previous generation (National Center for Health Statistics, 2007). In 2003, 83% of American older adults were non-Hispanic white; by 2030 that percentage will decrease to 72% (CDC & Merck Company, 2007). Unfortunately, the healthcare disparities that we have seen in the past with regard to ethnic and racial groups are not decreasing, but increasing. The 2007 National Health Disparities Report found that across all core measures, the number of measures of quality and access where disparities existed in 2000 to 2001 grew larger in 2004 to 2005 (Agency for Healthcare Research and Quality [AHRQ], 2008). How will the current system or a future system cope with this diverse group of seniors and their accompanying chronic conditions?

Multiple factors have produced the increasing number of individuals with chronic disease. Developments in the fields of public health, bacteriology, immunology, and pharmacology have led to a significant decrease in mortality from acute disease. Medical success has contributed, in part, to the unprecedented growth of chronic illness by extending life expectancy and by earlier detection of disease in general. Living longer, however, leads to greater vulnerability to the occurrence of accidents and disease events that can become chronic in nature. The client who may have died from a myocardial infarction in earlier years now needs continuing health care for heart failure. The cancer survivor has healthcare needs related to the iatrogenic results of life-saving treatment. The adolescent, who is a quadriplegic because of an accident, may live a relatively long life with our current rehabilitation efforts, but needs continuous preventive and maintenance care from the healthcare system. Children with cystic fibrosis have benefitted from lung transplantation, but need care for the rest of their lives. Therefore, many previously fatal conditions, injuries, and diseases have become chronic in nature.

Disease versus Illness

Although the terms, disease and illness, are often used interchangeably by healthcare professionals, there is a distinguishable difference between them. Disease refers to a condition that is viewed from a pathophysiologic model, such as an alteration in structure and function. Illness, on the other hand, is the human experience of symptoms and suffering, and refers to how the disease is perceived, lived with, and responded to by individuals and their families. Although it is important to recognize the pathophysiologic process of a chronic disease, understanding the illness experience is essential in providing holistic care.

> I put my elbows on my knees and let my forehead sink into my palms. I'm tired. Not just tired...weary. My husband's catheter went AWOL at one in the morning, and we've spent the rest of the night in the ER (How many nights does that make, now? How many hours?) Noise and cold and too-bright lights and too-bright student doctors. Repeating Bruce's history, over and over (Harleman, 2008).

This excerpt from an article chronicles part of the illness experience for this caregiver and her husband with multiple sclerosis. The illness experience is nursing's domain. Therefore, the focus of this book is on the illness experience of individuals and families, and not specific disease processes.

Acute Conditions versus Chronic Conditions

When an individual develops an acute disease, there is typically a sudden onset, with signs and symptoms related to the disease process itself. Acute diseases end in a relatively short time, either with recovery and resumption of prior activities, or with death.

Chronic illness, on the other hand, continues indefinitely. Although a welcome alternative to death in most, but not all cases, the illness is often seen as a mixed blessing to the individual and to society at large. In addition, the illness often becomes the person's identity. For example, an individual having any kind of cancer, even in remission, acquires the label of "that person with cancer" (see Chapter 3).

Chronic conditions take many forms, and there is no single onset pattern. A chronic disease can appear suddenly or through an insidious process, have episodic flare-ups or exacerbations, or remain in remission with an absence of symptoms for long periods. Maintaining wellness or keeping symptoms in remission is a juggling act of balancing treatment regimens while focusing on quality of life.

Defining Chronicity

Defining chronicity is complex. Many individuals have attempted to present an all-encompassing definition of chronic illness (Table 1-1). Initially, the characteristics of chronic diseases were identified by the Commission on Chronic Illness as all impairments or deviations from normal that included one or more of the following: permanency; residual disability; non-pathologic alteration; required rehabilitation; or a long period of supervision, observation, and care (Mayo, 1956). The National Conference on Care of the Long-Term Patient added a time dimension to these characteristics: chronic disease or impairment necessitating acute hospitalization exceeding 30 days, or medical supervision and rehabilitation of 3 months or longer in another care setting (Roberts, 1954).

The extent of a chronic disease further complicates attempts in defining the term. Disability may depend not only on the kind of condition and its severity, but also on the implications it holds for the person. A teenager may require greater adjustment than an older adult to the limitations necessitated by bone cancer. The degree of disability and altered life style, part of traditional definitions, may relate more to the client's *perceptions and beliefs* about the disease than to the disease itself.

Long-term and iatrogenic effects of some treatment may constitute chronic conditions in

TABLE 1-1

Definitions of Chronic Disease and Chronic Illness

Author	Definitions
Commission on Chronic Diseases (1956)	All impairments or deviations from normal that have one or more characteristics: are permanent, leave residual disability, are caused by nonreversible pathologic alteration, require special training of the patient for rehabilitation, and may be expected to require a long period of supervision, observation, or care
Feldman (1974) [summarized]	Ongoing medical condition with spectrum of social, economic, and behavioral complications that require meaningful and continuous personal and professional involvement [summarized]
Cluff (1981)	A condition not cured by medical intervention, requiring periodic monitoring and supportive care to reduce the degree of illness, maximize the person's functioning and their responsibility for self-care [summarized]
Curtin & Lubkin (1995)	Chronic illness is the irreversible presence, accumulation, or latency of disease states or impairments that involve the total human environment for supportive care and self-care, maintenance of function, and prevention of further disability

their own right, making them eligible to be defined as a chronic illness. For example, this situation is represented by the changes in lifestyle required of clients receiving hemodialysis for end-stage renal disease (ESRD). Life-saving procedures can create other problems. For instance, abdominal radiation that arrested metastatic intestinal cancer when an individual was 30 years of age can contribute to a malabsorption problem years later, so that continuous diarrhea results in a now cachectic and exhausted person. Chemotherapy or radiation given to a client for an initial bout with cancer may be an influencing factor in the development of leukemia years later.

Chronic illness, by its very nature, is never completely cured. Biologically the human body wears out unevenly. Medical advances cause older adults to need a progressively wider variety of specialized services for increasingly complicated conditions. In the words of Emanuel (1982), "Life is the accumulation of chronic illness beneath the load of which we eventually succumb" (p. 502).

Although definitions of chronic disease are important, from a nursing perspective, we are far more interested in how the illness is affecting the client and family. What is the illness experience of the client and family? Price (1996) suggests that the onus of defining chronic illness, and similarly, quality of life and comfort should be that of the client's, as only the client truly understands illness. However, that aside, the following definition of chronic illness is offered:

> Chronic illness is the irreversible presence, accumulation, or latency of disease states or impairments that involve the total human environment for supportive care and self-care, maintenance of function, and prevention of further disability (Curtin & Lubkin, 1995, pp. 6–7).

IMPACT OF CHRONIC ILLNESS

This section addresses the influence of chronic illnesses and their impact on society in general.

Other chapters in the book address the effect on the individual and family, for example, stigma, social isolation, and body image.

The Older Adult

Although chronic diseases and conditions exist in children, adolescents, and young and middle-aged adults, the bulk of these conditions occur in adults age 65 years and older. Julie Gerberding, Director of the CDC states "the aging of the US population is one of the major public health challenges we face in the 21st century" (CDC & Merck Company, 2007). In 2006 persons older than 65 years of age numbered 37.3 million, and represented 12.4% of Americans (Administration on Aging, 2007). Since 1900, the percentage of older Americans has tripled. By 2030 there will be 71.5 million adults in the United States who are older than age 65 years, nearly double the current number and roughly 20% of the US population (CDC & Merck Company, 2007). The longer life spans of Americans and the aging baby boomers are contributing to these demographic changes.

The *State of Aging and Health in America 2007* (CDC & Merck Company, 2007) reports that 80% of older Americans have at least one chronic health condition. The most frequently occurring conditions in 2004 to 2005 included hypertension (48%); diagnosed arthritis (47%); all types of heart disease (29%); any cancer (20%); diabetes (16%); and sinusitis (14%) (Administration on Aging, 2007). Medicare data document that 83% of all of their beneficiaries have at least one chronic condition (Anderson, 2005). However, 23% of Medicare beneficiaries with five or more conditions account for 68% of the program's funding (Anderson, 2005, p. 305).

A compounding factor in the physical health of older adults is the presence of depression, the occurrence of which is increasing in the older population. Himelhoch, Weller, Wu, Anderson, and Cooper (2004) analyzed data in a randomized sample of 1,238,895 Medicare recipients, with 60,382 of those clients meeting the criteria for a depressive syndrome. For each of eight chronic medical conditions, Medicare beneficiaries with a depressive syndrome were at least twice as likely to use emergency department services and medical inpatient hospital services as those without depression (Himelhoch et al., 2004, p. 512).

As people age, it is clear they will have more chronic conditions and will access, if their socioeconomic status permits, an acute care system. What will the needs of these aging adults mean to our healthcare delivery system? As mentioned previously, there is evidence of growing inequities in healthcare services that racial and ethnic minorities receive. Combine those inequities with being an older adult, and there is a significant population that will be without quality health care or perhaps any health care.

Lynn and Adamson (2003, p. 9) discuss a trajectory model of caring for older adults with serious chronic illnesses. The first trajectory is the "short period of evident decline." A chronic condition most typical of this trajectory is cancer. Individuals are treated initially, but when the illness becomes overwhelming, patients cease treatment and hospice care is a common end result of this trajectory.

The second trajectory is "long-term limitations with intermittent exacerbations and sudden dying." This type of trajectory is common with individuals who have organ system failure. Disease management, advance care planning, and mobilizing services to home are key to care. The last trajectory is "prolonged dwindling." Conditions typical of this trajectory are dementia, disabling stroke, and frailty (Lynn & Adamson, 2003, p. 9).

Lynn and Adamson's (2003) trajectory is different from how older adults with chronic illness were viewed previously. Typically there was a steep decline in health status, and older adults either got better or died. However, even the concept of dying has become less clear (p. 8). With more advanced technology and further developments in palliative care, there may not be an identified "time" that we can determine when a client is "terminally ill," and will thus move into the hospice trajectory. Lynn

and Adamson (2003) state that older adults with chronic illness should expect the following from a care system: correct medical treatment, reliable symptom relief, no gaps in care, no surprises in the course of care, customized care, consideration for family situation, and help as needed to make the best of every day (p. 15).

The Healthcare Delivery System

The current healthcare system was largely designed and shaped in the two decades following World War II (Lynn & Adamson, 2003). In 1946, Congress passed P.L. 79-725, the Hospital Survey and Construction Act, sponsored by Senators Lister Hill and Harold Burton. The Hill-Burton Act was designed to provide Federal grants to modernize hospitals that had become obsolete, owing to lack of capital investment throughout the Great Depression and World War II (1929 to 1945). The healthcare system was designed to provide acute, episodic, and curative care, and it was never intended to address the needs of individuals with chronic conditions. At the time, little, if any, thought was given to what "future patients" would look like. Generally, our present healthcare delivery system provides acute care effectively and efficiently. However, it is based on a component style of care in which each component or care setting of the system is reimbursed separately, that is, hospital, home care, physician visit. Each component of the healthcare system views the client through its narrow window of care. No one entity, practice, institution, or agency is managing the entire disease, and is certainly not managing the illness experience of the client and family. No one component is responsible for the overall care of the individual, only their own independent component of care. Typically this approach produces higher costs for the client.

The current healthcare delivery system is disease oriented. Clients need to fit within the "standards of care," or the algorithm of a specific disease. With diagnosis-related groups (DRGs), payment is predetermined according to diagnosis as opposed to how many services are used. Let's apply an older adult to this scenario: Mr. Jones, with several comorbidities, enters the acute care institution. His admitting diagnosis is pneumonia, but now his diabetes is flaring up along with his hypertension, and his kidneys are not working as well as they should. A specialty physician is treating each of his chronic conditions, but there is no coordinator of his care. He is taking multiple medications, and soon he becomes confused and incontinent. What does our acute care system do with this older adult with multiple chronic health problems? In addition, the focus of the acute care facility is the disease processes of this individual and not the illness experience of the patient and his elderly wife. How does our healthcare delivery system care for Mr. Jones and the multitude of others like him on the horizon?

Healthy People 2010

The effect of chronic disease across the United States has prompted a national approach to prevention and management of chronic disease. *Healthy People 2000* and now *Healthy People 2010* are the result of the influence of chronic disease, but they are also interventions to the problems of chronic illness.

The objectives of *Healthy People 2010* are based on two overarching goals: (1) increase the quality and years of healthy life; and (2) eliminate health disparities among subgroups of the population. These goals are being monitored through 467 objectives in 28 focus areas. Many of the objectives focus on interventions designed to reduce or eliminate illness, disabilities, and premature death among individuals and communities. Furthermore, many of the focus areas relate to chronic disease and/or prevention of chronic disease (Table 1-2).

Quality of Care

In 1996 the Institute of Medicine (IOM) initiated a focus on assessing and improving the quality of care in the United States. A number of documents and/or books have evolved from that initiative.

TABLE 1-2
Healthy People 2010 Focus Areas

Access to quality health services
Arthritis, osteoporosis, and chronic back disorders
Cancer
Chronic kidney disease
Diabetes
Disability and secondary conditions
Educational and community-based programs
Environmental health
Family planning
Food safety
Health communication
Heart disease and stroke
HIV
Immunization and infectious diseases
Injury and violence prevention
Maternal, infant, and child health
Medical product safety
Mental health and mental disorders
Nutrition and overweight
Occupational safety and health
Oral health
Physical activity and fitness
Public health infrastructure
Respiratory diseases
Sexually transmitted diseases
Substance abuse
Tobacco use
Vision and hearing

Source: Department of Health and Human Services. (2000). *Healthy People 2010. A systematic approach to health improvement.* Retrieved from http://www.health.gov/healthypeople/Document/html/uih/uih_2.htm

Perhaps the most known of those include *Crossing the Quality Chasm* (released in March of 2001) and *To Err is Human* (released in November of 1999). The intent of these documents and others was to improve the health outcomes of individuals in the nation. The IOM's definition of quality is "the degree to which health services for individuals and populations increased the likelihood of desired health outcomes and are consistent with current professional knowledge" (IOM, 2006). Since 2003, the AHRQ with the Department of Health and Human Services (DHHS) has reported on quality measures. The National Healthcare Quality Report (NHQR) examines 218 measures across four dimensions on quality that include effectiveness, patient safety, timeliness, and patient centeredness. The 2007 report focuses on 41 core measures from which three themes evolved:

- Healthcare quality continues to improve, but the rate of improvement has slowed;
- Variation in quality of health care across the nation is decreasing, but not for all measures;
- The safety of health care has improved since 2000, but more needs to be done (AHRQ, 2008a, p. 1).

Data across the country are contradictory as well. Although progress has been made in some areas, other areas have not seen any improvement. Data involving quality of care of those with chronic illness include the following:

- The percentage of heart attack patients who were counseled to quit smoking has increased from 42.7% in 20002001 to 90.9% in 2005. In addition, 48 states, Puerto Rico, and the District of Columbia all performed above 80% on this measure in 2005; however,
- In 2000, patients with diabetes in the worst performing state versus the best performing state were admitted to the hospital 7.6 times more often with their diabetes out of control. By 2004, this difference had doubled to 14 times. If all states had reached the level of the top four best performing states, at least 39,000 fewer patients would have been admitted for uncontrolled diabetes in 2004, with a potential cost savings of $216.7 million (AHRQ, 2008a, p. iv).

Certainly, these data demonstrate that as a nation we have much work to do to improve the quality of care that our clients receive. More

information is available in the AHRQ's annual reports including a data breakdown by individual states. In addition, AHRQ added *State Snapshots* to their website in 2005 (http://statesnapshots.ahrq.gov/snaps07/index.jsp). This Web site documents the quality measures of each individual state.

Health Disparities

The second goal of *Healthy People 2010* is to eliminate health disparities in a subgroup of the population based on characteristics such as race and ethnicity, sex, and income or education (Keppel, Bilheimer, & Gurley, 2007). Unfortunately, progress on this goal is slow. The publishing of the book *Unequal Treatment: Confronting Racial and Ethnic Disparities in Healthcare* (Smedley, Stith, & Nelson, 2003) opened the eyes of many to the inequities that minority populations may face in accessing and receiving health care. Of particular note were the disparities seen in cardiovascular health.

Not coincidentally, the first National Healthcare Disparities Report sponsored by AHRQ was released in the same year that *Unequal Treatment* was published. The fifth national report on health disparities (AHRQ, 2008b), released in February 2008, examines 42 measures of quality and 8 measures of access across a number of racial, ethnic, and socioeconomic priority groups and a comparison group. Three themes emerge from the data:

- Overall, disparities in healthcare quality and access are not getting smaller
- Progress is being made, but many of the biggest gaps in quality and access have not been reduced;
- The problem of persistent uninsurance is a major barrier to reducing barriers (AHRQ, 2008b, p. 1)

Although there has been some progress made, that is, disparity between black and white hemodialysis patients with adequate treatment has been eliminated, there are a number of areas where healthcare delivery disparities in the United States has worsened considerably. The biggest disparities include the following:

- Blacks had a rate of new AIDS cases 10 times higher than that of whites.
- The proportion of black children who were hospitalized because of asthma was almost four times higher than that of white children.
- Asian adults age 65 years and older were 50% more likely than whites to lack immunization against pneumonia.
- American Indians and Alaska Natives were twice as likely as whites to lack prenatal care in the first trimester.
- Hispanics had a rate of new AIDS cases more than 3.5 times higher than that of non-Hispanic whites.
- Poor children were more than 28% more likely than high income children to experience poor communication with their healthcare providers (AHRQ, 2008b, p. 8).

Culture

Illness belief systems form a cultural milieu that define one's attitudes about illness, both acute and chronic. Conceptions or misconceptions about the source of the disease, potential treatment, and possible outcomes are all influenced by these belief systems, and one's belief system is influenced by one's culture. Providing culturally competent care may be a daunting task; however, health care is not "one size fits all," and healthcare professionals must take the extra steps to ensure culturally competent care (see Chapter 12).

Another way to view culture is to consider chronic illness as a culture. Although we often believe that each disease process is "different," there are multiple tasks that are similar, although not the same, and illness experiences may look alike across diseases. Strauss (1975), and again with other colleagues (Strauss et al., 1984), was among the first researchers to recognize the similar issues

and tasks within the culture of chronic illness. Generally, the culture of chronic illness includes preventing and managing medical crises; managing a treatment regimen; controlling symptoms; the reordering of time; and social isolation. Nearly 25 years ago, Strauss and colleagues (1984) suggested that the basic strategy to cope with these issues was to normalize, not just to stay alive or keep their symptoms under control, but to live as normally as possible (p. 79).

A number of years ago when teaching a chronic illness practicum to graduate students, this author developed a mini-ethnography project of the individuals who the students were caring for that semester. Students were caring for clients with a variety of diseases—HIV, liver disease, heart failure, rheumatoid arthritis, and breast cancer. Using grand tour questions that had been developed as a class, students interviewed their clients over the course of the semester. During the final weeks of seminar after the practicum was completed, students compiled the data from all of the clients and looked at the themes that presented themselves. Clearly the class was able to see the culture of what it was like to have a chronic illness and to understand the vast number of similarities between individuals with totally different chronic conditions.

Social Influences

As a society we often stereotype individuals according to the color of their skin, their culture, and their ethnicity. Unfortunately we behave in a similar fashion with individuals with chronic conditions and disabilities (see Chapter 3). To this day there are some individuals who avoid others who may be in a wheelchair, have visible signs of disease (burns, paralysis, amputations, etc.), a diagnosis of AIDS, and so forth. Yes, the advertisements of department stores with individuals in wheelchairs may help, but as a nation, there is much progress to be made.

Publicly recognized individuals have stepped forward with stories about their own chronic conditions. The courage of these individuals to share their experiences and speak out for more comprehensive legislation to support those with chronic disease and increased research funding is admirable. Examples include Michael J. Fox and Muhammed Ali, with diagnoses of Parkinson's disease; Magic Johnson with his diagnosis of HIV; and the late Christopher and Dana Reeve, as advocates for spinal cord injury research.

Financial Impact

Healthcare spending in the United States grew 6.7% to $2.1 trillion, or $7026 per person in 2006 (Catlin, Cowan, Hartman, Heffler, & National Health Expenditure Accounts Team 2008), the most current year for which data are available. However, the good news is that the rate was only slightly higher than the 6.5% growth that was seen in 2005, which was the slowest growth since 1999. Currently, healthcare spending accounts for 16.0% of the gross domestic product (GDP), up from 15.9% in both 2004 and 2005. Despite growth in prescription drug spending and this slight increase in healthcare spending, most major health services and public payers experienced slower growth in 2006 (pp. 20–21).

Catlin and colleagues (2008) note several important findings, particularly with prescription drugs in 2006. After 6 years of slowed growth, prescription drug spending growth accelerated in 2006. This occurred at the same time as the implementation of Medicare Part D, which caused major shifts in the sources of funds that paid for drugs. These shifts and movement toward more enrollment in Medicare-managed care plans caused growth in Medicare's administrative and net cost of insurance to increase (p. 15). The impact of Medicare Part D on overall national healthcare spending in 2006 was modest; however, the public share of drug spending increased from 28% in 2005 to 34% in 2006, whereas the private share fell from 72% to 66% (p. 19).

As a nation, the United States continues to outspend other countries in the Organization for Economic Cooperation and Development (OECD) at a rate that is 2.5 times that of the median OECD country (Anderson, Frogner, & Reinhardt, 2007). However, with the highest healthcare spending rate, the United States continues to provide less access to healthcare resources when compared with the 29 industrialized countries in the OECD (p. 1481), as individuals of lower socioeconomic status and some minority groups have a more difficult time accessing healthcare resources.

CDC's National Center for Chronic Disease Prevention and Health Promotion has provided some quick facts about the economic burden of chronic disease in this country (Table 1-3). Included in this table are two major factors that contribute to chronic disease: obesity and tobacco use.

Using Medical Expenditure Panel Survey (MEPS) data, five conditions have been identified as the most costly conditions in the non-institutionalized population, and four of them are chronic conditions. The five conditions— heart disease, cancer, trauma-related disorders, mental disorders, and pulmonary conditions— ranked highest in terms of direct medical spending in 2000 and again in 2004 (Soni, 2007). These data are based on expenditures (what is paid for healthcare services), and does not include any indirect costs. Heart disease had the largest medical expenditures in 2004 with 10%, followed by cancer at 6.9%, trauma-related disorders at 6.5%, mental disorders at 5.8%, and pulmonary conditions at 5.4% (Soni, 2007).

Compounding chronic disease and the aging population is the issue of the uninsured. The long-term uninsured, versus those uninsured for short periods, is a significant population. MEPS data for 2002 to 2005 (most current available) demonstrate the following in the population younger than 65 years of age:

■ 17.4 million US residents younger than 65 years of age were uninsured for the entire 4-year period (2002 through 2005).
■ Those reporting fair/poor health were the most likely to be uninsured (11.2%) for the entire 4-year period.

TABLE 1-3

Quick Facts: Economic and Health Burden of Chronic Disease

Disease/Risk Factors	Morbidity (Illness)	Mortality (Death)	Direct Cost/Indirect Cost
Arthritis	Arthritis affects 1 in 5, or 46 million, US adults, making it one of the most common chronic conditions. More than 40%, or nearly 19 million, adults with arthritis are limited in their activities because of their arthritis. By 2030, nearly 67 million (25%) of US adults will have doctor-diagnosed arthritis. In addition, adults with arthritis-attributable activity limitation are projected to increase from 16.9 million (7.9%) to 25 million (9.3% of the US adult population) by 2030.	From 1979 to 1998, the annual number of arthritis and other related rheumatic conditions (AORC) deaths rose from 5537 to 9367. In 1998, the crude death rate from AORC was 3.48 per 100,000 population.	The total costs attributable to arthritis and other rheumatic conditions AORC in the United States in 2003 was approximately $128 billion ($80.8 billion in medical care expenditures and $47 billion in earnings losses). This equaled 1.2% of the 2003 US gross domestic product.
Cancer	About 1.3 million people in the United States are diagnosed with cancer each year.	Cancer is the second leading cause of death in the United States. In 2004, an estimated 553,000 people died of cancer.	The NIH estimated the overall costs for cancer in the year 2007 at $219 billion: of this amount, $89 billion for direct medical costs and $130 billion for indirect costs such as lost productivity.
Diabetes	More than 20.8 million Americans have diabetes, and about 6.2 million don't know that they have the disease.	Diabetes is the sixth leading cause of death. More than 200,000 people die each year of diabetes-related complications.	The estimated economic cost of diabetes in 2007 was $174 billion. Of this amount, $116 billion was the result of direct medical costs and $58 billion, indirect costs such as lost workdays, restricted activity, and disability caused by diabetes.
Heart disease and stroke	More than 80 million Americans currently live with a cardiovascular disease.	More than 870,000 Americans die of heart disease and stroke each year, which is about 2400 people dying each day.	The cost of heart disease and stroke in the United States in 2008 is projected to be more than $448 billion, including direct and indirect costs.

(Continued)

| TABLE 1-3 | | | |

Quick Facts: Economic and Health Burden of Chronic Disease (*Continued*)

Disease/Risk Factors	Morbidity (Illness)	Mortality (Death)	Direct Cost/Indirect Cost
Overweight/ obesity	In 2005 to 2006 more than 34% of adults aged 20 years or older, were obese. More than 125 million or 17.1% of children and adolescents 2 to 19 years of age are overweight.	The latest study from CDC scientists estimates that about 112,000 deaths are associated with obesity each year in the United States.	Direct health costs attributable to obesity have been estimated at $52 billion in 1995 and $75 billion in 2003. Among children and adolescents, annual hospital costs related to overweight and obesity more than tripled over the last two decades.
Tobacco	An estimated 45.3 million adults in the United States smoke cigarettes, even though this single behavior will result in death or disability for half of all regular users.	Tobacco use is responsible for approximately 438,000 deaths each year.	The economic burden of tobacco use is enormous: more than $96 billion in medical expenditures and another $97 billion in indirect costs.

Source: Centers for Disease Control and Prevention. National Center for Chronic Disease Prevention and Health Promotion. Retrieved on January 31, 2008 from http://www.cdc.gov/nccdphp/press/index.htm

■ Hispanics were disproportionately represented among the long-term uninsured. Although they represented only 15.7% of the US population during this period, they represented 40.1% of the long-term uninsured.

■ Individuals who were poor were disproportionately represented among the long-term uninsured. Although representing 13.2% of the population younger than age 65 years, they represented 25.6% of the long-term uninsured (Rhoades & Cohen, 2007).

In individuals older than 65 years of age, only 1% of noninstitutionalized adults did not have insurance coverage of some kind. In 2006, Medicare covered 94% of noninstitutionalized older adults (Administration on Aging, 2007). Medicare covers mostly acute care services and requires that beneficiaries pay nearly half of all of their healthcare expenses. Approximately 61% of those older than 65 years had some type of private health insurance, 7% had military-based health insurance, and 9% were covered by Medicaid (Administration on Aging, 2007).

When looking at the costs of chronic disease, one needs to identify the lost productivity of the individual and/or family affected, as well as the number of health resources used. The American Diabetes Association (ADA) has developed a model for diabetes that identifies lost productivity as well as the monetary costs. Through a prevalence-based model utilizing epidemiologic data, healthcare costs, and economic data, a cost of diabetes model was developed. The total estimated cost for diabetes in 2007 was $174 billion dollars, with $116 billion in medical expenditures and $58 billion in decreased productivity, either by the individual or the family caregiver (American Diabetes Association, 2008).

Of note are the costs that are *not* included in the $174 billion. Those include: healthcare system administrative costs, over-the-counter medications, care provided by nonpaid caregivers, excess medical costs associated with undiagnosed diabetes, and so forth (p. 1).

In summary, the financial impact of chronic disease is large. With the changing demographics of the population and the incidence of chronic disease, the impact will increase.

INTERVENTIONS

Chronic disease is an issue that is all encompassing, such that interventions from many sources will be needed to "make a difference." What follows are examples of what the United States is doing to eliminate the impact of chronic disease.

Professional Education

One of the challenges in chronic disease care and management is educating healthcare professionals about caring for those individuals. The differences are vast between caring for a person with an acute illness on a short term basis, and caring for those over the "long haul" with a chronic condition. The WHO has developed a document outlining the steps to prepare a healthcare workforce for the 21st century that can appropriately care for individuals with chronic conditions. The WHO document calls for a "transformation" of healthcare training to better meet the needs of those individuals with chronic conditions. The document, *Preparing a healthcare workforce for the 21st century: The challenge of chronic conditions* (2005b), has the support of the World Medical Association, the International Council of Nurses, the International Pharmaceutical Federation, the European Respiratory Society, and the International Alliance of Patients' Organizations.

The competencies delineated by the WHO were identified with a process that included an extensive document/literature review and international expert agreement (p. 14). All competencies were based on addressing the needs of patients with chronic conditions and their family members from a longitudinal perspective, and focused on two types of "prevention" strategies: initial prevention of the chronic disease; and secondly, prevention of complications from the condition (p. 18).

The five competencies include: patient-centered care; partnering; quality improvement; information and communication technology; and public health perspective (see Table 1-4). At first glance, the competencies don't seem unique. However, in an acute care healthcare delivery system, these concepts aren't as prominent. Clients are

TABLE 1-4

WHO Core Competencies

Patient-centered care
    Interviewing and communicating effectively
    Assisting changes in health-related behaviors
    Supporting self-management
    Using a proactive approach
Partnering
    Partnering with patients
    Partnering with other providers
    Partnering with communities
Quality improvement
    Measuring care delivery and outcomes
    Learning and adapting to change
    Translating evidence into practice
Information and communication technology
    Designing and using patient registries
    Using computer technologies
    Communicating with partners
Public health perspective
    Providing population-based care
    Systems thinking
    Working across the care continuum
    Working in primary health care–led systems

Source: World Health Organization. (2005b). *Preparing a Health Care Workforce for the 21st Century: The Challenge of Chronic Conditions* (p. 20). Geneva, Switzerland: WHO.

in and out of the care system quickly, and there is less need for implementation of these concepts.

Chronic Disease Practitioner Competencies

From another point of view, the National Association of Chronic Disease Directors (NACDD) has developed competencies for chronic disease practice. This organization was founded in 1988 to link the directors of chronic disease programs in each state and US territory. These competencies assist state and local healthcare programs to develop both competent workforces and effective programs. The NACDD document is based on domains, with individual competencies within each domain. Several of the domains address the WHO competencies (i.e, partnering, evidence-based interventions). Furthermore, the NACDD has developed an assessment tool for practitioners to gauge their level of proficiency in each of the seven domains. Table 1-5 lists the competencies for chronic disease practitioners.

Resources

Since the publication of the previous edition of this book, two of the entities that provided education about chronic disease and recommendations for practice (and were referenced in the prior edition) are no longer in business. The Partnership for Solutions, jointly funded by the Robert Wood Johnson Foundation and Johns Hopkins University, no longer exists, as the Robert Wood Johnson Foundation is not providing funding. The other group that no longer exists is the National Chronic Care Consortium. Their Web site states "the consortium went out of business the summer of 2003." Both of these organizations provided leadership in caring for those with chronic illness.

Institute of Medicine

In 2007, the IOM charged an ad hoc committee with the task of determining the healthcare needs of an aging America, and, more importantly, developing recommendations to address those needs. On April 14, 2008, the IOM report, *Retooling for an Aging America: Building the Health Care Workforce*, was released to the public. This report suggests a three-pronged approach that includes the following: (1) enhance the geriatric competence of the entire workforce, (2) increase the recruitment and retention of geriatric specialists and caregivers, and (3) improve the way care is delivered (IOM, 2008).

The report states a well-known fact: little attention is paid to educating healthcare professionals about caring for older adults. The committee recommends that healthcare professionals be required to demonstrate their competence in caring for older adults as a criterion for licensure and certification. More stringent training standards would be implemented for direct-care providers by increasing existing federal training requirements and establishing state-based standards. And finally, since informal caregivers continue to play important roles in the care of older adults (with and without chronic illness), training opportunities should also be available for them (IOM, 2008).

Currently only a small percentage of the healthcare workforce specializes in caring for older adults. The IOM report recommends that financial incentives be provided to increase the number of geriatric specialists in every health profession. Incentives would include an increase in payments for clinical services, development of awards to increase the number of faculty in geriatrics, and the establishment of programs that would provide loan forgiveness, scholarships, and direct financial incentives for individuals to become specialists in geriatrics. For the direct-care workers in long-term care facilities that typically have high levels of turnover and job dissatisfaction, the recommendation is to improve job desirability, improve supervisory relationships and provide opportunities for career growth. In addition, the report recommends that state Medicaid programs increase pay for direct care workers and provide access to fringe benefits (IOM, 2008).

TABLE 1-5

National Association of Chronic Disease Directors Competencies for Chronic Disease Practice

Domain 1—Build Support
Chronic disease practitioners establish strong working relationships with stakeholders, including other programs, government agencies, and nongovernmental lay and professional groups, to build support for chronic disease prevention and control.

Domain 2—Design and Evaluate Programs
Chronic disease practitioners develop and implement evidence-based interventions and conduct evaluation to ensure on-going feedback and program effectiveness.

Domain 3—Influence Policies and Systems Change
Chronic disease practitioners implement strategies to change the health-related policies of private organizations or governmental entities capable of affecting the health of targeted populations.

Domain 4—Lead Strategically
Chronic disease practitioners articulate health needs and strategic vision, serve as a catalyst for change and demonstrate program accomplishments to ensure continued funding and support within their scope of practice.

Domain 5—Manage People
Chronic disease practitioners oversee and support the optimal performance and growth of program staff as well as themselves.

Domain 6—Manage Programs and Resources
Chronic disease practitioners ensure the consistent administrative, financial, and staff support necessary to sustain successful implementation of planned activities and build opportunities.

Domain 7—Use Public Health Science
Chronic disease practitioners gather, analyze, interpret, and disseminate data and research findings to define needs, identify priorities, and measure change.

Source: National Association of Chronic Disease Directors. Competencies for chronic disease. Retrieved April 17, 2008 from www.chronicdisease.org/files/public/complete_draft_Competencies_for_Chronic_Disease_Practice.pdf

Lastly, improving models of care for older adults needs to occur. The report envisions three key principles in improving care: (1) the healthcare needs of older adults need to be addressed comprehensively, (2) services need to be provided efficiently, and (3) older adults need to be encouraged to be active partners in their own care. Because no one model of care will be appropriate for all persons, the IOM recommends that Congress and public and private foundations significantly increase support for research and programs that promote development of new models of care (IOM, 2008).

Healthy People 2010

All 467 objectives of *Healthy People 2010* were examined in 2005 as part of the midcourse review.

On the basis of an evaluation of each objective and comments received from the public as part of the review, 28 objectives were deleted because data were not available or because of a change in science (*Healthy People 2010: Midcourse Review, 2005*). Overall, 29 objectives met the target; 138 objectives moved toward the target; 40 objectives demonstrated mixed progress (in their subobjectives); 17 objectives were unchanged from the baseline; and 57 objectives moved away from the target.

The midcourse review of focus area 12, heart disease and stroke, is described as one example. The goal of focus area 12 is to improve cardiovascular health and quality of life through prevention, detection, and treatment of risk factors; early identification and treatment of heart attacks and strokes; and prevention of recurrent cardiovascular events. There are 16 sub-objectives in this focus area. Overall, one objective met or exceeded the target; six moved toward the target; one demonstrated no change; one demonstrated mixed progress; one moved away from the target; and six could not be assessed (see Table 1-6).

Centers for Disease Control and Prevention Programs

The CDC has provided both leadership and funding in developing state-based programs nationwide. Programs have been developed to look at both risk factors and prevention of disease, as well as examine ways to prevent complications and delay death resulting from chronic disease. One example of CDC's work is with diabetes.

The CDC's programs with diabetes encompass several components and include: promoting effective state programs, monitoring the burden and translating science, providing education and sharing expertise, supporting primary prevention, and targeting populations at risk. What follows is a brief description of what each of these components is providing.

Diabetes. *Promoting Effective State Programs.* In 2007 the CDC provided funding for capacity building to 22 states, 8 current or former US territories, and the District of Columbia for diabetes prevention and control programs. In addition, the CDC provided funding for basic implementation of programs in the other 28 states. These state programs identify the disease burden in their states, develop and evaluate new prevention strategies, establish partnerships, increase awareness of prevention and control opportunities, and improve access to quality care (CDC Diabetes, 2008).

Monitoring the Burden and Translating Science. CDC analyzes data from several national sources, including the Behavioral Risk Factor Surveillance System. The translating of these data into quality practice is implemented with the assistance of other research partners, managed care organizations, and community health centers (CDC Diabetes, 2008).

Providing Education and Sharing Expertise. Another component of the CDC's work is providing education. The National Diabetes Education Program (NDEP) is sponsored by both the CDC and the National Institutes of Health (NIH). The NDEP comprises more than 200 public and private partners to increase knowledge about diabetes. In addition, CDC is working to target populations at risk (CDC Diabetes, 2008).

Supporting Primary Prevention. The Diabetes Prevention Program (DPP) was a CDC clinical trial demonstrating that sustained lifestyle changes could reduce the progression to type 2 diabetes among adults who were at high risk. The results from this study were so compelling that the study was ended a year early (CDC Diabetes, 2008).

Targeting Populations at Risk. The CDC has developed primary prevention programs for those most at risk for diabetes in five states. The CDC is working in communities with American Indians and Alaska Natives to develop culturally appropriate interventions for those populations (CDC Diabetes, 2008).

REACH. The CDC's Racial and Ethnic Approaches to Community Health (REACH) 2010 program is a community-based public health program that is working to eliminate health disparities in 40 communities of color across the United States (Liburd, Giles, & Mensah, 2006). Within these 40 communities, the CDC supports local coalitions in designing, implementing, and evaluating community-driven strategies to eliminate health disparities. The coalitions use local data to develop individual community based plans. As an example, the Bronx Health REACH project developed a seven-point advocacy agenda intended to eliminate the root causes of health disparities in the southwest Bronx. Their coalition is working to achieve "universal health insurance, an end to segregation in healthcare facilities based on insurance status, accountability for state uncompensated care fund,

TABLE 1-6

Heart Disease and Stroke: Midcourse Review of Objectives Met

Category	Objective numbers	Description
Objectives that exceeded the target		No objectives exceeded the target
Objectives that met the target	12-14	High blood cholesterol levels: 17%
		17% of persons 20 years of age and older had high total blood cholesterol levels (down from 21% in 1988 to 1994)
Objectives that moved toward their target	12-1	Coronary heart disease death rate
		Death rate dropped from 203/100,000 to 180/100,000 (target is 162)
	12-7	Stroke death rate
		Death rate from 62/100,000 to 56/100,000 (target is 50)
	12-10	High blood pressure control
		64% of the population achieved control in blood pressure (target is 68%)
	12-11	Action to help control blood pressure
		93% of the population took action to control high blood pressure (target is 98%)
	12-13	Mean total blood cholesterol levels
		Total cholesterol levels were reduced from 206 to 203 (target is 199)
	12-15	Blood cholesterol screening
		73% of adults 18 and older had cholesterol screenings up from 67% (target is 80%)
Objectives that demonstrated no change	12-12	Blood pressure monitoring for those with high blood pressure remained constant at 90% (target is 95%)
Objectives that moved away from their target	12-6b	Heart failure hospitalizations for persons aged 75 to 84
	12-9	Proportion of persons aged 20 and older with high blood pressure
Objectives that could not be assessed	12-2	Measure knowledge of heart attack symptoms and calling 911
	12-3a	Receipt of artery-opening therapy
	12-3b	Use of percutaneous intervention within 90 minutes
	12-4	Cardiopulmonary resuscitation training
	12-8	Knowledge of early stroke
Objectives that remain developmental	12-5	Out-of-hospital care for cardiac arrest
	12-16	LDL cholesterol levels in CHD patients

Source: Healthy People 2010. (2005). Midcourse Review. Retrieved March 6, 2007 from http://www.cdc.gov/DHDSP/library/hp2010/objectives.htm

culturally competent care for greater health work-force diversity, an expansion of public health education, and environmental justice" (Calman, 2005, p. 491).

Agency for Healthcare Research and Quality

AHRQ sponsors a number of programs that are working to reduce or eliminate health disparities. The reason that these programs are mentioned is because, as previously noted, 80% of US healthcare dollars are spent on chronic disease. Therefore, healthcare inequities largely involve chronic care.

The Federal Collaboration on Health Disparities Research (FCHDR) is identifying and supporting research priorities for cross-agency collaboration to hasten the elimination of health disparities. The Health Disparities Roundtable is a public-private partnership on research and policy. The Disparity Reducing Advances Project is identifying strategies for bringing health gains to poor and underserved populations. The Think Cultural Health website offers the latest resources and tools to promote cultural competency. The AHRQ National Health Plan Collaborative wants to reduce disparities among 87 million enrollees in health plans. The AHRQ Learning Partnership to Decrease Disparities in Pediatric Asthma identifies areas of need and then makes the case to state governments for further action on asthma disparities. The AHRQ Hispanic Diabetes Disparities Learning Network in Rural and Urban Community Health Clinics focuses on diabetes in adult Hispanics (AHRQ, 2008).

Evidence-Based Practice

In recent years, issues of quality and safety for patients have come to the forefront, with an emphasis on improving health care. The IOM book, *Health Professions Education: A Bridge to Quality* (Greiner & Knebel, 2003) lists five essential competencies for quality care, and one of those

is "employ evidence based practice" (Greiner & Knebel, 2003).

The evidence-based practice movement had its beginnings in the 1970s with Dr. Archie Cochrane, a British epidemiologist. In 1972, he published a book that criticized physicians for not conducting rigorous reviews of evidence to make appropriate treatment decisions. Cochrane was a proponent of randomized clinical trials, and in his exemplar case noted that thousands of low birthweight premature infants died needlessly while at the same time there were several randomized clinical trials (RCTs) that had been conducted on the use of corticosteroid therapy, but the data had never been reviewed or analyzed. After review, these studies demonstrated that use of this therapy reduced infant deaths significantly. Cochrane died in 1988, but as a result of his influence and call for systematic review of the literature, the Cochrane Center was launched in Oxford, England, in 1992. It is known as the Cochrane Library Database, currently the most sophisticated database available of current research that supports practice.

However, it is accepted knowledge that evidence-based practice does not rely on RCTs alone. A number of definitions have been brought forth, but Porter-O'Grady's succinct definition makes the most sense. "Evidence based practice is simply the integration of the best possible research to evidence with clinical expertise and with patient needs. Patient needs in this case refer specifically to the expectations, concerns , and requirements that patients bring to their clinical experience" (Porter-O'Grady, 2006, p. 1).

DiCenso, Guyatt, and Ciliska (2005) add that clinical expertise is "our ability to use clinical skills and past experience to identify the health state of patients or populations, their risks, their preference and actions, and the potential benefits of interventions" (p. 5).

As healthcare professionals examine the evidence to improve the care of their clients, there are a number of sources for reference. The following agencies and organizations are just a sample of the resources available:

- Agency for Healthcare Research and Quality (AHRQ)—the United State's premier evidence-based practice agency: //www.ahrq.gov
- Cochrane Library: www.cochrane.org
- Task Force on Community Preventive Services: www.thecommunityguide.org
- US Preventive Services Task Force: www.ahrq.gov/clinic/uspstfab.htm
- Veterans Evidence-Based Research Dissemination Implementation Center (VERDICT): www.verdict.research.va.gov/
- National Guideline Clearinghouse: www.guideline.gov
- British Medical Journal & United Health Foundation: www.clinicalevidence.com

Legislation

National surveys of 1238 physicians, 1663 Americans, and a convenience sample of 155 policy makers were asked their perceptions of how well the current healthcare delivery system addresses the needs of individuals with chronic conditions (Anderson, 2003). Compared with the public and the physicians, policymakers were more pessimistic about the healthcare system. A majority of all three groups agreed that it is somewhat or very difficult for individuals with chronic conditions to obtain adequate care (p. 437).

Changing public policy continues to be a primary intervention in assisting clients and their families with chronic conditions. Institution of national policies and the financing of prevention and health promotion need to occur. In addition, until healthcare professionals are able to make a difference in the agency maze and the financing of that maze, clients will continue to have difficulty accessing the chronic long-term care that they need (see Chapter 23).

Research

Although research on chronicity continues to increase, there is a continuing need to demonstrate new paradigms of caring for those with chronic illness. What follows are examples of studies that may be useful in caring for those with chronic illness.

Advanced Practice Nursing Interventions

McCauley, Bixby, and Naylor (2006) designed an RCT that examined the effectiveness of advanced practice nurse (APN) interventions in increasing length of time between hospital discharge and readmission or death, reducing readmissions, and decreasing overall healthcare costs in clients with heart failure (HF). Their original work looked at a one-month intervention, but follow-up deemed that the duration was far too short. Their latest study looked at a nursing home care intervention at 3 months and included APNs with more HF experience. Thus they were able to demonstrate improved outcomes for up to 1 year after the acute episode of HF. Interventions focused on individualized patient assessment, enhanced patient-provider communication, targeted interventions to improve self-management, and improved access to resources. Although the primary focus of the study was HF, most clients had multiple, active comorbid conditions that complicated their HF and put them at risk for poor outcomes. The study produced statistically significant results and demonstrated that the APNs were effective in reducing rehospitalizations related to these comorbid conditions (McCauley et al., 2006).

Another nursing intervention study with patients with HF was carried out by Sisk and colleagues (2006). An RCT was conducted with HF patients in four hospitals in Harlem, New York, working with a mostly black or Hispanic population of 406 adults. During a 12-month intervention, bilingual nurses counseled patients on diet, medication adherence, and self-management of symptoms through an initial visit and then regularly scheduled follow-up phone calls, and contact with their physicians as well. The outcome measures of the study were re-hospitalizations and self-reported functioning. Both outcome measures had better results and were significantly different than the "usual care" clients (Sisk et al., 2006).

Hamner (2005) published a state-of-the-science review of studies of interventions in which nurses played a major role in the outcomes of patients with HF. Hamner categorized the research as (1) home-based nursing interventions, (2) nurses in pivotal roles in multidisciplinary interventions that extended to the home, (3) heart failure clinics, and (4) telephone- or technology-based nursing interventions. The home-based intervention studies included five RCTs with 569 patients. There were mixed results, with some of the studies showing improved self-care behavior, whereas others did not; some of the studies showed decreased re-hospitalization rates and others did not.

In the multidisciplinary intervention studies, more positive results were obtained in the studies (mostly RCTs, again) of 1879 patients. Results demonstrated decreased lengths of stay, decreased admissions and re-admissions, decreased costs, decreasing mortality, longer event-free periods and improved quality of life (QOL) (Hamner, 2005).

Ten studies focusing on an extended role of nursing in HF clinics demonstrated convincing evidence that HF clinics that included a strong nursing role are effective in reducing hospital admission and emergency department visits, decreasing mortality, improving self-care and QOL, and reducing costs. Only one study in this group did not show positive outcomes (Hamner, 2005).

In the last grouping of four studies on technology- and/or telephone-based home intervention, there were few positive outcomes. Two studies found decreased emergency department visits and one showed increased patient satisfaction, but there were few positive results in studies that included 700 patients (Hamner, 2005).

Health Promotion

Typically, interventional studies of chronic illness have focused on symptom management—what nursing intervention(s) can be performed to alleviate a physical symptom. From this author's perspective, that approach views chronic illness through a disease model, or a medical model, and does not address the whole person. Such research is important in the care of those with chronic disease, but there may be another way to view chronic disease, and that is through a wellness lens. Stuifbergen (2006) suggests that it makes sense to develop and test interventions to promote health rather than control the disease of persons with chronic conditions: in other words, conceptualizing health within illness. Three of her studies demonstrate the possibilities of this concept.

An RCT including 113 women with multiple sclerosis operationalized a two-phase intervention program, the Wellness Program for Women with MS, with lifestyle-change classes for 8 weeks and follow-up telephone calls for 3 months. Participants were then followed over an 8-month period. The experimental group had statistically significant differences in self-efficacy for health behaviors, health-promoting behaviors, and the mental health and pain scales of the SF-36 (Stuifbergen, Becker, Blozis, Timmerman, & Kullberg, 2003).

In two small studies of clients with HF, 19 clients reported increased self-perceived health and increased use of health-promoting behaviors (Clark et al., 2006). The intervention used with these clients was modeled after the Wellness Program for Women with MS.

The Future

In 2005, the Surgeon General's Office disseminated a document entitled *Call to Action to Improve the Health and Wellness of Persons with Disabilities* (Smeltzer, 2007). This document spoke to the need of ensuring that individuals with disabilities can access comprehensive health care so that they can live productive lives (p. 189). Smeltzer (2007) suggests that the amount of research examining individuals with disabilities and appropriate interventions to enhance their health outcomes has not kept pace with the increasing number of individuals with disabilities. Although we know that individuals with disabilities may have acquired their disability from multiple causes, chronic disease is the major cause/proponent of most of the disabilities.

The IOM (2008) in their report on *Retooling for an Aging America,* suggests that more research is needed that addresses the effective use of the workforce to care for older adults and how to increase both the size and the capabilities of that workforce. In addition, the IOM report recommends that more support be provided for technologic advances that could enhance the capacity to care for older adults.

A growing patient population includes those with chronic critical illness. This population consists of individuals who cross over from acute to chronic critical illness with a syndrome of significant, characteristic derangements of metabolism, neuroendocrine, neuropsychiatric, and immunologic function

(Nelson et al., 2004, p. 1527). Often these individuals make the transition to a chronic condition after having a tracheotomy for failure to wean from mechanical ventilation. How do we assist this population in maintaining QOL? What nursing interventions assist in better outcomes for these chronically ill patients?

OUTCOMES

This chapter has included data from a number of national reports, each with a list of recommendations and benchmarks to improve health outcomes of the population. Perhaps the best known is *Healthy People 2010.* Although we have made progress in meeting some of the benchmarks for chronic disease, much progress is required. Caring for the client and family with chronic disease will continue to be an on-going challenge.

STUDY QUESTIONS

1. What factors and influences have led to the increased incidence of chronic disease in the United States?
2. What factors should be considered in defining chronicity?
3. How can we better prepare healthcare professionals to care for those with chronic disease? To care for older adults with chronic disease?
4. What changes does the healthcare delivery system need to embrace to better care for those with chronic disease?
5. Compare and contrast chronic disease and chronic illness.
6. What action does the United States need to take to decrease healthcare disparities?
7. What should the nursing research foci be related to chronic disease?

INTERNET RESOURCES

British Medical Journal & United Health Foundation: www.clinicalevidence.com
Cochrane Library: www.cochrane.org
National Guideline Clearinghouse: www.guideline.gov
Task Force on Community Preventive Services: www.thecommunityguide.org
Think Cultural Health: www.thinkculturalhealth.org
US Preventive Services Task Force: www.ahrq.gov/clinic/uspstfab.htm
Veterans Evidence-Based Research Dissemination Implementation Center (VERDICT): verdict.uthscsa.edu/verdict/default.htm

REFERENCES

Administration on Aging (2007). *A Profile of Older Americans: 2007.* Washington, D.C.: US Department of Health and Human Services.

Agency for Healthcare Research and Quality (2008a). *National Healthcare Quality Report 2007.* Rockville, MD: US Department of Health and Human Services. AHRQ Pub. No. 08–0040.

Agency for Healthcare Research and Quality. (2008b). *National Healthcare Disparities Report 2007.* Rockville, MD: U.S. Department of Health and Human Services. AHRQ 08–0041.

American Diabetes Association. (2008). Economic costs of diabetes in the U.S. for 2007 [Electronic version]. *Diabetes Care, 31(3),* 1–20.

Anderson, G.F. (2005). Medicare and chronic conditions [Electronic version]. *New England Journal of Medicine, 343(3),* 305–309.

Anderson, G.F. (2003). Physician, public, and policymaker perspectives on chronic conditions. *Archives of Internal Medicine, 163,* 437–442.

Anderson, G.F., Frogner, B.K., & Reinhardt, U.E. (2007). Health spending in OECD countries in 2004: An update [Electronic version]. *Health Affairs, 26(5),* 1481–1489.

Calman, N. (2005). Making health quality a reality: *The Bronx takes action* [Electronic version]. *Health Affairs, 24(2),* 491–498.

Catlin, A., Cowan, C., Hartman, M., Heffler, S., & the National Health Expenditure Accounts Team. (2008). National health spending in 2006: A year of change for prescription drugs [Electronic version]. *Health Affairs, 27(1),* 14–29.

Centers for Disease Control and Prevention & the Merck Company Foundation. (2007). *The State of Aging and Health in America 2007.* Whitehouse Station, NJ: The Merck Company Foundation.

Centers for Disease Control and Prevention. National Center for Chronic Disease Prevention and Health Promotion. (2008a). Retrieved April 10, 2008, from http://www.cdc.gov/nccdphp/overview.htm

Centers for Disease Control and Prevention. National Center for Chronic Disease Prevention and Health Promotion (2008b). Retrieved January 31, 2008, from http://www.cdc.gov/nccdphp/press/index.htm

Centers for Disease Control and Prevention. National Center for Chronic Disease Prevention and Health Promotion. Diabetes 2008. Retrieved April 17, 2008, from http://www.cdc.gov/diabetes

Clark, A.P., Stuifbergen, A., Gottlieb, N., Voelmeck, W., Darby, D., & Delville, C. (2006). Health promotion in heart failure: A paradigm shift: *Holistic Nursing Practice, 20(2),* 73–79.

Curtin, M., & Lubkin, I. (1995). What is chronicity? In I. Lubkin (Ed.) *Chronic illness: Impact and interventions* (3rd ed.). Sudbury, MA: Jones & Bartlett.

DiCenso, A., Guyatt, G., & Ciliska, D. (2005). *Evidence-based nursing: A guide to clinical practice.* St. Louis: Elsevier Mosby.

Emanuel, E. (1982). We are all chronic patients. *Journal of Chronic Diseases, 35,* 501–502.

Greiner, A., & Knebel, E. (Eds.). (2003). *Health professional education: A bridge to quality.* Washington, DC: National Academies Press.

Hamner, J. (2005). State of the science: Posthospitalization nursing interventions in congestive heart failure [Electronic version]. *Advances in Nursing Science, 28(2),* 175–190.

Harleman, A. (2008, January & February). My other husband. *AARP Magazine,* 74–78.

Healthy People 2010: Midcourse Review (2005). Retrieved March 6, 2007, from http://www.healthypeople.gov/data/midcourse/default.htm

Himelhoch, S., Weller, W.E., Wu, A.W., Anderson, G.F., & Cooper, L.A. (2004). Chronic medical illness, depression and use of acute medical services among medicare beneficiaries [Electronic version]. *Medical Care, 42,* 512–521.

Institute of Medicine. (2008). *Retooling for an aging America: Building the health care workforce.* Washington, DC: National Academies Press.

Institute of Medicine (2006). Crossing the quality chasm: The IOM health care quality initiative. Retrieved May 6, 2008, from http://www.iom.edu/CMS/8089.aspx?printfriendly=true

Keppel, K., Bilheimer, L., & Gurley, L. (2007). Improving population health and reducing health care disparities [Electronic version]. *Health Affairs, 26(5),* 1281–1292.

Liburd, L.C., Giles, W., & Mensah, M. (2006). Looking through a glass, darkly: Eliminating health disparities. Preventing Chronic Disease [serial online]

2006 July. Retrieved January 31, 2008, from http://www.cdc.gov/pcd/issues/2006/jul/05_0209.htm

Lynn, J. & Adamson, D.M. (2003). *Living well at the end of life: Adapting healthcare to serious chronic illness in old age.* Santa Monica, CA: RAND.

Mayo, L. (Ed.). (1956). *Guides to action on chronic illness.* Commission on Chronic Illness. New York: National Health Council.

McCauley, K.M., Bixby, M.B., & Naylor, M. (2006). Advanced practice nurse strategies to improve outcomes and reduce cost in elders with heart failure [Electronic version]. *Disease Management, 9*(5), 302–310.

National Association of Chronic Disease Directors. Competencies for Chronic Disease Practice. Retrieved April 17, 2008 from www.chronicdisease.org/i4a/pages/index.cfm?pageid=3290

National Center for Health Statistics. (2008). *Health, United States, 2007.* Hyattsville, MD: NCHS.

Nelson, J.E., Meier, D.E., Litke, A., Natale, D.A. Siegel, R.E. & Morrison, R.S. (2004). The symptom burden of chronic critical illness [Electronic version]. *Critical Care Medicine, 32*(7), 1527–1534.

Porter-O'Grady, T. (2006). A new age for practice: Creating the framework for evidence. In Malloch, K., Porter-O'Grady, T. (Eds.) *Introduction to evidence-based practice in nursing and health care.* Sudbury, MA: Jones & Bartlett.

Price, B. (1996). Illness careers: The chronic illness experience. *Journal of Advanced Nursing, 24,* 275–279.

Rhoades, J.A., & Cohen, S.B. (2007). *The long-term uninsured in America, 2002–2005: Estimates for the U.S. population under age 65.* Statistical Brief #183. Rockville, MD: Agency for Healthcare Research and Quality. Retrieved April 15, 2008, from http://www.meps.ahrq.gov/mepsweb/date_files/publications/st183/stat183.pdf

Roberts, D. (1954). The overall picture of long-term illness. Address given at a conference on problems of long-term aging. School of Public Health, Harvard University, June 1954. Subsequently published in *Journal of Chronic Diseases,* February 1955, 149–159.

Sisk, J.E., Hebert, P.L., Horowitz, C.R., McLaughlin, M.A., Wang, J.J. & Chassin, M.R. (2006). Effects of nurse management on the quality of heart failure care in minority communities [Electronic version]. *Annals of Internal Medicine, 145*(4), 273–283.

Smedley, B.D., Stith, A.Y., & Nelson, A.R. (2003). *Unequal treatment: Confronting racial and ethnic disparities in health care.* Washington, DC: The National Academies Press.

Smeltzer, S.C. (2007). Improving the health and wellness of persons with disabilities: A call to action too important for nursing to ignore. *Nursing Outlook, 55,* 189–195.

Soni, A. (2007). *The Five Most Costly Conditions, 2000–2004: Estimates for the U.S. Civilian Noninstitutionalized Population.* Statistical Brief #167. Rockville, MD: Agency for Healthcare Research and Quality. Retrieved April 8, 2007, from http://www.meps.ahrq.gov/mepsweb/data_files/publications/st167/stat167.pdf

Strauss, A. (1975). *Chronic illness and the quality of life.* St. Louis: Mosby.

Strauss, A., Corbin, J., Fagerhaugh, S., Glaser, B., Maines, D., Suczek, B., et al. (1984). *Chronic illness and the quality of life* (2nd ed.). St. Louis: Mosby.

Stuifbergen, A.K. (2006). Building health promotion interventions for persons with chronic disability conditions [Electronic version]. *Family Community Health, 29*(Suppl. 1), 28–34.

Stuifbergen, A.K., Becker, H., Blozis, S., Timmerman, G., & Kullberg, V. (2003). A randomized clinical trial of a wellness intervention for women with multiple sclerosis [Electronic version]. *Archives of Physical Medicine and Rehabilitation, 84,* 467–476.

World Health Organization. (2005a). *Preventing chronic disease: A vital investment.* Geneva, Switzerland: WHO.

World Health Organization. (2005b). *Preparing a health care workforce for the 21st century: The challenge of chronic conditions.* Geneva, Switzerland: WHO.

Yach, D., Hawkes, C., Gould, C.L.O., & Hofman, K. (2004). The global burden of chronic diseases: Overcoming impediments to prevention and control [Electronic version]. *Journal of the American Medical Association, 291*(21), 2616–2622.

2

Illness Behavior

Pamala D. Larsen

Illness is the night-side of life, a more onerous citizenship. Everyone who is born holds dual citizenship, in the kingdom of the well and in the kingdom of the sick. Although we all prefer to use only the good passport, sooner or later each of us is obligated, at least for a spell, to identify ourselves as citizens of that other place.

Susan Sontag, *Illness as Metaphor*, 1988, p. 3

INTRODUCTION

Society establishes both formal and informal guidelines that influence the behavior of its members. The behavior of an individual with a chronic condition is shaped by these societal influences as well. The individual who fully recovers from an illness returns to prior behaviors and roles. However, when there is only partial recovery or continuing illness, as with a chronic disease, the individual has to modify or adapt previous behavior and roles to accommodate societal expectations, their own expectations, and their health status. This chapter provides an overview of the illness experience and corresponding behavior demonstrated by those with chronic illness. It is not meant to be a comprehensive review of the entire body of knowledge, which is vast.

Historical Perspectives

Disease involves not only the body, but it also affects one's relationships, self-image, and behavior. The social aspects of disease may be related to the pathophysiologic changes that are occurring, but may be independent of them as well. The very act of diagnosing a condition as an illness has consequences far beyond the pathology involved (Conrad, 2005).

> When a veterinarian diagnoses a cow's condition as an illness, he does not merely by diagnosis change the cow's behavior...but when a physician diagnoses a human's condition as an illness, he changes the man's behavior by diagnosis: a social state is added to a biophysiological state by assigning the meaning of illness to disease (Freidson, 1970, p. 223).

The earliest concept of illness behavior was described in a 1929 essay by Henry Sigerist. His essay described the "special position of the sick" (cited in Young, 2004). Talcott Parsons developed this concept further and described the "sick role" in his 1951 work, *The Social System*.

FH chronic

Sick Role

Sickness has typically been viewed by sociologists as a form of deviant behavior (Cockerham, 2001, p. 157). This view was corroborated by Parsons' development of the sick role. Parsons, a proponent of structural–functionalist principles, viewed health as a functional prerequisite of society. From Parsons' point of view, sickness was dysfunctional and was a form of social deviance (Williams, 2005). From this functionalist viewpoint, social systems are linked to systems of personality and culture to form a basis for social order (Cockerham, 2001, p. 160). Parsons viewed sickness as a response to social pressure that permitted the avoidance of social responsibilities. Anyone could take on the role he identified; therefore, the role was achieved through failure to keep well.

The four major components of the sick role include:

■ The person is exempt from normal social roles.
■ The person is not responsible for his/her condition.
■ The person has the obligation to want to become well.
■ The person has the obligation to seek and cooperate with technically competent help (Williams, 2005, p. 124).

The Impaired Role

Gordon (1966) developed the impaired role in response to the sick role. He saw the sick role as being more applicable to individuals with acute illness and injuries. When the sick role is applied to long-term chronic illness, the role is less useful. A more appropriate role for those with chronic illness is the "impaired" role (Gordon, 1966). Although less well known than the sick role, it better addresses the needs of those with chronic illness.

Gordon (1966) identified behaviors, responses, and expectations of several socioeconomic groups

toward illnesses that differed in both severity and duration. He found, among all groups, that prognosis was the major factor in defining someone as "sick," and that once someone was so defined, behaviors were consistent with Parsons' model. When prognosis worsened, all groups encouraged increased exemption from social responsibility. Socioeconomic groups varied in terms of who was defined as sick, with members from lower socioeconomic groups equating sickness with functional incapacity.

Gordon identified two illness role statuses. The first was the sick role, as previously defined by Parsons, which was a valid role when the prognosis was grave and uncertain. The second role, which Gordon called the impaired role, was considered appropriate for conditions in which the prognosis was known and was not grave. When individuals were seen in the impaired role, "normal" social expectations and responsibilities were expected (Gordon, 1966). In other words, if society did not consider the individual "sick," it was expected that the individual return to normal behavior, within the limitations of the condition.

The impaired role assumes the following characteristics:

■ The individual has an impairment that is permanent.
■ The individual does not give up normal role responsibilities, but is expected to maintain normal behavior within the limits of the health condition. Modification of life situations may be necessitated by the disability.
■ The individual does not have to "want to get well," but rather is encouraged to make the most of remaining capabilities.

Inherent in the impaired role is the attitude that retaining sick role behaviors prevents the individual from managing their own care. However, once the impaired role is accepted, activities that help maintain control of the condition, prevent complications, lead to resumption of role responsibilities, and result in full realization of potentialities are acceptable. The impaired role incorporates rehabilitation concepts and maximization of wellness.

The impaired role, sometimes called the "at-risk" role, is seen as a transitional state, one in which individuals make changes in a variety of role behaviors in which they engaged before the illness. This role has some obligations, such as carrying out the medical regimen, but requires much less reduction in other social roles than does the sick role. One important difference between the two roles is that the impaired role is associated with more uncertainty than is the sick role.

Using Parsons' work as a basis, Mechanic (1962) proposed the concept of illness behavior as the way in which given symptoms may be differently perceived, evaluated, and acted (or not acted) upon by different persons (p. 189). His work in this area was initiated because he believed it was essential to understand the influence of norms, values, fears, and expected rewards and punishments on how an individual with illness acts. Mechanic's latest definition defines illness behavior as the "varying ways individuals respond to bodily indications, how they monitor internal states, define and interpret symptoms, make attributions, take remedial actions and utilize various sources of formal and informal care" (Mechanic, 1995, p. 1208).

Around the time of Mechanic's earlier work, Kasl and Cobb (1966) identified three types of health-related behavior: illness behavior, health behavior, and sick role behavior:

> Health behavior is any activity undertaken by a person believing himself to be healthy, for the purpose of preventing disease or detecting it in an asymptomatic stage.
>
> Illness behavior is any activity, undertaken by a person who feels ill, to define the state of his health and to discover a suitable remedy. Sick-role behavior is the activity undertaken, for the purpose of getting well, by those who consider themselves ill.

McHugh and Vallis (1986) suggest that perhaps instead of categorizing behavior as health-related, illness-related, or sick-role–related that it makes more sense to look at illness behavior on a continuum. By doing this, the term illness behavior can be broadly defined, and this characterization is more helpful, since the distinction between health and illness behaviors is arbitrary at times (p. 8).

Throughout the chronic illness literature, the term illness behavior is used in different ways and with different meanings. It has been used synonymously with the "sick role" (Turk & Salovey, 1995). Pilowsky (1986) supports the notion that patients who present with illness behaviors that are not congruent with the physical illness exhibit "abnormal" illness behavior. These behaviors would include excessive or inadequate response to symptoms, including but not limited to hypochondriasis, somatization, and denial of illness (Kirmayer & Loper, 2006).

Displaying extreme behavior over the result of a minor health issue, for instance, an ingrown toenail, may be termed abnormal illness behavior. But how do we as healthcare professionals describe behavior as normal or abnormal when it is not we who are diagnosed with the chronic condition and have the resulting illness experience?

Influences to Illness Behavior and Roles

Illness behavior is shaped by sociocultural and social-psychological factors (Mechanic, 1986). What follows in this section are examples of these factors.

Culture of Poverty

The culture of poverty (see Chapter 12) influences the development of social and psychological traits among those experiencing it. These traits include dependence, fatalism, inability to delay gratification, and a lower value placed on health (Cockerham, 2001, p. 123). The poor, who have to work to survive, often deny sickness unless it brings functional incapacity (Helman, 2007). Different cultures may define and interpret health and illness in a variety of ways (see Chapter 12).

Demographic Status

Marital status may influence illness behavior as well. In general, married individuals require fewer services because they are healthier, but utilize other services because they are more attuned to preventive care (Thomas, 2003). Searle, Norman, Thompson, and Vedhara (2007) examined the influence of the illness perceptions of clients' significant others and their impact on client outcomes and illness perceptions. Differences in illness representations of significant others and clients have shown to influence psychological adaptation in chronic fatigue syndrome and Addison's disease (cited in Searle et al., 2007). Searle and colleagues sought to understand illness representations in clients with type 2 diabetes and their partners. However, in this study, almost without exception, there was agreement between the illness representations of patients and their partners. Another aim of the study was to determine the influence of the partner or significant other on the clients' illness representation. There was some evidence to suggest that partners' representations did partially mediate clients' representations on exercise and dietary behaviors (Searle et al., 2007).

Gender may influence illness behavior and "help-seeking" behavior in chronic conditions. Sociologic analysis has suggested that women are more likely than men to seek medical help (Bury, 2005). Morbidity rates demonstrate that women are more likely to be sick than men and thus seek more professional medical help (p. 55). Lorber (2000) states that women are not more fragile than men, but are just more self-protective of their health status.

Increasing age often brings chronic conditions and disability. However, older individuals in poor health (as measured by medicine's standard measures) often do not see themselves in this way. What may influence older adults' perceptions of their illness and subsequent behavior may not even be considered by healthcare professionals as "relevant." Kelley-Moore, Schumacher, Kahana, and Kahana (2006) identified that cessation of driving and receiving home health care were two markers that self-identified older adults' illness perceptions, causing them to consider themselves disabled.

Past Experience

One's learning, socialization, and past experience, as defined by their social and cultural background, mediate illness behavior. Past experiences of observing one's parents being stoic, going to work when they were ill, avoiding medical help, all influence their children's future responses. If children see that "hard work" and not giving in to illness pays off with rewards, they will assimilate those experiences and mirror them in their own lives. Elfant, Gall, and Perlmuter (1999) evaluated the effects of avoidant illness behavior of parents on their adult children's adjustment to arthritis. Even after several decades, children's early observations of their parents' illness behaviors appears to affect their own adjustment to arthritis. Those clients whose parents avoided work and other activities when ill with a minor condition reported greater severity of arthritis and its limitations, depression, and helplessness when compared with clients whose parents did not respond to minor illness with avoidance (p. 415).

In another vein, how parents respond to their children's health complaints may later influence how the children, as adults, cope with illness. Whitehead and colleagues, and (1994) studied the influence of childhood social learning on the adult illness behavior of 383 women aged 20 to 40 years of age. Illness behavior was measured by frequency of symptoms, disability days, and physician visits for menstrual, bowel, and upper respiratory symptoms. Findings included that childhood reinforcement of menstrual illness behavior significantly predicted adult menstrual symptoms and disability days, and childhood reinforcement of cold illness behavior predicted adult cold symptoms and disability days. The study's data supported the hypothesis that specific patterns of illness behavior are learned during childhood through parental reinforcement and modeling, and that these behaviors continued into adulthood (p. 549).

Illness Representations

Clients and their families do not simply develop their own illness beliefs and perceptions within a vacuum, but they are molded by everyday social interactions (Marks, Murray, Evans, Willig, Woodall, & Sykes, 2005). Social representation theory is concerned about how societal belief systems influence and shape interpretations of illness of clients and their families. A classic study by Herzlich in 1973 (Marks et al., 2005) used social representation theory as a framework in a sample of French adults. The individuals considered activity to be the defining part of health and illness. If you were active, you were healthy. If you were inactive, it meant you were ill. Herzlich described three lay reactions to illness:

■ Illness as destructive: The experience of those actively involved in society

■ Illness as liberator: The experience of those with excessive social obligations

■ Illness as an occupation: The experience of those who accept illness and feel they must contribute to its alleviation (Marks et al., 2005, p. 231).

Levanthal, Levanthal, and Cameron (2001) describe five attributes of illness representations. These include:

■ The identity of the threat or the symptoms that define it

■ The time line for development and duration of the disease, treatment regimen, and time needed for cure, treatment, or death

■ The causes of the threat (internal or external)

■ The anticipated and experienced consequences of the disease

■ The controllability of the condition (Levanthal et al., 2001, p. 22)

According to Levanthal and colleagues these attributes form the basis of lay models of illness and

guide and shape how we select and use coping strategies (p. 22).

IMPACT AND ISSUES RELATED TO ILLNESS BEHAVIOR

As we describe illness behavior, it is important to reiterate the difference between the terms disease and illness. Disease is the pathophysiology, the change in body structure or function that can be quantified, measured, and defined. Disease is the objective "measurement" of symptoms.

Illness is what the client and family experience. It is what is experienced and "lived" by the client and family, and includes the "meaning" the client gives to that experience (Helman, 2007). Both the meaning given to the symptoms and the client's response, or behavior, are influenced by the client's background and personality as well as the cultural, social, and economic contexts in which the symptoms appear (p. 126).

The Illness Experience

The diagnosis of a chronic disease and subsequent management of that disease brings unique experiences and meanings of that process to both the client and family. The biomedical world disregards illness and its meaning and prefers to think of the disease. Disease can be quantified and measured, and it can be considered a "black and white" concept. Disease fits into our medical model framework. Illness, and its meaning, does not fit into a neat little box; it is not a black and white concept, but consists of many shades of gray and is difficult to measure and categorize. Kleinmann, who has written since the 1970s about illness behavior and its meaning, becomes concerned that researchers have "reduced sickness to something divorced from meaning in order to avoid the hard and still unanswered technical questions concerning how to actually go about measuring meaning and objectivizing and quantitating its effect on health status and illness behavior" (Kleinmann, 1985, p. 149). While realizing the importance of this scientific work, Kleinmann sees it as "detrimental to the understanding of illness as human experience, since they redefine the problem to subtract that which is mostly innately human, beliefs, feelings…" (p. 149).

The common sense self-regulation model (Leventhal et al., 2001) seeks to explain that individual illness perceptions influence coping responses to an illness. This perspective explains that clients construct their own illness representations to help them make sense of their illness experience. It is these representations that form a basis for appropriate or inappropriate coping responses (Leventhal et al., 2001). Stuifbergen and colleagues (2006) used a convenience sample of 91 women with fibromyalgia to explore their illness representations. Overall, the women had fairly negative perceptions of their illness. Emotional representations explained 41% of the variance in mental health scores. Using the model of Levanthal and colleagues (2001), less emotional distress predicted more frequent health behaviors and more-positive mental health scores; whereas those women who perceived their fibromyalgia to have more serious consequences and as less controllable, were more likely to have higher scores on the Fibromyalgia Impact Questionnaire (p. 359).

Price (1996) describes individuals with a chronic disease as those developing an illness career that responds to changes in health, his or her involvement with healthcare professionals, and the psychological changes associated with pathology, grief, and stress management (p. 276). This illness career is dynamic, flexible, and goes through different stages of adaptation as the disease itself may change.

Loss of Self

Charmaz (1983) coined the phrase, loss of self, with her research in the 1980s, interviewing individuals with chronic illness through a symbolic interactionist perspective. The influences to the loss of self develop from the chronic condition(s) and the illness experience. Charmaz describes clients' illness experience as living a restricted life, experiencing social isolation, being discredited, and burdening others. Slowly the individual with chronic illness feels their self-image disappear: a loss of self, without the development of an equally valued new one (p. 168).

In another study of 40 men with chronic illness, Charmaz (1994) describes different identity dilemmas than with women. Charmaz sees these men as "preserving self." As men come to terms with illness and disability, they preserve self by limiting the effect from illness in their lives. They intensify control over their lives. Many assume that they can recapture their past self, and they try to do so. They may devote vast amounts of energy to keeping their illness contained and the disability invisible to maintain their masculinity. At the same time, they often maintain another identity at home … thus a public identity and a private identity to preserve self (p. 282).

Moral Work

Townsend, Wyke, and Hunt (2006) in their qualitative study describe the moral dimension of the chronic illness experience. Their work speaks to the fact that moral work is integral to the illness, similar to the biographical and everyday "work" of Corbin and Strauss (1988) . The participants in their study spoke about the need to demonstrate their moral worth as individuals, that it was their moral obligation to manage symptoms alongside their daily life (p. 189).

Devalued Self

In a qualitative study of Chinese immigrant women in Canada, Anderson (1991) describes how these women with type 1 diabetes have a devalued self, not only from the disease but also because of dealing with being marginalized in a foreign country where they do not speak the language. Similar to the "loss of self" described by Charmaz, Anderson speaks of women who need to reconstruct a new self. Influencing this devalued self are the interactions with healthcare professionals. Interactions with care providers, which were frequently negative in nature, added additional sources of stress to further devalue these women.

Continuity and Discontinuity

Secrest and Zeller (2007) describe the continuity and discontinuity of self following stroke. Although similar to the "loss of self" concept of Charmaz, Secrest and Zeller use these terms from gerontology literature, specifically Atchley's continuity theory of normal aging. They see continuity and discontinuity as dimensions of quality of life (Secrest & Zeller, 2007).

Who Legitimizes Chronic Illness?

With some illnesses, especially when symptoms are not well defined and diagnostic tests may be ambiguous, receiving legitimization from the physician or other healthcare professionals may be difficult and frustrating. Denial of opportunity to move into the sick role leads to "doctor hopping," placing clients in problematic relationships in which they must "work out" solutions alone (Steward & Sullivan, 1982). As a result, symptomatic persons may be left to question the truth of their own illness perceptions.

As examples, two current chronic conditions often defy diagnosis and are slow to respond to treatment. Chronic fatigue syndrome (CFS) and fibromyalgia are typically seen as diseases of young women. In both diseases there is uncertainty with respect to etiology, treatment, and prognosis. They have been contested illnesses, in that some question their existence (Asbring, 2001). Without legitimatization from physicians or the healthcare system, these clients are labeled as hypochondriacs or malingerers. Some of these clients are referred to psychologists or psychiatrists when a physical diagnosis cannot be made and diagnostic tests results are normal.

When a diagnosis is finally made, the client frequently shows an initial somewhat joyous response to having a name for the recurrent and troublesome symptoms. This reaction results from the decrease in stress over the unknown. These clients have an enormous stake in how their illnesses are understood. They seek to achieve the legitimacy necessary to elicit sympathy and avoid stigma, and to protect their own self-concept (Mechanic, 1995).

Asbring (2001) identifies two themes from her qualitative study in which women with CFS or fibromyalgia were interviewed. She describes an earlier identity partly lost, and coming to terms with a new identity. Asbring uses the term "identity transformation" in the women she interviewed. However, she also saw illness gains in these women. The illness and its limitations provided the women with time to think and reflect on their lives and perhaps rearrange priorities. Therefore, the illness experience of these women may be seen as a paradox with both losses and gains (p. 318).

Larun and Malterud (2007) examined 20 qualitative studies in a meta-ethnography about the illness experiences of individuals with CFS to summarize the illness experiences of the individuals as well as the physicians' perspectives. Across studies, clients spoke of being "controlled and betrayed by their bodies" (pp. 22–23). Although physical activities were mostly curtailed, individuals spoke of the mental fatigue that affected memory and concentration, and conversations that were hard to follow, and several clients felt that their learning abilities had decreased (p. 24). One of the themes that emerged was stories about *bodies which no longer held the capacity for social involvement.* For some individuals the most distressing part of the illness were the negative responses from family members, the workplace, and their physicians, who *questioning the legitimacy of their illness behavior* because of the dynamic symptoms of CFS (p. 25). Thus their physicians' beliefs about CFS influenced the clients' perceptions of the disease and thereby their illness experience. To summarize, the researchers' analysis determined that clients' sense of identity becomes more or less invalid and that a change in identity of the individuals was experienced.

CASE STUDY

Ms. Janet Brown is a 36-year-old woman, who was recently diagnosed with fibromyalgia. She has been a client at the clinic where you work for several years, calling in every few weeks and/or having frequent appointments. Typically her clinical symptoms have been vague; however, she has often seemed frantic about them. Her recent diagnosis initially seemed to make her be more content and settled. However, now it seems that she is escalating in her behavior and talking about no one caring about her (including her family), that your clinic does not "understand" her, and is just generally being unreasonable on the phone and in person.

Discussion Questions

1. How do you make sense of this client's illness behavior? Is it abnormal?
2. What strategies might you use to deal with this client?
3. How could you apply the frameworks for practice mentioned in this chapter to this client situation?

Professional Responses to Illness Behavior and Roles

Healthcare professionals generally expect those entering the acute hospital setting to conform to sick role behaviors. Most people entering the hospital for the first time are quickly socialized and expected to cooperate with treatment, to recover, and to return to their normal roles. Provider expectations and client responses are in line with social expectations and fit with the traditional medical model of illness as acute and curable. When clients are compliant and cooperative, healthcare professionals communicate to them that they are "good patients" (Lorber, 1981). When clients are less cooperative, the staff may consider them problematic.

But the percentage of individuals with chronic illness entering hospitals is increasing, and these conditions cannot be cured. Such admissions occur when symptoms flare or acute illnesses are superimposed. Many of these individuals have had their chronic illnesses for long periods and have had prior hospital experiences. Multiple contacts with the health care system result in loss of the "blind faith" that the individual once had in that system. Individuals with chronic illness are seeking a different kind of relationship with health care professionals (Thorne & Robinson, 1988). The extent to which a client with chronic illness is included in the formulation of his or her treatment plan will likely influence the assumption of responsibility for it and, ultimately, its success (Weaver & Wilson, 1994).

Being in Gordon's "impaired" role is integral to the daily lives of the chronically ill. Although willing to delegate some responsibility for care to healthcare professionals, they prefer to retain as much control of their regimens as possible. These clients have developed their own competence over time dealing with their illnesses, and they have come to expect acknowledgment of that competence in their health care relationships (Thorne & Robinson, 1988).

Thorne's (1990) study of individuals with chronic illness and their families found that their relationships with healthcare professionals evolved from what was termed "naive trust" through "disenchantment" to a final stage of "guarded alliance." She proposed that the "rules" that govern these relationships should be entirely different for acute and chronic illness. Although assuming sick role dependency may be adaptive in acute illness, where medical expertise offers hope of a cure, it is not so in chronic illness. Chronically ill individuals are the "experts" in their illnesses and should have the ultimate authority in managing those illnesses over time.

When individuals with chronic illness are hospitalized, they view the situation quite differently from the healthcare professionals with whom they interact. Clients with multiple chronic disorders may focus on maintaining stability of quiescent conditions to prevent unnecessary symptomatology, whereas staff are more likely to focus on managing the current acute disorder (Strauss, 1981). In addition, clients who have had multiple prior admissions are more likely to use their hospital savvy to gain what they want or need from the system. During hospitalization, these individuals may demand certain treatments, specific times for treatment, or routines outside of hospital parameters. They may keep track of times that various routines occur or complain about or report actions of the staff as a means to an end they consider important. All of these demands increase staff work and stress, and frequently the client is labeled a "problem patient" (Lorber, 1981).

In a grounded theory study in the United Kingdom, Wilson, Kendall, and Brooks (2006) explored how patient expertise is viewed, interpreted, defined, and experienced by both clients and healthcare professionals. With nursing playing a key role in empowering clients with chronic disease to self-manage their conditions, knowing how that client expertise is viewed (by the care provider) is extremely important. Generally, in this study of 100 healthcare professionals (physicians, nurses, physical therapists), the nurses found the expert patients to be more threatening than other healthcare professionals did. The nurses had issues with accountability, perceived threats to their professional power, and potential litigation. The data from the study demonstrated that the nurses lacked a clear role definition and distinct expertise in working with patients with chronic disease and were unable to work in a flexible partnership with self-managing patients (p. 810).

Lack of Role Norms for Individuals with Chronic Illness

Chronic illnesses require that a variety of tasks be performed to fulfill the requirements of both the medical regimen and the individual's personal lifestyle. Despite residual disability that limits activity, society does not identify the chronically ill as individuals who are experiencing illness. Assuming sick role behaviors is discouraged. These individuals enter and remain in the impaired role, but implicit behaviors for this role are not well defined by society, leading to a situation of role ambiguity. Given this lack of norms, influences on the client include the degree of disability (with different attributes of disability producing different consequences), visibility of the disability (the lower the visibility, the more normal the response), self-acceptance of the disability (resulting in others' reciprocating with acceptance), and societal views of the disabled as either economically dependent or productive. Without role definition, whether disability is present or not, individuals are unable to achieve maximum levels of functioning. Individuals must adapt their definitions of themselves to their limitations, and to what the anticipated future imposes on them by the chronic condition (Watt, 2000).

INTERVENTIONS

There is no magic list of interventions to assist and support clients and their families with their illness experience. Our current healthcare system with its acute care focus, fix and cure model, and a prescription for each symptom, does not fit with caring for individuals long term. These clients do not need their illness behavior "fixed: or "cured," but instead need a healthcare professional that will listen and understand the illness experience and not the disease process. What follows are suggestions that assist and support clients and their families.

Frameworks and Models for Practice

Caring for a client with chronic illness requires a framework or model for practice that differs from that of caring for those with acute, episodic disease. The frameworks that follow are examples, and are not intended to be all-inclusive.

These frameworks and models should not be confused with the disease management models discussed in Chapter 19. Disease management models address the physical symptoms of the condition. Some of those models assign an algorithm to the condition where clients receive certain "care" when their blood work is at an inappropriate level, or their symptoms "measure" a certain degree of seriousness. These models manage the disease, but not the illness. Illness frameworks and models address the illness experience of the individual and family that occurs as a result of changing health status.

Chronic Illness and Quality of Life

In the early 1960s, Anselm Strauss, working with Barney Glaser, a social scientist, and Jeanne Quint Benoliel, a nurse, interviewed dying patients to ascertain what kind of "care" was needed for these clients (Corbin & Strauss, 1992). As a result of those early interviews, Strauss et al. (1975/1984) published a rudimentary framework that addressed the issues and concerns of individuals with chronic illness. Although the term "trajectory" was coined at that time, it did not become fully developed until 20 years later. His framework was simple, but it was an early attempt to examine the illness experience of the individual and family as opposed to the disease perspective. If care professionals could better understand the illness experience of clients and families, perhaps more appropriate care would be provided. Basic to this care was understanding the key problems that include:

- The prevention of medical crises and their management if they occur
- Controlling symptoms

- Carrying out of prescribed medical regimens
- Prevention of, or living with, social isolation
- Adjustment to changes in the disease
- Attempts to normalize interactions and lifestyle
- Funding—finding the necessary money
- Confronting attendant psychological, marital, and familial problems (Strauss et al., 1984, p. 16)

After identifying the key problems of the individual and family with chronic illness, what followed were basic strategies, family and organizational arrangements, and the consequences of those arrangements (Strauss et al., 1984, p. 17).

The Trajectory Framework

From the work of Strauss and colleagues in the 1960s and 1970s, the trajectory framework was further refined in the 1980s. Corbin and Strauss (1992) developed this framework so that nurses could: (1) gain insight into the chronic illness experience of the client; (2) integrate existing literature about chronicity into their practice; and (3) provide direction for building nursing models that guide practice, teaching, research, and policymaking (p. 10).

A trajectory is defined as the course of an illness over time, plus the actions of clients, families and healthcare professionals to manage that course (Corbin, 1998, p. 3). The illness trajectory is set in motion by pathophysiology and changes in health status, but there are strategies that can be used by clients, families, and healthcare professionals that shape the course of dying and thus the illness trajectory (Corbin & Strauss, 1992). Even if the disease may be the same, each individual's illness trajectory is different, and takes into account the uniqueness of each individual (Jablonski, 2004). Shaping does not imply that the ultimate course of the disease will be changed or the disease will be cured, merely that the illness trajectory may be shaped or altered by actions of the individual and family so that the disease course is stable, fewer exacerbations occur, and symptoms are better controlled (Corbin & Strauss, 1992).

Within the model, the term "phase" indicates the different stages of the chronic illness experience for the client. There are nine phases in the trajectory model, and although it could be conceived as a continuum, it is not linear. Clients may move through these phases in a linear fashion, regress to a former phase, or plateau for an extended period. In addition, having more than one chronic disease influences movement along the trajectory as well. Another term used in the model is biography. A client's biography consists of previous hospital experiences, and useful ways of dealing with symptoms, illness beliefs, and other life experiences (White & Lubkin, 1998).

The initial phase of the trajectory model is the pretrajectory phase, or preventive phase, in which the course of illness has not yet begun; however, there are genetic factors or lifestyle behaviors that place an individual at risk for a chronic condition. An example would be the individual who is overweight, has a family history of cardiac disease and high cholesterol, and does not exercise.

During the trajectory phase, signs and symptoms of the disease appear and a diagnostic workup may begin. The individual begins to cope with implications of a diagnosis. In the stable phase, the illness symptoms are under control and management of the disease occurs primarily at home. A period of inability to keep symptoms under control occurs in the unstable phase. The acute phase brings severe and unrelieved symptoms or disease complications. Critical or life-threatening situations that require emergency treatment occur in the crisis phase. The comeback phase signals a gradual return to an acceptable way of life within the symptoms that the disease imposes. The downward phase is characterized by progressive deterioration and an increase in disability or symptoms. The trajectory model ends with the dying phase characterized by gradual or rapid shutting down of body processes (Corbin, 2001, pp. 4–5).

Chronic Illness and the Life Cycle

Rolland's (1987) illness trajectory model encompasses three phases: (1) crisis, (2) chronic, and (3) terminal. The crisis phase has two subphases consisting of the symptomatic period prior to diagnosis; and the period of initial adjustment just after diagnosis.

The chronic phase is the period between the beginning of treatment and the terminal phase. Rolland (1987) was one of the first authors to describe chronic illness, and in this case the chronic phase, as the "long haul," the day to day living with chronic illness. Lastly, the terminal phase is divided into the preterminal phase, where the client and family acknowledge that death is inevitable, and the period following death (Jablonski, 2004, p. 54).

Shifting Perspectives Model of Chronic Illness

This model resulted from work of Thorne and Paterson (1998), who analyzed 292 qualitative studies with chronic physical illness that were published from 1980 to 1996. Of these, 158 studies became a part of a metastudy in which client roles in chronic illness were described. The work of Thorne and Paterson reflects the "insider" perspective of chronic illness as opposed to the "outsider" view, the more traditional view. This change in perspective is a shift from the traditional approach of patient-as-client to one of client-as-partner in care (p. 173). Results from the metastudy also demonstrated a shift away from focusing on loss and burden, and an attempt to view health within illness.

Analysis of these studies led to the development of the Shifting Perspectives Model of Chronic Illness (Paterson, 2001). The model depicts chronic illness as an ongoing, continually shifting process where people experience a complex dialectic between the world and themselves (p. 23). Donnelly (1993) first spoke of individuals with chronic illness living in the "dual kingdoms of the well and the sick" (p. 6). Paterson's model considers both the "illness" and the "wellness" of the individual (Paterson, 2003). The illness-in-the-foreground perspective focuses on the sickness, loss, and burden of the chronic illness. This is a common reaction of those recently diagnosed with a chronic disease. The overwhelming consequences of the condition, learning about their illness, considerations of treatment, and long-term effects contribute to putting the illness in the foreground. The disease becomes the individual's identity.

Illness-in-the-foreground could also be a protective response by the individual and be used to conserve energy for other activities. However, it could be used to maintain their identity as a "sick" person, or because it is congruent with their need to have sickness as their social identity and receive secondary gains (Paterson, 2001).

With wellness-in-the-foreground, the "self" is the source of identity and not the disease (Paterson, 2001, p. 23). The individual is in control and not the disease. It does not mean, though, that the individual is physically well, cured, or even in remission of the disease symptoms. The shift occurs in the individual's thinking that allows the individual to focus away from the disease. However, any threat that cannot be controlled will transition the individual back to the illness-in-the-foreground perspective. Threats could be disease progression, lack of ability to self-manage the disease, stigma, or interactions with others (Paterson, 2001).

Lastly, neither the illness perspective nor the wellness perspective is right or wrong, but each merely reflects the individual's unique needs, health status, and focus at the time (Paterson, 2001). In Paterson's research published in 2003, one of her study participants was concerned that those reading about the Shifting Perspectives Model might interpret the two perspectives as "either/or," that one has to have either wellness or illness in the foreground. This individual states:

> I think there is danger when researchers think there is a right way to have a chronic illness. There is only one way... the one you choose at the moment . . . generally I live in the orange. If red is illness and yellow

represents wellness, then I like to be a blend of both things . . . in the orange . . . It is not a good idea for me to be completely yellow because then I forget that I have MS and I do stupid things that I pay for later. And if I am totally in the red, I am too depressed to do anything (Paterson, 2003, p. 990).

Dealing with Dependency

Miller (2000) discusses dependency in individuals with chronic illness and links it with the sense of powerlessness that these individuals often confront. Chronic illness is fraught with unpredictable dilemmas. Even when an acute stage is past, the client's energy for recovery may be sapped by the uncertainty about the future course of the illness, the effectiveness of medical regimens, and the disruption of usual patterns of living. Awareness of behavioral responses and when they occur can help the professional avoid premature emphasis on independence until the client can collaborate in working toward a return to normal roles (see Chapter 11).

Miller (2000) recommends several strategies for decreasing clients' feelings of powerlessness as they work toward independence:

1. Modifying the environment to afford clients more means of control
2. Helping clients set realistic goals and expectations
3. Increasing clients' knowledge about their illness and its management
4. Increasing the sensitivity of health professionals and significant others to the powerlessness imposed by chronic illness
5. Encouraging verbalization of feelings

Utilizing knowledge of illness roles in planning interventions allows the healthcare professional to maximize time spent with the client. One such intervention that could benefit from integrating knowledge of illness roles is teaching (see Chapter 14). The client who is still in the highly dependent phase cannot benefit from teaching. As

▌ EVIDENCE-BASED PRACTICE BOX

A sample of 23 people in their early fifties was recruited from a community health survey in Scotland. All participants had four or more chronic illnesses. Through interviews, the aim of the study was to identify how individuals with multiple chronic illnesses negotiate their daily lives. They shared with the researchers that they had a moral obligation to manage their symptoms as well as manage their daily lives. Many talked about the importance of paid employment, and some considered being unemployed a "loss." Others continued with the employment despite considerable risks to their health. Being employed was important to participants' identities. "The participants faced moral concerns as they tried to be 'responsible' patients, living 'normal' lives. The ability to manage illness alongside social obligations in daily life was framed as a sense of duty" (p. 190). The findings of this study demonstrate that recognizing and understanding the constant dilemmas that those with chronic illness face is critical in working with these clients. Controlling the disease and its accompanying symptoms may not always be your clients' priority, but it may be your priority. This mismatch in priorities needs to be recognized.

Source: Townsend, A., Syke, S., & Hunt, K. (2006). Self-managing and managing self: Practical and moral dilemmas in accounts of living with chronic illness. *Chronic Illness, 2,* 185–194.

improvement in physical status occurs, emphasis on the desire to return to normal roles creates motivation to learn about the condition and necessary procedures for maximizing health. As the client moves into the impaired role and becomes aware of the necessity to maximize remaining potential, teaching provides a highly successful tool both in the hospital and at home.

Self-Management

The participants in the study of Kralick, Koch, Price, and Howard (2004) identified self-management as a process that they initiated to bring about order in their lives. This is in sharp contrast to how most healthcare professionals describe self-management in a structured patient education program that assists clients in adhering to their medical regimen. The participants saw self-management as creating a sense of order, and a process that included four themes: (1) recognizing and monitoring the boundaries; (2) mobilizing the resources; (3) managing the shift in self-identity; and (4) balancing, pacing, planning, and prioritizing (pp. 262–263). Kralick

and colleagues suggest that self-management is a combination of a process by clients and families and a structure of patient education.

The Women to Women project has been instrumental in helping women with chronic illness in rural states manage their illnesses. Through a computer intervention model that provides education, support groups, and fosters self-care, women have successfully managed their illness responses (Sullivan, Weinert, & Cudney, 2003).

Clients with chronic illness use multiple techniques to manage symptoms, maintain social roles, be the "good patient" and maintain some degree of normality. Townsend, Wyke, and Hunt (2006) describe the moral obligation of individuals to both self-manage their symptoms and manage their self. Although individuals are trying to manage both symptoms and social roles, the priority is always given to behaviors that typify a "normal" life and identity management over managing the symptoms of the disease (p. 193).

Critical to working with clients and families in self-managing both their disease and their illness is appropriate client–healthcare provider communication. Thorne, Harris, Mahoney, Con, and McGuiness (2004) interviewed clients with end-stage renal disease, type 2 diabetes, multiple sclerosis, and fibromyalgia to determine what clients perceived as priorities. Across all diseases, the concepts of courtesy, respect, and engagement were important. Certainly courtesy and respect are fairly clear in their meaning. Engagement was described by clients as an extension of courtesy and respect. An example would be a healthcare professional engaged with a client in problem solving and care management, and there would be a feeling of teamwork and working together (p. 301). Such communication enhanced their relationships with clients.

Research

Do we understand and can we place in an appropriate context the meaning of illness for our clients? Why do some individuals ignore symptoms and refuse to seek medical advice, while others with the same condition seek immediate care and relief from their "social roles" at the slightest symptom. A relatively minor symptom in one individual causes great distress, whereas more serious health conditions in others cause little concern.

Stuifbergen and colleagues (2006) suggest that it is unclear from the literature how illness perceptions change over time and how specifically these perceptions are influenced. These researchers believe that if illness perceptions can be altered, then interactions with those in a positive manner could be encouraged.

Mechanic (1986/1995) asks a question that is still pertinent today. What are the processes or factors that cause individuals exposed to similar stressors to respond differently and present unique illness behavior? There is such variation in how individuals perceive their health status, seek or not seek medical care, and function in their social and work roles. What causes these differences?

OUTCOMES

Illness behavior is not deviant or need to be fixed. However, we need to support our clients and understand the lived experience of the illness. As healthcare professionals, we are efficient and effective working within the disease model. However, the client lives in the illness model. Because nursing is an art and a science, there is a strong "fit" with the illness model. The best outcome for clients with chronic illness would be the healthcare professional supporting and assisting the client through the illness experience.

STUDY QUESTIONS

1. Differentiate between health and illness behavior and give examples of each.
2. Describe the "fit" of the sick role and "impaired" role with someone with chronic obstructive pulmonary disease (COPD). With metastatic cancer.
3. How do healthcare professionals influence the illness behavior of clients and families?
4. How could you apply each of the frameworks for practice described in this chapter to your own population of clients with chronic illness?
5. What influences your own illness behaviors?

6. Using this chapter as a guide, how would you support and work with an individual that has either CFS or fibromyalgia? How do your own past experiences influence your practice with these clients?
7. Dealing with "expert" patients can be difficult. Often your own "power" as a healthcare professional is threatened. How do you deal with "expert" patients?
8. There are no norms for individuals with long-term illness. What does this mean and how does it apply to your population of clients with chronic illness?

REFERENCES

Anderson, J.M. (1991). Immigrant women speak of chronic illness: The social construction of the devalued self. *Journal of Advanced Nursing, 16,* 710–717.

Asbring, P. (2001). Chronic illness—a disruption in life: Identity transformation among women with chronic fatigue syndrome and fibromyalgia. *Journal of Advanced Nursing, 34* (3), 312–319.

Bury, M. (2005). *Health and illness.* Cambridge, UK: Polity Press.

Charmaz, K. (1983). Loss of self: A fundamental form of suffering in the chronically ill. *Sociology of health and illness, 5*(2), 168–195.

Charmaz, K. (1994). Identity dilemma of chronically ill men. *The Sociological Quarterly, 35*(2), 269–288.

Cockerham, W.C. (2001). The sick role. In *Medical sociology* (8th ed.) (pp. 156–178). Upper Saddle River, NJ: Prentice-Hall.

Conrad, P. (2005). *The sociology of health and illness: Critical perspectives* (7th ed.). New York: Worth Publishers.

Corbin, J. (1998). The Corbin & Strauss chronic illness trajectory model: An update. *Scholarly Inquiry for Nursing Practice, 12*(1), 33–41.

Corbin, J. (2001). Introduction and overview: Chronic illness and nursing. In R. Hyman & J. Corbin (Eds.), *Chronic illness: Research and theory for nursing practice* (pp. 1–15). New York, NY: Springer.

Corbin, J.M., & Strauss, A. (1988). *Unending work and care: Managing chronic illness at home.* San Francisco: Jossey-Bass.

Corbin, J., & Strauss, A. (1992). A nursing model for chronic illness management based upon the trajectory framework. In P. Woog (Ed.), *The chronic illness trajectory framework: The Corbin and Strauss nursing model.* (pp. 9–28). New York: Springer.

Donnelly, G. (1993). Chronicity: Concept and reality. *Holistic Nursing Practice, 8,* 1–7.

Elfant, E., Gall, E., & Perlmuter, L.C. (1999). Learned illness behavior and adjustment to arthritis [Electronic version]. *Arthritis Care and Research, 12*(6), 411–416.

Freidson, E. (1970). *Profession of medicine.* New York: Dodd, Mead.

Gordon, G. (1966). *Role theory and illness: A sociological perspective.* New Haven, CT: College and University Press.

Helman, C.G. (2007). *Culture, health and illness* (5th ed.). London: Arnold.

Jablonski, A. (2004). The illness trajectory of end-stage renal disease dialysis patients. *Research and Theory for Nursing Practice: An International Journal, 18*(1), 51–72.

Kasl, S.V., & Cobb, S. (1966). Health behavior, illness behavior, and sick-role behavior. *Archives of Environmental Health, 12,* 531–541.

Kelley-Moore, J.A., Schumacher, J.G., Kahana, E., & Kahana, B. (2006). When do older adults become "disabled"? Social and health antecedents of perceived disability in a panel study of the oldest old. *Journal of Health and Social Behavior, 47,* 126–141.

Kirmayer, L.J., & Looper, K.J. (2006). Abnormal illness behavior: Physiological, psychological, and social dimensions of coping with distress [Electronic version]. *Current Opinion in Psychiatry, 19,* 54–60.

Kleinmann, A. (1985). Illness meanings and illness behavior. In S. McHugh & M. Vallis (Eds.), *Illness behavior: A multidisciplinary model* (pp. 149–160). New York: Plenum.

Kralick, D., Koch, T., Price, K., & Howard, N. (2004). Chronic illness management: Taking action to create order [Electronic version]. *Journal of Clinical Nursing, 13,* 259–267.

Larun, L., & Malterud, K. (2007). Identify and coping experiences in chronic fatigue syndrome: A synthesis of qualitative studies [Electronic version]. *Patient Education and Counseling, 69,* 20–28.

Leventhal, H., Leventhal, E.A., & Cameron, L. (2001). Representations, procedures, and affect in illness self-regulation: A perceptual-cognitive model. In Baum, A., Revenson, T.A., & Singer, J.E. (Eds.), *Handbook of health psychology.* (pp. 19–47). Mahwah, NJ: Lawrence Erlbaum Associates.

Lorber, J. (2000). Gender and health. In P. Brown (Ed.), *Perspectives in Medical Sociology* (3rd ed., pp. 40–70). Prospect Heights, IL: Waveland Press.

Lorber, J. (1981). Good patients and problem patients: Conformity and deviance in a general hospital. In P. Conrad & R. Kern (Eds.), *The sociology of health and illness: Critical perspectives.* New York: St. Martin's.

Marks, D.F., Murray, M., Evans, B., Willig, C., Woodall, C., & Sykes, C. (2005). *Health psychology: Theory, research and practice* (2nd ed.). Thousand Oaks, CA: Sage.

McHugh, S., & Vallis, M. (1986). Illness behavior: Operationalization of the biopsychosocial model. In S. McHugh & M. Vallis (Eds.), *Illness behavior: A multidisciplinary model* (pp. 1–32). New York: Plenum.

Mechanic, D. (1962). The concept of illness behavior. *Journal of Chronic Diseases, 15,* 189–194.

Mechanic, D. (1986). The concept of illness behavior: Culture, situation, and personal predisposition. *Psychological Medicine, 16,* 1–7.

Mechanic, D. (1995). Sociological dimensions of illness behavior. Social Science and Medicine, *41*(9), 1207–1216.

Miller, J.F. (2000). *Coping with chronic illness: Overcoming powerlessness* (3rd ed.). Philadelphia: F.A. Davis.

Parsons, T. (1951). The social system. New York: The Free Press.

Paterson, B. (2001). The shifting perspectives model of chronic illness. *Journal of Nursing Scholarship, 33*(1), 21–26.

Paterson, B. (2003). The koala has claws: Applications of the shifting perspectives model in research of chronic illness. *Qualitative Health Research, 13*(7), 987–994.

Pilowsky, I. (1986). Abnormal illness behavior: A review of the concept and its implications. In S. McHugh & T.M. Vallis (Eds.), *Illness behavior: A multidisciplinary model* (pp. 391–408). New York: Plenum.

Price, B. (1996). Illness careers: The chronic illness experience. *Journal of Advanced Nursing, 24,* 275–279.

Rolland, J.S. (1987). Chronic illness and the life cycle: A conceptual framework. *Family Process, 26,* 203–221.

Searle, A., Norman, P., Thompson, R., & Vedhara, K. (2007). Illness representations among patients with type 2 diabetes and their partners: Relationships with self-management behaviors [Electronic version]. *Journal of Psychosomatic Research, 63*(2), 175–184.

Secrest, J., & Zeller, R. (2007). The relationship of continuity and discontinuity, functional ability, depression, and quality of life over time in stroke survivors. *Rehabilitation Nursing, 32*(4), 158–164.

Sontag, S. (1988). *Illness as metaphor.* Toronto: Collins Publishers.

Steward, D.C., & Sullivan, T.J. (1982). Illness behavior and the sick role in chronic disease: The case of multiple sclerosis. Social science and medicine, 16, 1397–1404.

Stuifbergen, A., Phillips, L., Voelmeck, W., & Browder, R. (2006). Illness perceptions and related outcomes among women with fibromyalgia syndrome [Electronic version]. *Women's Health Issues, 16,* 353–360.

Strauss, A. (1981). Chronic illness. In P. Conrad & R. Kern (Eds.), *The sociology of health and illness: Critical perspectives.* New York: St. Martin's.

Strauss, A., & Glaser, B. (1975). *Chronic illness and the quality of life.* St. Louis: Mosby.

Strauss, A., Corbin, J., Fagerhaugh, S., Glaser, B., et al. (1984). *Chronic illness and the quality of life* (2nd ed.). St. Louis: Mosby.

Sullivan, T., Weinert, C., & Cudney, S. (2003). Management of chronic illness: Voices of rural women. *Journal of Advanced Nursing, 44*(6), 566–574.

Thomas, R. (2003). *Society and health: Sociology for health professionals.* New York: Kluwer.

Thorne, S.E. (1990). Constructive noncompliance in chronic illness. *Holistic Nursing Practice, 5*(1), 62–69.

Thorne, S.E., Harris, S.R., Mahoney, K., Con, A., & McGuinness, L. (2004). The context of health care communication in chronic illness [Electronic version]. *Patient Education and Counseling, 54*(3), 299–306.

Thorne, S.E., & Paterson, B. (1998). Shifting images of chronic illness. *Image, 30* (2), 173–178.

Thorne, S.E., & Robinson, C.A. (1988). Reciprocal trust in health care relationships. *Journal of Advanced Nursing, 13,* 782–789.

Townsend, A., Wyke, S., & Hunt, K. (2006). Self-managing and managing self: Practical and moral dilemmas in accounts of living with chronic illness. *Chronic Illness, 2,* 185–194.

Turk, D.C. & Salovey, P. (1995). Cognitive-behavioral treatment of illness behavior. In P.M. Nicassio & T.W. Smith (Eds.), *Managing chronic illness: A biopsychosocial perspective* (pp. 245–284). Washington, DC: American Psychological Association.

Watt, S. (2000). Clinical decision-making in the context of chronic illness. *Health Expectations, 3,* 6–16.

Weaver, S.K. & Wilson, J.F. (1994). Moving toward patient empowerment. *Nursing and Health Care, 15*(9), 380–483.

White, N., & Lubkin, I. (1998). Illness trajectory. In I. Lubkin & P. Larsen (Eds.), *Chronic illness: Impact and interventions* (4th ed.) (pp. 53–76). Sudbury, MA: Jones & Bartlett.

Whitehead, W.E., Crowell, M.D., Heller, B.R., Robinson, J.C., Schuster, M.M., & Horn, S. (1994). Modeling and reinforcement of the sick role during childhood predicts adult illness behavior. *Psychosomatic Medicine, 56,* 541–550.

Williams, S.J. (2005). Parsons revisited: From the sick role to…? [Electronic version]. *Health, 9,* 123–144.

Wilson, P.M., Kendall, S., & Brooks, F. (2006). Nurses' responses to expert patients: The rhetoric and reality of self-management in long term conditions: A grounded theory study [Electronic version]. *International Journal of Nursing Studies, 43,* 803–818.

Young, J.T. (2004). Illness behavior: A selective review and synthesis. *Sociology of Health and Illness, 26*(1), 1–31.

3

Stigma

Diane L. Stuenkel and Vivian K. Wong

*My car came to a stop at the intersection.
I looked around me at all the people in the other
cars, but no one there was like me. They were
apart from me, distant, different. If they looked
at me, they couldn't see my defect. But if they
knew, they would turn away. I am separate and
different from everybody that I can see in every
direction as far as I can see. And it will never be
the same again.*

Client with new diagnosis of cancer

INTRODUCTION

This chapter demonstrates how the concept of
stigma has evolved and is a significant factor in
many chronic illnesses and disabilities. It also
explores the relationship of stigma with the concepts of prejudice, stereotyping, and labeling.
Because stigma is socially constructed, it varies
from setting to setting. In addition, individuals and
groups react differently to the stigmatizing process.
Those reactions must be taken into consideration
when planning strategies to improve the quality of
life for individuals with chronic illnesses.

Although stigmatizing is common, not all
individuals attach a stigma to their disease or disability. This chapter does not assume that all who
come in contact with those who are disabled or
chronically ill devalue them; rather, it insists that
each of us examine our values, beliefs, and actions
carefully.

The *Merriam Webster Dictionary On-Line*
(2007) defines stigma as a "mark of shame or discredit, an identifying mark or characteristic." The
Merriam Webster Thesaurus On-Line (2007) explains
stigma as a mark of guilt or disgrace. Goffman
(1963) traced the historic use of the word stigma to
the Greeks, who referred to "bodily signs designed
to expose something unusual and bad about the
moral status of the signifier" (p. 1). These signs were
cut or burned into a person's body as an indication of being a slave, a criminal, or a traitor. Notice
the moral and judgmental nature of these stigmas.
The disgrace and shame of the stigma became
more important than the bodily evidence of it.
Labeling, stereotyping, separation, status loss, and
discrimination can all occur at the same time and
are considered components of the stigma (Link &
Phelan, 2001).

Theoretical Frameworks: Stigma, Social Identity, and Labeling Theory

Society teaches its members to categorize persons by common defining attributes and characteristics (Goffman, 1963). Daily routines establish the usual and the expected. When we meet strangers, certain appearances help us anticipate what Goffman called "social identity." This identity includes personal attributes, such as competence, as well as structural ones, such as occupation. For example, university students usually tolerate some eccentricities in their professors, but stuttering, physical handicaps, or diseases may bestow a social identity of incompetence. Although this identity is not based on actuality, it may be stigmatizing.

One's social identity may include: (1) physical activities, (2) professional roles, and (3) the concept of self. Anything that changes one of these, such as a disability, changes the individual's identity and, therefore, potentially creates a stigma (Markowitz, 1998). Goffman (1963) used the idea of social identity to expand previous work done on stigma. His theory defined stigma as something that disqualifies an individual from full social acceptance. Goffman argued that social identity is a primary force in the development of stigma, because the identity that a person conveys categorizes that person. Social settings and routines tell us which categories to anticipate. Therefore, when individuals fail to meet expectations because of attributes that are different and/or undesirable, they are reduced from accepted people to discounted ones—that is, they are stigmatized.

Goffman recognized that people who had stayed in a psychiatric institute or a prison were labeled. To label a person as different or deviant by powers of the society is applying a stigma (Goffman, 1963). In general, labeling theory is the way that society labels behaviors that do not conform to the norm. For instance, an individual experiencing constant drooling or the leakage of food that requires frequent wiping of the mouth may be considered deviant. The difficulty in swallowing may be labeled by society as deviant

behavior, despite the fact that tremor and dyskinesias associated with Parkinson's disease may be the cause (Miller, Noble, Jones & Burn, 2006).

During the two decades following Goffman's work in the 1960s, extensive criticism arose concerning the impact and long-term consequences of stigma on social identity. In the area of mental illness, critics resisted the theory that stigma could contribute to the severity and chronicity of mental illness. In a series of studies, Link proposed a modified labeling theory that asserted that labeling, derived from negative social beliefs about behavior, could lead to devaluation and discrimination. Ultimately, these feelings of devaluation and discrimination could lead to negative social consequences (Link, 1987; Link et al., 1989; Link et al., 1997). Those who are labeled with mental illness often are excluded from social activities and discriminated against when they do participate.

In 1987, Link compared the expectations of discrimination and devaluation and the severity of demoralization among clients with newly diagnosed mental illness, repeat clients with mental illness, former clients with mental illness, and community residents (Link, 1987). He found that both new and repeat clients with mental illness scored higher on measures of demoralization and discrimination than community residents and former mentally ill clients. Further, he demonstrated that high scores were related to income loss and unemployment.

In 1989, Link and colleagues tested a modified labeling theory on a similar group of clients with newly diagnosed mental illness, repeat clients with mental illness, former clients, untreated clients, and community residents who were well (Link et al., 1989). They found that all groups expected clients to be devalued and discriminated against. They also found that, among current clients, the expectation of devaluation and discrimination promoted coping mechanisms of secrecy and withdrawal. Such coping mechanisms have a strong effect on social networks, reducing the size of those networks to persons considered to be safe and trustworthy.

In 1997, Link and colleagues tested modified labeling theory in a longitudinal study that compared the effects of stigma on the well-being of clients who had mental illness and a pattern of substance abuse to determine the strength of the long-term negative effects of stigma and whether the effects of treatment have counter-balancing positive effects (Link et al., 1997). They found that perceived devaluation and discrimination, as well as actual reports of discrimination, continued to have negative effects on clients even though clients were improved and had responded well to treatment. They concluded that healthcare professionals attempting to improve quality of life for clients with mental illness must contend initially with the effects of stigma in its own right to be successful.

Fife and Wright (2000) studied stigma using modified labeling theory as a framework in individuals with HIV/AIDS and cancer. They found that stigma had a significant influence on the lives of persons with HIV/AIDS and with cancer. However, they also found that the nature of the illness had few direct effects on self-perception, whereas the effects on self appeared to relate directly to the perception of stigma. Their findings suggested that stigma has different dimensions, which have different effects on self. Rejection and social isolation lead to diminished self-esteem. Social isolation influences body image. A lack of sense of personal control stems from social isolation and financial insecurity. Social isolation appears to be the only dimension of stigma that affects each component of self.

Camp, Finlay, and Lyons (2002) questioned the inevitability of the effects of stigma on self based on the hypothesis that, in order for stigma to exert a negative influence on self-concept, the individuals must first be aware of and accept the negative self-perceptions, accept that the identity relates to them, and then apply the negative perceptions to themselves. A study of women with long-term mental health problems found that these women did not accept negative social perceptions as relevant to them. Rather, they attributed the negative perceptions to deficiencies among those who stigmatized them. These researchers found no evidence of the passive acceptance of labels and negative identities. These women appeared to avoid social interactions where they anticipated feeling different and excluded, and formed new social networks with groups in which they felt accepted and understood. Whereas they acknowledged the negative consequences of mental illness, there did not appear to be an automatic link between these consequences and negative self-evaluation. Factors that contributed to a positive self-evaluation included membership in a supportive in-group, finding themselves in a more favorable circumstance than others with the same problems, and sharing experiences with others who had knowledge and insight about mental illness.

In summary, stigma, defined as discrediting another, arises from widely held social beliefs about personality, behavior, and illness, and is communicated to individuals through a process of socialization. When individuals display the condition that engenders the mark of discredit, they may experience social devaluation and discrimination. Stigma clearly attaches to individuals with mental illness as well as individuals with infectious and terminal diseases. Stigma may produce changes in perception of body image, social isolation, rejection, loss of status, and perceived lack of personal control. However, there is some evidence to suggest that stigma does not attach universally to individuals with marked behavior or conditions. Some individuals appear resistant to stigma, identifying flaws in the society conveying the negative beliefs. These individuals share experiences with others who have knowledge of and sensitivity to being stigmatized and benefit from the ability to perceive themselves as equal to or better off than others with the same condition.

Unique Aspects of Stigma

There are special circumstances in which stigma can be perceived with enhanced distinction. Individuals who lack a fully-developed sense of personal identity and who are reliant upon external sources to reinforce their internal sense of worthiness may be uniquely prone to a sense of stigma. Adolescence can be used as an example. There are aspects of society that tend to be highly valued by individuals, and when that society communicates stigma, the stigmatizing beliefs are uniquely powerful. Religion and culture are examples, as well as issues concerning self-infliction and punishment.

The task of developing a stable, coherent identity is one of the most important tasks of adolescence (Erikson, 1968). To successfully complete this task, the adolescent must be able to utilize formal operational thinking within a context of expanded social experiences to evolve a sense of self that integrates not only the similarities, but also the differences observed between him- or herself and others. Social interactions and messages from the sociocultural environment about what is desirable and what is not desirable guide and direct the adolescent toward an identity that incorporates desired similarities and rejects undesired differences. The influences and preferences of peers become important as the adolescent seeks acceptance of this newly developed sense of identity. The skill of labeling and stigmatizing individuals with intolerable differences is wielded with frightening force and sometimes terrible consequences. The Columbine High School (Colorado) massacre in 1999 is an example:

> Eric and Dylan seemed to relish their roles as outsiders....It wasn't that they were labeled that way. It's what they chose to be. That choice invited taunting by a group of jocks...known bullies throughout the school....Some of the jocks and their friends pushed Eric into lockers. They called him 'faggot'...Jessica defined Columbine this way...."There's basically two classes of people. There's the low and the high. The low [people] stick together and the high [people] make fun of the low and you just deal with it (Bartels & Crowder, 1999).

Culture may determine stigma as well. For some conditions, such as traumatic brain injury (Simpson, Mohr, & Redman, 2000), HIV/AIDS (Heckman, Anderson, Sikkema, Kochman et al., 2004), and epilepsy (Baker, Brooks, Buck, & Jacoby, 2000), stigma and social isolation cross cultural boundaries. On the other hand, in a study of attitudes about homelessness in 11 European cities, Brandon, Khoo, Maglajlie, and Abuel-Ealeh (2000) found marked differences in attitudes between countries, with high levels of stigma predominating in former Warsaw Pact countries. A determination of racial and/or cultural inferiority of a minority group by a dominant group may result in racism, discrimination, and stigma (Weston, 2003; Williams, 1999).

Religion may also play a role in stigma. In a study of five large religious groups in London that examined attitudes about depression and schizophrenia, it was found that fear of stigma among non-white groups was prevalent, and particularly the fear of being misunderstood by white healthcare professionals not of the same religious group (Cinnirella & Loewenthal, 1999).

Actual physical or mental disability is not solely responsible for social reaction. The incorporation of children with "special needs" (often children with delayed or slowed mental development) into mainstream education has forced the reevaluation of long-held beliefs and stereotypes that have stigmatized these children in the past (Waldman, Swerdloff, & Perlman, 1999). The label produces the negative response from nonlabeled people, rather than some aberrant or inadequate behavior producing it. Therefore, the label and associated stigma of a disability or disease exclude individuals from social interaction while their intellectual or physical handicaps alone may or may not (Link et al., 1997).

Most stigmas are perceived as threatening by and to others. Criminals and social deviants are stigmatized because they create a sense of anxiety by threatening society's values and safety. Similarly, encounters with sick and disabled individuals also cause anxiety and apprehension, but

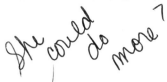

in a different way. The encounter destroys the dream that life is fair. Sick people remind us of our mortality and vulnerability; consequently, physically healthy individuals may make negative value judgments about those who are ill or disabled (Kurzban & Leary, 2001). For example, some sighted individuals may regard those who are blind as being dependent or unwilling to take care of themselves, an assumption that is not based on what the blind person is willing or able to do. Individuals with AIDS are often subjected to moral judgment. Those with psychiatric illness have been stigmatized since medieval times (Keltner, Schwecke, & Bostrom, 2003). As a result, these individuals deal with more than their symptomatology; on a daily basis they contend with those who perceive them as less worthy or valuable: They possess a stigma.

Some individuals are stigmatized because the behavior or difference is considered to be self-inflicted and, therefore, less worthy of help. Alcoholism, drug-related problems, and mental illness are frequently included in this category (Crisp et al., 2000; Ritson, 1999). HIV, AIDS, and hepatitis B are examples of infectious diseases in which the mode of infection is considered to be self-inflicted as a result of socially unacceptable behavior; therefore, affected individuals are stigmatized (Halevy, 2000; Heckman et al., 2004).

In the past, the words shame and guilt were used to describe a concept similar to stigma—a perceived difference between a behavior or an attribute and an ideal standard. From this perspective, guilt is defined as self-criticism, and shame results from the disapproval of others. Guilt is similar to seeing oneself as discreditable. Shame is a painful feeling caused by the scorn or contempt of others. For example, a person with alcoholism may feel guilty about drinking and also feel ashamed that others perceive his or her behavior as less than desirable.

Therefore, the concept of deviance versus normality is a social construct. That is, individuals are devalued because they display attributes that some call deviant (Kurzban & Leary, 2001).

At Columbine High School, some teens, labeled jocks, stigmatized other teens who were considered as "low" and therefore "expected" to be taunted (Bartels & Crowder, 1999). Indeed, old age, which will one day characterize all of us, is often stigmatized (Ebersole, Hess, Touhy, & Jett, 2005). Furthermore, because stigma is socially defined, it differs from setting to setting. Use of recreational drugs, for instance, may be normal in one group and taboo in another.

Whenever a stigma is present, the devaluing characteristic is so powerful that it overshadows other traits and becomes the focus of one's personal evaluation (Kurzban & Leary, 2001). This trait, or differentness, is sufficiently powerful to break the claim of all other attributes (Goffman, 1963). As an example, the fact that a nurse has unstable type 1 diabetes may cancel her/his remaining identity as a competent health professional. The stigma attached to a professor's stutter may overshadow academic competence.

The extent of stigma resulting from any particular condition cannot be predicted. Individuals with a specific disease do not universally feel the same degree of stigma. On the other hand, very different disabilities may possess the same stigma. In writing about individuals with mental illness, Link et al. (1997) described variations in symptomology among them; however, individuals without mental illness did not take those variations into account. All individuals who were disabled were seen as sharing the same stigma—mental illness—regardless of their capabilities or severity of their illness. That is, people responded to the mental illness stereotype rather than to the person's actual physical and mental capabilities.

Similarly, Herek, Capitanio, and Widaman (2003) reported on the stigmatizing effects of the label of HIV/AIDS. They found that those individuals who reported a perceived reduction in the level of stigma attached to HIV/AIDS overall, generally expressed negative feelings toward people with AIDS and favored a name-based reporting system such as that used by the public health department for other communicable diseases.

Types of Stigma

Stigma is a universal phenomenon and every society stigmatizes. Goffman (1963) distinguished among three types of stigma. The first is the stigma of physical deformity. The actual stigma is the deficit between the expected norm of perfect physical condition and the actual physical condition. For example, many chronic conditions create changes in physical appearance or function. These changes frequently create a difference in self- or other-perception (see Chapter 6). Changes of this kind also occur with aging. The normal aging process creates a body far different from the television commercial "norm" of youth, physical beauty, and leanness, although this norm is changing slowly to include mature and elderly individuals as changes in the demographics of the population occur.

The second type of stigma is that of character blemishes. This type may occur in individuals with AIDS, alcoholism, mental illness, or homosexuality. For example, individuals infected with HIV face considerable stigma because many believe that the infected person could have controlled the behaviors that resulted in the infection (Halevy, 2000; Heckman et al., 2004; Herek, Capitanio, & Widaman, 2003; Weston, 2003). Likewise, individuals with eating disorders such as anorexia nervosa fear being stigmatized (Stewart, Keel, & Schiavo, 2006). The fear of stigma can be a major barrier to seeking treatment.

The third type of stigma is tribal in origin and is known more commonly as prejudice. This type of stigma originates when one group perceives features of race, religion, or nationality of another group as deficient compared with their own socially constructed norm. Most healthcare professionals agree that prejudice has no place in the healthcare delivery system. Although some professionals display both subtle and overt intolerance, others strive to treat persons of every age, race, and nationality with sensitivity. However, prejudice against individuals with chronic illnesses exists as surely as racial or religious prejudice.

The three types of stigma may overlap and reinforce each other (Kurzban & Leary, 2001).

Individuals who are already socially isolated because of race, age, or poverty will be additionally hurt by the isolation resulting from another stigma. Heukelbach and Feldmeier (2006) stated that scabies infestations are associated with poverty in undeveloped countries, which contributes to the stigmatization of both diagnosis and treatment. Those who are financially disadvantaged or culturally distinct (that is, stigmatized by the majority of society) will suffer more stigma should they become disabled. Poor women with HIV feared the stigma associated with HIV/AIDS more than dying of the disease (Abel, 2007).

More recently, psychologists and sociologists have built on Goffman's theory to address the concepts of felt stigma and enacted stigma (Jacoby, 1994; Scambler, 2004). Felt stigma is the internalized perception of being devalued or "not as good as" by an individual. It may be related to fears of having others treat one as different or of being labeled by others, even though the stigmatizing attribute is not known or outwardly apparent. The other component of felt stigma is shame (Scambler, 2004). Individuals view themselves as discreditable. The quote at the beginning of this chapter is an example of a client experiencing felt stigma.

Enacted stigma, on the other hand, refers to behaviors and perceptions by others toward the individual who is perceived as different. Enacted stigma is the situational response of others to a visible, overt stigmatizing attribute of another (Jacoby, 1994; Scambler, 2004). Hesitating or failing to shake hands with a person who has vitiligo, a dermatologic condition characterized by hypopigmentation of the skin, is an example of enacted stigma.

Stigma is prevalent in our society and, once it occurs it endures (Link et al., 1997). If the cause of stigma is removed, the effects are not easily overcome. An individual's social identity has already been influenced by the stigmatizing attribute. A person with a history of alcoholism or mental illness continues to carry a stigma in the same way that a former prison inmate does.

Chronic Disease as Stigma

Individuals with chronic illness present deviations from what many people expect in daily social interchanges. In general, most people do not expect to meet someone with an electronic voice-box following treatment for laryngeal cancer. Both the cancer and the assistive device may not be readily visible, but once the person begins to speak, the individual is at risk of being labeled as "different" by others.

American values contribute to the perception of chronic illness as a stigmatizing condition. That is, the dominant culture emphasizes qualities of youth, attractiveness, and personal accomplishment. The work ethic and heritage of the western frontier provide heroes who are strong, conventionally productive, and physically healthy. Television and magazines demonstrate, on a daily basis, that physical perfection is the standard against which all are measured, yet these societal values collide with the reality of chronic disease. A discrepancy exists between the realities of a chronic condition, such as arthritis or AIDS, and the social expectation of physical perfection.

A disease characteristic or one having an unknown etiology, may contribute to the stigma of many chronic illnesses. In fact, any disease having an unclear cause or ineffectual treatment is suspect, including Alzheimer's disease (Jolley & Benbow, 2000) and anxiety disorders (Davies, 2000). Clients with Alzheimer's disease also may be stigmatized because of perceptions relating to their level of decision making competence (Werner, 2006). Diseases that are somewhat mysterious and at the same time feared, such as leprosy, are often felt to be morally contagious.

Stigma can be associated with inequitable treatment, although the relative severity of such inequitable treatment often varies with the degree of severity of the stigmatized condition. For example, public policy about HIV/AIDS has acted both to increase accessibility to treatment and potentially to limit the civil rights of the stigmatized individuals (Herek et al., 2003). In addition, the shame, guilt, and social isolation of some stigmatized individuals may lead to inequitable treatment for their families. Because of the secrecy associated with being HIV-positive, affected clients and family members may not be able to access needed mental health, substance abuse rehabilitation, or infectious disease therapies (Salisbury, 2000).

So far, this chapter has defined stigma and presented a framework for understanding stigma as a social construct. All types of stigma share a common tie: In every case, an individual who might have interacted easily in a particular social situation may now be prevented from doing so by the discredited trait. The trait may become the focus of attention and potentially turn others away.

IMPACT OF STIGMA

Stigma has an impact on both the affected individual and those persons who do not share the particular trait. Responses to stigma vary and will be discussed from the perspective of the person living with stigma, the lay person, and the health-care professional.

The Individual Living With Stigma

Stigmatized individuals respond to the reactions of others in a variety of ways. They are often unsure about the attitudes of others and, therefore, may feel a constant need to make a good impression. Individuals living with stigma each and every day may choose to accept society's or others' view of them, or choose to reject others' discrediting viewpoints. Culture may limit the coping choices that are available, particularly in relation to disclosing a mental illness. In a study of West Indian women coping with depression, Schreiber, Stern, and Wilson (2000) found that "being strong" was the culturally sanctioned behavior for depression, rather than disclosure.

Passing

Passing oneself off as "normal" is one strategy used by individuals living with a stigmatizing condition. Pretending to have no disability or a less

CASE STUDIES

Case Study #1

Natalie Johnson is a 52-year-old, divorced, administrative assistant for the local school district. She began experiencing increasing fatigue, vision disturbances, and global muscle weakness approximately 6 years ago. After a lengthy and anxiety-producing year of testing, she was diagnosed with multiple sclerosis 3 weeks ago. Her disease course has been primary-progressive, and she anticipates that she will not be able to work much longer. She is thankful that the union contract provides healthcare benefits that include long-term care insurance. Her primary concern at this stage is mobility and maintaining her independence for as long as possible.

Discussion Questions

1. What type of stigma is Ms. Johnson at risk for? How would you assess this client's self-perception of stigma?
2. What strategies would you use to reduce the effects of stigma for this client?
3. You approach Ms. Johnson about sending an intake nurse to her home to do an initial home environment assessment and to get her established with the local home healthcare agency. How can healthcare professionals break down the barriers of stigma among the healthcare team?
4. What behaviors by Ms. Johnson would suggest that she does or does not label herself as stigmatized?

Case Study #2

Angel Martinez is a 19-year-old college student who was diagnosed with epilepsy at age 8. He works part-time at the bookstore on campus and lives in a fraternity house. His seizures are well-controlled by medications. He was treated for mild depression following the death of his twin sister in a motor vehicle accident 9 months ago. Mr. Martinez is concerned that his employer and fraternity brothers will "find out" about his depression and has avoided refilling the prescription for an antidepressant medication.

Discussion Questions

1. What suggestions could you give to the healthcare team to facilitate a culturally appropriate assessment?
2. Are there any specific "labels" that Mr. Martinez may apply to himself? Are there any specific "labels" that the healthcare team may apply, thereby creating the barrier of stigma?
3. What stigmatizing situations might arise for Mr. Martinez in the workplace? In the community?
4. What are the benefits and costs of increasing client participation in healthcare delivery? How does increasing client participation affect the stigma that Mr. Martinez may feel?
5. What strategies might lessen the stigma that Mr. Martinez perceives?

stigmatic identity (Dudley, 1983; Goffman, 1963; Joachim & Acorn, 2000) may be an option if the stigmatizing attribute is not readily visible. Passing is a viable option for those with felt stigma associated with conditions such as type 2 diabetes or a positive AIDS antibody test but no symptoms. The process of passing may include the concealment of any signs of the stigma. Some individuals refuse to use adaptive devices, such as hearing aids, because this tells others of their disability. Another

Diabetics

example is the abused client who provides reasonable explanations for bruises, swelling, and injuries. The practice of "passing" may significantly impair the health-seeking behavior of the abused individual, particularly where sociocultural barriers to disclosure exist (Bauer, Rodriguez, Quiroga, & Flores-Ortiz, 2000).

Covering

Because of the potential threat and anxiety-provoking nature of disclosing a stigmatizing difference, most people deemphasize their differentness. This response, called covering, is an attempt to make the difference seem smaller or less significant than it really is (Goffman, 1963). Covering involves understanding the difference between visibility and obtrusiveness; that is, the condition is openly acknowledged, but its consequences are minimized. Persons with special dietary requirements may deny the importance of maintaining the restriction in a social situation, even though they follow it. The goal is to divert attention from the defect, create a more comfortable situation for all, and minimize the risk of experiencing enacted stigma.

Humor, used in a skillful and light-hearted manner by the stigmatized individual, may decrease the anxiety of others and avoid an awkward encounter. This form of covering neutralizes the anxiety-producing subject; therefore, it is no longer taboo and can more easily be managed.

Disregard

A person's first response to enacted stigma may be disregard. In other words, they may choose not to reflect on or discuss the painful incidents. Well-adjusted individuals who are comfortable with their identity, have dealt with stigma for a long time, and choose not to respond to the reaction of others, may disregard it (Dudley, 1983).

Another example is provided by wheelchair athletes. These athletes disregard perceptions that their disabilities prohibit them from participating

in strenuous, athletic endeavors. Any person who has observed these well-conditioned athletes racing their wheelchairs up hills in competitive meets may find it difficult to consider them discredited.

Going public with a serious medical diagnosis is another example of disregard by acting in the face of negative consequences. One positive aspect of going public is the potential for assertive political action and social change. Celebrities such as Muhammed Ali, Earvin (Magic) Johnson, Michael J. Fox, and the late Christopher and Dana Reeve, among others, have captured public attention and acted positively to reduce enacted stigma by disclosing their personal struggles with a variety of conditions.

Resistance and Rejection

Similar to disregard, resistance, and rejection are additional strategies used in response to stigma (Dudley, 1983). Individuals may speak out and challenge rules and protocol if their needs are not met. More recently, Franks, Henwood, and Bowden (2007) noted that resisting and rejecting were strategies used by maternal mental health clients. These disadvantaged mothers outright rejected or actively resisted the judgments of professionals who held negative opinions. Broader societal misconceptions, such as all teen mothers are on welfare, also were rejected. The use of resistance or rejection can be used to preserve or bolster a more positive self-identity and effect larger societal changes.

Isolation *my patient*

Human beings have a proclivity for separating themselves into small subgroups because staying with one's own group is easier, requires less effort, and, for some individuals, is more congenial. However, this separation into groups tends to emphasize differences rather than similarities (Link et al., 1989) (see Chapter 5).

Closed interaction from within may enhance one's feelings of normality because the individual is surrounded by others who are similar (Camp, Finlay, & Lyons, 2002). This feeling of normality characterized "The Trenchcoat Mafia" at Columbine High School (Bartels & Crowder, 1999). The process of isolation can occur any time outsiders are seen as threatening or are reminders that the world is different from the in-group.

Staying with like-others may be a source of support, but some individuals with a disability or chronic illness may feel more comfortable when they are surrounded by nondisabled individuals. A young woman, disabled since birth, feels better around nondisabled people because she has always considered herself normal. Her attitude reminds us to use caution when making assumptions about the perceptions of others.

Information Management

In addition to the stigmatized individual, family members often acquire a secondary stigma as a result of association (Goffman, 1963) and must deal with their own responses to situations of enacted stigma. Mothers who are HIV positive expend significant effort to protect their children from the negative effects of disclosure of their HIV status (Sandelowski & Barroso, 2003). Likewise, family members who care for persons with AIDS share the stigma of AIDS and are discredited, resulting in rejection, loss of friends, and harassment (Gewirtz & Gossart-Walker, 2000; Salisbury, 2000).

Information management is used by both the individual and loved ones in dealing with felt and enacted stigma. The world may be divided into a large group of people to whom they tell nothing and a small group of insiders who are aware of the stigmatizing condition. Healthcare professionals may use information management in an attempt to lessen the likelihood of stigma for a client. For example, listing a diagnosis of Hansen's disease or mycobacterial neurodermatitis then gives the client the option of revealing the alternate name of leprosy, with its accompanying historical stigma.

The Lay Person: Responses to and Effects of Stigma

Responses of an individual to a stigmatized person vary with the particular stigma and the individual's past conditioning. Because society specifies the characteristics that are stigmatized, it also teaches its members how to react to that stigma. Differences between groups based on nationality and culture have been found in attitudes toward those with disabilities (Brandon et al., 2000; Cinnirella & Loewenthal, 1999). Just as children learn to interact with others who are culturally different by watching and listening to those around them, they also learn how to treat chronically ill or disabled individuals by incorporating societal judgments. Sadly, these reactions are often negative.

Devaluing

People may believe that the person with the stigma is less valuable, less human, or less desired. Unfortunately, many of us practice more than one kind of discrimination and, by so doing, effectively reduce the life chances of the stigmatized individual (Goffman, 1963). Devaluing results in enacted stigma as demonstrated by those who categorize individuals as inferior or even dangerous. Use of words such as cripple or moron also represent a devaluing of individuals.

Stereotyping

Categories simplify our lives. Instead of having to decide what to do in every situation, we can respond to categories of situations. Stereotypes are a negative type of category. They are a social reaction to ambiguous situations and allow us to react to group expectations rather than to individuals. When individuals meet those with physical impairments, expectations are not clear (Katz, 1981). People often are at a loss as to how to react, so placing the individual with chronic illness in a stereotyped category reduces the ambiguousness toward him or her and makes the situation more comfortable for those doing the stereotyping. Much less effort is required to sustain a bias than is required to reconsider or alter it.

Using stereotypes to understand individuals decreases our attention to other positive characteristics (Hynd, 1958). Categorizing tends to make one see the world as a dichotomy. For example, people are categorized as either mentally delayed or not, even though mental capabilities exist on a continuum, with all of us falling somewhere along the line.

Responses such as scapegoating and ostracizing people with AIDS have increased the impact of this disease and delayed treatment (Distabile, Dubler, Solomon, & Klein, 1999; Rehm & Franck, 2000; Salisbury, 2000). These responses also impede appropriate health education aimed at prevention.

Labeling

The label attached to an individual's condition is crucial and influences the way we think about that individual. The diagnosis of AIDS is a powerful label, possibly resulting in the loss of relationships and jobs. People with learning disabilities may not mind being called slow learners, but may be startled by being called mentally retarded (Dudley, 1983). Their response indicates that they see this latter term as a negative label.

Professional Responses: Attitudes and Perceptions of Stigma

In the United States, most healthcare professionals share the American dream of achievement, attractiveness, and a cohesive, healthy family. These values influence our perceptions of individuals who are disabled, chronically ill, or otherwise considered "less than normal." Although the factors that contribute to these individual differences vary, the consequences of stigma associated with chronic illnesses are similar in different health conditions and cultures (Van Brakel, 2006).

Attitudes

It is not surprising that society's values and definitions of stigma affect the attitudes of healthcare professionals. Attitudes can be changed by interactions with clients and chronically ill acquaintances (Sandelowski & Barroso, 2003). Students' confidence in clients' ability to cope with a disease increased with professional experience. In a similar manner, knowing someone with a chronic disease increased positive attitudes. When healthcare professionals (general practitioners, nurses, and counselors) were asked about their perceptions of depression among older adults, they agreed that the older adults displayed embarrassment and shame when disclosing feelings of depression. Older adults were perceived as reluctant to seek mental health services because depression was identified as a stigma. Whether these perceptions of the healthcare professionals are consistent with those of the older adults will require further examination (Murray et al., 2006).

Perceptions

Healthcare professionals' perceptions of stigma affect care outcomes. Liggins and Hatcher (2005) studied the stigma of mental illness in the hospital setting. Labeling a client as mentally ill had a negative impact on both the client and the healthcare professional. Clients believed that they were ignored or treated differently because they had mental illness. They feared how the healthcare professional would respond to them. The healthcare professional showed disbelief toward physical ailments because the client had "mental disease." Healthcare providers also assumed that mental illness was associated with an unpredictable behavior that may affect the healthcare professional–patient relationship (Liggins & Hatcher, 2005). Clearly, interventions to reduce perceptions of stigma and episodes of enacted stigma in the hospital setting are needed.

The attitude of the healthcare worker is vital in reducing the stigma associated with chronic illness. Healthcare professionals who are non-judgmental, empathic, and knowledgeable were observed to reduce the perception of stigma in a specialized HIV/AIDS unit. Stigma was minimized when nurses and other interdisciplinary team members identified themselves with the behaviors of the clients, held a positive view of the disease, and reached consensus in the delivery of appropriate care (Hodgson, 2006).

Another study of medical students' perspectives of illness disclosed a surprising aspect of stigma. Medical students revealed a high level of concern over the perception of social stigma attached to their own personal health problems and the resulting professional jeopardy they might encounter upon disclosure (Roberts, Warner, & Trumpower, 2000).

Healthcare professionals potentially display all the reactions and responses toward discredited individuals that lay persons do. Therefore, caregivers need a thorough understanding of these responses if we are to overcome the effects of stigmatizing behavior or to eliminate it outright. Understanding the concept of stigma increases one's ability to plan interventions for clients with chronic illnesses (Joachim & Acorn, 2000).

INTERVENTIONS: COPING WITH STIGMA OR REDUCING STIGMA

A chronic illness or disability imposes various constraints on an individual's life. The stigma of a specific disorder adds additional burdens, often far greater than those caused by the disorder itself (Joachim & Acorn, 2000). Individuals with chronic conditions usually receive medical treatment, but few interventions may be directed at reducing the effects of the associated stigma.

Helping others to manage the effects of stigma is not simple and should be approached with care. At best, change will be slow and uneven. However, consistent and knowledgeable interventions aimed specifically at reducing the impact of stigma are as crucial as those that reduce blood pressure or chronic pain. The following section discusses

appropriate strategies the healthcare provider can employ in his or her practice to address the issue of stigma.

Healthcare Professional and Client Interactions

The healthcare professional who is aware of his or her own biases, beliefs, and behaviors has already begun to mitigate the effects of stigma for the client and family members. Being aware of the societal context and implications that a diagnosis of chronic illness carries with it enables the healthcare professional to work with the client to develop strategies to prevent, reduce, or cope with potentially stigmatizing conditions.

Professional Attitudes: Cure versus Care

Traditionally, the goal of healthcare has been to cure the client. Because chronic illness is now more prevalent than infectious disease or acute illness, this criterion of success may be inappropriate. Cure is neither essential nor necessary in order that the client benefit. Instead, caring, demonstrated by valuing and assisting, should be the criterion. With the increasing number of people with chronic illnesses, professionals must learn to accept those characteristics accompanying chronic illness: an indeterminate course of disease, relapses, and multiple treatment modalities. Cost containment is a central focus in healthcare delivery. Providers must not lose sight, however, of health policy considerations that include ideas of personhood and equitable health care sensitive to the reality of stigmatizing chronic illness (Gewirtz & Gossart-Walker, 2000; Roskes, Feldman, Arrington, & Leisher, 1999; Salisbury, 2000).

The Mutual Participation Model

The manner in which health care is delivered may increase or decrease the effects of stigma. Encouraging a client's participation in healthcare decision making is an outward demonstration of respect and regard for that person. Establishing the client as a partner in setting goals demonstrates one's acceptance and valuing of the individual. On the other hand, when healthcare professionals make decisions regarding treatment or goals without consulting a client, they reinforce the person's feeling of being discredited or discreditable. Therefore, any mode of care delivery that increases client participation enhances that person's perception of self-worth and reduces the effects of stigma. The mutual participation model is the model of choice in managing chronic diseases because it enhances the client's feelings of self-worth. The client is responsible for long-term disease management, and the healthcare professional is responsible for helping the client help himself or herself.

Mutual participation divides power evenly between professional and client and leads to a relationship that can be mutually satisfying. In other words, the client should be as satisfied with the recommendations and decisions as the provider is. In addition, each party depends on the other for information culminating in a satisfactory solution. The client needs the provider's experience and expertise; the provider needs not only the client's history and symptoms but his or her priorities, expectations, and goals. Sometimes a choice between treatments with relatively equal mortality rates is necessary—for example, surgery or radiation for cancer treatment. The professional can offer expert knowledge regarding long-term effects of radiation and changes in body image due to surgery. The client must decide the relative value of side effects of the alternative proposed treatments. Because the "right" decision depends on the individual, input from both client and healthcare provider is necessary to produce a course of action that is mutually acceptable.

When healthcare professionals become more comfortable with allowing clients a greater range of participation and decision making, the relationship decreases some of the stigmatizing effects of the disability. Health professionals must create an atmosphere in which individuals with chronic conditions not only are expected to cooperate, but are encouraged to express their concerns, observations, expectations, and limitations. Together, they explore alternative strategies and decide on one that is agreeable to both. When a client's priorities and goals are valued and incorporated into the regimen, an increased sense of acceptance emerges. Therefore, the respect and regard for clients demonstrated by this model provide effective tools to counteract some stigmatizing effects of illness.

Healthcare professionals who establish a therapeutic relationship with their client are ideally situated to assess their client's perceptions of felt or enacted stigma. Asking open ended questions to ascertain how the client perceives himself or herself, the meaning of the disease to the client, and types of interactions with others may elicit valuable information. Family members and significant others may be included in the assessment as well.

It is particularly important to distinguish between nonparticipation and nonacceptance when caring for stigmatized individuals. Nonparticipation is an abstinence from social activities that is based on limitations caused by a disability or illness. Nonacceptance, on the other hand, is a negative attitude—a resistance or reluctance on the part of the nondisabled person to admit the disabled person to various kinds and degrees of social relationships (Ladieu-Leviton, Adler, & Dembo, 1977). A person with a disability who chooses not to join a camping trip is a nonparticipant; the physical disability serves as the basis for that person's decision not to participate. Deciding not to invite that person to join the group, whether or not participation is possible, is nonacceptance; it preempts the person's choice and is a form of enacted stigma.

Commonly, individuals without a disability cannot accurately estimate the limits of potential participation for those with a disease or disability— a key point for healthcare professionals to remember. Typically, the physical limitations imposed by a disability are overestimated by others. If nondisabled individuals incorrectly assume that a disabled individual is not able to participate, that is a form of nonacceptance. Such nonacceptance is created by the difference between the degree of participation that is actually possible and the degree assumed possible by those who are not disabled. If the difference can be resolved, nonacceptance ceases to be a problem.

The remedy for this dilemma is simple. Nondisabled individuals can simply indicate that they want the disabled individual to participate, leaving to him or her the decision of whether to become involved. Perhaps the individual with the disability would like to participate, but in a different way. For example, the young adult who has juvenile arthritis may not regret being unable to go fishing if he or she can go along and spend time socializing with friends. Healthcare professionals can encourage their clients to look for these opportunities to participate as they are able.

Family members or significant others who are involved in the client's care must not be forgotten. An ethnographic study of immediate family members of burn survivors explored the perceptions of stigma (Rossi, Vila Vda, Zago, & Ferreria, 2005). The stigma associated with the burn and the accompanying feelings of loss of control affected both the client and the family. The family had fears of facing the reactions from society, which encompassed feelings of sadness, anger, denial, resignation, and/or anxiety. Some family members expressed feelings of shame when living with someone whose role and appearance changed due to the burn injuries. Thus, it is imperative that the perceptions of both the stigmatized person and the family are assessed.

Client-Centered Interventions

Strategies to Increase Self-Worth

Societal norms and values are a major determinant of an individual's sense of self-esteem and self-worth. The person who does not possess the expected attribute is quite aware of this discredit as an equal and desired individual in society. In addition, individuals with chronic conditions may find their own deformities or failings decrease their self-respect. That is, not only do stigmatized individuals have to deal with the responses

of others (enacted stigma), but some experience strong negative feelings about their own self-worth (felt stigma). These internalized perceptions may be more difficult to deal with than the illness or disability itself. Examples of negative feelings were described by 60 study participants with epilepsy. More than half of the participants experienced feelings of shame, fear, worry, and low self-esteem, and one-fourth had the perception of stigma (de Souza & Salgado, 2006).

In another study, obese individuals and their family members noted both stigmatization and discrimination on the basis of weight. They reported being constantly reminded by family members, peers, healthcare providers, and strangers that they were inferior as compared to those who were not obese (Rogge, Greenwald, & Golden, 2004). In an attempt to change self-perception of stigma, Abel (2007) utilized an intervention of emotional writing disclosure for women with HIV. Women who participated in the intervention had more positive scores on the Stigma Scale tool at the end of the 12-week pilot study than women in the control group. This journaling strategy may be one way the healthcare provider can help individuals change their internal perception of stigma.

With these internalized negative perceptions, some people with chronic illness choose to conceal the disclosure of the disease. When 14 people with a diagnosis of multiple sclerosis and their families were interviewed, it was found that the disease was purposefully concealed or selectively disclosed to shield from social judgment or to enhance social belonging at work (Grytten & Maseide, 2005). In describing studies of clients with cerebral palsy, cancer, facial deformity, arthritis, and multiple sclerosis, Shontz (1977) noted that the personal meaning of the disability to each client was uniformly regarded as crucial. For example, individuals who feel valuable because they are healthy and physically fit usually experience feelings of worthlessness if they contract a chronic condition. But people with diabetes will never be without a regimen and the necessary paraphernalia; visually impaired individuals will never see normally again. Therefore, the individuals' reactions and ability to accommodate these discrepancies determine their attitudes of worth and value.

In contrast, some individuals with chronic conditions can accept deviations from expected norms and feel relatively untouched. They have reordered life's priorities; no longer is the absence of disease or disability their major criterion for self-worth. Rather, an alternative ideology evolves to counter the "standard" ideologies. A strong sense of identity protects them, and they are able to feel acceptable in the face of the stigma (Goffman, 1963).

This identity belief system, also called cognitive belief patterns, refers to a person's perspective. It includes one's perceptions, mental attitudes, beliefs, and interpretations of experiences (Link et al., 1997). Individuals who are stigmatized by the major society may believe and perceive that their groups are actually superior or at least preferable. These belief patterns offer protection from the stigmatized reactions of others. Yet, being in a specific cultural or ethnic group does not always provide protection against stigma in certain diseases. In fact, the stigma of having a mental illness is even more prominent among some ethnic groups. A literature review by Gary (2005) found that African Americans, Asian Americans, Hispanic Americans, and Indian Americans all perceived stigma related to mental illness in addition to the prejudice and discrimination already experienced due to the affiliation with their particular ethnic group.

Cognitive belief patterns help individuals with chronic illnesses achieve identity acceptance and protection in the face of stigmatizing conditions. For example, after extensive cancer surgery, clients may consciously tell themselves that they are full human beings because the missing part was diseased or useless. The body, although disfigured, is now healthy and totally acceptable. Similarly, wheelchair athletes take pride in their superb physical condition and competitiveness. That is, one's perception of self-worth influences one's reactions to disease or disability. An individual's question,

"Am I worthwhile?" is answered by determining his or her own values and perspective. Therefore, clients' definitions of themselves are crucial factors in self-satisfaction (see Chapter 7).

Support Groups

Goffman (1963) used the term *the own* for those who share a stigma. Those who share the same stigma can offer the "tricks of the trade," acceptance, and moral support to a person living with stigma. Self-help or support groups are examples of persons who are the own. Alcoholics Anonymous (AA), for instance, provides a community of the own as well as a way of life for its members. Members speak publicly, demonstrating that people with alcoholism are treatable, not terrible, people.

Groups composed of people with similar conditions can be formal or informal and are enormously helpful. First, peer groups can be used to explore all of the potential response options discussed previously, such as resisting and passing. Second, problem-solving sessions in these groups explore possible solutions to common situations (Dudley, 1983). Finally, others who share the stigma provide a source of acceptance and support for both the individuals with the chronic condition and their families. Maternal mental health clients developed and implemented an ongoing support group in consultation with a healthcare professional (Franks et al., 2007). These women were able to promote and sustain their group for a 12-month period.

O'Sullivan (2006) reported on a unique twist to the self-help group. A Barcelona, Spain radio program is planned and implemented by persons with mental illness. The program seeks to inform, educate, and break down the stigma and stereotypes associated with mental illness. Benefits to the participants included an increase in self-esteem and more positive self-perception.

A word of caution is needed. Sometimes stigmatized individuals feel more comfortable with nonstigmatized individuals than with like others as a result of a closer identity with the former. For example, not all women respond positively to Reach to Recovery groups; some may feel more discomfort than support. Reputable online support groups present another option for people with the technologic equipment and skills to access these resources. The ability to control the encounter with like others from a safe haven may be appealing to many clients. The "best" solution varies from individual to individual.

Other Considerations

Other points for the healthcare professional to consider are issues of "inclusion" and "exclusion," and how they impact stigma. Technology and assistive devices are significant factors because they underline the fact that "quality of life" is not a static entity. Not many years ago, electric wheelchairs were not readily available. Now such wheelchairs exist, in pediatric to bariatric sizes, as well as electric scooters that allow mobility for clients with a variety of conditions. Formerly, a person with paralyzed arms could only type slowly with a stick fastened to a headband; now there are increasingly accurate voice-activated home computers that type as the person speaks. In the same vein, a person whose speech is unintelligible to most others can press symbols on a display board that produces full sentences spoken in a nonrobotic, smooth human voice. The savvy healthcare professional will attend to technologic advances and assist clients in obtaining necessary aids to promote full functioning of the individual.

To that end, the opportunity to hire personal assistants is also important. Having such assistance allows individuals with severe disabilities to have a far richer life than those without such help. Many disability advocates are pressing for public money that is currently spent on nursing homes and other institutions to be redirected to enable individuals who are disabled or chronically ill to live in their own homes (see Chapter 23). Maintaining function and independence may lessen the impact of both felt and enacted stigma.

Developing Supportive Others

Supportive others are persons (professional and nonprofessional) who do not carry the stigmatizing trait but are knowledgeable and offer sensitive understanding to individuals who do carry it. These people are called the wise by Goffman (1963) and are accorded acceptance within the group of stigmatized individuals. Desired behaviors are simply the ones two friends or acquaintances would use. The stigmatized person must be seen and treated as a full human being—viewed as more than body changes or orthopedic equipment, seen as a person who is more than a stigmatized condition.

The AIDS epidemic has added to the impetus for the development of groups of supportive others. In many cities, the model of care for those with AIDS depends on volunteer, community-based groups that supply food, transportation, in-home care, acceptance, and support. This community network is an adjunct to hospital care and provides a vivid example of wise others who are essential to the care of these clients.

Implications for Professional Practice

One way an individual can become wise is by asking straightforward, sensitive questions, such as inquiring about the disabled person's condition. Many individuals with disabilities would welcome the opportunity to disclose as much or as little as they wish, because that would mean that the disability was no longer taboo. For example, the disabled person may prefer that others ask about a cane or a walker rather than ignore it. This opportunity allows the disabled individual to reply with whatever explanation he or she wishes. Therefore, the disability is acknowledged, not ignored. It goes without saying that these questions should be asked after a beginning relationship is established, as opposed to being asked out of idle curiosity.

The process of becoming wise is not simple; it may mean offering oneself and waiting for

■ EVIDENCE-BASED PRACTICE BOX

This chapter has dealt primarily with adults' perceptions of stigma and interventional strategies that healthcare providers can use to both raise awareness of and to decrease the incidence of stigma. To decrease the cycle of stigma throughout society, it is necessary to begin with the next generation. Indeed, raising awareness and decreasing stigma for children with mental illness is a goal of the US Surgeon General. A study by Watson et al. (2005) offers some insight into adolescents' attitudes and thought processes regarding people with mental illness, and suggests strategies appropriate for the adolescent population.

Purpose: To explore the dimensions of mental illness stigma relevant to adolescents and to determine the effects of demographic factors (race, gender, age, familiarity with mental illness).

Sample: Students at two suburban Chicago high schools (N = 415). The sample was 53% female, 79% caucasian, 40% stated that they had a family member with mental illness, and 24% self-identified as having a mental illness.

Method: The 24-item Attitudes Toward Serious Mental Illness Scale-Adolescent Version (ATSMI-AV) was used. Factor analyses were conducted and t tests were done to examine differences in ratings by demographic factors.

Findings: Males scored significantly higher ($t = 5.21$, $p = .00$) on both the Threat and Categorical Thinking factors. The Freshmen/Sophomore students scored significantly higher ($t = 3.38$, $p = 0.00$) on the Social Control/Concern factor than did the Junior/Senior group of students. Students with a family history of mental illness had statistically significantly higher scores on the Social Control/Concern factor and lower scores for Categorical Thinking than those students who did not indicate a family history.

Conclusions: Findings supported previous research indicating a connection between more positive attitudes and interaction with people with mental illness. Strategies targeting categorical by assisting adolescents to view people with mental illness as individuals may be a first step in raising awareness and decreasing enacted stigma.

Source: Watson, A., Miller, F., & Lyons, J. (2005). Adolescent attitudes toward serious mental illness. *The Journal of Nervous and Mental Disease, 193*(11), 769–772.

validation of acceptance. Healthcare professionals who encounter individuals with chronic illness cannot prove themselves as wise immediately. Validation requires consistent behavior by the professional that is sensitive, knowledgeable, and accepting. Being wise is not a new role for nurses or other caring healthcare professionals. Nurses have traditionally worked in medically underserved areas with discredited persons and are accustomed to treating clients as individuals, not as conditions. Nurses often assume the predominant role of gatekeepers to the healthcare delivery system for many devalued individuals. Often, clients with chronic illnesses receive effective and efficient care from these nurses and other healthcare professionals, who have great opportunities to perform the role of the wise.

Another strategy healthcare professionals can use to acquire real-life knowledge about individuals with a particular illness is to increase their interaction with people who have the disorder (Heijenders & Van Der Meij, 2006). In addition to increasing exposure to and interaction with people who have a particular stigmatizing condition, Corrigan and Penn (1999) suggest that it is important for healthcare professionals to be exposed to people who are successfully coping with a condition; those who have recovered from mental illness, who are in remission, or who have been successfully rehabilitated. This knowledge can enable them to offer not only sensitive understanding and practical suggestions to chronically ill individuals, but also hope. Nurses who work with AIDS clients, for instance, have the opportunity to find out which behavior is really effective and can learn about outcomes and clients' reactions. This information is extremely valuable as providers advocate for similar clients and their families.

Implications for Professional Education

Healthcare professionals' attitudes are representative of general societal views and so can be expected to include prejudices. Because healthcare professionals have prolonged relationships with chronically ill individuals, the impact of these prejudices can be great. Programs to teach professional staff to identify and correct preconceived and often unconscious notions of categories and stereotypes deserve high priority (Dudley, 1983).

Providing intensive staff education for the purpose of reducing stigma perception by all employees in any particular agency is beneficial. In addition, professional staff are then in a position to practice role model behavior and to give information to help nonprofessional staff treat clients in an accepting manner.

One study of stigma-promoting behaviors provides ideas for healthcare professionals who wish to change their attitudes (Dudley, 1983). In Dudley's study, the most frequent stigma-promoting behaviors included the following: staring, denial of opportunities for clients to present views, inappropriate language in referring to clients, inappropriate restrictions of activities, violation of confidentiality, physical abuse, and ignoring clients. Inservice days that focus on both didactic presentation of communication strategies and role-playing specific scenarios would be a first step to eliminating situations of enacted stigma in the workplace.

One way to increase visibility and heighten awareness about the impact of stigma is to encourage structured contact between healthcare professionals and affected individuals (Joachim & Acorn, 2000). This approach should be preceded by group work with a knowledgeable leader who can help identify and work through attitudes and reactions. For example, many nursing students do not like skilled nursing facilities (SNFs) because older adults are seen as unappealing. A gerontology nurse specialist spent time with such a group of students before they began working in the SNF. She showed slides of faces etched with character and told stories of interesting experiences these individuals had that helped the students see the elderly as human beings. A group discussion between the specialist and students confronted myths and stereotypical thinking regarding the stigma of aging. As a result, these students had a more positive experience at the SNF.

Knowledgeable preparation for contact with stigmatized individuals does not solve all problems; it is, however, one way to expose stigmatized reactions such as stereotypes, to examine them, and to provide information to caregivers. The group sessions described here may be appropriate for both nonprofessional and professional caregivers in the community or in agencies.

Implications for Community Education Programs

Educational programs that reduce the effects of stigma can be shared with the community at large. Many organizations, such as the American Cancer Society and the American Diabetes Association, provide speakers or literature for the community. Schools, scout troops, and church groups are ideal settings for sensitive introductions of individuals who have many positive values and characteristics but do not meet normal health expectations. For instance, individuals with AIDS have been the focus of group discussions in which children learn to see these people simply as other human beings. Educational programs, such as those that dispel the fears about mental illness, reduce the stigmatizing effects of that disease (Link et al., 1989).

Much of the stigma attached to chronic conditions still pervades society's attitudes and policies (Herek et al., 2003); yet, situations have changed. In the 1970s, an unprecedented and multilayered surge of activism grew among individuals with disabilities and their advocates and resulted in significant social and structural change. Individuals with disabilities began to speak out by publishing magazines, creating movies and videos, and organizing political action on both the local and national levels. Their actions greatly influenced a landmark change, namely, the Americans with Disabilities Act (ADA), which was signed into law in 1990. This legislation requires the government and the private sector to provide disabled individuals with opportunities for jobs, education, access to transportation, and access to public buildings.

The media can also be influenced to present a more positive portrayal of people with chronic conditions. Providers and others can write to television networks that show individuals with disabilities functioning well and commend them for these portrayals.

Mass media campaigns designed to increase awareness of certain conditions or risk factors for disease can backfire in terms of preventing or reducing stigma. Clients with lung cancer not only perceived stigma of cancer in general (such as fear of disclosure, financial impact,

body image changes, and effects on family and social relationships), but also the stigma that is associated with smoking and the shame of a self-inflicted disease, regardless of whether they stopped smoking or had never smoked. They experienced fear related to death as depicted by the mass media, families and friends avoiding contact, and being looked upon as being "dirty" in relation to smoking (Chapple, Ziebland, & McPherson, 2004).

Another study identified methods of health communication that were designed to increase public awareness but actually had the opposite effect of increasing public stigma (Wang, 1998). The health communication approaches conveyed individuals with obvious disabling characteristics with the accompanying message, "Don't be like this." Awareness was heightened at the expense of furthering the stigma of the disabled individual. Healthcare professionals who volunteer to serve on executive boards of healthcare agencies or support agencies can offer guidance to those developing marketing campaigns, public service announcements, and community education materials.

Recent social changes have suggested that internalization of stigma based on prevailing social norms may be changing for some health problems. Rehabilitation programs for substance abuse are now commonly covered by health insurance, in part as a result of active consumer demand, evidencing a change of social attitude (Garfinkel & Dorian, 2000). The impact of stigmatizing conditions in women's health, such as abortion and breast cancer with mastectomy, has been reduced (Bennett, 1997). These changes are, perhaps, evidence that visibility and disclosure may have a positive impact on the process of negative stereotyping.

OUTCOMES

Determining client outcomes, like many of the psychosocial concepts associated with chronic illnesses, is difficult. Some clients may be stigmatized on a regular basis but have been able to overcome the personal feelings associated with it. Therefore, client outcomes of stigma might be the *lack* of other common psychosocial effects of chronic illness. For example:

1. The client is *not* socially isolated, but is continuing his or her daily and normal activities without difficulty.
2. The client's self-esteem remains high despite the chronic illness and accompanying physical symptoms.
3. Healthy relationships continue with family, friends, and supportive others.
4. The client is *not* depressed and interacts appropriately with others.

STUDY QUESTIONS

1. Compare and contrast the concepts of felt stigma and enacted stigma. Are these two concepts mutually exclusive?
2. How does the process of labeling by others influence the perception of felt stigma and incidences of enacted stigma?
3. Advanced practice nurses can implement strategies to decrease incidences of enacted stigma in society. What might the advanced practice nurse do in each of the following roles to decrease stigma: nurse administrator, nurse educator, clinician?
4. As a change agent in your practice setting, what strategies can you readily implement to increase awareness of stigma among administrators, healthcare professionals, and support staff?
5. What strategies can you readily implement to decrease the perceptions of stigma by your clients?
6. Discuss the similarities and differences among prejudice, stereotyping, and labeling. What is the relationship to stigma?

INTERNET RESOURCES

Mental Health Issues

US Department of Health and Human Services stigma homepage: www.mentalhealth.samhsa.gov/stigma
Stigma.org links to mental health Web sites: www.stigma.org
National Health Awareness Campaign: www.nostigma.org
National Alliance on Mental Illness Stigma Busters: www.nami.org/Hometemplate.cfm

HIV/AIDS Issues

HRSA Care Action—Providing HIV/AIDS Care in a Changing Environment: hab.hrsa.gov/publications/august2003.htm
Stigma, Discrimination, and Attitudes to HIV & AIDS: www.avert.org/aidsstigma

REFERENCES

Abel, E. (2007). Women with HIV and stigma. *Family and Community Health, 30*(Suppl 1), 104–106.

Baker, G.A., Brooks, J., Buck, D., & Jacoby, A. (2000). The stigma of epilepsy: A European perspective. *Epilepsia, 41*(1), 98–104.

Bartels, L., & Crowder, C. (1999). Fatal friendship. *Denver Rocky Mountain News.* Retrieved from www.rockymountainnews.com

Bauer, H., Rodriguez, M., Quiroga, S., & Flores-Ortiz, Y. (2000). Barriers to health care for abused Latina and Asian immigrant women. *Journal of Health Care for the Poor and Underserved, 11*(1), 33–44.

Bennett, T. (1997). Women's health in maternal and child health: Time for a new tradition? *Maternal and Child Health Journal, 1*(3), 253–265.

Brandon, D., Khoo, R., Maglajlie, R., & Abuel-Ealeh, M. (2000). European snapshot homeless survey: Result of questions asked of passers-by in 11 European cities. *International Journal of Nursing Practice, 6*(1), 39–45.

Camp, D.L., Finlay, W.M.L., & Lyons, E. (2002). Is low self-esteem an inevitable consequence of stigma? An example from women with chronic mental health problems. *Social science and medicine, 55*(5), 823–834.

Chapple, A., Ziebland, S., & McPherson, A. (2004). Stigma, shame, and blame experienced by patients with lung cancer: Qualitative study. *British Medical Journal, 328*(7454), 1470.

Cinnirella, M., & Loewenthal, K.M. (1999). Religion and ethnic group influences on beliefs about mental illness: A qualitative interview study. *British Journal of Medical Psychology, 72*(4), 505–524.

Corrigan, P., & Penn, D. (1999). Lessons from social psychology on discrediting psychiatric stigma. *American Psychology, 54*(9), 765–776.

Crisp, A., Gelder, M., Rix, S., Meltzer, H., et al. (2000). Stigmatization of people with mental illness. *British Journal of Psychiatry, 177*, 4–7.

Davies, M.R. (2000). The stigma of anxiety disorders. *International Journal of Clinical Practice, 54*(1), 44–47.

de Souza, E.A., & Salgado, P.C. (2006). A psychosocial view of anxiety and depression in epilepsy. *Epilepsy and Behavior, 8*(1), 232–238.

Distabile, P., Dubler, N., Solomon, L., & Klein, R. (1999). Self-reported legal needs of women with or at risk for HIV infection. The HER Study Group. *Journal of Urban Health, 76*(4), 435–447.

Dudley, J. (1983). *Living with stigma: The plight of the people who we label mentally retarded.* Springfield, IL: Charles C. Thomas.

Ebersole, P., Hess, P., Touhy, T., & Jett, K. (2005). *Gerontological nursing and healthy aging.* St. Louis: Mosby.

Erikson, E. (1968). *Identity: Youth in crisis.* New York: W.W. Norton.

Fife, B., & Wright, E. (2000). The dimensionality of stigma: A comparison of its impact on the self of persons with HIV/AIDS and cancer. *Journal of Health and Social Behavior, 41*(1), 50–67.

Franks, W., Henwood, K., & Bowden, G. (2007). Promoting maternal mental health: Women's strategies for presenting a positive identity and the implications for mental health promotion. *Journal of Public Mental Health, 6*(2), 40–51.

Garfinkel, P.E., & Dorian, B.J. (2000). Psychiatry in the new millennium. *Canadian Journal of Psychiatry, 45*(1), 40–47.

Gary, F.A. (2005). Stigma: Barrier to mental health care among ethnic minorities. *Issues in Mental Health Nursing, 26*(10), 979–999.

Gewirtz, A., & Gossart-Walker, S. (2000). Home-based treatment for children and families affected by HIV and AIDS. Dealing with stigma, secrecy, disclosure, and loss. *Child and Adolescent Psychiatry Clinics of North America, 9*(2), 313–330.

Goffman, E. (1963). *Stigma: Notes on management of spoiled identity.* Englewood Cliffs, NJ: Prentice-Hall.

Grytten, N., & Maseide, P. (2005). What is expressed is not always what is felt: Coping with stigma and the embodiment of perceived illegitimacy of multiple sclerosis. *Chronic Illness, 1*(3), 231–243.

Halevy, A. (2000). AIDS, surgery, and the Americans with Disabilities Act. *Archives of surgery, 135*(1), 51–54.

Heckman, T.G., Anderson, E.S., Sikkema, K.J., Kochman, A., et al. (2004). Emotional distress in nonmetropolitan persons living with HIV disease enrolled in a telephone-delivered, coping improvement group intervention. *Health Psychology, 23*(1), 94–100.

Heijnders, M., & Van Der Meij, S. (2006). The fight against stigma: An overview of stigma-reduction strategies and interventions. *Psychology, Health & Medicine, 11*(3), 353–363.

Herek, G.M., Capitanio, J.P., & Widaman, K.F. (2003). Stigma, social risk, and health policy: Public attitudes toward HIV surveillance policies and the social construct of illness. *Health Psychology, 22*(5), 533–540.

Heukelbach, J., & Feldmeier, H. (2006). Scabies. *The Lancet, 367*, 1767–1774.

Hodgson, I. (2006). Empathy, inclusion and enclaves: The culture of care of people with HIV/AIDS and nursing implications. *Journal of Advanced Nursing, 55*(3), 283–290.

Hynd, H.M. (1958). *On shame and the search for identity* (3rd ed.). New York: Harcourt Brace Jovanovich.

Jacoby, A. (1994). Felt versus enacted stigma: A concept revisited. *Social science and medicine, 8*(2), 269–274.

Joachim, G. & Acorn, S. (2000). Stigma of visible and invisible chronic conditions. *Journal of Advanced Nursing, 32*(1), 243–248.

Jolley, D.J., & Benbow, S.M. (2000). Stigma and Alzheimer's disease: Causes, consequences, and a constructive approach. *International Journal of Clinical Practice, 54*(2), 117–119.

Katz, I. (1981). *Stigma: A social psychological analysis.* Hillsdale, NJ: Lawrence Erlbaum Associates.

Keltner, K., Schwecke, L., & Bostrom, C. (2003). *Psychiatric nursing* (4th ed.). St. Louis: Mosby.

Kurzban, R. & Leary, M.R. (2001). Evolutionary origins of stigmatization: The functions of social exclusion. *Psychological Bulletin, 127*(2), 187–208.

Ladieu-Leviton, G., Adler, D., & Dembo, T. (1977). Studies in adjustment to visible injuries: Social acceptance of the injured. In R. Marinelli & A. Dell Orto (eds.), *The psychological and social impact of the physical disability.* New York: Springer.

Liggins, J., & Hatcher, S. (2005). Stigma toward the mentally ill in the general hospital: A qualitative study. *General Hospital Psychiatry, 27*(5), 359–364.

Link, B.G. (1987). Understanding labeling effects in the area of mental disorders: An assessment of the effects of expectations of rejection. *American Sociological Review, 52*(1), 96–112.

Link, B.G., Cullen, F.T., Struening, E., Shrout, P.E., et al. (1989). A modified labeling theory approach to mental disorders: An empirical assessment. *American Sociological Review, 54*(3), 400–423.

Link, B.G., Struening, E.L., Rahav, M., Phelan, J.C., et al. (1997). On stigma and its consequences: Evidence from a longitudinal study of men with dual diagnoses of mental illness and substance abuse. *Journal of Health and Social Behavior, 38*(2), 177–190.

Link, B.G., & Phelan, J.C. (2001). Conceptualizing stigma. *Annual Review of Sociology, 27*, 363–385.

Markowitz, F.E. (1998). The effects of stigma on the psychological well-being and life satisfaction of persons with mental illness. *Journal of Health and Social Behavior, 39*, 335–347.

Merriam Webster Dictionary and Thesaurus OnLine (2007). Retrieved on November 10, 2007 from www.m-w.com

Miller, N., Noble, E., Jones, D., & Burn, D. (2006). Hard to swallow: Dysphagia in Parkinson's disease. *Age and Ageing, 35*(6), 614–618.

Murray, J., Banerjee, S., Byng, R., Tylee, A., Bhugra, D., & Macdonald, A. (2006). Primary care professionals' perceptions of depression in older people: A qualitative study. *Social Science and Medicine, 63*(5), 1363–1373.

O'Sullivan, M. (2006). Making radio waves. *A Life in the Day, 10*(2), 6–8.

Rehm, R.S., & Franck, L.S. (2000). Long-term goals and normalization strategies of children and families affected by HIV/AIDS. *Advances in Nursing Science, 23*(1), 69–82.

Ritson, E.B. (1999). Alcohol, drugs, and stigma. *International Journal of Clinical Practice, 53*(7), 549–551.

Roberts, L.W., Warner, T.D., & Trumpower, D. (2000). Medical students' evolving perspectives on their personal health care: Clinical and educational implications of a longitudinal study. *Comprehensive Psychiatry, 41*(4), 303–314.

Rogge, M.M., Greenwald, M., & Golden, A. (2004). Obesity, stigma, and civilized oppression. *Advances in Nursing Science, 27*(4), 301–315.

Roskes, E., Feldman, R., Arrington, S., & Leisher, M. (1999). A model program for the treatment of mentally ill offenders in the community. *Community Mental Health Journal, 35*(5), 461–472.

Rossi, L.A., Vila Vda, S., Zago, M.M. & Ferreira, E. (2005). The stigma of burns perceptions of burned patients' relatives when facing discharge from hospital. *Burns, 31*(1), 37–44.

Salisbury, K.M. (2000). National and state policies influencing the care of children affected by AIDS. *Child and Adolescent Psychiatry Clinics of North America, 9*(2), 425–449.

Sandelowski, M., & Barroso, J. (2003). Motherhood in the context of maternal HIV infection. *Research in Nursing and Health, 26,* 470–482.

Scambler, G. (2004). Reframing stigma: Felt and enacted stigma and challenges to the sociology of chronic and disabling conditions. *Social Theory and Health, 2,* 29–46.

Schreiber, R., Stern, P.N., & Wilson, C. (2000). Being strong: How black West-Indian Canadian women manage depression and it's stigma. *Journal of Nursing Scholarship, 32*(1), 39–45.

Shontz, E. (1977). Physical disability and personality: Theory and recent research. In R. Marinelli & A. Dell Orto (Eds.), *The psychological and social impact of physical disability.* New York: Springer.

Simpson, G., Mohr, R., & Redman, A. (2000). Cultural variations in the understanding of traumatic brain injury and brain injury rehabilitation. *Brain Injury, 14*(2), 125–140.

Stewart, M., Keel, P., & Schiavo, R.S. (2006). Stigmatization of anorexia nervosa. *International Journal of Eating Disorders, 39*(4), 320–325.

VanBrakel, W.H. (2006). Measuring health-related stigma: A literature review. *Psychology of Health and Medicine, 11*(3), 307–334.

Waldman, H.B., Swerdloff, M., & Perlman, S.P. (1999). Children with mental retardation: Stigma and stereotype images are hard to change. *ASDC Journal of Dentistry for Children, 66*(5), 343–347.

Wang, C. (1998). Portraying stigmatized conditions: Disabling images in public health. *Journal of Health Communication, 3*(2), 149–159.

Werner, P. (2006). Lay perceptions regarding the competence of persons with Alzheimer's disease. *International Journal of Geriatric Psychiatry, 21,* 674–680.

Weston, H.J. (2003). Public honor, private shame, and HIV: Issues affecting sexual health service delivery in London's South Asian communities. *Health and Place, 9*(2), 109–117.

Williams, D.R. (1999). Race, socioeconomic status, and health. The added effects of racism and discrimination. *Annals of the New York Academy of Science, 896,* 173–188.

4

Adaptation

Pamala D. Larsen and Faye I. Hummel

INTRODUCTION

Persons with chronic illness chart a life-course to successfully navigate the challenges that are inherent within themselves, their relationships, or the setting in which they find themselves. Throughout the course of their illness, individuals must rely on a healthcare system in which pharmaceuticals, machines, and a wide array of technology to manage and cure disease and injury have become the hallmarks of quality health care. Although the disease focus may be appropriate intermittently during the trajectory of a chronic illness to meet the physical demands of the individual, this perspective does not meet the social, psychological, and emotional needs of clients with chronic conditions. In other words, the disease focus of the healthcare system does not and cannot manage the illness experience of the client and family.

Early work by Visotsky, Hamburg, Goss, and Lebovits (1961) posed some initial questions regarding adaptation in their study of clients with polio. They asked their clients how it was possible to deal with this stressor, polio, and what coping behavior(s) could predict a favorable outcome (Stanton & Revenson, 2007). Nearly fifty years later, we are still asking the same questions.

Although we have made progress in understanding certain components of adaptation, many questions remain answered.

The lens for viewing chronic illness is determined by numerous variables within the person as well as how the healthcare professional views the chronic condition. The elderly woman with arthritis who has been socialized to the primacy of medicine in the health care arena may rely solely on her physician prescribed pharmaceutical treatment of her joint pain and fatigue. On the other hand, a young man with Hepatitis C gathers information from a wide variety of sources regarding the treatment and management of his chronic condition and maintains control of his treatment plan.

Similarly, the adaptation mechanism of the elderly woman and the young man may be very different as well. Each individual brings to the illness their own uniqueness, whether it be personality traits, past experiences, culture, or values, to influence the adaptation process in their own way.

Defining Adaptation

The terms adjustment and adaptation are used interchangeably in the literature (Stanton & Revenson, 2007) and will be in this chapter as well. The term adaptation means that there is an event, or something that is unusual or different that is perceived as a stressor to the individual that dictates a reaction, a change, or a behavior by the individual. Sharpe and Curran (2006) define adjustment as a response to a change in the environment that allows an organism to become more suitably adapted to that change (p. 1154).

An early description of adjustment (and a continuing one) is the absence of a diagnosed psychological disorder, psychological symptoms, or negative mood (Stanton, Revenson, & Tennen, 2007). Even in Visotsky's study in 1961 with clients with polio, there was a movement to discount that definition. Yes, it may be a part of adjustment, but it is only one indicator of it.

Adjustment to illness has been operationalized as good quality of life, well-being, vitality, positive affect, life satisfaction, and global self-esteem (Sharpe & Curran, 2006). Conversely, Adjustment Disorder is defined as "the development of clinically significant emotional or behavioral symptoms in response to an identifiable stressor or stressor" (APA, 1997, p. 623).

There is little consistency in the literature in defining adaptation or adjustment. Each author/researcher defines adaptation or adjustment differently based on their own theoretical framework or outcome measurement.

This chapter provides a brief overview of adaptation in individuals with chronic illness. With entire books devoted to coping and adaptation, the depth in this chapter is limited. However, classic sources and models are included, along with interventions appropriate for individuals and families with chronic illness.

IMPACT

Conceptualization of Adaptation

Stanton and Revenson (2007) have identified five attributes of adjustment: (1) chronic illness necessitates adjustment in multiple life domains; (2) there are positive and negative indicators of adjustment; (3) adjustment is dynamic; (4)

adjustment can be described only within the context of each unique individual; and (5) heterogeneity is the rule rather than the exception in adjustment. Each of these concepts are further described.

Chronic Illness Necessitates Adjustment in Multiple Life Domains

We know from caring for clients that adjustment is more than just physical, but includes adjustment that crosses interpersonal, cognitive, emotional, and behavioral domains. Adjustment is a holistic event in the client, with all domains being interrelated. Therefore, a change in one domain may affect adjustment in another domain (Stanton & Revenson, 2007; Stanton, Collins, & Sworowski, 2001; Stewart, Ross, & Hartley, 2004). Cognitive adaptation might involve a personal self-evaluation. Adaptation in the behavioral domain includes returning to work or resuming the role of the "breadwinner" of the family. Anxiety, in the emotional domain, may affect the ability to socialize, in the interpersonal domain, or influence blood pressure, in the physical domain. Emotional adaptation could be the absence of depression, and interpersonal adaptation may be the willingness to be "social" again. Again, each domain may affect the other.

Adjustment Involves Both Positive and Negative Outcome Dimensions

Typically we think of outcomes of chronic illness as being negative, as evidenced by distress, psychological dysfunction, relationships in disarray, and so forth. As stated previously, one definition of positive adjustment is the absence of a psychological disorder. However, there may be a positive side of chronic illness as well.

It's not unusual to hear individuals with chronic illness say "having this disease has been the best thing that ever happened to me . . . it made me wake up to see what was important." There may be positive aspects of chronic disease, but how this occurs, we don't know. Folkman, Moskowitz, Ozer, and Park (1997), in their study of HIV-positive and HIV-caregiving partners of men with AIDS, found that although study participants reported high levels of depressive symptoms, they also demonstrated positive morale and positive states of mind when compared with general population norms.

One possible way to describe these paradoxical findings is a concept titled response shift. Sprangers and Schwartz (2000) coined this phrase to describe a change in the meaning of one's self-evaluation of a target construct as a result of (1) change in an individual's internal standards of measurement, (2) change in the individual's values, or (3) reconceptualization of the target construct (p. 12).

Although anecdotally we consider negative outcomes of chronic illness more common, research demonstrates that positive adjustment may more accurately represent the adjustment experience of most individuals with chronic disease (Stanton & Revenson, 2007). By focusing solely on psychopathology, a negative aspect of adjustment, one will have a limited understanding of adjustment.

Adjustment Is a Dynamic Process

Adjustment to chronic illness is neither linear nor lockstep (Stanton & Revenson, 2007, p. 568). As exacerbations occur, as in rheumatoid arthritis or multiple sclerosis, the cancer recurs, and the physical limitations of heart failure increase; each change requires a re-adjustment or re-adaptation. In addition, changes may not be limited to changes in one's physical condition that affect adaptation, but changes in the rest of the individual's life. Perhaps a spouse loses his/her job, a child is seriously injured, a parent is no longer able to care for themselves; all of these factors affect the adaptation of the client with chronic illness.

Adjustment Can Be Viewed Only from Within the Context of the Individual

There is variability in adaptation, and that is to be expected. From the context of the individual,

the physical symptoms, the functional changes, and the uncertainty, may or may not be pertinent to that individual. Each stressor of the illness has a different relevance for each individual, and as a result will elicit a different reaction from each individual. The context of each individual is different, whether it be their age, gender, ethnicity, or social status. The 35-year-old married woman with three grade-school-aged children with newly diagnosed breast cancer has a different context than the 80-year-old woman whose family is raised. Although that is an extreme example, the variation that exists among individuals cannot be understated.

Heterogeneity Is the Rule, Not the Exception

Anecdotally we know that if we put 20 women of the same age with the same stage of breast cancer and same prognosis in a room, each of those individuals will adapt to their chronic condition differently. Some will be considered by most as "well-adjusted," whereas others might be considered maladjusted. The remaining individuals may fall somewhere in the middle. The person's individual determinants and uniqueness as a person affect the ability of the individual to adapt to the illness. Although commonalities exist among individuals with chronic illness, there is significant variability as well.

Differences in individual adjustment abound in the literature. Helgeson, Snyder, and Seltman (2004) in a study of women with breast cancer from 4 to 55 months after diagnosis found that 43% of the sample evidenced high and stable psychological quality of life, 18% had a somewhat lower quality of life, 26% evidenced low psychological functioning, and 12% had an immediate and substantial decline in psychological function.

Dew and colleagues (2005) identified five groups of distinct distress profiles in heart transplantation patients over several years. Groups evidenced: (1) consistently low distress; (2) consistent, significant levels of distress; (3) high distress for the initial 3 months; (4) high distress at 3 years; and (5) fluctuating distress.

Models

As researchers, we have a broad goal to understand the process of adaptation, predict outcomes, and by having predictive ability, be able to modify interventions to meet the needs of our clients. A model that is able to perform all those activities is preferred for practice; however, a perfect model does not exist at this time. What follows are sample models from the literature.

Medical Model

The medical model provides a framework for the assumptions about the nature of health and illness. The client becomes a complex set of anatomic parts and interrelated systems. Anatomic, physiologic, and/or biochemical failures translate into etiologies of ill health, thus promoting a disease-oriented approach to care. This theoretical perspective of chronic illness is reflected in the language and actions of healthcare professionals who refer to "the diabetic in room 328," rather than to Mrs. Sanchez.

Pathophysiology, pharmacotherapy, and high technology are emphasized and become prominent in the diagnosis and intervention of all illness and disease, albeit acute or chronic. Antonovsky (1979) considered the medical model a dichotomous model. If pathology is present, then there is illness, and wellness or health is not possible. Explanatory assumptions and theories are used for determining the cause of symptoms, and uniformity of causality and treatment of disease is inferred.

The biomedical paradigm tends to medicalize all human conditions in which symptoms can be controlled and cured with biomedical strategies. This model reduces the individual to a disease and fails to recognize the human aspects and experiences of the individual who happens to have a chronic illness (Sakalys, 2000), and diminishes social and cultural explanation of disease (Mirowsky & Ross, 2002). Physical complaints and signs or symptoms of disease become the hallmarks of interaction and discourse within the healthcare arena.

The relationship between the healthcare professional and the client with chronic illness is one of objectivity, biological pathology, diagnosis, and signs and symptoms, all of which require medical interventions. Healthcare professionals tend to shield themselves from the human aspects of chronic illness, while their skill sets, techniques, and procedures become the focus of interaction with the client (Freeth, 2007). Power and expertise are held exclusively by the healthcare system, and the interactions between the healthcare professional and the client are directive and unbalanced. The individual with chronic illness becomes disempowered to engage in his/her own healthcare decisions and relies solely on the healthcare professional.

The medical model is insufficient in providing health care to individuals with chronic illness (Waisbond, 2007), and it fails to acknowledge the breadth and depth of the illness experience. This model does not acknowledge the person with the chronic condition, who holds knowledge and expertise about the factors that influence his/her physical symptoms of chronic disease, in other words, the expert patient. For example, at the end of the month, Mrs. Jones becomes anxious that she will not have enough money to purchase her prescriptions for her hypertension. Although she is able to financially manage, Mrs. Jones' stress and worry exacerbate her hypertension. Mrs. Jones does not inform her physician that the probable cause of her elevated blood pressure is related to her stress. The physician responds to Mrs. Jones' hypertension with a change of medication to manage her symptoms. The quantification of all signs and symptoms of disease fails to address the total illness experience of the individual. With increased attention to genetic research and gene technologies, the biomedical theories of disease will be continue to be reinforced, with less emphasis on the individual's social context and experiences (Dixon-Woods, 2001).

Despite the limitations of the biomedical model for adaptation, its usefulness is apparent during the acute phase of chronic illness. Although the focus of the biomedical model is limited to disease and organic dysfunction, this model is central for adaptation to chronic illness, particularly at the time of diagnosis when individuals and families are overwhelmed with a new diagnosis and sorting out the facts about the illness. In addition, during periods of illness exacerbations, the medical model helps to explain signs and symptoms and may provide a source of retreat and relief, depending on the stage of the chronic illness. There are times when individuals and families need current information about the chronic illness, signs and symptoms, the anticipated trajectory of the illness course, the array of treatment modalities, and traditional as well as alternative strategies. The biomedical model is the foundation for evidence based health care practice and provides the gold standard for treatment and intervention. As a consequence, the medical model provides measurable goals for treatment and client outcomes relative to morbidity and mortality.

Lazarus and Folkman Model

Although there are other stress and coping models, none are more well-known than the one developed by Richard Lazarus and Susan Folkman (1984). Their model, a cognitive-phenomenological theory of stress, views adaptation to chronic illness through adapting to stressors. It is a transactional model of stress and coping, meaning that antecedent variables, such as personality traits, past experiences, and disease and treatment variables, act via mediating variables, such as coping strategies, to produce outcomes, and, in this case, adaptation. Stressors are mediated by primary appraisal, which is the individual's gauge of the significance and importance of the stressor. Primary appraisal is influenced by the background, experiences, culture, ethnicity, and personality of the individual, and is, therefore, characterized by stability across situations (Folkman, Lazarus, Gruen, & DeLongis, 1986).

The second step of the model is secondary appraisal of the situation. The individual asks the question, "what can I do about this situation," and this leads to the coping strategies used to manage the stressor. Secondary appraisal is influenced by the physical and social environment and may be context specific (Stewart et al., 2004). To adapt involves applying the coping strategies that are most appropriate to the situation. Individuals use both problem-focused coping and emotion-focused coping. Originally it was presumed by Lazarus and Folkman that the goal was for all individuals to utilize problem-focused coping, and that emotion-focused coping yielded poor adaptation to the stressor, in this case the illness. However, work over the last 20 years has supported that there is a place for emotion-focused coping as well as problem-focused coping (Stewart et al.).

Engel's Biopsychosocial Model

Clearly a model that could address both the biological and psychosocial aspects of chronic disease would be a preferred one for health care. Engel (1977) was perhaps one of the earliest authors of such a model. The main theme of the model is the influence of biologic, psychological, and social influences on the disease process. Engel's model outlined three ways in which a psychosocial factor could influence a health outcome: direct, indirect, and moderating. A direct effect would be a belief or value of the client that would preclude him or her from a specific medical intervention. An indirect effect would be defined through a mediational process (Stewart et al., 2004). An example would be an individual's current symptoms, for instance nausea and vomiting, decreasing their motivation to participate in a prescribed exercise regimen, and thereby decreasing physical functioning. A moderating effect alters the causal relationship between a psychosocial factor and a health outcome.

Livneh and Antonak Model

Livneh and Antonak (1997), working from previous models, proposed that variables that were associated with chronic illness could be organized into four main categories: (1) disability-related (e.g., type of condition, terminal vs. nonterminal); (2) sociodemographic factors of the individual (e.g., gender, age, ethnicity); (3) individual differences or personality (e.g., coping strategies, locus of control, personal meaning of the condition); and (4) social and environmental factors (e.g., social support, stigma). The interactions of these classes of variables significantly affected adaptation.

Livneh and Antonak (1997) also saw the adaptation process as different from adaptation. They theorized that the process of adaptation was fluid and dynamic, whereas adaptation status was the end result or outcome of the process (Stewart et al., 2004).

Moos and Holahan Model

Stewart and colleagues (2004) suggest that an ideal model for adaptation should address four criteria: (1) the reciprocal influences of biological, psychological, social, and behavioral variables of the client and the disease process; (2) be sufficiently broad to apply to clients with a wide range

of chronic illnesses and conditions; (3) be able to address the influences of culture, gender, ethnicity, and life stage of the client; and (4) be able to predict the level of client adaptation, which will then lead to appropriate interventions for the client.

Currently a search of the literature does not identify any "ideal" models that can meet the preceding criteria. Moos and Holahan (2007), however, have developed a simple model that provides a framework to view adaptation. Because of its ease of use and understanding, more detail will be provided on this model.

Moos and Holahan's framework (Figure 4-1) is a way of conceptualizing coping, and integrating it into a broader model. According to the model, there are five sets of factors that are associated with the selection of appropriate coping skills and the resulting health-related outcomes; in this case, adaptation. The model includes three factors that influence cognitive appraisal: (1) personal resources (Panel I); (2) health-related factors (Panel II); and (3) the social and physical context (Panel III). Cognitive appraisal (Panel IV) then dictates what adaptive

FIGURE 4-1

Conceptual Model of the Determinants of Health-Related Outcomes of Chronic Illness and Disability.

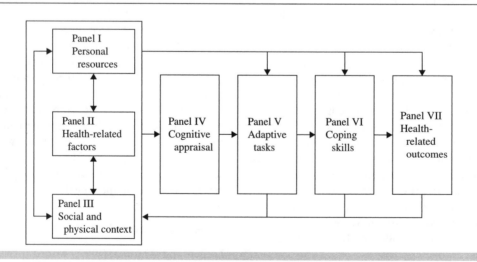

Source: Moos, R.H., & Holahan, C.J. (2007). Adaptive tasks and methods of coping with illness and disability. In E. Martz & H. Livneh (Eds.). *Coping with chronic illness and disability* (pp. 107–128). New York: Springer.

tasks (Panel V) need to be accomplished. Lastly, Panels I through V mediate the choice of coping skills (Panel VI) leading to Panel VII, the outcome.

Personal Resources

This is a broad category that includes intellectual ability, ego and self-confidence, religion, and prior health-related and coping experiences. Demographic characteristics, such as age, gender, ethnicity, culture, and education are included in this category as well. Personal resources also include personality, which may be viewed as a risk factor or protective factor (Stanton et al., 2007), locus of control, optimism, and autonomy. Individuals who have a more internal locus of control, higher self-confidence and self-efficacy, and a stronger sense of coherence are more likely to rely on problem-solving and other aspects of approach coping (Moos & Holahan, 2007, p. 110).

Ethnic group membership is associated with many psychological processes such as identity, group pride, and discrimination (Stanton et al., 2007). Each ethnic group or culture may have different values and beliefs that affect illness perceptions that, in turn, may affect adaptation (see Chapter 12) (Cohen & Welch, 2000). For some cultures, chronic disease and disability may induce stigma so that adaptation is not possible.

Zauszniewski, Chung, and Krafcik (2001) found greater resourcefulness in coping strategies among African American older adults with chronic illness than among white older adults. Degazon (1995), when exploring ethnic identification and coping strategies, found a significant relationship between the ethnic group with which the individual identified and the coping strategy used. Religion was key to coping with chronic illness for many African American older adults (Chin, Polonsky, Thomnas, & Nerney, 2000). Loeb (2006) categorized coping strategies of African American older adults as: (1) dealing with it, (2) engaging in life, (3) exercising, (4) seeking information, (5) relying on God, (6) changing dietary patterns, (7) medicating, (8) self-monitoring, and (9) self-advocacy.

Although these studies looked at coping specifically, the relationship of coping with adaptation is uncertain. In addition, it is clear that little is known about the implications of culture and ethnicity in disease-related adaptation (Stanton et al., 2007).

The uniqueness of each individual influences how the chronic condition is appraised, what coping strategies are used, and how and if adaptation can be achieved. For instance, pessimists report higher levels of hostility and depression on the day before coronary artery bypass graft surgery than do optimists (Maes, Levanthal, & DeRidder, 1996). Clients who are optimists tend to cope in a more active, problem-oriented way, as opposed to pessimists who tend to use more avoidant or passive ways of coping. It is not clear how specifically these personality traits influence and affect coping. Carver, Scheier, and Weintraub (1989) have noted that the impact of personality characteristics on coping is modest, and that coping preferences exist independent of personality factors. Although coping preferences could be viewed as personality attributes, they may influence coping indirectly through their impact on appraisal (Maes et al., 1996).

Socioeconomic class affects health outcomes directly and through environmental mechanisms, including access to care and risky and protective health behaviors (Stanton et al., 2007). Although it can be conceptualized as a determinant of adaptation, the pattern is not unidirectional (p. 570). Chronic conditions often influence work patterns and work disability. Work-related disability and loss of a job can decrease an individual's socioeconomic status.

Health-Related Factors

These factors include the type of onset and progression of the chronic condition, the location of symptoms, the prognosis, and the type of disability. Disease and treatment-related factors are often considered exogenous variables in adaptation (Stanton et al., 2001). A disease factor could be the stigma that the individual (and or family) associates with the condition. Other disease factors could include a change in body image, declining mobility, extreme fatigue, and so forth. However, the existence and impact of disease factors may actually be influenced significantly by other determinants, such as ethnicity, socioeconomic status, and social support. Many studies do not reveal significant relationships of disease-related factors with adjustment (Stanton et al., 2001). For instance, disease stage of a chronic condition is related inconsistently to adjustment (van't Spijker, Trijsburg, & Duivenvorrden, 1997).

Not only do the characteristics of the disease contribute, but also the treatment characteristics may contribute to the appraisal of the disease-related event. Surgery, monitoring of physical symptoms (e.g. blood glucose), diet, radiation, chemotherapy, and all of the side effects of treatment are important components in how the client appraises the situation.

Social and Physical Context

This context includes the relationships between the individuals with the chronic disease: their family members, caregivers, and social network. A supportive social context can enhance self-efficacy, transforming appraisal of a health condition as a challenge rather than a threat, and enhance reliance on approach coping (Rohrbaugh et al., 2004). When family members or friends do not convey interest, individuals with serious chronic conditions may avoid talking about their problem and be less likely to cope with the illness-related demands (Norton, Manne, Rubin, Hernandez, et al., 2005).

In general, social support is related to positive adaptation in several chronic diseases (Stanton et al., 2001). However, studies differ in how social support is conceptualized. Social support has been used as a coping strategy, a coping resource in the environment, and considered dependent on personality attributes and coping of the individual (Schreurs & deRidder, 1997). Clearly, interpersonal relationships can both aid and hinder adaptation to chronic illness. For women in particular, interpersonal relationships are vital components of women's adjustment to major stressors (Revenson, 1994).

Cognitive Appraisal

Appraising the illness is the first step in deciding the adaptive tasks that need to be accomplished. This is also the step in the adaptation process where the illness is appraised as either a challenge or a threat. How the illness is appraised, whether it is controllable or threatening, determines appropriate adaptive tasks and subsequent coping strategies. Using Lazarus and Folkman's model, primary appraisal of the "threat" or "event" includes the appraisal of harm or loss that has already occurred, or threatened harm or loss (Folkman & Greer, 2000), and includes an evaluation of its personal significance (Walker, Jackson, & Littlejohn, 2004). Secondary appraisal occurs when one assesses the situation's controllability and compares to one's available coping resources.

The individual who appraises their diagnosis of colon cancer as a death sentence will make very different decisions regarding treatment than another individual who sees hope. These two individual's appraisals, coping and adjustment, will be very different.

Adaptive Tasks

The model of Moos and Holahan (2007) identified seven adaptive tasks. Three of the seven tasks are related to the health condition and its treatment, and the other four are more general and could apply to all life crises and transitions, not just chronic illness. The tasks include (1) managing symptoms, (2) managing treatment, (3) forming relationships with health care providers, (4) managing emotions, (5) maintaining a positive self-image, (6) relating to family members and friends, and (7) preparing for an uncertain future (Moos & Holahan, 2007, pp. 112–114).

During football practice in the summer before his senior year in high school, Jack, the star quarterback on the local high school team, collapsed on the field and was taken to the emergency room of the nearest hospital. Jack soon learned that his significant weight loss and increasing fatigue over the preceding year were caused by diabetes. There must be some mistake Jack kept telling himself; after all, only old people get this illness. "Why me"? Jack asked himself over and over. Jack had worked hard throughout high school, both in the class-room and on the football field to increase his chances of getting a full-ride scholarship to the university of his choice. He was acutely aware his parents were not financially able to send him to college, so Jack knew it was up to him; his athletic ability was his ticket out of his small, rural town. "What does this mean"? "I know I'll never be able to play football again. That's it, no college for me." Jack was discharged home the next morning after the nurse had given

him detailed instructions on how to manage his newly diagnosed diabetes. He became despondent and depressed, and he refused to acknowledge or discuss his concerns, questions, and fears with his parents, much less his friends. Jack didn't want anyone to know that he was going to be sidelined and that his hopes and dreams for the future had been dashed by this illness called diabetes.

Discussion Questions

1. What is adaptation for Jack, and how can you as his nurse assist him in this process?
2. What information could you provide to both Jack and his parents to help him understand that he is not "sidelined" for life?
3. What are Jack's personal resources, health-related factors, and social and physical factors that are contributing to his cognitive appraisal of the situation?

Coping

Moos and Holahan (2007) identify eight categories of coping skills: (1) logical analysis and the search for meaning, (2) positive reappraisal, (3) seeking guidance and support, (4) taking problem-solving action, (5) cognitive avoidance or denial, (6) acceptance and resignation, (7) seeking alternative rewards, and (8) emotional discharge.

Logical Analysis and the Search for Meaning. This set of skills may include drawing on past experiences, mentally rehearsing potential actions and positive self-talk that you've handled tough situations like this before. Likely the individual will need educational programs to learn about their condition, possible treatment, and consequences.

With appropriate education and the facts, a logical analysis can then be accomplished.

Taylor's cognitive adaptive theory (1983) suggests that the process of adjustment reflects a search for meaning in the experience, an endeavor for control of the situation, and an attempt to restore self-esteem. In Taylor's study of breast cancer patients, clients needed to find meaning in their illness before moving on to adaptive tasks. Many individuals with chronic illness experience exacerbations, remissions, unpredictability of pain, and uncertainty, which means their adjustment is dynamic. As such, these individuals find themselves redefining the meaning that they have ascribed to the illness. Meaning is generated from one's experience and is understood in terms of one's responses to those experiences (Fife, 1995).

According to Janoff-Bulman and Frantz, (1997), finding meaning in chronic illness takes two forms. The first reflects an effort to determine if an event makes sense and often attributes causal factors to the event, and the second form of finding meaning reflects the value of the experience to the individual.

Pakenham (2007), using Taylor's (1983) work as a basis, examined "sense making" in individuals living with multiple sclerosis (MS), and the relationship between sense making and positive and negative adjustment outcomes. With 408 persons with MS and 232 caregivers, six factors emerged from a factor analysis of the Sense Making Scale (SMS). They included redefined life purpose, acceptance, spiritual perspective, luck, changed values and priorities, and causal attribution. Results supported the hypothesis that the sense making dimensions that afforded a realistic sense of controllability and predictability or that preserved self-worth were related to better adjustment; whereas those dimensions that entailed viewing illness as fully random and uncontrollable, or that did not preserve self-worth were related to poorer adjustment (p. 386).

Positive Reappraisal. These are cognitive strategies by which the individual accepts the reality of the situation, but reframes it in a different light (Moos & Holahan, 2007, p. 115). Strategies might include positive self-talk, altering values and priorities, and focusing on something good emerging from the chronic illness.

Seeking Guidance and Support. This category of skills includes obtaining education about the health condition, and it may be used in connection with logical analysis. Related coping skills entail seeking emotional help and support from family, friends, and caregivers (Moos & Holahan, 2007).

Taking Problem-Solving Action. These skills involve taking action. Skills may involve learning how to control physical symptoms, planning their daily treatment regimen or minimizing the

appearance of side effects of a treatment (Moos & Holahan, 2007).

Cognitive Avoidance or Denial. These strategies minimize the seriousness of a situation or perhaps even deny that it exists. These self-protective responses may temporarily assist an individual to "get through" a tough time and prevent feeling overwhelmed (Moos & Holahan, 2007).

Acceptance and Resignation. Acceptance may involve admitting to a health problem and being resigned to the changes it presents. If this is a terminal illness, the individual may be consciously accepting the inevitable (Moos & Holahan, 2007).

Seeking Alternative Rewards. Responses in this area redirect one's energy and activities in other directions. Attempts are made to replace the losses that are associated with the illness (Moos & Holahan, 2007).

Emotional Discharge. This category includes the venting of emotions, perhaps crying or screaming out, or using jokes to help displace distress (Moos & Holahan, 2007).

Overview of Coping

Richard Lazarus's 1966 book, *Psychological Stress and Coping*, was probably the initial scholarly work that expanded how coping was conceptualized. Since that time, the coping literature has increased significantly, with researchers undertaking studies to understand why some individuals fare better than others when encountering stress in their lives (Folkman & Moskowitz, 2004). Coping is a process that unfolds in the context of a situation or condition that is appraised as personally significant, and as taxing or exceeding the individual's resources for coping (Lazarus & Folkman, 1984). The coping process is initiated in response to the individual's appraisal that important goals have been harmed, lost, or threatened (Folkman & Moskowitz, 2004). What we have learned in the last 40 or more years is that coping is a complex, multidimensional process that is sensitive both to the environment and its demands and resources, and to personality traits that influence the appraisal of stress, in this case chronic illness, and the resources for coping (Folkman & Moskowitz, 2004). Coping is not a stand-alone concept or phenomenon, but embedded in a complex, dynamic stress process that involves the person, the environment, and the relationship between them.

Lazarus and Folkman (1984) described problem-focused coping strategies and emotion-focused coping strategies. Problem-focused strategies were to alter person–environment relationships, and the purpose of emotion-focused strategies was to regulate internal states. Initially problem-focused strategies were seen as "better," or could influence health outcomes in a more positive manner. However, since Lazarus and Folkman posited their original work, that view has changed. Emotion-focused coping strategies may specifically assist in developing and sustaining a sense of psychological well-being, despite unfavorable circumstances (Folkman & Greer, 2000).

Other theorists have used different terms to describe coping. In addition to problem-focused and emotion-focused coping, meaning-focused coping has been identified as a type of coping in which cognitive strategies are used to manage the meaning of the situation (Folkman & Moskowitz, 2004).

Shaw uses the terms passive coping, which includes avoidance, and active coping, which is nonavoidance coping (Shaw, 1999). This two-factor structure of coping is incorporated into the coping framework as an antecedent to the behavioral intention to cope as well as carrying out the coping behavior. It is likely that individuals may have a number of coping responses at their disposal, although each individual may have their own preferred styles based on their personality attributes (Shaw, 1999).

It is argued that there needs to be a better integration of the perspectives of coping and social support. Studies seem to focus on either social support or on coping, and not the integration of the two concepts (Schreurs & deRidder, 1997). Studying that relationship may be helpful in understanding adaptation to chronic illness.

Another issue in studying coping is that the coping strategy needs to be evaluated in the specific context in which it is used (Folkman & Moskowitz, 2004). Coping strategies are not inherently good or bad, but instead their effectiveness depends on the context in which they are used. Evaluation of the effectiveness of coping requires first, to have the appropriate outcomes selected, and second, attention must be paid to the fit between the coping and the situation (p. 754).

Adaptation/Adjustment

What do we know about adaptation? It is a complex construct (like coping), it is multidimensional, and it is a holistic concept. However, it is rarely measured holistically in studies. Consensus does exist regarding the centrality of an individual's appraisal of their adjustment, it's *their* adjustment and their perception, not the healthcare professional's (Stanton et al., 2001).

We also understand that emotionally supportive relationships set the stage for positive adjustment, whereas criticism, social constraints, and social isolation impart risk (Stanton et al., 2007). Active approach-oriented coping strategies manage disease-related challenges and may bolster adjustment, whereas concerted efforts to avoid disease-related thoughts and feelings are predictors of distress (p. 578). Two basic conclusions come from the descriptive research literature: Most individuals appear to "adjust" well to chronic illness; and there is considerable variability in adjustment both across studies and across individuals within single studies (Stanton et al., 2001).

Maes and colleagues (1996) believe that definitions of adjustment are too simplistic, as many studies operationalize adjustment in terms of psychological outcomes and neglect the medical, cognitive, or social outcomes. Positive adjustment is not merely the absence of pathology. Typical indicators of adjustment in research are both positive and negative affect and represent two very different dimensions. Therefore, using only depressive symptoms to indicate adjustment will yield only a partial picture of adjustment (Stanton et al., 2001). Maes and colleagues posit that although anxiety and depression are important markers of adjustment, perhaps assessment of everyday life behaviors and activities may be much more relevant (p. 243).

One variable that was studied in the 1970s with Kobasa's work and into the early 1990s with Pollack, is the concept of hardiness. Brooks (2003) analyzed 125 articles published from 1966 to 2002 to determine the significance of hardiness in adaptation. This "personal resource," within Moos and Holahan's framework, demonstrated a significant relationship to psychological, psychosocial, and physiologic adaptation. Higher levels of hardiness had positive outcomes in clients with chronic illness (p. 11).

How coping is related specifically to adjustment has not been clearly described (Sharpe & Curran, p. 1154). Intellectually we believe that coping strategies do contribute to adaptation, and may be a mediator, but probably interact with other factors in contributing to adaptation (Stanton & Revenson, 2007).

Berg and Upchurch (2007) have advanced a model that speaks to dyadic coping and adjustment. Their development–contextual model of couples coping with chronic illness views chronic illness as affecting the adjustment of both the client and the spouse such that coping strategies enacted by the patient are related to those enacted by the spouse and vice versa.

INTERVENTIONS

The literature provides an abundance of descriptive studies measuring coping and/or adaptation, but few interventional studies exist. It appears that we can measure coping or adaptation, but that we are unable to conceptualize those results into interventions or ways in which we can help clients better cope with or adapt to chronic illness.

Stanton and Revenson (2007) suggest that we improve the interpersonal context of our clients by teaching them to develop and maintain social ties, recognize and accept others' help and emotional encouragement, or change their appraisals of the support they are receiving. Psychosocial interventions are directed toward individual-level change and may include cognitive-behavioral interventions, educational, and interpersonal support components. Support groups may provide emotional support as well as an educational focus. The education is expected to strengthen one's sense of control over the disease, reduce feelings of confusion, and enhance decision making (p. 221). The peer support provides emotional support and thus enhances self-esteem, minimizes aloneness, and may re-enforce coping strategies.

An earlier study that is still referred to frequently in the literature is that of Folkman and colleagues (1991) coping effectiveness training with HIV-positive men. This interventional study based on Lazarus and Folkman's stress and coping theory was effective in increasing the quality of life in these men. The training included (1) appraisal training to disaggregate global stressors into specific coping tasks, (2) coping training to tailor application of strategies, and (3) social support training.

Nurses may be wise to capitalize on a client's religious beliefs and partner with clergy to effect adaptation (Loeb, 2006). Programs related to health education and screening, support groups and physical activity that are based in a church may be helpful. Barg and Gullatte (2001) explain that church-based health programming can frame health information in a way that may better fit with a client's view of life, that is, their relationship with God.

Pakenham's study (2007), described earlier in this chapter, highlights the need for practitioners to facilitate clients' cognitive processing of the implications and meaning of their illness.

Perhaps a blend of cognitive-restructuring strategies, client-centered approaches, and existential approaches may be helpful to the client and family.

Cognitive-Behavioral Strategies

Cognitive-behavioral strategies can be used to teach coping skills to clients with chronic illness (Folkman & Moskowitz, 2004). Sharpe and Curran (2007) have also encouraged the use of cognitive-behavioral treatments (CBTs), as the research literature is clear that CBT is effective in managing psychological distress associated with illness. Such programs include strategies with the aim of facilitating a realistic, but optimistic, attitude toward illness and/or facilitating more-adaptive coping strategies. Programs typically include education about the illness, goal setting and pacing, relaxation strategies and attention diversion skills, cognitive therapy, communication skills, and management of high-risk situations (such as exacerbations of the illness).

Emotional Intelligence

Emotional intelligence describes the ability to understand, perceive, use, and manage the emotions of self and others (McKenna, 2007). Emotional intelligence training includes six spheres of emotional competence: emotional openness/adaptation; the impact on and of others; self-esteem/identity; management of stress; communication skills/social functioning; and goal management and motivation. It is suggested that emotional self-management can affect the adjustment of individuals with chronic illness and this can be enabled by the use of emotional intelligence techniques by healthcare professionals (p. 551).

Self-Management Programs

Self-management programs based on enhancing self-efficacy are highly successful in reducing symptoms and encouraging behavior change in many chronic illnesses (Newman, 2006). Self-efficacy could be considered a personal context variable and thus may be a determinant in the appraisal of the illness, the coping strategies used by the individual, and the outcome (the physical, emotional, and social adaptation). Although self-efficacy is task- and situation-specific, programs that encourage that concept could influence adaptation.

Self-Help Groups

As common as self-help and self-support groups are for those with chronic illness, the research literature should be clearer as to their value. Unfortunately, that is not the case. Anecdotal articles exist, but there are few research-based articles. In addition, research commonly looks at such support groups for a short period—6, 10, 12, and 15 weeks—whereas a chronic illness can be present for 30, 40, or 50 years. Therefore, the outcome that we might see in such studies is greatly diminished as the studies demonstrate outcomes at one point in time.

Dibb and Yardley (2006) investigated the role that social comparison might play in adaptation using a self-help group as the context. Social comparison proposes that individuals with similar problems compare each other's health status. Often this comparison occurs within self-help groups, which consist of individuals with similar circumstances. It has been suggested that downward comparison, where comparison is made with a person who is doing less well, will initiate positive affect as it increases self-esteem. Conversely, upward comparison with a person doing less well, may result in hope (p. 1603). Results of the study with 301 clients with Ménière's disease demonstrated that positive social comparison was associated with better adjustment after controlling for other baseline variables, whereas negative social comparison was associated with worse adjustment over time.

Positive Life Skills

In a sample of 187 HIV-infected women, a positive life skills workshop was effective in increasing antiretroviral adherence, improving mental well-being, and reducing stress (Bova, Burwick, & Quinones, 2008). The workshop consisted of 10 weekly sessions with 6 to 15 women in each group. Workshop facilitators shared a vision of a safe, positive, and respectful environment for women to learn and experience. Part of the workshop involved reframing negative meanings.

OUTCOMES

Stanton, Collins, and Sworowski (2001) in their summary of the literature suggest five conceptualizations of *positive* adjustment: (1) successful performance of various adaptive tasks that accompany chronic disease, (2) absence of a psychological disorder, (3) relatively low experience of negative affect and/or high experience of positive affect, (4) optimal behavioral/functional status, and (5) appraisals of satisfaction or well-being in various life domains (p. 388). Some of these are easily "measured." For example, absence or presence of a psychological disorder could be ascertained with a degree of certainty. However, other conceptualizations cannot. An example is the appraisal of satisfaction. Does having an individual score high in life satisfaction or life well-being on a questionnaire accurately measure adjustment? How would optimal behavioral/functional status be measured? Furthermore, if we consider adjustment/adaptationas dynamic, could someone have positive adaptation today, but not tomorrow?

We have a long way to go in understanding, effecting, and measuring adaptation. With the increasing numbers of older adults and chronic disease, continuing research and study needs to be accomplished in this area.

EVIDENCE-BASED PRACTICE BOX

Loeb (2006) utilized a focus group to identify the coping strategies used by 28 community-dwelling African American older adults with multiple chronic conditions. Participants' ages ranged from 55 to 89 with 69% being female. Focus group size ranged from 3 to 10 participants. Nine categories of coping strategies were identified and included: (1) dealing with it; (2) engaging in life; (3) exercising; (4) seeking information; (5) relying on God; (6) changing dietary patterns; (7) medicating; (8) self-monitoring; and (9) self-advocacy. Clients exhibited both emotion-focused and problem-focused coping. The "dealing with it" category included feeling fortunate to have lived a long life, reframing health problems as annoyances and maintaining a positive attitude. Problem-focused coping was evident in the "engaging in life" category. The health-related coping strategies, exercising, changing dietary patterns and medicating, involved action-based problem-focused coping. For the participants in this study, religion and relying on God were strong concepts. Loeb suggests that healthcare professionals capitalize on clients' strong religious beliefs by partnering with clergy or churches to deliver health programs, screening programs, and support groups.

Source: Loeb, S. (2006). African American older adults coping with chronic health conditions. *Journal of Transcultural Nursing, 17*(2), 139–147.

STUDY QUESTIONS

1. Why is adaptation to chronic illness important to the client and family with chronic illness?
2. Describe how different personal resources could affect adaptation.
3. Compare and contrast the key concepts of the models discussed in this chapter. What are the overlaps in these models? What are the missing elements in these models that would facilitate adaptation?
4. "Finding meaning" was a concept discussed in depth in this chapter. Why is this a necessary component of the adaptation process?

Or, if you do not think it is, explain your reasoning.
5. Apply the adaptation framework of Moos and Holahan to one of your clients with chronic illness. What fits and does not fit?
6. From your perspective, what is social support's relationship to adaptation? What is your experience with the role of social support in the adaptation in your clients?
7. Develop a generic teaching plan that would address adaptation to chronic illness. What are key points that could then be individualized to clients?

REFERENCES

American Psychiatric Association. (1997). *Diagnostic and statistical manual IV (DSM-IV)*. New York: APA.

Antonovsky, A. (1979). *Health, stress, and coping*. San Francisco: Jossey-Bass.

Barg, F.K., & Gullatte, M.M. (2001). Cancer support groups: Meeting the needs of African Americans with cancer. *Seminars in Oncology Nursing*, 17, 171–178.

Berg, C.A., & Upchurch, R. (2007). A developmental-contextual model of couples coping with chronic illness across the adult life span [Electronic version]. *Psychological Bulletin*, 133(6), 920–954.

Bova, C., Burwick, T.N., & Quinones, M. (2008). Improving women's adjustment to HIV infection: Results of the positive life skills workshop project [Electronic version]. *Journal of the Association of Nurses in AIDS Care*, 19(1), 58–65.

Brooks, M. (2003). Health-related hardiness and chronic illness: A synthesis of current research [Electronic version]. *Nursing Forum*, 38(3), 11–20.

Carver, C.S., Scheier, M.F., & Weintraub, J.K. (1989). Assessing coping strategies: A theoretically based approach. Journal *of Personality and Social Psychology*, 56, 267–283.

Chin, M.H., Polansky, T.S., Thomas, V.D., & Nerney, M.P. (2000). Developing a conceptual framework for understanding illness and attitudes in older, urban African Americans with diabetes. *Diabetes Educator*, 26, 439–449.

Cohen, J.A., & Welch, L.M. (2000). Attitudes, beliefs, values and culture as mediators of stress. In V. Rice (Ed.). *Handbook of stress, coping and health: Implications for nursing research, theory and practice* (pp. 335–366). Thousand Oaks, CA: Sage.

Degazon, C.E. (1995). Coping, diabetes, and the older African American. *Nursing Outlook*, 43(6), 254–259.

Dew, M.A., Myaskovsky, L., Switzer, G.E., DiMartini, A.F., Schulberg, H.C. & Kormos, R.L. (2005). Profiles and predictors of the course of psychological distress across four years after heart transplantation [Electronic version]. *Psychological Medicine*, 35, 1215–1227.

Dibb, B., & Yardley, L. (2006). How does social comparison within a self-help group influence adjustment to chronic illness? A longitudinal study. *Social Science and Medicine*, 63, 1602–1613.

Dixon-Woods, A. (2001). Writing wrongs? An analysis of published discourses about the use of patient information leaflets. *Social Science & Medicine*, 52, 1432–1437.

Engel, G.L. (1977). Need for a new medical model. *Science*, 196, 129–136.

Fife, B. (1995). The measurement of meaning in illness. *Society, Science and Medicine, 40*(8), 1021–1028.

Folkman, S., Chesney, M., McKusick, L., Ironson, G., Johnson, D., & Coates, T.J. (1991). Translating coping theory into intervention. In J. Eckenrode (Ed.). *The social context of coping* (pp. 239–259). New York: Plenum.

Folkman, S., & Greer, S. (2000). Promoting psychological well-being in the face of serious illness: When theory, research, and practice inform each other. *Psycho-Oncology, 9,* 11–19.

Folkman, S., & Moskowitz, J.T. (2004). Coping: Pitfalls and promise. *Annual Review of Psychology, 55,* 745–774.

Folkman. S., Lazarus, R.S., Gruen, R.J., & DeLongis, A. (1986). Appraisal, coping, health status, and psychological symptoms. *Journal of Personality and Social Psychology, 50*(3), 571–579.

Folkman, S., Moskowitz, J.T., Ozer, E.M., & Park, C.L. (1997). Positive meaningful events and coping in the context of HIV/AIDS. In B.H. Gottlieb (Ed.). *Coping with chronic stress* (pp. 293–314). New York: Plenum.

Freeth, R. (2007). Working within the medical model. *Healthcare Counselling & Psychotherapy Journal, 7*(4), 3–7.

Helgeson, V.S., Snyder, P., & Seltman, H. (2004). Psychological and physical adjustment to breast cancer over 4 years: Identifying distinct trajectories of change [Electronic version]. *Health Psychology, 23,* 3–15.

Janoff-Bulman, R., & Frantz, C.M. (1997). The impact of trauma on meaning: From meaningless world to meaningful life. In M. Power & C.R. Brewin (Eds.). *The transformation of meaning in psychological therapies* (pp. 91–106). New York: Wiley.

Lazarus, R.S., & Folkman, S. (1984). *Stress appraisal and coping.* New York: Springer.

Livneh, H., & Antonak, R.F. (1997). *Psychoscial adaptation to chronic illness and disability.* Gaithersburg, MD: Aspen.

Loeb, S. (2006). African American older adults coping with chronic health conditions [Electronic version]. *Journal of Transcultural Nursing, 17*(2), 139–147.

Maes, S., Levantha, H., & DeRidder, D. (1996). Coping with chronic diseases. In M. Zeidner & N.S. Endler (Eds.). *Handbook of coping: Theory, research, applications* (pp. 221–251). New York: Wiley.

McKenna, J. (2007). Emotional intelligence training in adjustment to physical disability and illness [Electronic version]. *International Journal of Therapy and Rehabilitation, 14*(12), 551–556.

Mirowsky, J., & Ross, C. (2002). Measurement for a human science [Electronic version]. *Journal of Health and Social Behavior, 43,* 152–170.

Moos, R.H., & Holahan, C.J. (2007). Adaptive tasks and methods of coping with illness and disability. In E. Martz & H. Livneh (Eds.). *Coping with chronic illness and disability* (pp. 107–128). New York: Springer.

Newman, A. (2006). Self-efficacy. In I. Lubkin & P. Larsen (eds.). *Chronic illness: Impact and interventions* (6th ed.) (pp. 105–120). Sudbury, MA: Jones & Bartlett.

Norton, T.R., Manne, S.L., Rubin, S., Hernandez, E., et al. (2005). Ovarian cancer patients' psychological distress: The role of physical impairment, perceived unsupportive family and friend behavior, perceived control, and self-esteem [Electronic version]. *Health psychology, 24,* 143–152.

Pakenham, K.I. (2007). Making sense of multiple sclerosis [Electronic version]. *Rehabilitation psychology, 52*(4), 380–389.

Revenson, T. (1994). Social support and marital coping with chronic illness. *Annals of Behavioral Medicine, 16,* 122–130.

Rohrbaugh, M.J., Shoham, V., Coyne, J.C., Cranford, J.A., Sonnega, J.S., & Nicklas, J.M. (2004). Beyond the "self" in self-efficacy: Spouse confidence predicts patient survival following heart failure. *Journal of Family Psychology, 18,* 184–193.

Sakalys, J.A. (2000). The political role of illness narratives. *Journal of Advanced Nursing, 31*(6), 1469–1475.

Schreurs, K.M.G., & de Ridder, D.T.D. (1997). Integration of coping and social support perspectives: Implications for the study of adaptation to chronic diseases [Electronic version]. *Clinical Psychology Review, 17,* 89–112.

Sharpe, L., & Curran, L. (2006). Understanding the process of adjustment to illness [Electronic version]. *Social Science & Medicine, 62,* 1153–1166.

Shaw, C. (1999). A framework for the study of coping illness behavior and outcomes. *Journal of Advanced Nursing, 29*(5), 1246–1255.

Sprangers, M.A.G., & Schwartz, C.E. (2000). Integrating response shift into health-related quality-of-life research: A theoretical model. In C.E. Schwartz &

M.A.G. Sprangers (Eds.). *Adaptation to changing health: Response shift in quality-of-life research* (pp. 11–23). Washington, DC: American Psychological Association.

Stanton, A.L., Collins, C.A., & Sworowski, L.A. (2001). Adjustment to chronic illness: Theory and Research. In A. Baum, T.A. Revenson & J.E. Singer (Eds.). *Handbook of health psychology* (pp. 387–403). Mahwah, NJ: Lawrence Erlbaum.

Stanton, A.L., & Revenson, T.A. (2007). Adjustment to chronic disease: Progress and promise in research. In H.S. Friedman & R.C. Silver (Eds.). *Foundations of health psychology* (pp. 203–233). New York: Oxford.

Stanton, A.L., Revenson, T.A., & Tennen, H. (2007). Health psychology: Psychological adjustment to chronic disease [Electronic version]. *Annual Review of Psychology, 58*, 565–592.

Stewart, K.E., Ross, D., & Hartley, S. (2004). Patient adaptation to chronic illness. In T.J. Boll, J.M. Raczynski, & L.C. Leviton (Eds.). *Handbook of clinical health psychology, Vol 2, Disorders of behavior and health* (pp. 405–421) Washington, DC: American Pychological Association.

Taylor, S.E. (1983). Adjustment to threatening events: A theory of cognitive adaption. *American Psychologist, 38*, 1161–1173.

van't Spijker, A., Trijsburg, R.W., & Duivenvorrden, H.J. (1997). Psychological sequelae of cancer diagnosis: A meta-analytical review of 58 studies after 1980 [Electronic version]. *Psychosomatic medicine, 59*, 280–293.

Visotsky, H.M., Hamburg, D.A., Goss, M.E., & Lebovits, B.Z. (1961). Coping behavior under extreme stress: Observations of patients with severe poliomyelitis. *Archives of General Psychiatry, 5*, 27–52.

Waisbond, S. (2007). Beyond the medical-informational model: Recasting the role of communication in tuberculosis control [Electronic version]. *Social Science & Medicine, 65*(10), 2130–2134.

Walker, J.G., Jackson, J.J., & Littlejohn, G.O. (2004). Models of adjustment to chronic illness: Using the example of rheumatoid arthritis [Electronic version]. *Clinical Psychology Review, 24*, 461–488.

Zauszniewski, J.A., Chung, C., & Krafcik, K. (2001). Social cognitive factors predicting the health of elders. *Western Journal of Nursing Research, 23*, 490–503.

5

Social Isolation

Diana Luskin Biordi and Nicholas R. Nicholson

INTRODUCTION

Most of us actively seek human companionship or relationships. The lives of hermits or cloistered, solitary existences are extraordinary because they so vividly remind us that, usually, life is richer for the human contact we share. As valuable as life may be when we engage in a variety of relationships, time reserved for solitude is also necessary as we seek rest or contemplative opportunity in "our own space." The weaving together of individual possibilities for social engagement or solitude develops a certain uniqueness and texture in personal and community relationships. These distinctive personal configurations of engagement and disengagement have consequences for our work and social lives. It is critical, therefore, that healthcare professionals understand the value of social engagement and of solitude.

Isolation: A Working Definition

"Belonging" is a multidimensional social construct of relatedness to persons, places, or things, and is fundamental to personality and social well being (Hill, 2006). If belonging is connectedness, then social isolation is the distancing of an individual, psychologically or physically, or both, from his or her network of desired or needed relationships with other persons. Therefore, social isolation is a loss of place within one's group(s). The isolation may be voluntary or involuntary. In cognitively intact persons, social isolation can be identified as such by the isolate.

The literature portrays social isolation as typically accompanied by feelings related to loss or marginality. Apartness or aloneness, often described as solitude, may also be a part of the concept of social isolation, in that it is a distancing from one's network, but this state may be accompanied by more positive feelings and is often voluntarily initiated by the isolate. Some researchers debate whether apartness should be included in, or distinguished as a separate concept from, social isolation. As seen in the literature that follows, social isolation has several definitions and distinctions, dependent upon empirical research and the stance of the observer.

When Is Isolation a Problem?

Social isolation ranges from the voluntary isolate who seeks disengagement from social intercourse for a variety of reasons, to those whose isolation is involuntary or imposed by others. Privacy or being alone, if actively chosen, has the potential for enhancing the human psyche. On the other hand, involuntary social isolation occurs when an individual's demand for social contacts or communications exceeds the human or situational capability of others. Involuntary isolation is negatively viewed because the outcomes are the dissolution of social exchanges and the support they provide for the individual or their support system(s). Some persons, such as those with cognitive deficits, may not understand their involuntary isolation, but their parent, spouse, or significant other may indeed understand that involuntary social isolation can have a negative and profound impact on the caregiver and care recipient.

When social isolation is experienced negatively by an individual or his or her significant other, it becomes a problem that requires management. In fact, according to much of the literature, only physical functional disability ranks with social isolation in its impact on the client and the client's social support network (family, friends, fellow workers, and so forth). Therefore, social isolation is one of the two most important aspects of chronic illness to be managed in the plan of care.

Distinctions of Social Isolation

Social isolation is viewed from the perspective of the number, frequency, and quality of contacts; the longevity or durability of these contacts; and the negativism attributed to the isolation felt by the individual involved. Social isolation has been the subject of the humanities for hundreds of years. Who has not heard of John Donne's exclamation, "No man is an island," or, conversely, the philosophy of existentialism—that humans are ultimately alone? Yet the concept of social isolation has been systematically researched during only the last 50 years. Unlike some existentialists and social scientists, healthcare professionals, with their problem-oriented, clinical approach, tend to regard social isolation as negative rather than positive.

The Nature of Isolation

Isolation can occur at four layers of the social concept. The outermost social layer is community, where one feels integrated or isolated from the larger social structure. Next is the layer of organization (work, schools, churches), followed by a layer closer to the person, that is, confidantes (friends, family, significant others). Finally, the innermost layer is that of the person, who has the personality, the intellectual ability, or the senses with which to apprehend and interpret relationships (Lin, 1986).

In the healthcare literature, the primary focus is on the clinical dyad, so the examination of social isolation tends to be confined to the levels of confidante and person, and extended only to the organization and community for single clients, one at a time. For the healthcare professional, the most likely relationships are bound to expectations of individually centered reciprocity, mutuality, caring, and responsibility. On the other hand, health policy literature tends to focus on the reciprocity of community and organizations to populations of individuals, and so it deals with collective social isolation.

At the level of the clinical dyad, four patterns of social isolation or interaction have been identified; although these were originally formulated with older adults in mind, they can be analogized easily to younger persons by making them age-relative:

1. Persons who have been integrated into social groups throughout their lifetime
2. The "early isolate," who was isolated as an adult but is relatively active in old age
3. The "recent isolate," who was active in early adulthood but is not in old age
4. The "lifelong isolate," whose life is one of isolation

Feelings that Reflect Isolation

Social isolation can be characterized by feelings of boredom and marginality or exclusion (Weiss, 1973). Boredom occurs because of the lack of validation of one's work or daily routines; therefore, these tasks become only busy work. Marginality is the sense of being excluded from desired networks or groups. Other feelings ascribed to social isolation include loneliness, anger, despair, sadness, frustration, or, in some cases, relief.

Description and Characteristics of Social Isolation

The existence of social isolation increases our awareness of the need for humans to associate with each other in an authentic intimate relationship, whether characterized by caring or some other emotion, such as anger. When we speak of social isolation, we think first of the affected person; then we almost immediately consider that individual's relationships. This chapter will demonstrate that, as a process, social isolation may be a feature in a variety of illnesses and disabilities across the life cycle.

As an ill person becomes more aware of the constricting network and declining participation, he or she may feel sadness, anger, despair, or reduced self-esteem. These emotions factor into a changed social and personal identity, but are also separate issues for the person who is chronically ill. Moreover, depending on their own emotional and physical needs, friends and acquaintances may drop out of a person's social support system until only the most loyal remain (Tilden & Weinert, 1987). Families, however, are likely to remain in the social network. As the social network reaches its limitations, it may itself become needful of interventions, such as respite care for the parents of a child who is chronically ill or support groups for the siblings of children with cancer (Heiney et al., 1990).

Social Isolation versus Similar States of Human Apartness

Social isolation has been treated as a distinct phenomenon, or it has been combined or equated with other states relating to human apartness. The literature is replete with a variety of definitions of social isolation, many of which are interrelated, synonymous, or confused with other distinct but related phenomena.

Social Isolation and Alienation

Social isolation and alienation have been linked together or treated as synonymous in much of the healthcare literature, although these two concepts differ from one another. Alienation encompasses powerlessness, normlessness, isolation, self-estrangement, and meaninglessness (Seeman, 1959). Powerlessness refers to the belief held by an individual that one's own behaviors cannot elicit the results one desires or seeks. In normlessness, the individual has a strong belief that socially unapproved behaviors are necessary to achieve goals. Isolation means the inability to value highly held goals or beliefs that others usually value. Self-estrangement has come to mean the divorce of one's self from one's work or creative possibilities. Finally, meaninglessness is the sense that few significant predictions about the outcomes of behavior can be made. Thus, one can see that isolation is only one psychological state of alienation. However, authors frequently merge the finer points of one or more of the five dimensions of alienation and call the result isolation.

Social Isolation and Loneliness

Although social isolation is typically viewed today as a deprivation in social contacts, Peplau and Perlman (1986) suggest that it is loneliness, not social isolation, that occurs when an individual perceives her or his social relationships as not containing the desired quantity or quality of social contacts. In an even more subtle distinction, Hoeffer (1987) found that simply the perception of relative social isolation was more predictive of loneliness than actual isolation. Loneliness has been referred to as an alienation of the self and is sometimes seen as global, generalized, disagreeable, uncomfortable, and more terrible than anxiety (Austin, 1989). Loneliness differs from depression in that in loneliness, one attempts to integrate oneself into new relationships, whereas in depression, there is a surrendering of oneself to the distress (Weiss, 1973).

Nonetheless, loneliness does relate to social isolation. In fact, loneliness is the one concept most invoked when social isolation is considered (Dela Cruz, 1986; Hoeffer, 1987; Mullins & Dugan, 1990; Ryan & Patterson, 1987). However, to use social isolation and loneliness as interchangeable terms can be confusing. To maintain clarity, loneliness should be considered the subjective emotional state of the individual, whereas social isolation is the objective state of deprivation of social contact and content (Bennet, 1980). Therefore, loneliness refers to the psychological state of the individual, whereas social isolation relates to the sociologic status. Although it is true that social isolation might lead to loneliness, loneliness is not, in itself, a necessary condition of social isolation. Both conditions can exist apart from each other.

Peplau and Perlman's view of loneliness is distinct from the current North American Nursing Diagnosis Association's (NANDA's) nursing diagnosis of social isolation (Carpenito-Moyet, 2006). The NANDA diagnosis extends from the person to include the possibility that a group could also experience a "need or desire for increased involvement with others but is unable to make that contact". Attached to that must be feelings of rejection or aloneness, insecurity, or lack of meaningful relationships. In the NANDA definition, the model combines psychological feelings with the sociologic state of isolation, and thus blurs the distinctions so carefully treated by others. As will be demonstrated in this chapter, social isolation becomes cause, process, or response, depending on analysis and circumstances. The complex sets of variables that figure into social isolation lend themselves to a variety of assessments, diagnoses, and interventions: Loneliness is only one aspect of social isolation.

Social Isolation and Aloneness

Tightly linked with social isolation is the need for social support, which is the social context or environment that facilitates the survival of human beings (Lin, 1986) by offering social, emotional, and material support needed and received by an individual, especially one who is chronically ill. Although social support literature has focused on the instrumental and material benefits of support, recent literature on social isolation relates isolation more to the negative feeling state of aloneness. This feeling is associated with deficits in social support networks, diminished participation in these networks or in social relationships, or feelings of rejection or withdrawal.

Social Isolation as a Nursing Diagnosis

Social isolation is defined by NANDA (Carpenito-Moyet, 2006) as a state in which a person or group experiences or perceives a need or desire for increased involvement with others but is unable to make that contact. The NANDA definition has moved beyond the person to the possibility that a group experiences social isolation. Yet, the defining characteristics are those of a *person's* subjective feelings of aloneness. In the current NANDA definition, only one of the major characteristics must be present for the diagnosis, and several minor characteristics are further described. Four major characteristics are noted: insecurity in social situations, a lack of meaningful relationships, expressed feelings of rejection, and a desire for contact with more people. Of the 12 minor characteristics, most relate to uncommunicativeness, whether in affect or decision making, or expressions of withdrawals. These are mostly personal characteristics, and although some may be generalizable to a group, it might be difficult to do so.

In the NANDA description, social isolation is a *cause* for loneliness, but it is not a response of loneliness. Related to social isolation are several other factors, for example, diseases, social situations, or secondary sequelae to social factors or environments. The current nursing diagnosis of social isolation, combining as it does both psychological and sociologic states of isolation for both persons and groups, requires systematic empirical bases for refined distinctions of isolation. Nurses should continue to build on earlier studies (see Lien-Gieschen, 1993, for a validation study of major identifying characteristics of social isolation in the older adult) to empirically identify and distinguish the truly defining characteristics of social isolation. As it presently stands now, the nursing diagnosis of social isolation is rather holistic and resonates strongly with earlier dimensions of the concepts of alienation and loneliness. Carpenito-Moyet (2006) suggests that nurses change diagnoses from social isolation to the diagnosis of loneliness or risk for loneliness, which is conceptually a clearer approach. However, the sociologic reality of social isolation remains, and can require intervention in its own right.

PROBLEMS AND ISSUES OF SOCIAL ISOLATION

Regardless of how social isolation occurs, the result is that basic needs for authentic intimacy remain unmet. Typically this is perceived as alienating or unpleasant, and the social isolation that occurs can lead to depression, loneliness, or other social and cognitive impairments that then exacerbate the isolation.

Several predisposing reasons for social isolation have been proposed: status-altering physical disabilities or illnesses; frailties associated with advanced age or developmental delays; personality or neurologic disorders; and environmental constraints, which often refer to physical surroundings but are also interpreted by some to include diminished personal or material resources (Tilden & Weinert, 1987).

The Isolation Process

A typical course of isolation that evolves as an illness or disability becomes more apparent is the change in social network relationships. Friends or families begin to withdraw from the isolated individual or the individual from them. This process may be slow or subtle, as with individuals with arthritis, or it may be rapid, as with the person with AIDS. Unfortunately, the process of isolation may not be based on accurate or rational information. For example, one woman with cancer reported that, at a party, she was served her drink in a plastic cup while everyone else had glasses (Spiegel, 1990).

Individuals with serious chronic illnesses come to perceive themselves as different from others and outside the mainstream of ordinary life (Williams & Bury, 1989). This perception of being different may be shared by others, who may then reject them, their disability, and their differentness. Part of this sense of being different can stem from the ongoing demands of the illness. For example, social relationships are interrupted because families and friends cannot adjust the erratic treatment to acceptable social activities. From such real events, or from social perceptions, social isolation can occur, either as a process or as an outcome.

Individuals with chronic illness often face their own mortality more explicitly than do others. For example, unmarried or younger clients with cancer express a loss of meaning in life, suggested to be due to cancer's threat to their lives as they grapple with the meaning of life; they may withdraw from their networks or the networks may withdraw from them (Noyes et al., 1990; Weisman & Worden, 1977; Woods, Haberman, & Packard, 1993).

Even if death does not frighten those with chronic illness, it frequently frightens those in their social networks, which leads to guilt, and can lead to strained silences and withdrawal. In the case of individuals with cancer (Burnley, 1992; House, Landis, & Umberson, 1988; Reynolds & Kaplan, 1990) or heart disease (Kaplan et al., 1988; Orth-Gomer, Unden, & Edwards, 1988), social support is significant to their survival. For those who lack this social support, social isolation is not merely a metaphor for death but can hasten it.

Social Isolation and Stigma

Social isolation may occur as one effect of stigma. Many persons will risk anonymity rather than expose themselves to a judgmental audience.

Because chronic illnesses can be stigmatizing, the concern about the possibility of revealing a discredited or discreditable self can slow or paralyze social interaction (see Chapter 3). In a study examining chronic sorrow in HIV-positive patients, stigma created social isolation. Women with children, particularly African American women, were more stigmatized and isolated than gay men because others perceived the women as associated with "dirty sex," contagion, and moral threat (Lichtenstein, Laska, & Clair, 2002). Therefore, social roles and the robustness of network support affect social isolation.

The individual with chronic illness or their families grapple with how much information about the diagnosis they should share, with whom, and when (Gallo et al., 1991). If the illness is manageable or reasonably invisible, its presence may be hidden from all but a select few, often for years. Parents of children with chronic illnesses were reported to manage stressful encounters and uncertainty by disguising, withholding, or limiting information to others (Cohen, 1993), an action that may add to limiting their social network. Jessop and Stein (1985) found that invisible illnesses of chronically ill children led to greater difficulty in social interactions because of the uncertainty of ambiguity (disagreement about revealing or passing, or what courses of action to take). For example, parents of a child with cystic fibrosis may tell a teacher that the child is taking pills with meals because of a digestive disease (Cohen, 1993).

As siblings of children with cancer deal with the isolation of their brother or sister, they became vulnerable to being socially isolated themselves (Bendor, 1990). Social isolation not only burdens those with chronic illness, it also extends into family dynamics and requires the healthcare professional to consider how the family manages. Nurses must explicitly plan for the isolation in families with children who are chronically ill (Tamlyn & Arklie, 1986). Thus, with social isolation being a burden for the family, it requires the healthcare professional to consider how the family manages the illness and the isolation.

Where the stigmatized disability is quite obvious, as in the visibility of burn scars or the odor of colitis, the person who is chronically ill might venture only within small circles of understanding individuals (Gallo et al., 1991). Where employment is possible, it will often be work that does not require many social interactions, such as night work or jobs within protected environments (sheltered workshops, home offices). Regardless of what serves as reminders of the disability, the disability is incorporated into the isolate's sense of self; that is, it becomes part of his or her social and personal identity.

Social Isolation and Social Roles

Any weakening or diminishment of relationships or social roles might produce social isolation for individuals or their significant others. Clients who lose family, friends, and associated position and power are inclined to feelings of rejection, worthlessness, and loss of self-esteem (Ravish, 1985). These feelings become magnified by the client's culture if that culture values community (Litwin & Zoabi, 2003; Siplic & Kadis, 2002). An example of social isolation of both caregiver and care recipient occurred in a situation of a woman whose husband had Alzheimer's disease. The couple had been confined for more than 2 years in an apartment in a large city, from which her confused husband frequently wandered. Her comment, "I'm not like a wife and not like a single person either," reflected their dwindling social network and her loss of wifely privileges but not obligations. This ambiguity is common to many whose spouses are incapacitated. Moreover, after a spouse dies, the widow or widower often grieves as much for the loss of the role of a married person as for the loss of the spouse.

The loss of social roles can occur as a result of illness or disability, social changes throughout the life span (e.g., in school groups, with career moves, or in unaccepting communities), marital dissolution (through death or divorce), or secondary to ostracism incurred by membership in a "wrong" group. The loss of social roles and the resultant isolation of the individual have been useful analytic devices in the examination of issues of the aged, the widowed, the physically impaired, or in psychopathology.

The Older Adult and Social Isolation

Older age, with its many losses of physical and psychological health, social roles, mobility, economic status, and physical living arrangements, can contribute to decreasing social networks and increasing isolation (Creecy, Berg, & Wright, 1985; Howat, Iredell, Grenade, Nedwetzky, & Collins, 2004; Ryan & Patterson, 1987; Trout, 1980; Victor et al., 2002). This will become even more of an issue as the number of older adults are expected to increase arithmetically and proportionately in the next two decades (Fowles & Greenberg, 2003). The prevalence of social isolation in older adults has been approximated now to be at 2–20% and even as high as 35% in assisted-living arrangements (Greaves & Farbus, 2006).

Social isolation has been linked with confusion, particularly in older adults with chronic illness. But when the socially isolated are also immobilized, the combination of isolation and immobilization can lead to greater impairments, such as perceptual and behavioral changes (e.g., confusion, noncompliance, or time distortions) (Stewart, 1986). Physical barriers (such as physical plant designs) or architectural features (such as heavy doors) also contribute to social isolation or homeboundedness (DesRosier, Catanzaro, & Piller, 1992). All of these limits contribute to social isolation in ways that motivation alone cannot easily overcome.

Social isolation has been shown to be a serious health risk for older adults (Findlay, 2003), with studies indicating a relationship between all-cause mortality, (Ceria et al., 2001), coronary disease (Eng, Rimm, Fitzmaurice, & Kawachi, 2002), and cognitive impairments (Barnes, Mendes de Leon, Wilson, Bienias, & Evans, 2004; Holtzman et al., 2004; Zunzunegui, Alvarado, Del Ser, & Otero, 2003). In a converse finding, older adults with extensive social networks were protected against dementia (Fratiglioni, Wang, Ericsson, Maytan, & Winblad, 2000; Fratiglioni, Paillard-Borg, & Winblad, 2004; Seidler, Bernhardt, Nienhaus, & Frolich, 2003; Wang, Karp, Winblad, & Fratiglioni, 2002). And, as described earlier, although low social engagement may not be a form of social isolation per se, it is a psychological isolator and thus a risk factor in social isolation (Howat et al., 2004). For example, depressive symptoms in older adults were shown to be decreased by social integration (Ramos & Wilmoth, 2003). Isolated older adults were shown to have increased risk for coronary heart disease (Brummett et al., 2001; Eng et al., 2002) and death related to congestive heart failure was predicted by social isolation (Murberg, 2004). Similarly, post-stroke outcomes, for example, strokes, myocardial infarction, or death, were predicted by pre-stroke isolation (Boden-Albala, Litwak, Elkind, Rundek, & Sacco, 2005). Isolated women before a diagnosis of breast cancer, when compared with socially integrated women, were found to have a 66% increase in all-cause mortality (Kroenke, Kubzansky, Schernhammer, Holmes, & Kawachi, 2006). Quality of life among breast cancer survivorship is impacted negatively by social isolation (Michael, Berkman, Colditz, Holmes, & Kawachi, 2002). Finally, and perhaps most relevant to health and cost outcomes, socially isolated older adults were found to be four to five times more likely to be re-hospitalized within the year (Mistry et al., 2001).

The extent and nature of a social network (Litwin, 1997; Wenger, Davies, Shahtahmasebi, & Scott, 1996) from local to community, and integrated to contained, as well as the positive or negative nature of the social relationships in the social network, impact health as well as social isolation (Seeman, 2000; Wenger, 1997). In fact, the quality of the social relationship may have more impact than the number of ties (Pinquart & Sorensen, 2001), which suggests that a few solid relationships may be more beneficial than many ties of poor quality.

CASE STUDY

Dorothy is a 77-year-old woman who is also your charming nextdoor neighbor. She has a wonderful attitude, and loves to visit to gossip about the little things. She just has a way of telling stories. Dorothy's busy social life and calendar also make her memorable. She often jokes that she is the queen of the dance at the senior center and has to beat away the gentlemen with a stick.

Dorothy is very active in the community and at the local senior center, which include volunteering for a service driving other older adults to their appointments in her late husband's car, bowling regularly, and being president of the walking club. In addition, Dorothy knits. You have lost count of the number of hand-knit sweaters she has made for you.

One day, just as you suddenly realize that you haven't seen Dorothy for quite a while, you receive a telephone call from her son saying that Dorothy had fallen down the stairs and will be in the hospital for some time with arm injuries, which will also require a move to skilled rehab for even more time. He asks if you can look in on the house from time to time: of course you agree.

When Dorothy returns home, months later, she is helped by her son and other medical personnel because she now has a walker. A week goes by and you haven't seen Dorothy, so you go over to her house to look in on her. There you find that her bed is now in the downstairs living room and that Dorothy is extremely afraid of going up the stairs because of the injury she had sustained. In more conversation with her, you discover that she quit the bowling league and resigned her position in the walking club. She assures you that she will still walk. However, she states unhappily that the doctor has taken her driver's license away and she just doesn't know what to do about all those older adults who need her services to ride to

their appointments. As she is saying this, you remember seeing her son and a tow truck at her house a few days earlier, and the tow truck took away her car.

You also notice that her calendar is completely empty except for doctor's appointments. You offer to write in her social outings because you thought that she hadn't had time to do so with all the recent commotion. But Dorothy responds that she is now a little more frail and she feels she shouldn't keep so busy. Knitting by herself is still fun, but it's becoming more and more difficult to complete the sweaters since she "has the visiting nurses coming in twice a day for wound changes, not to mention the nerve damage" that she has suffered from the fall. You jokingly parry with her about how much the gentlemen must miss her at the senior center. Dorothy replies that she doesn't seem to fit in at the senior center, since it's difficult to get there and she doesn't really know what's going on there anymore. On the way out Dorothy assures you that another sweater is right around the corner.

A few more weeks go by and one day, as you arrive home in the early afternoon, you can see Dorothy through the window, sitting in her bed. You go over to say hello, and when she answers the door you notice she is wearing nightclothes. Dorothy is also crying, saying that she is losing touch with everybody because she cannot leave her house. This is making her so sad that she now cries regularly and wonders what is the point of living.

Discussion Questions

1. How would you define Dorothy's current condition? What are some of the factors that contributed to Dorothy's current condition? If her condition worsens what is she at risk for developing?

(Continued)

CASE STUDY (*Continued*)

2. If you were Dorothy's nurse during a clinic visit, what services might you recommend for her? Who might you contact to help with Dorothy's plan of care?
3. What other information would be helpful for you to know to intervene on Dorothy's behalf? What assessments are most important to perform on Dorothy? Recommend an intervention to help with Dorothy's condition.
4. If you were going to devise a research study examining older adults who are socially isolated list the following: your study question(s), the independent variables, the dependent variables, and the proposed study design.

Although much of the current research in social isolation with older adults has used community-dwelling adults, one growing segment of study has been in settings of assisted-living arrangements, which is one of the fastest growing segments of senior housing (Hawes, Phillips, Rose, Holan, & Sherman, 2003). In assisted-living settings where there are many internal (to the setting) social networks, life satisfaction, quality of life, and perception of home were positively reported (Street, Burge, Quadagno, & Barrett, 2007). Assisted living has the potential to focus on health promotion and function maintenance, such as the identification of social isolation and appropriate interventions (Resnick, 2007).

Strictly speaking, social isolation is not confined to a place. The socially isolated are not necessarily homebound or place-bound, although that is typically the case. That being said, however, environments that are removed (such as rural locations) or those not conducive to safety (such as high-crime areas) can contribute to social isolation (Klinenberg, 2001). Social isolation as a function of location has been demonstrated, particularly for the older adult in urbanized settings, in a number of countries other than the United States (Klinenberg, 2001; Russell & Schofield, 1999). In these cases, elderly individuals cannot leave their homes because of lack of transportation or for fear of assault, so they increasingly isolate themselves from others. This situation is intensified by distrust, socioeconomic status, or locale, and it is worse if the older adult has a chronic illness compounding their constraints. Vehicular driving

cessation may be an eventual reality as one ages. Limited or no driving confines activities outside the home (Marottoli et al., 2000) and thus limits interactions with others for the older adult.

One objective of planned senior housing is to provide individuals with a ready-made social network within a community (Lawton, Kleban, & Carlson, 1973; Lawton, Greenbaum, & Liebowitz, 1980; Lawton, Moss, & Grimes, 1985), although this objective is not always met. However, the frail elderly are found to be less interactive with more mobile, healthier older adults, possibly because healthier older adults have few extra resources to expend on others who may have even fewer resources, or they may have better health and networks that are incongruent with, and less likely to cross, those of the frail elderly (Heumann, 1988).

Nursing home residents with chronic illness or sensory impairments tend to be more isolated than others. In England, for instance, those in residential care who are ill or disabled are considered socially dead, impoverished by the inactive nature of institutionalization and unable to occupy any positive, valued role in the community (Watson, 1988). Stephens and Bernstein (1984) found that older, sicker residents were more socially isolated than healthier residents. The investigators found that family and longer-standing friendships served as better buffers to social isolation than did other residents. Impressionistically, however, the number of research citations about social isolation in England and Ireland, as well as in other European countries seems to have increased from the two previous decades in contrast to the research in social isolation in the United States. More recent social isolation research in the United States focuses on policy that seems to incorporate the socially isolated individual into more viable social networks.

Social Isolation and Culture

As globalization and sensitivity to United States multiculturalism increases, with its concurrent absorption of multiethnic, multilingual, and multi-religious individuals into yet other cultures, there is an overlap into mainstream healthcare systems. This is especially true of cultural groups that have not assimilated into the dominant culture. Language differences and traditional living arrangements may impede social adaptation. In addition, many immigrants, especially those who are chronically ill, are less able to engage in support networks, given their long working hours, low-paying jobs, lack of health insurance, and changes in family life-styles and living arrangements. Changes may occur over the second and third generations, but this is less true where the immigrants' home cultures are geographically close, such as Mexican Americans who live along the United States–Mexican border, or have reminders of traditions that are more visible (Jones, Bond, & Cason, 1998).

An extensive literature review on health care and its relationship with culture demonstrated two overarching issues: (1) The definitions of culture are conceptually broad and/or indistinct, and (2) mainstream health care struggles to integrate these multicultural groups with varying degrees of success. When one speaks of "culture," many concepts are mixed, even confused (Habayeb, 1995). The dominant white society in the United States and its healthcare system is secular, individualistic, technology- and science-oriented, and tends to be male dominated (Borman & Biordi, 1992; Smith, 1996). Other European-based cultures have similar situations. Social isolation must be viewed from the client's cultural definition of the number, frequency, and quality of contacts, the longevity

or durability of these contacts, and the negativism attributed to the isolation felt by the individual involved.

Studies done during the last decade indicate how women, minority groups, the poor, and so forth, have not received the same care as the dominant male caucasian middle or upper classes (Fiscella et al., 2000). Fortunately, current cultural healthcare literature indicates a greater awareness of cultural groups and their values. One factor that may be influencing this change is that during the last two decades, other healthcare providers, including nurses, psychologists, case managers, and a variety of technical support personnel, have made significant advances in providing higher quality health care to formerly disenfranchised groups (Biordi, 2000).

Many ethnic and religious groups in the United States value community closeness, family kinship, geographic proximity, and social communication. They seek acknowledgment of their right to mainstream or alternative care (Cheng, 1997; Helton, 1995; Keller & Stevens, 1997; Kim, 1998; Kreps & Kreps, 1997). The task of attempting to deliver "tailored" culturally competent care to so many groups is overwhelming and lacks an integrating strategy that appeals across all groups. One can now find a large number of articles providing hints, tips, or insights into cultural groups targeting mainstream healthcare providers.

Social Components of Social Isolation

Mere numbers of people surrounding someone does not cure negative social isolation; an individual can be socially isolated even in a crowd if one's significant social network is lost. This situation is true for such groups as those living or working in sheltered-care workshops, residents in long-term care facilities, or people in prisons. What is critical to social isolation is that, because of situations imposed on them, individuals perceive themselves as disconnected from meaningful discourse with people important to them.

Associated with social isolation is reciprocity or mutuality, that is, the amount of give and take that can occur between isolated individuals and their social networks. Throughout the years, much evidence has accumulated to indicate that informal networks of social support offer significant emotional assistance, information, and material resources for a number of different populations. These support systems appear to foster good health, help maintain appropriate behaviors, and alleviate stress (Cobb, 1979; DiMatteo & Hays, 1981; Stephens & Bernstein, 1984).

Examining reciprocity in the relationships of social networks focuses not only on social roles and the content of the exchange, but also on the level of agreement between the isolated person and his or her "others" in the network (Goodman, 1984; Randers, Mattiasson, & Olson, 2003). The incongruence between respondents in a social network regarding their exchanges can help alert the healthcare professional to the level of emotional or material need or exhaustion that exists in either respondent. For example, the senior author observed, during a home visit by a nurse, that a homebound older woman complained that her children had done very little for her. However, it was discovered that the children visited every day, brought meals, shopped for their mother, and managed her financial affairs. In this case, the elderly mother felt isolated despite her children's visits and assistance.

Demographics and Social Isolation

Few studies focus directly on demographic variables and social isolation; typically, this topic is embedded in other research questions across a variety of illnesses. Nevertheless, when these disparate studies are taken together, the impact of demographics on social isolation in the individual with chronic illness is evident. Issues of gender, marital status, family position and context, and socioeconomic standing (such as education or employment) have been shown to affect social isolation.

Socioeconomic Factors

Changes in socioeconomic status, such as employment status, have been correlated with social isolation. The lack of employment of both caregiver and care recipient, cited in much of the caregiver literature, can have an adverse effect. A study of caregivers of frail elderly veterans noted that these caregivers are more at risk for physical, emotional, and financial strain than are other populations, because disabled elderly veterans receive fewer long-term care services than do other elderly populations (Dorfman, Homes, & Berlin, 1996).

Unemployment of the older adult is just one component of the maturational continuum; parents worry about the potential for employment and insurance for their children who have chronic illnesses (Cohen, 1993; Wang & Barnard, 2004). Lower income status, especially when coupled with less education, negatively influences health status and is associated with both a limiting social network and greater loneliness, which, in turn, impacts health status and social isolation (Cox, Spiro, & Sullivan, 1988; Williams & Bury, 1989). For instance, almost half of the head-injured clients in one study could not work, which then affected their families' economic status and increased their social isolation (Kinsella, Ford, & Moran, 1989).

In addition to problems of employment potential, there are economic and social concerns over the costs incurred by health care, employment discrimination, subsequent inability to secure insurance, and loss of potential friendship networks at work—all of which are factors in increasing social isolation or reducing social interactions. In fact, economics exaggerates the costs of chronic illness. People with disabilities suffer disproportionately in the labor market, which then affects their connections with family and community social networks (Christ, 1987). This is particularly evident in the examination of those with mental illness and their social isolation (Chinman, Weingarten, Stayner, & Davidson, 2001; Melle, Friis, Hauff, & Vaglum, 2000).

General Family Factors

As chronic illness persists, and given tasks must be managed, relationships are drained, leaving individuals with chronic illness at high risk for social isolation (Berkman, 1983; Tilden & Weinert, 1987). When isolation does occur, it can be a long-term reality for the individual and their family. However, if there is social support and involvement, people with chronic illnesses tend toward psychological well-being. Particularly important is the adequacy, more than the availability, of social relationships (Wright, 1995; Zimmer, 1995).

There is evidence that social isolation does not necessarily occur in every situation. In fact, the negative impact of social isolation on families with children who are chronically ill has been questioned. One study, which used a large community-based, random sample, found that families with children who are chronically ill did not experience a greater degree of social isolation than those with healthy children, nor did they function differently, except for modest increases in maternal dysfunction (Cadman et al., 1991). Cadman and his associates argue that prior studies were subject to biases because the families in those studies were in the clinic populations of the hospital or agency. By definition, such populations were receiving care for illnesses or responses to illnesses and hence were experiencing an unusual aggregate of problems, which is why they were at the clinic or hospital. Therefore, such families were not representative families of those throughout the community.

In another study, classroom teachers evaluated children with cancer or sickle cell disease with a matched sample of controls. The authors found that the children who were chronically ill were remarkably resilient in the classroom setting, although those who survived their brain tumors and could attend regular classes were perceived as more sensitive and isolated (Noll et al., 1992). On the other hand, adolescents with chronic illnesses have been marginalized, which predisposes them to feelings of isolation and low self-worth (DiNapoli & Murphy, 2002).

Similarly, some studies of older adults found that isolation did not always occur as they aged (Victor et al., 2002). Although childless older individuals tend to be more socially isolated than those with children, when adult children live nearby, older people frequently interact with at least one of them (Mullins & Dugan, 1990). Interestingly, older African American women, even if they lived alone, tended to have more visits from their children than did older African American men; the difference was not explained by needs, resources, or child/gender availability (Spitz & Miner, 1992). It is also interesting to note that older people tend to be less influenced by their children than by contacts with other relatives, friends, and associates (Berkman, 1983; Ryan & Patterson, 1987). One study found no relationship between the elders' emotional well-being and the frequency of interaction with their children (Lee & Ellithorpe, 1982).

Findings indicate that in every group from age 30 to older than 70 years of age, it was primarily those with the fewest social and community ties who were nearly three times as likely to die as those with more ties (Berkman, 1983). In other words, maintaining social contacts enhanced longevity. These individuals tended to be widowers or widows and lacked membership in formal groups (Berkman, 1983), thereby limiting their social contacts. In another study, the older adults who lived in senior housing complexes showed little difference in friendship patterns and life satisfaction (Poulin, 1984). Both of these studies found that living alone, being single, or not having family does not necessarily imply social isolation. Rather, if older people have social networks, many developed throughout a lifetime, and if these networks remain available to them, they are provided with support when needed (Berkman, 1983).

Gender and Marital Status

Typically, women have more extensive and varied social networks than do men (Antonucci, 1985). However, if one spouse is chronically ill, married couples spend more time together and less time with networks and activities outside the home (DesRosier, Catanzaro, & Piller, 1992; Foxall, Eckberg, & Griffith, 1986; Smith, 2003). Although gender differences in caregiving occur (Miller, 1990; Tilden & Weinert, 1987), women caregivers indicate greater isolation, increased loneliness, and decreased life satisfaction than do men. Yet both genders show psychological improvement if social contacts, by telephone or in person, increase (Foxall et al., 1986).

Although women caregivers may have professional, community, and social networks to aid them in coping with their disabled spouses, over time, they reduce their links to these potential supports. Physical work, social costs and barriers, preparation time for care and outings, and other demands of caregiving become so extreme that women curtail access to and use of support networks external to home. As these caregivers narrow their use of social networks, they unwittingly isolate their chronically ill spouse as well. Although women reported needing personal or psychological time alone for relief, the subject of their isolation, the person with chronic illness, also became their greatest confidante as the pair struggles in their joint isolation (DesRosier et al., 1992).

Illness Factors and Social Isolation

Chronic illness is multidimensional, and persons who are chronically ill or their networks must assume a variety of tasks: managing treatment regimens, controlling symptoms, preventing and managing crises, reordering time, managing the illness trajectory, dealing with healthcare professionals, normalizing life, preserving a reasonable self-image, keeping emotional balance, managing social isolation, funding the costs of health care, and preparing for an uncertain future (Strauss et al., 1984) (see Chapter 2). As people with chronic illnesses struggle to understand their body failure and maintain personal and social identities, they may become fatigued, sicker, or lose hope more readily. Should this happen, they may more easily withdraw from their social networks.

It has been suggested that isolation not only influences the individual's social network (Newman et al., 1989), but also can lead to depression and even suicide (Lyons, 1982; Trout, 1980), particularly in the elderly (Frierson, 1991). Women whose illnesses required more physical demands on themselves and greater symptom management reported greater depression but no effect on their relationship with their partner. Women who had concerns about the meaning of their illness reported greater marital distress and lower satisfaction with their family network (Woods, Haberman, & Packard, 1993).

Persons with the HIV or AIDS had psychological effects that depended not only on the diagnosis, but also on the age of the person. Older individuals showed significant differences in a number of variables, including social isolation (Catalan, 1998). In addition, HIV-negative men who cared for their partners or friends often lived in social isolation with their care recipients (Mallinson, 1999).

In the case of individuals with severe head injuries, it was not the chronic physical disability that disrupted family cohesion as much as the resulting social impairment (Kinsella et al., 1989). The greatest burden identified was social isolation brought on by the impaired self-control of the head-injured person and their inability to learn from social experience. However, the social isolation was particularly burdensome for the families, because the head injury reduced the client's capacity for recognition of and reflection on the deficiencies in social relationships and precluded formation of new close relationships. Consequently, although friendships and employment possibilities were reduced for the client, the real impact was felt by the constrained family (Kinsella et al., 1989).

Healthcare Perspectives

People with chronic illnesses struggle to understand their body failure and its effect on their activities and lives (Corbin & Strauss, 1987). In doing so, they also struggle to maintain their sense of personal and social identity, often in the face of altered self-image and enormous financial, psychological, and social obstacles. If individuals with chronic illness lose hope or become otherwise incapacitated, they may withdraw from their social networks, isolating themselves and others important to them.

Frequently, the daily management of illness means working with healthcare professionals who often do not recognize the inconspicuous but daily struggles of the person's realities of a "new" body, the issues of care, and the development of a new self-identity (Corbin & Strauss, 1987; Dropkin, 1989; Hopper, 1981).

With the advent of high technology, the aging of the population, and changes in economics, chronic illness has begun to assume major proportions in the United States. Concomitantly, the literature contains more articles describing various chronic illnesses, the strategies used to manage them, and issues of social and psychological well-being, including social isolation. More recently, the literature has been extended to consider how chronic illnesses and related technologies are impacted by cultural variety.

The impact of prevailing paradigms of care interventions held by various constituencies is evident. For example, most healthcare professionals still see clients only episodically, using the medical model of "cure" and within the model of the dominant healthcare system. But, in the case of children with cancer, the child focuses on the meaning of his or her impairment (which varies by age); the parents focus first on the immediate concern with their child's longevity and cure and later on the impairment and long-term effects; the healthcare professional focuses on client survival; the mental health professional focuses on identifying and minimizing impact, impairments, and social barriers; and the public (third-party payers, employers, schoolmates, partners) focuses on contributions and cost. All of these views center on the interaction and exchange, as well as the specific responsibilities and obligations, incurred by the various networks that touch them. Interactions are intensified by the potential withdrawal of any party from the network (Christ, 1987).

Given the variety of care-versus-cure paradigms, the real, daily micro-impositions of chronic illness on social identity and social networks are often lost. The compassion felt by many healthcare professionals is evident in the increasing number of articles available and the attempts to present evidence of the isolation felt by clients and their networks. Nevertheless, these articles may not be explicit; therefore, the proposed interventions for the isolate are unclear, irrelevant, or even discouraging. For example, when discussing facial disfigurement, one article noted that the healthcare professional expected evidence of the client's image integration as early as 1 week postsurgery (Dropkin, 1989). That same article suggested and reiterated that, although the surgery was necessary for removal of the cancer, the resulting defect was confined to a relatively small aspect of the anatomy and that the alteration in appearance or function did not change the person (Dropkin, 1989). Both points of emphasis are added. The terminology and the interventions in this article focused on the acute postoperative period and did not take into account what disfigured clients were likely to feel later than 1 week post-surgery or that the word defect gives a strong clue to the understanding that the disfiguring surgery is obvious and emotionally charged toward the negative.

For a clearer view of the impact of such surgery as seen by the client, Gamba and colleagues (1992) asked postsurgical patients, grouped by the extent of their facial disfigurement, questions about their self-image, relationship with their partner and social network, and overall impact of the therapy. Those with extensive disfigurement reported that it was "like putting up with something undesirable" (p. 221), and many patients were unable to touch or look at themselves. Those with extensive disfigurement also reported more social isolation, poor self-image, and/or a worsened sexual relationship with their partner, even though they maintained satisfactory relationships with their children. In another study, reported in the Gamba article, half of the individuals who underwent hemi-mandibulectomy for head and neck cancers became social recluses, compared with 11% of patients who had laryngectomies. As can be seen, in more than one study, respondents attached a negative meaning to their disfiguring surgery and its results.

Such findings take into account the client's personal meaning of illness and treatment and their effects on social isolation, demonstrating that the isolating treatment or illness (e.g., disfigurement) often is not associated with objective disability. In fact, others have found that the degree of isolation is not directly proportional to the extent of disability (Creed, 1990; Maddox, 1985; Newman et al., 1989). It is important that healthcare professionals not ignore or discount the meaning of illness to the client, regardless of any professional opinion about objective disability or the desirability of treatment.

INTERVENTIONS: COUNTERACTING SOCIAL ISOLATION

In social isolation, the interventions of choice need to remain at the discretion of the client or caregiver. As can be seen from this chapter, writers focus largely on definitions and correlates of social isolation and relatively less on interventions. When interventions are reported, they often relate to the aggregate, such as the policy-related interventions of community housing. The results of many of these larger-scale interventions have been noted in this chapter. Other interventions are mentioned herein, although the list is not all-inclusive.

Because the situation of each person with chronic illness is unique, interventions can be expected to vary (see Holley 2007, for examples). Nonetheless, certain useful techniques and strategies can be generalized (Dela Cruz, 1986). Basically, these strategies require that a balance of responsibilities be developed between the

healthcare professional and the client, with the following aims:

1. Increasing the moral autonomy or freedom of choice of the isolate
2. Increasing social interaction at a level acceptable to the client
3. Using repetitive and recognizable strategies that are validated with the client, which correlate to reducing particular isolating behaviors

The approach to interventions can also be matched, layer by layer, to the social layering model presented earlier in this chapter, that is, from community, to organization, to network, to person. Therefore, interventions might be cast as ranging from community-based empowerment (transportation-system improvements, for example), work-related enhancements (computer telecare), network and family support group enhancements (nursing), case management, neighborhood watches, or client-professional clinical treatments or care. Examples of these are discussed in this chapter.

Another point to remember is that evaluation is a key principle in any problem-solving system, such as the evaluation found in the nursing process. Throughout the assessment and intervention phases, the healthcare professional should explicitly consider how effective the intervention is or was. The effect of cultural and social differences should be taken into account. The willingness and flexibility to change an ineffective strategy is the mark of the competent professional.

Assessment of Social Isolation

When social isolation occurs, a systematic assessment can help determine proposed interventions, which the professional must validate with the client before taking action. Guiding people, rather than forcing them to go along with interventions, requires the healthcare professional to offer a rationale for the proposed interventions. One must ask if one is giving reasonable rationales, assurances, or support. At the same time, the professional should remember that some cultures value the authority and the expertise of other family members over that of the individual. Consequently, the healthcare professional may have to provide a rationale for suggested interventions to the ranking authority within the support group. Frequently, this is a male figure, often older, who is considered most deserving of any explanation. Other cultures may be matriarchal, so it would be a woman who is the ranking authority.

The key to assessing social isolation is to observe for three distinct features: (1) negativity, (2) involuntary, other-imposed solitude, and (3) declining quality and numbers within the isolate's social networks. Social isolation must be distinguished from other conditions such as loneliness or depression, both often accompanied by anxiety, desperation, self-pity, boredom, and signs of attempts to fill a void, such as overeating, substance abuse, excessive shopping, or kleptomania. In addition, loneliness is often associated with losses, whereas depression is frequently regarded as anger turned inward. Because social isolation, loneliness, and depression can all be destructive, the healthcare professional must be resourceful in assessing which issue predominates at any particular point in time.

Properly conducted, an assessment yields its own suggestions for responsive intervention. For instance, the assessment may indicate that the client is a lifelong isolate and that future isolation is a desired and comfortable life style. In this case, the professional's best intervention is to remain available and observant but noninterfering.

If, on the other hand, the client has become isolated and wants or needs relief, then the intervention should be constructed along lines consistent with his or her current needs and history. In a study designed to be culturally sensitive, Norbeck and associates (1996) applied a standardized intervention using designated individuals for person-to-person and telephone contacts for pregnant African American women who lacked social support networks. Their study showed significantly reduced low-birth-weight infants.

In another example, if the healthcare professional discovers that a support network is lax in calling or contacting a client, the provider can help the client and support network rebuild bridges to each other. Keep in mind that there are usually support groups to which those in a social network can be referred for aid. As an illustration, if the network is overwhelmed, information can be provided about respite programs. Interventions such as these will help members of the social network maintain energy levels necessary to help their chronically ill relative or friend.

Assessment typically involves the clinical dyad of caregiver and client. It is at this level that assessment is critical to the development of appropriate and effective interventions. Without an adequate and sensitive assessment, interventions are likely to be ineffective or incomplete.

Measurement of Social Isolation

The major issue in measuring social isolation in instrumentation is that the instrumentation does not fully capture the conceptual definition of social isolation. For example, social isolation, as described in this chapter, has no specific instrument of measurement. Some researchers have used instruments that define social isolation as an extreme lack of social networks or support, whereas others use a group of questions that purport to measure social isolation.

A review of the literature found that the two most commonly used and reported research measures were the Lubben Social Network Scale (LSNS) (Lubben, 1988) and the Berkman-Syme Social Network Index (SNI) (Berkman & Syme, 1979). Both of these tools measure, essentially, the amount of contact one has with others.

The SNI was cited in 209 articles and the LSNS was cited in 38 articles found in MEDLINE, CINAHL, EMBase, and PSYCinfo. The SNI is a nontheoretical summed aggregation of several items that examined a range of social ties and networks and how they directly affected people. Both the importance and the number of social contacts are aggregated into four weighted sources. The weighting is cumbersome and potentially error prone, therefore, making it less appealing to researchers and clinicians. Nevertheless, it is useful for secondary data analysis and remains a popular choice.

The Lubben Social Network Scale was developed to measure social networks among older adults (Lubben, 1988) and is somewhat based on the SNI and its original questionnaire. The LSNS has 10 equally weighted items, which place individuals into four quartiles with a cut-off score for social isolation. Reliability and validity have been examined (Lubben, 1988; Lubben & Gironda, 1996; Rubenstein, Josephson, & Robbins, 1994)). The LSNS is typically administered prospectively during data collection, and is difficult to use in secondary data analysis, although this has been attempted (Lubben, Weiler, & Chi, 1989). Lubben has developed several other scales, most of which are still undergoing psychometric testing.

Given the state of the science, it is suggested that when measuring social isolation, the researcher choose from the SNI or LSNS dependent upon one's research purpose and question, and also use semi-structured interviews or questionnaires to confirm a diagnosis of social isolation. Once social isolation is identified in an older adult, it is important to use evidence-based recommendations as interventions to decrease negative health-related consequences.

Management of Self: Identity Development

The need for an ongoing identity leads an individual to seek a level where he or she can overcome, avoid, or internalize stigma and, concomitantly, manage resulting social isolation. Social networks can be affected by stigma. Managing various concerns requires people who are chronically ill to develop a new sense of self consistent with their disabilities. This "new" life is intertwined with the lives of members of their social networks, which may now include both healthcare professionals and other persons with chronic illnesses. Lessons

must be learned to deal with new body demands and associated behaviors. Consequently, the individual with chronic illness must redevelop an identity with norms different from previous ones.

The willingness to change to different and unknown norms is just a first step, one that often takes great courage and time. For instance, one study indicated that clients with pronounced physical, financial, and medical care problems following head and neck surgery exhibited prolonged social isolation 1 year post-surgery (Krouse, Krouse, & Fabian, 1989). Although no single study has indicated the time necessary for such identity transformations, anecdotal information suggests that it can last several years, and indeed, for some, it is a lifelong experience.

Identity Transformation

Clarifying how networks form and function is a significant contribution to the management of the struggles of the client who is chronically ill and isolated. The perceptive healthcare worker should know that much of the management done by the chronically ill and their networks is not seen or well-understood by healthcare professionals today (Corbin & Strauss, 1987). However, we can use Charmaz's findings as guides for assessing the likely identity level of the individual as we try to understand potential withdrawal or actual isolation.

Charmaz (1987), using mostly middle-aged women, developed a framework of hierarchical identity transformations that is useful in diagnosing a chronically ill individual's proclivity to social networking and in discovering which social network might be most appropriate. This hierarchy of identity takes into account a reconstruction toward a desired future self, based on past and present selves, and reflects the individual's relative difficulty in achieving specific aspirations. Charmaz's analysis progresses toward a "salvaged self" that retains a past identity based on important values or attributes while still acknowledging dependency.

Initially, the individual takes on a supernormal identity, which assumes an ability to retain all previous success values, social acclamation, struggles, and competition. At this identity level, the individual who is chronically ill attempts to participate more intensely than those in a non-impaired world despite the limitations of illness. The next identity level that the person moves to is the restored self, with the expectation of eventually returning to the previous self, despite the chronic illness or its severity. Healthcare workers might identify this self with the psychological state of denial, but in terms of identity, the individual has simply assumed that there is no discontinuation with a former self. At the third level, the contingent personal identity, one defines oneself in terms of potential risk and failure, indicating the individual still has not come to terms with a future self but has begun to realize that the supernormal identity will no longer be viable. Finally, the level of the salvaged self is reached, whereby the individual attempts to define the self as worthwhile, despite recognizing that present circumstances invalidate any previous identity (Charmaz, 1987).

Not only does social isolation relate to stigma; it can develop as an individual loses hope of sustaining aspirations for a normal or supernormal self, which are now unrealistic. As persons who are chronically ill act out regret, disappointment, and anger, their significant others and healthcare professionals may react in kind, perpetuating a downward spiral of loss, anger, and subsequent greater social isolation. The idea of identity hierarchies thus alerts the caregiver to a process in which shifts in identity are expected.

The reactions, health advice, and the experiences of the individuals with chronic illness must be taken into account in managing that particular identity, and also the various factors that help shape it. Both the social network and adapted norms now available play a role at each stage in identity transformation. At the supernormal identity level, individuals who are chronically ill were in only limited contact with healthcare professionals but presumably in greater contact with

healthier individuals who acted as their referents; at the level of the salvaged self, a home health agency typically was used (Charmaz, 1987).

Integrating Culture into Health Care

Isolation, by its very definition, must include a cultural screening through which desired social contacts are defined. When one speaks of social isolation among unique ethnic groups, the number, type, and quality of contact must be sifted through a particularistic screen of that person's culture. Not only the clients, but also the provider's communication patterns, roles, relationships, and traditions are important elements to consider for both assessment and intervention (Barker, 1994; Cheng, 1997; Groce & Zola, 1993; Kim, 1998; Hill, 2006; Margolin, 2006; Treolar, 1999; Welch, 1998).

Some feel that matching culturally similar providers to clients would be a way to meet needs with effective interventions (Welch, 1998). However, healthcare educators and service providers recognize the issues of a smaller supply of providers and the greater numbers of clients in a struggling dominant healthcare system coping with multiculturalism. To meet supply and demand issues, as well as cultural needs, the idea of cultural competence is being promoted. Education about cultures is being advanced as the key to effective interventions that intersect the values of two disparate groups of individuals (Davidhizar, Bechtel, & Giger, 1998; Jones, Bond, & Cason, 1998; McNamara et al., 1997; Smith, 1996). Cultural education not only results in outcomes of culturally relevant compliance (Davidhizar et al., 1998) but also helps alleviate the isolation of individuals with chronic illness (Barker, 1994; Hildebrandt, 1997; Treolar, 1999).

For those who find that such culturally based education is unavailable, and assuming there are more groups and more traditions than can possibly be understood by a single healthcare provider, a fail-safe strategy remains. This approach requires the provider to approach each person, regardless of their cultural milieu, with respect and dignity, in an explicit good-faith effort to inquire, understand, and be responsive to the client's culture, needs, and person. The provider must set aside prejudices and stereotypes and instead use an authentic sensitive inquiry into the client's beliefs and well-being (Browne, 1997; Treolar, 1999).

By seeking to understand differences, one can find pleasure in the differences and move beyond them to enjoy the similarities of us all. This approach is undergirded by a culture of "caring," and moves toward a model of actively participating groups exchanging concerns of identity, egalitarianism, and needed care (Browne, 1997; Catlin, 1998; Keller & Stevens, 1997; Treolar, 1999). In so doing, social isolation can be managed within the context most comfortable to the client, who is the raison d'être of the healthcare professional.

Respite

The need for respite has been cited as one of the greatest necessities for isolated ill older adults and their caregivers, many of whom are themselves elderly (Miller, 1990; Subcommittee on Human Services, 1987). Its purpose is to relieve caregivers for a period of time so that they may engage in activities that help sustain them or their loved ones, the care recipients. Respite involves four elements: (1) purpose, (2) time, (3) activities, and (4) place. The time may be in short blocks or for a longer (but still relatively short-term) period, both of which temporarily relieve the caregiver of responsibility. Activities may be practical, such as grocery shopping; psychological, such as providing time for self-replenishment or recreation; or physical, such as providing time for rest or medical/nursing attention.

Respite may occur in the home or elsewhere, such as senior centers, day care centers, or long-term care facilities. Senior centers usually accommodate persons who are more independent and flexible, often offering social gathering places and events, meals, and health assessment/exercise/maintenance activities. Day care centers typically host individuals with more diminished

functioning. Other places, such as long-term care facilities, manage clients with an even greater inability to function.

Finally, respite may be delivered by paid or unpaid persons who may be friends, professionals, family, employees, or neighbors. Although many care recipients welcome relief for their caregiver, some may fear abandonment. The family caregiver and professional must work together to assure the care recipient that he or she will not be abandoned (Biordi, 1993). Therefore, the professional has a great deal of latitude in using the four elements to devise interventions tailored to the flexible needs of an isolated caregiver and care recipient.

Support Groups and Other Mutual Aid

Support groups, or even peer counselors (Holley, 2007), have been identified for a wide variety of chronic illnesses and conditions, such as breast cancer (Reach to Recovery), bereavement (Widow to Widow), and alcoholism (Alcoholics Anonymous), or for other conditions such as multiple sclerosis (MS) or blindness. These groups or individuals assist those with chronic illness or disabilities to cope with their illness and the associated changes in identities and social roles of their chronic illness or disability. Such counseling can help enhance one's self-esteem, provide alternative meanings of the illness, suggest ways to cope, assist in specific interventions that have helped others, or offer services or care for either the isolate or caregiver (Holley, 2007). Almost every large city or county has lists of resources that can be accessed: health departments, social work centers, schools, and libraries. Even the telephone book's yellow pages can assist in finding support groups or other resources. The Internet, or World Wide Web, is also a source of information about support groups and resource listings. Some resources list group entry requirements or qualifications. Because of their variety and number, support groups are not always available in every community, so healthcare professionals may find themselves in the position of developing a group. Therefore, as part of a community assessment, the healthcare professional should not only note the groups currently available, but also identify someone who might be willing to develop a needed group. The healthcare professional also may have to help find a meeting place, refer clients to the group, assist clients in discussing barriers to their care, and, if necessary, develop structured activities (such as exercise regimens for arthritic individuals). In addition, the use of motivational devices, such as pictures, videos, audio recordings, reminiscence, or games, may be helpful in developing discussion. Demonstrations of specific illness-related regimens, such as exercises, clothing aids, or body mechanics, are also useful to support groups.

Professionals should be alert to problems the isolate may have in integrating into groups, such as resistance to meeting new people, low self-esteem, apprehension over participation in new activities, or the problems of transportation, building access, and inconvenient meeting times (Matteson, McConnell, & Linton, 1997).

Social activity groups are one way of integrating isolated institutionalized individuals or of reversing hospital-induced confusion; such groups could be recreational therapy groups or those developed particularly to address a special interest (e.g., parents facing the imminent death of a child). Given the limited financial resources typical of most persons who are chronically ill, support groups that are not costly to the chronically ill or their families are more likely to be welcomed.

Spiritual Well-Being

For many, religious or spiritual beliefs offer an important social connection and give great meaning to life. Spiritual well-being typically affirms the unity of the person with his or her environment, often expressed in oneness with his or her god(s) (Matteson et al., 1997). Consequently, assuring isolates some means of connection to their religious support may help them find newer meaning in life or illness and provide them with other people with

whom to share that meaning. The healthcare professional should assess the meaning of spirituality or religion to the individual, the kind of spiritual meeting place he or she finds most comforting, and the types of religious support available in the community. Religious groups range from formal gatherings to religiously aided social groups.

Frequently, the official gathering places of religious or spiritual groups, for example, churches, temples, or mosques, have outreach or social groups that will make visits, arrange for social outings, or develop pen pals or other means of human connectedness. The nurse or other healthcare professional may have to initiate contact with these groups to assist in developing the necessary outreach between them and the isolate.

Rebuilding Family Networks

Keeping, or rebuilding, family networks has much to offer. However, families that have disintegrated may have a history of fragile relationships. The healthcare professional must assess these networks carefully to develop truly effective interventions.

The professional must also take into account the client's type of isolation (lifelong vs recent) and the wishes of the isolate: With whom (if anyone) in the family does the isolate wish contact? How often? What members of the family exist or care about the isolate? What is their relationship to the isolate—parent, sibling, child, friend-as-family, other relative? The professional can then make contact with the individuals indicated to be most accommodating to the isolate, explain the situation, make future plans to bring them and the isolate together, and afterward assess the outcome. However, it may not be possible to bring uninterested family members back into the isolate's social network.

For family members who are interested and willing, rebuilding networks means the professional must take into account the location or proximity of family members to the isolate. If they live near each other, and because a "space of one's own" is a critical human need, a balance of territorial and personal needs must be managed if the isolate is to be reintegrated. Should the isolate and family agree to live together, the family's physical environment will require assessment for safety, access, and territorial space. Not only are factors such as sleeping space and heat and ventilation important, but personal space and having one's own possessions are as important to the family members as they are to the ill person. Teaching the family and isolate how to respect each other's privacy (such as by getting permission to enter a room or look through personal belongings, speaking directly to one another, and so forth) is a way to help them bridge their differences.

Understanding Family Relationships

The nature of the relationship between family and isolate must be understood. The family's meanings and actions attached to love, power, and conflict, and observations of the frequency of controlling strategies by various individuals will inform the professional of potential interventions. For example, some clients who live alone were found to be more likely to be satisfied with support when they were feeling depressed, whereas clients living with others were more satisfied with supporters who cared about them (Foxall et al., 1994). Recalling the earlier example, the elderly woman's use of guilt with an otherwise accommodating family informed the nurse about interventions most likely to succeed.

In some families, love is thought to indicate close togetherness, whereas, in other families, love is thought to provide members with independence. Love and power can be developed and thought of either as a pyramidal (top-down) set of relationships or as an egalitarian circle. Conflict may be a means of connection or of distancing and can be expressed by shouting and insults or by quiet assertion.

Community Resources to Keep Families Together

Using community resources, such as support groups, is a way to help keep a family together. Families draw on each other's experiences as models for coping. For example, families in which there is a child with cancer find ways to help their child cope with the isolation induced by chemotherapy. When necessary, the healthcare professional may wish to refer the isolate and family to psychiatric or specialty nurses, counselors, psychiatrists, or social workers to help them overcome their disintegration. Successful implementation of the wide range of family-related interventions requires sensitive perceptions of the needs not only of the isolate, but also of the various family members with whom that individual must interact. (See the intervention research noted in the boxed evidence-based practice section of this chapter.)

Two interesting community resources that could help alert families to potential problem situations for isolates are the post office and newspaper delivery services. If these delivery persons observe a build-up of uncollected mail or newspapers, they can call or check the house to see if there is an older adult isolate in distress. Families who are concerned about their isolated family member can provide their post office, regular mail carrier, or news delivery service with information about the isolate that can be used in the event of a problem. Nurses and social workers can also contact mail and news services or help families make these contacts. This intervention can be expanded to include any regular visitor, such as a rental manager, janitor, or neighbor, who might be willing to check on the welfare of the isolate.

In some communities, employees at banks and stores also react to older individuals who may be isolated. Should there be unusual financial activities or changes in shopping patterns, the individual can be contacted to make sure that everything is satisfactory. Although, in some communities, mail and newspaper services and banks and stores are not involved with people in their areas, these resources are valuable and should be expanded throughout the country.

Communication Technologies

Telephone

The telephone is a method used to counteract the effects of place-boundedness. However, findings are equivocal (Kivett, 1979; Praderas & MacDonald, 1986). Still, the telephone is considered almost a necessity in reducing the isolation of a place-bound individual. In literature other than that of the socially isolated, nurses using telephone contact reduced health problems and costs of readmission for patients (Norbeck, 1996).

Computers

For many persons, including homebound older adults or people with disabilities, computers have helped offset social isolation and loneliness through features such as access to the Internet, which allows the person to reach family and friends or to find new friends, activities, and other common interests. Computers can also be used to provide fun activities, such as computerized games. In the United States, computers are more widely available than elsewhere, and more so among those-withn higher socioeconomic status and the more highly educated. Increasingly, on-line groups offer support, such as that described for breast cancer patients (Hoybye, Johansen, & Tjornhoj-Thomsen, 2005).

▌ EVIDENCE-BASED PRACTICE BOX

Methodologically rigorous, evidence-based practice research about social isolation is difficult to find. One such study, however, is that reported by Fyrand and colleagues. This study examines the effect of a social network intervention on 264 women participants with rheumatoid arthritis (RA). Participants were randomized into three groups, that is, one intervention and two control groups. These were labeled as the Intervention Group, the Attention Control Group, and the No-Treatment Control Group.

The *research questions* guiding this study were: "To what extent, if any, will network intervention influence (1) the total size of the patients' social network, (2) the amount of the patients' daily emotional support, and (3) the patients' social functioning . . . " (Fyrand, 2003, p. 72). The *intervention* in this study consisted of two separate, but related sessions, (1) a Preparatory Assessment session and (2) the Network Meeting. If the participants were randomized into the attention control group, they were given the opportunity to attend a single 2-hour meeting in which they were presented information about RA from a panel of experts who also responded to their questions about RA. The third control group had no intervention or meeting.

Three *findings* indicated that (1) the intervention group experienced a statistically significant increase in their social network size, (2) at Time 2 in the study, emotional social support was higher for the intervention group, and (3) less social dysfunction occurred in the intervention group.

The *intervention* basically assessed a patient participant's social network and then helped the patient and the social network to assist the patient in socially functional problem solving about the illness. Through the meeting process in the intervention group, a change in attitude was observed when the patient developed an increased awareness of the need for social network members. In addition, the network members often would share problems about their own

(Continued)

EVIDENCE-BASED PRACTICE BOX *(Continued)*

lives, which normalized any feelings of stigma experienced by the patient. The authors call this a "response shift," where both parties change their self-evaluation and make a concerted effort to support each other (p. 83).

During the preparatory assessment session, three important areas were covered: (1) information about the research project, (2) the relationship between health and social networks, and (3) how the patient experienced chronic illness. During this 2-hour preparatory assessment, the researchers mapped the participant's present social network. The social network map helped the participants to obtain a deeper analysis of the makeup of their social networks, and allowed the researcher and participant to make decisions about which member of the network should be invited to the network meeting (the second element of this intervention). In this initial preparatory session, participant patients also discussed, in depth, how their chronic disease (RA) impacted their life. As feelings were explored, researchers took great care to ensure that the participants had adequate time and attention regarding these important topics.

The network meeting consisted of network members, typically the friends and family who were listed in the preparatory assessment, getting together to problem solve. An average of seven network members, in addition to a network research therapist, attended for an average of 2 hours. The research network therapist acted as a leader and catalyst of the group, mobilizing the participant and the group of network members to dialogue about the participant patient's problem-solving process. The group leader opened the meeting with the expectations of the meeting and a presentation of the topics that were deemed important, as derived from the preparatory meeting. The general goal for the group was to share how they viewed the participant's life with RA and to describe their hopes and expectations of the meetings. The goal for the participant was to elicit free discussion of those topics that were of highest importance . A consensus was formed within the group about how to best solve the problems raised, with the further intention to develop trust and involvement between members of the network. In addition to the participant learning how to best present problems to social network members, the aim of the network meeting was to help the participant and members change dysfunctional network behaviors. The researchers suggested that, by clustering the network members and the participant together in a single room, the network and participant would better sense their collective power and the participant could re-bond with any hitherto damaged social network relationships.

This article lays out a sensible intervention that targets social network members. Through a pair of relatively short meetings, the researchers created an exportable, effective intervention that reduced social isolation and rehabilitated, to some extent, dysfunctional social networks. Furthermore, not only is this intervention brief, but it also does not require technology that requires extra training. It does require that the network therapist should be a professional, such as a nurse, social worker, or psychologist, who is skilled in group therapy and mapping social networks. Therefore, this cost-effective intervention can be easily conducted in a variety of settings with a variety of patients who have social networks willing to meet together for a minimum of only 4 hours.

Source: Fyrand, L. (2003). The effect of social network intervention for women with rheumatoid arthritis. *Family Process, 42*(1), p. 71.

Advances in computer technology have created special attachments, such as cameras, breath tubes, or special keyboards and font sizes, which customize computers to the needs of the isolated or disabled, including those with visual impairment (Imel, 1999; Salem, 1998). In parts of the United States, outreach efforts are increasing, as projects aim to reduce the social isolation of the homebound by providing computers and Internet access to caregivers and care receivers. The use of information and other communication technologies has been helpful in alleviating barriers to the return to work for those with spinal cord injuries and the resulting disabilities (Bricout, 2004). Telework permitting home based work is a technology with proven effects for those with mobility or transportation limitations, or those whose illnesses or disabilities necessitate rest periods incompatible with typical work environments. Computers have also been used to relieve isolation or loneliness, and assist in the management of chronic illness and support groups located in rural environments (Clark, 2002; Hill & Weinert, 2004; Johnson & Ashton, 2003; Weinert, Cudney, & Winters, 2005).

Whether connecting with the Internet, using word processing, corresponding via e-mail, taking classes, and so on, computers also allow isolates to actively fill many hours of otherwise empty time, bringing a measure of relief to tedium while expanding their intellectual and social lives. The caveat, of course, is that the use of the computer, and especially the Internet, could itself be an isolating factor for many individuals. This creates a danger of virtual reality overrunning actual reality, in which case, isolates compound their isolation. That having been said, however, the computer offers many more advantages than disadvantages in the possibilities for overcoming some elements of isolation.

Touch

In cultures where touch is important, families and professionals must learn the use and comfort of touch. American studies indicate that the elderly are the least likely group to be touched, and yet they find touch very comforting. Pets may be useful alternatives to human touch and human interaction; pet therapy is increasingly used as an intervention in families, communities, and in group settings such as nursing homes (Banks, 1998; Collins, Fitzgerald, Sachs-Ericsson, Scherer, Cooper, & Boninger, 2006). Feeling loved and having it demonstrated through touch can do much to reduce isolation and its often concomitant lowered self-esteem. Because some individuals find touch uncomfortable, professionals must assess (by simply asking or observing flinching, grimacing, or resignation) the family's or isolate's responsiveness to touch.

Behavior Modification

Behavior modification is a technique that is best used by skilled professionals. It involves the systematic analysis of responses and their antecedent cues and consequences; the use of cognitive therapy to change awareness, perceptions, and behaviors; and the specification of realistic, measurable goals or actual behaviors. In addition, reward structures and understanding support persons are necessary in the definition of the problem and its solution. Consistency is needed to develop stable patterns of responses. The time frame of such modification can vary with the problem.

Behavior modification is particularly useful for addressing specific problems, for example, the isolate who is fearful of going outside the house. It is also an important intervention when the environment can be held stable, such as in an institutional setting. Matteson and colleagues (1997) note that where groups are small or the motivation intense, successful behavioral interventions have been instituted for the socially isolated in institutions as well as in the home.

■ OUTCOMES

Ideally, the reduction of social isolation and the maintenance of the integrity of the person who is chronically ill and his or her caregiver(s) are preferred outcomes of interventions. However, so many factors can affect social isolation, its assessment, and intervention, that it is difficult to draw simple linear relationships between structure, process, and outcomes. As shown throughout this chapter, a professional must be sensitive to, and prioritize, interventions within the cultural milieu in which the client and support network reside.

Handling the emotionally charged issues surrounding every social isolate requires that professionals recognize in their clients, as well as in themselves, those values that most drive their relationships, and build solutions that best deliver culturally and personally competent care toward a better life for their clients.

STUDY QUESTIONS

1. Is loneliness the same thing as social isolation? Why or why not?
2. How might the distance that a manually powered or an electrically powered wheelchair can go relate to social isolation?
3. List six characteristics that might incline a client to social isolation. What criteria did you use to develop these characteristics?
4. Suppose another healthcare professional said about a very new client, "Oh, we must make certain that Mrs. Jones has company. She's a widow, you know." With regard to social isolation, what arguments could you make, pro or con, about this statement?
5. Develop at least five questions you could adapt to assess and validate social isolation in a client. Consider how you might approach identity levels, actual isolation, network assessment, and feelings of the isolate. Add other priorities as you wish, but offer rationales for each of them.
6. Name three community resources you could use to reduce the social isolation of clients.
7. What two principles should guide a healthcare professional when developing any

intervention with an isolated client? Why are these important?

8. Suppose a client said to you, "I have had arthritis in my fingers and hands for a long time now. I simply can't do what I used to do. I now have new handles for my kitchen cabinets because the knobs hurt my hands, and new clothes especially made for people like me who can't work buttons. My daughter was shopping and she saw them and told me about them. Now I feel better when I get together with them to see my grandchildren." At what stage of identity might you expect this client to be? Why? Is this person an isolate? Explain your answer.

9. A gay teenager is your client. He has recently "come out" and is now depressed because his schoolmates shun him, his parents are going through a grief reaction to his announcement, and he has few other friends who share his interests or sexual orientation. Is he at risk for social isolation? Loneliness? How would you assess his social network? What interventions, if any, would you recommend? Explain your answers.

REFERENCES

Antonucci, T. (1985). Social support: Theoretical advances, recent findings, and pressing issues. In I.G. Sarason & B.R. Sarason (Eds.), *Social support: Theory, research, and application*. Boston: Martinus Nyhoff.

Banks, M.R. (1998). *The effects of animal-assisted therapy on loneliness in an elderly population in long-term care facilities*. Louisiana State University Health Sciences Center School of Nursing.

Austin, D. (1989). Becoming immune to loneliness: Helping the elderly fill a void. *Journal of Gerontological Nursing, 15*(9), 25–28.

Barker, J.C. (1994). Recognizing cultural differences: Health care providers and elderly patients. *Gerontology & Geriatric Education, 15*(1), 9–21.

Barnes, L.L., Mendes de Leon, C.F., Wilson, R.S., Bienias, J.L., & Evans, D.A. (2004). Social resources and cognitive decline in a population of older African Americans and whites. *Neurology, 63*(12), 2322–2326.

Bendor, S. (1990). Anxiety and isolation in siblings of pediatric cancer patients: The need for prevention. *Social Work in Health Care, 14*(3), 17–35.

Bennet, R. (1980). *Aging, isolation, and resocialization.* New York: VanNostrand Reinhold.

Berkman, L. (1983). The assessment of social networks and social support in the elderly. *Journal of the American Geriatrics Society, 31*(12), 743–749.

Berkman, L.F., & Syme, S.L. (1979). Social networks, host resistance, and mortality: A nine-year follow-up study of Alameda County residents. *American Journal of Epidemiology, 109*(2), 186–204.

Biordi, D. (2000). Research agenda: Emerging issues in the management of health and illness. *Seminars for Nurse Managers, 8,* 205–211.

Biordi, D. (1993). [In-home care and respite care as self-care] Unpublished data.

Boden-Albala, B., Litwak, E., Elkind, M.S., Rundek, T., & Sacco, R.L. (2005). Social isolation and outcomes post stroke. *Neurology, 64*(11), 1888–1892.

Borman, J., & Biordi, D. (1992). Female nurse executives: Finally, at an advantage. *Journal of Nursing Administration, 22*(9), 37–41.

Bricout, J.C. (2004). Using telework to enhance return to work outcomes for individuals with spinal cord injuries. *Neurorehabilitation, 19*(2), 147–159.

Browne, A.J. (1997). The concept analysis of respect applying the hybrid model in cross-cultural settings. *Western Journal of Nursing Research, 19*(6), 762–780.

Brummett, B.H., Barefoot, J.C., Siegler, I.C., Clapp-Channing, N.E., Lytle, B.L., Bosworth, H.B., et al. (2001). Characteristics of socially isolated patients with coronary artery disease who are at elevated risk for mortality. *Psychosomatic Medicine, 63*(2), 267–272.

Burnley, I.H. (1992). Mortality from selected cancers in NSW and Sydney, Australia. *Social Science and Medicine, 35*(2), 195–208.

Cadman, D., Rosenbaum, P., Boyle, M., & Offord, D. (1991). Children with chronic illness: Family and parent demographic characteristics and psychosocial adjustment. *Pediatrics, 87*(6), 884–889.

Carpenito-Moyet, L.J. (2006). Social Isolation. In L.J. Carpenito-Moyet, *Nursing diagnosis: Application to clinical practice* (11th ed.), 734–736.

Catalan, J. (1998). Mental health problems in older adults with HIV referred to a psychological medicine unit. *AIDS Care: Psychological and Socio-medical Aspects of AIDS/HIV, 10*(2), 105–112.

Catlin, A.J. (1998). Editor's choice. When cultures clash, comments on a brilliant new book. *The spirit catches you and you fall down.* New York: Farrar, Straus, and Giroux.

Ceria, C.D., Masaki, K.H., Rodriguez, B.L., Chen, R., Yano, K., & Curb, J.D. (2001). The relationship of psychosocial factors to total mortality among older Japanese-American men: The Honolulu heart program. *Journal of the American Geriatrics Society, 49*(6), 725–731.

Charmaz, K. (1987). Struggling for a self: Identity levels of the chronically ill. In J. Roth & P. Conrad (Eds.), *Research in the sociology of health care.* Greenwich, CT: JAI Press.

Cheng, B.K. (1997). Cultural clash between providers of majority culture and patients of Chinese culture. *Journal of Long Term Home Health Care, 16*(2), 39–43.

Chinman, M.J., Weingarten, R., Stayner, D., & Davidson, L. (2001). Chronicity reconsidered: Improving person-environment fit through a consumer-run service. *Community Mental Health Journal, 37*(3), 215–229.

Christ, G. (1987). Social consequences of the cancer experience. *The American Journal of Pediatric Hematology/Oncology, 9*(1), 84–88.

Clark, D.J. (2002). Older adults living through and with their computers. *Computers, Informatics, Nursing, 20*(3), 117–124.

Cobb, S. (1979). Social support and health through the life course. In M.W. Riley (Ed.), *Aging from birth to death.* Boulder, CO: Westview Press.

Cohen, M. (1993). The unknown and the unknowable—Managing sustained uncertainty. *Western Journal of Nursing Research, 15*(1), 77–96.

Collins, D., Fitzgerald, S., Sachs-Ericsson, N., Scherer, M., Cooper, R., & Boninger, M. (2006). Psychosocial well-being and community participation of service dog partners. *Disability and Rehabilitation, 1*(1), 41–48.

Corbin, J., & Strauss, A. (1987). Accompaniments of chronic illness: Changes in body, self, biography, and biographical time. In J. Roth & P. Conrad (Eds.), *Research in the sociology of health care.* Greenwich, CT: JAI Press.

Cox, C., Spiro, M., & Sullivan, J. (1988). Social risk factors: Impact on elders' perceived health status. *Journal of Community Health Nursing, 5*(1), 59–73.

Creecy, R., Berg, W., & Wright, L. (1985). Loneliness among the elderly: A causal approach. *Journal of Gerontology, 40*(4), 487–493.

Creed, F. (1990). Psychological disorders in rheumatoid arthritis: A growing consensus? *Annual Rheumatic Disorders, 49*, 808–812.

Davidhizar, R., Bechtel, G.L., & Giger, J.N. (1998). Model helps CMs deliver multicultural care: Addressing cultural issues boosts compliance. *Case Management Advisor, 9*(6), 97–100.

Dela Cruz, L. (1986). On loneliness and the elderly. *Journal of Gerontological Nursing, 12*(11), 22–27.

DesRosier, M., Catanzaro, M., & Piller, J. (1992). Living with chronic illness: Social support and the well spouse perspective. *Rehabilitation Nursing, 17*(2), 87–91.

DiMatteo, M.R., & Hays, R. (1981). Social support and serious illness. In B.H. Gottlieb (Ed.), *Social networks and social support.* Beverly Hills, CA: Sage.

DiNapoli, P., & Murphy, D. (2002).The marginalization of chronically ill adolescents. *The Nursing Clinics of North America, 37*(3), 565–572.

Dorfman, L., Homes, C., & Berlin, K. (1996). Wife caregivers of frail elderly veterans: Correlates of caregiver satisfaction and caregiver strain. *Family Relations, 45*, 46–55.

Dropkin, M. (1989). Coping with disfigurement and dysfunction. *Seminars in Oncology Nursing, 5*(3), 213–219.

Eng, P.M., Rimm, E.B., Fitzmaurice, G., & Kawachi, I. (2002). Social ties and change in social ties in relation to subsequent total and cause-specific mortality and coronary heart disease incidence in men. *American Journal of Epidemology, 155*(8), 700–709.

Findlay, R. (2003). Interventions to reduce social isolation amongst older people: Where is the evidence? *Aging & Society, 23*, 647–658.

Fiscella, K., Franks, M., Gold, M., & Clancy, D. (2000). Social support, disability, and depression:

A longitudinal study of rheumatoid arthritis. *Journal of the American Medical Association, 283*, 2579–2584.

Fitzpatrick, R., Newman, R., Archer, R., & Shipley, M. (2000). Inequalities in racial access to health care. *Journal of the American Medical Association, 284*(16), 2053.

Fowles, D., & Greenberg, S. (2003). *A profile of older Americans: 2003.* Retrieved November 10, 2007, from www.aoa.gov/prof/statistics/profile/2003/2003profile.pdf

Foxall, M., Barron, C., Dollen, K., Shull, K., et al. (1994). Low vision elders: Living arrangements, loneliness, and social support. *Journal of Gerontological Nursing, 20*, 6–14.

Foxall, M., Eckberg, J., & Griffith, N. (1986). Spousal adjustment to chronic illness. *Rehabilitation Nursing, 11*, 13–16.

Fratiglioni, L., Paillard-Borg, S., & Winblad, B. (2004). An active and socially integrated lifestyle in late life might protect against dementia. *Lancet Neurol, 3*(6), 343–353.

Fratiglioni, L., Wang, H.X., Ericsson, K., Maytan, M., & Winblad, B. (2000). Influence of social network on occurrence of dementia: A community-based longitudinal study. *Lancet, 355*(9212), 1315–1319.

Frierson, R.L. (1991). Suicide attempts by the old and the very old. *Archives of Internal Medicine, 151*(1), 141–144.

Fyrand, L. (2003). The effect of social network intervention for women with rheumatoid arthritis. *Family Process, 42*(1), 71.

Gallo, A.M., Breitmayer, B.J., Knafl, K.A., & Zoeller, L.H. (1991). Stigma in childhood chronic illness: A well sibling perspective. *Pediatric Nursing, 17*(1), 21–25.

Gamba, A., Romano, M., Grosso, I., Tamburini, M., Cantu, G., Molinari, R., et al. (1992). Psychosocial adjustment of patients surgically treated for head and neck cancer. *Head and Neck, 14*(3), 218–223.

Goodman, C. (1984). Natural helping among older adults. *Gerontologist, 24*(2), 138–143.

Greaves, C.J., & Farbus, L. (2006). Effects of creative and social activity on the health and well-being of socially isolated older people: Outcomes from a multi-method observational study. *Journal of the Royal Society of Health, 126*(3), 134–142.

Groce, N.E., & Zola, I. (1993). Multiculturalism, chronic illness, and disability. *Pediatrics, 91*(5), 32–39.

Habayeb, G.L. (1995). Cultural diversity: A nursing concept not yet reliably defined. *Nursing Outlook, 43*(5), 224–227.

Hawes, C., Phillips, C.D., Rose, M., Holan, S., & Sherman, M. (2003). A national survey of assisted living facilities. *The Gerontologist, 43*(6), 875–882.

Heiney, S., Goon-Johnson, K., Ettinger, R., & Ettinger, S. (1990). The effects of group therapy on siblings of pediatric oncology patients. *Journal of Pediatric Oncology Nursing, 7*(3), 95–100.

Helton, L.R. (1995). Intervention with Appalachians: Strategies for a culturally specific practice. *Journal of Cultural Diversity, 2*(1), 20–26.

Heumann, L. (1988). Assisting the frail elderly living in subsidized housing for the independent elderly: A profile of the management and its support priorities. *Gerontologist, 28*, 625–631.

Hildebrandt, E. (1997). Have I angered my ancestors? Influences of culture on health care with elderly black South Africans as an example. *Journal of Multicultural Nursing and Health, 3*(1), 40–49.

Hill, D.L. (2006). Sense of belonging as connectedness, American Indian worldview and mental health. *Archives of Psychiatric Nursing, 20*(5), 210–216.

Hill, W.G., & Weinert, C. (2004). An evaluation of an online intervention to provide social support and health education. *Computers, Informatics, Nursing, 22*(5), 282–288.

Hoeffer, B. (1987). A causal model of loneliness among older single women. *Archives of Psychiatric Nursing, 1*(5), 366–373.

Holley, U.A. (2007). Social isolation: A practical guide for nurses assisting clients with chronic illness. *Rehabilitation Nursing, 32*(2), 51–56.

Holtzman, R.E., Rebok, G.W., Saczynski, J.S., Kouzis, A.C., Wilcox Doyle, K., & Eaton, W.W. (2004). Social network characteristics and cognition in middle-aged and older adults. *The Journals of Gerontology, Series B, Psychological Sciences and Social Sciences, 59*(6), P278–284.

Hopper, S. (1981). Diabetes as a stigmatized condition: The case of low income clinic patients in the United States. *Social Science and Medicine, 15*, 11–19.

House, J., Landis, K., & Umberson, D. (1988). Social relationships and health. *Science, 241*, 540–544.

Howat, P., Iredell, H., Grenade, L., Nedwetzky, A., & Collins, J. (2004). Reducing social isolation amongst older people implications for health professionals. *Geriaction, 22*(1), 13–20.

Hoybye, M.T., Johansen, C., & Tjornboj-Thomsen, T. (2005). Online interaction: Effects of storytelling in an internet breast cancer support group. *Psychooncology, 14*(3), 211–220.

Imel, S. (1999) *Seniors in cyberspace. Trends and issues alerts.* Washington, DC: Office of Educational Research and Improvement (ED). EDD00036.

Jessop, D., & Stein, R. (1985). Uncertainty and its relation to the psychological and social correlates of chronic illness in children. *Social Science and Medicine, 20*(10), 993–999.

Johnson, D., & Ashton, C. (2003). Effects of computer-mediated communication on social support and loneliness for isolated persons with disabilities. *American Journal of Recreational Therapy, 2*(3), 23–32.

Jones, M.D., Bond, M.L., & Cason, C.L. (1998). Where does culture fit in outcomes management? *Journal of Nursing Care Quality, 13*(1), 41–51.

Kaplan, G., Salonen, J., Cohen, R., Brand, R., et al. (1988). Social connections and mortality from all causes and from cardiovascular disease: Prospective evidence from Eastern Finland. *American Journal of Epidemiology, 128*(2), 370–380.

Keller, C.S., & Stevens, K.R. (1997). Cultural considerations in promoting wellness. *Journal of Cardiovascular Nursing, 11*(3), 15–25.

Kim, L.S. (1998). Long term care for the Korean American elderly: An exploration for a better way of services. *Journal of Long Term Home Health Care, 16*(2), 35–38.

Kinsella, G., Ford, B., & Moran, C. (1989). Survival of social relationships following head injury. *International disability studies, 11*(1), 9–14.

Kivett, V. (1979). Discriminators of loneliness among the rural elderly: Implications for interventions. *Gerontologist, 19*(1), 108–115.

Klinenberg, E. (2001). Dying alone: The social production of urban isolation. *Ethnography, 2*(4), 501–531.

Kreps, G., & Kreps, M. (1997). Amishing "medical care." *Journal of Multicultural Nursing & Health, 3*(2), 44–47.

Kroenke, C.H., Kubzansky, L.D., Schernhammer, E.S., Holmes, M.D., & Kawachi, I. (2006). Social networks, social support, and survival after breast cancer diagnosis. *Journal of Clinical Oncology, 24*(7), 1105–1111.

Krouse, J., Krouse, H., & Fabian, R. (1989). Adaptation to surgery for head and neck cancer. *Laryngoscope, 99*, 789–794.

Lawton, M., Greenbaum, M., & Liebowitz, B. (1980). The lifespan of housing environments for the aging. *Gerontologist, 20,* 56–64.

Lawton, M., Kleban, M., & Carlson, D. (1973). The inner-city resident: To move or not to move. *Gerontologist, 13,* 443–448.

Lawton, M., Moss, M., & Grimes, M. (1985). The changing service need of older tenants in planned housing. *Gerontologist, 25,* 258–264.

Lee, G.R., & Ellithorpe, E. (1982). Intergenerational exchange and subjective well-being+ among the elderly. *Journal of Marriage and the Family, 44,* 217–224.

Lichtenstein, B., Laska, M.K., & Clair, J.M. (2002). Chronic sorrow in the HIV-positive patient: Issues of race, gender, and social support. *AIDS Patient Care and STDs, 16*(1), 27–38.

Lien-Gieschen, T. (1993). Validation of social isolation related to maturational age: Elderly. *Nursing diagnosis, 4*(1), 37–43.

Lin, N. (1986). Conceptualizing social support. In N. Lin, A. Dean, & W. Ensel (Eds.), *Social support, life events, and depression.* New York: Academic Press.

Litwin, H., & Zoabi, S. (2003). Modernization and elder abuse in an Arab-Israeli context. *Research on Aging, 25*(3), 224–246.

Litwin, H. (1997). Support network type and health service utilization. *Research on Aging, 19*(3), 274–299.

Lubben, J. (1988). Assessing social networks among elderly populations. *Family Community Health, 11*(3), 42–52.

Lubben, J., & Gironda, M. (1996). Assessing social support networks among older people in the United States. In H. Litwin (Ed.), *The social networks of older people: A cross-national analysis* (pp. 144). Westport, Connecticut: Praeger.

Lubben, J., Weiler, P., & Chi, I. (1989). Gender and ethnic differences in the health practices of the elderly poor. *Journal of Clinical Epidemiology, 42*(8), 725–733.

Lyons, M.J. (1982). Psychological concomitants of the environment influencing suicidal behavior in middle and later life. Dissertation Abstracts International, *43,* 1620B.

Maddox, G.L. (1985). Intervention strategies to enhance well-being in later life: The status and prospect of guided change. *Health Services Research, 19,* 1007–1032.

Mallinson, R.K., (1999). The lived experiences of AIDS-related multiple losses by HIV-negative gay men. *Journal of the Association of Nurses in AIDS Care, 10*(5), 22–31.

Margolin, S. (2006). African American youths with internalizing difficulties: Relation to social support and activity involvement. *Children and Schools, 28*(3), 135–144.

Marottoli, R.A., deLeon, C.F.M., Glass, T.A., Williams, C.S., Cooney, L.M. & Berkman, L.F. (2000). Consequences of driving cessation: Decreased out-of-home activity levels. *Journal of Gerontology Series B: Psychological Sciences and Social Sciences, 55*(6), S334–340.

Matteson, M.A., McConnell, E.S., & Linton, A. (1997). *Gerontological nursing: Concepts and practice* (2nd ed). Philadelphia: Saunders.

McNamara, B., Martin, K., Waddel, C., & Yuen, K. (1997). Palliative care in a multicultural society: Perceptions of health care professionals. *Palliative Medicine, 11*(5), 359–367.

Melle, I., Friis, S., Hauff, E., & Vaglum, P. (2000). Social functioning of patients with schizophrenia in high income welfare societies. *Psychiatric Services, 51*(2), 223–228.

Michael, Y.L., Berkman, L.F., Colditz, G.A., Holmes, M.D., & Kawachi, I. (2002). Social networks and health-related quality of life in breast cancer survivors: A prospective study. *Journal of Psychosomatic Research, 52*(5), 285–293.

Miller, B. (1990). Gender differences in spouse caregiver strain: Socialization and role explanations. *Journal of Marriage and the Family, 52,* 311–322.

Mistry, R., Rosansky, J., McGuire, J., McDermott, C., Jarvik, L., & UPBEAT Collaborative Group. (2001). Social isolation predicts rehospitalization in a group of older American veterans enrolled in the UPBEAT program. *International Journal of Geriatric Psychiatry, 16*(10), 950–959.

Mullins, L., & Dugan, E. (1990). The influence of depression, and family and friendship relations, on residents' loneliness in congregate housing. *Gerontologist, 30*(3), 377–384.

Murberg, T.A. (2004). Long-term effect of social relationships on mortality in patients with congestive heart failure. *International Journal of Psychiatry in Medicine, 34*(3), 207–217.

Newman, S.P., Fitzpatrick, R., Lamb, R., & Shipley, M. (1989). The origins of depressed mood in rheumatoid arthritis. *The Journal of Rheumatology, 16*(6), 740–744.

Noll, R., Ris, M.D., Davies, W.H., Burkowski, W., et al. (1992). Social interactions between children with cancer or sickle cell disease and their peers: Teacher ratings. *Developmental and Behavioral Pediatrics, 13*(3), 187–193.

Norbeck, J., DeJoseph, J., & Smith, R. (1996). A randomized trial of an empirically derived social support intervention to prevent low birthweight among African-American women. *Social Science and Medicine, 43*, 947–954.

Noyes, R., Kathol, R., Debelius-Enemark, P., Williams, J., et al. (1990). Distress associated with cancer as measured by the illness distress scale. *Psychosomatics, 31*(3), 321–330.

Orth-Gomer, K., Unden, A., & Edwards, M. (1988). Social isolation and mortality in ischemic heart disease: A 10-year follow-up study of 150 middle aged men. *Acta Med Scan, 224* (3), 205–215.

Peplau, L.A., & Perlman, D. (Eds.). (1986). *Loneliness: A sourcebook of current theory, research, and therapy.* New York: John Wiley & Sons.

Pinquart, M., & Sorensen, J. (2001). Influences on loneliness in older adults: A meta-analysis. *Basic and Applied Social Psychology, 23*(4), 245–266.

Poulin, J. (1984). Age segregation and the interpersonal involvement and morale of the aged. *Gerontologist, 24*(3), 266–269.

Praderas, K., & MacDonald, M. (1986). Telephone conversational skills training with socially isolated, impaired nursing home residents. *Journal of Applied Behavior Analysis, 19*(4), 337–348.

Ramos, M., & Wilmoth, J. (2003). Social relationships and depressive symptoms among older adults in southern Brazil. *Journal of Gerontology, Series B, Psychological Sciences and Social Sciences, 58*(4), S25361.

Randers, I., Mattiasson A., & Olson T.H. (2003). The "social self": The 11th category of integrity—implications for enhancing geriatric nursing care. *Journal of Applied Gerontology, 22*(2), 289–309.

Ravish, T. (1985). Prevent isolation before it starts. *Journal of Gerontological Nursing, 11*(10), 10–13.

Resnick, B. (2007). Assisted living: The perfect place for nursing. *Geriatric Nursing, 28*(1), 7–8.

Reynolds, P., & Kaplan, G. (1990). Social connections and risk for cancer: Prospective evidence from the Alameda County study. *Behavioral Medicine, 16*(3), 101–110.

Rubenstein, L.Z., Josephson, K.R., & Robbins, A.S. (1994). Falls in the nursing home. *Annals of Internal Medicine, 121*(6), 442–451.

Russell, C., & Schofield, T. (1999). Social isolation in old age: A qualitative exploration of service providers' perceptions. *Ageing and Society, 19*(1), 69–91.

Ryan, M., & Patterson, J. (1987). Loneliness in the elderly. *Journal of Gerontological Nursing, 13*(5), 6–12.

Salem, P. (1998). Paradoxical impacts of electronic communication technologies. Paper presented at the International Communication Association/National Communication Association Conference, Rome, Italy, July 15–17, 1998.

Seeman, M. (1959). On the meaning of alienation. *American Sociological Review, 24*, 783–791.

Seeman, T.E. (2000). Health promoting effects of friends and family on health outcomes in older adults. *American Journal of Health Promotion, 14*(6), 362–370.

Seidler, A., Bernhardt, T., Nienhaus, A., & Frolich, L. (2003). Association between the psychosocial network and dementia—A case-control study. *Journal of Psychiatric Research, 37*(2), 89–98.

Siplic F., & Kadis, D. (2002). The psychosocial aspect of aging. *Socialno Delo, 41*(5), 295–300.

Smith, J.W. (1996). Cultural and spiritual issues in palliative care. *Journal of Cancer Care, 5*(4), 173–178.

Spiegel, D. (1990). Facilitating emotional coping during treatment. *Cancer, 66*, 1422–1426.

Spitz, G., & Miner, S. (1992). Gender differences in adult child contact among Black elderly parents. *Gerontologist, 43*, 213–218.

Stephens, M., & Bernstein, M. (1984). Social support and well-being among residents of planned housing. *Gerontologist, 24*, 144–148.

Stewart, N. (1986). Perceptual and behavioral effects of immobility and social isolation in hospitalized orthopedic patients. *Nursing Papers/Perspectives in Nursing, 18*(3), 59–74.

Strauss, A., Corbin, J., Fagerhaugh, S., Glaser, B., et al. (1984). *Chronic illness and the quality of life* (2nd ed.). St. Louis: Mosby.

Street, D., Burge, S., Quadagno, J., & Barrett, A. (2007). The salience of social relationships for resident well-being in assisted living. *The Journals of Gerontology, Series B, Psychological Sciences and Social Sciences, 62*(2), S129–134.

Subcommittee on Human Services of the Select Committee on Aging: U.S. House of Representatives.

(1987). Exploding the myths: Caregiving in America (Committee Print No. 99–611). Washington, DC: U.S. Government Printing Office.

Tamlyn, D., & Arklie, M. (1986). A theoretical framework for standard care plans: A nursing approach for working with chronically ill children and their families. *Issues in Comprehensive Pediatric Nursing, 9,* 39–45.

Tilden, V., & Weinert, C. (1987). Social support and the chronically ill individual. *Nursing Clinics of North America, 22*(3), 613–620.

Treolar, L.L. (1999). People with disabilities—the same, but different: Implications for health care practice. *Journal of Transcultural Nursing, 10*(4), 358–364.

Trout, D. (1980). The role of social isolation in suicide. *Suicide and life threatening behavior, 10,* 10–22.

Victor, C., Scambler, S.J., Shah, S., Cook D.G., Harris, T., Rink, E., et al. (2002). Has loneliness amongst older people increased? An investigation into variations among cohorts. *Ageing and Society, 22*(5), 585–597.

Wang, K.W., & Barnard, A. (2004). Technology-dependent children and their families: A review. *Journal of Advanced Nursing, 45*(1), 34–46.

Wang, H.X., Karp, A., Winblad, B., & Fratiglioni, L. (2002). Late-life engagement in social and leisure activities is associated with a decreased risk of dementia: A longitudinal study from the Kungsholmen Project. *American Journal of Epidemiology, 155*(12), 1081–1087.

Watson, E. (1988). Dead to the world. *Nursing Times, 84*(21), 52–54.

Weinert, C., Cudney, S., & Winters, C. (2005). Social support in cyberspace: The next generation. *Computers, Informatics, Nursing, 23*(1), 7–15.

Weisman, A.D., & Worden, J.W. (1976–1977). The existential plight in cancer: Significance of the first 100 days. *International Journal of Psychiatry in Medicine, 7,* 1–15.

Weiss, R.S. (1973). *Loneliness: The experience of emotional and social isolation.* Cambridge, MA: Massachusetts Institute of Technology Press.

Welch, C.M. (1998). The adult health and development program: Bridging the racial gap. *International Electronic Journal of Health Education, 1*(3), 178–181.

Wenger, G.C. (1997). Social networks and the prediction of elderly people at risk. *Aging and Mental Health, 1*(4), 311.

Wenger, G.C., Davies, R., Shahtahmasebi, S., & Scott, A. (1996). Social isolation and loneliness in old age: Review and model refinement. *Aging & Society, 16,* 333–358.

Williams, S., & Bury, M. (1989). Impairment, disability, and handicap in chronic respiratory illness. *Social Science and Medicine, 29*(5), 609–616.

Woods, N., Haberman, M., & Packard, N. (1993). Demands of illness and individual, dyadic, and family adaptation in chronic illness. *Western Journal of Nursing Research, 15*(1), 10–30.

Wright, L. (1995). Human development in the context of aging and chronic illness: The role of attachment in Alzheimer's disease and stroke. *International Journal of Aging and Human Development, 44,* 133–150.

Zimmer, M. (1995). Activity participation and well being among older people with arthritis. *Gerontologist, 351,* 463–471.

Zunzunegui, M.V., Alvarado, B.E., Del Ser, T., & Otero, A. (2003). Social networks, social integration, and social engagement determine cognitive decline in community-dwelling Spanish older adults. *The Journals of Gerontology, Series B, Psychological Sciences and Social Sciences, 58*(2), S93–S100.

6

Body Image

Diana Luskin Biordi

INTRODUCTION

Of all the prisms through which culture can be viewed, body image is one of the most prevalent and profound. From the abstracts of beauty, sexuality, and community to the tangibles of health, mobility, and communication, the idea of the perfect body prevails. Against that culturally normed model of the perfect body, one forms an image of one's own body that is reflective of the culture and social interactions. The perfect body changes from culture to culture and across time. Models of ancient Greeks, for example, show muscular young men and women with broad shoulders, small waists, and narrow pelvises, whereas today, in America, waif-like thinness with body tone prevails as the model for women, and defined muscularity is the definition for men. When and how an individual differs from the cultural norm requires social and emotional management to explain the differences. Therefore, individuals use a frame of reference for their own bodies, which is shaped by the prevailing body norm of the culture, and perhaps, by subcultures within the larger culture. If one's body image differs from the body norm, social and physical rationalizations come into play. Insofar as those rationalizations themselves are exaggerated from

yet other norms, healthcare interventions may be required.

A person's frame of reference is his or her mental image of their physical self, that is, body image, which people use when referring to themselves. Individual body images may change over time, depending on life tasks such as learning one's gender role, performing a job or sport, creating a family, body or brain chemistry and structure, or aging. In chronic illness, body image is both a modifier of, and is modified by, the illness. Chronic illness, in its capacity to change the body, typically necessitates revisitations to one's body image. These revisitations are modified by the psychology of the individual and their perceptions of an ideal. That is, the individual will have to decide, consciously or unconsciously, whether to persevere in meeting an ideal body image (the culturally defined perfect body), reformulate or readjust the ideal to conform to one's own attributes, or reject the ideal.

Significant research in body image has occurred only recently, despite being the subject of the literature since the late 1800s. In fact, since 2004, an entire journal is devoted to *Body Image* (by Elsevier). In nursing, there appears to be a large gap from an initial spate of studies in the 1970s to those of the 1990s, with a substantial increase in research over the last decade. Most of the literature examining body image is found in practice disciplines such as nursing, medicine (e.g., neurology), bioengineering, psychology, and vocational counseling. This literature focuses on neurologic and psychological studies of person and gender, and in health, on studies of chronic illness (particularly, cancer), and most recently, in bariatrics and on obesity. In addition, plastic surgery or reconstruction is an interest of, or has been used by, a number of persons for cosmetic reasons and/or as interventions because of illness, accidents, obesity, or other treatments (see Frederick, Lever, & Peplau, 2007). If only because of the current emphasis on youth and beauty in American culture and because one of the national Leading Health Indicators (LHI) in *Healthy People 2010* is overweight and obesity, the research on body image is expected to increase.

Definitions of Body Image

Body image is defined and referred to in two ways. The most prevalent is the psychological, in which body image is the mental image of one's physical self, including attitudes and perceptions of one's physical appearance, state of health, skills, and sexuality. Recently, a new phrase, body schema, has been re-introduced into the literature, referring to the same definition of body image as that just described.

Body image is how one perceives one's own body, including its attractiveness, and how that body image influences interactions and others' reactions. Therefore, body image is not only the way people perceive themselves but, equally important, the way they think others see them. Consequently, body image is a major delimiter of social interactions, and as such has a profound effect on physical health, social interaction, psychological development, and interpersonal relationships. Moreover, because body image is conceptual, even if it is expressed inferentially, as in anorexia nervosa, most of the literature describes body image from information taken from cognitively intact, communicative human beings. Issues of profoundly retarded individuals and their body images, for example, are more likely examined from the perspective of others as they regard the person's body and whether it deviates from norms, as well as the reactions of others to the person.

The second way in which body image is used is more neurologic and technical. In this definition, body image has been shown to relate to the association of brain areas, particularly the *motor cortex,* with portions of the body, such as the limbs or lips. Particular parts of the brain are also associated with the sense of the body in space and that the self is localized, or embodied, within body borders (Blanke, 2007). Embodiment is important to the models of the self or self-consciousness, and also, more tangibly, of body parts properly belonging to one's person. Abnormalities in embodiment can lead to such distress as "amputation desire or amputation envy," when persons are profoundly frustrated by their sense that one of their body parts (limbs) does not "belong" to them, and actively seek its removal to satisfy their sense of body embodiment (Mueller, 2008). Voluntary movement of body limbs, or sensations, often of pain, have been shown to be linked to limbs, teeth, or breasts, when certain brain areas or neurons are invoked. Thus body image is defined and discussed in the theory, empiricism, and language of brain, neuropathology, neurology, anatomy, and/or physiology (Lewis, 1983; Mueller, 2007–2008; Ramachandran, 2004; Ramachandran & Rogers-Ramachandran, 2007).

The literature on body image also refers to body image in two other ways. First, body image is conceptualized as a *final product* or end state, a state of being, for example, "Charles's body image is that of a muscular young man." Second, body image can be portrayed as a *process,* in a continuous examination by its incumbent or others, whereby one's body is defined and redefined. In both of these conceptualizations, there are a number of factors that influence body image. Furthermore, the attitudes and perceptions about one's body guide evaluation and investment in body image, which affect physical and psychosocial functioning. Attitudes about body image are related to one's self-esteem, interpersonal functioning, eating and exercise patterns, self-care activities, and sexual behaviors (Cash & Fleming, 2002; Peelen & Downing, 2007).

In summary, body image is theorized as conceptual and neurologic, each concept feeding into the other. Body image is one's perception of one's body and its interactions with others, as well as having a sense of ownership and boundaries of one's body, the image of which is constructed psychologically and through the neurologic system of the brain, through proprioception (the sense of the body in space), vision, and the vestibular system. Body image can be thought of as both a process and an end product, and one's body image affects physical and psychosocial functioning.

Historical Foundations of Body Image

Although body image has been discussed in the literature since the 1880s, not until Schilder first presented his work in 1935 did a new understanding of this concept arise. In his book, *The Image and Appearance of the Human Body*, Schilder (1950) explored the dimensions of body image and stated, "The image of the human body means the picture of our own body which we form in our mind, that is to say the way in which the body appears to ourselves" (p. 11). He believed that the perception of one's body is based on a three-dimensional image that comprises physiologic, psychological, and social experiences.

Schilder's work affected several subsequent researchers, even into the twenty-first century. Critiquing Schilder's broad and complex theory, Cash and Pruzinsky (1990) claim that Schilder's chief contribution was not just the idea of body image, but that the idea that body image has "central pertinence not only for the pathologic but also everyday events of life" (p. 9). Subsequently, Cash and Pruzinsky (2002) claim that Schilder also "single handedly moved the study of body

image beyond the exclusive domain of neuropathology" (p. 4).

Most current discussions now view body image as having a perceptual component, a psychological component, and a social component (Cash & Fleming, 2002; Thompson & Gardner, 2002; Thompson & Van Den Berg, 2002). For example, with regard to eating and weight disorders, the perceptual component is the accuracy of the person's body size estimation, the psychological component is the person's attitudes or feelings toward their own body, and the social component might be the cultural context in which body image is assessed.

Like others, Thompson and Gardner (2002), and Cash and Fleming (2002) argue that body image is not a simple perceptual phenomenon, but is highly influenced by cognitive, affective, attitudinal, and other variables. Thompson has been attributed as the impetus in the 1990s to a more clinically and physiologically based concept of body image, particularly in examining eating disorders (Cash & Pruzinsky, 2002). Building on his work, research later focused on cultural overlays, including feminist critiques of the 1990s, and lately, the effects of family or ethnicity, on body image. The most recent work of the 2000s is again refocusing on physiologic bases of body image, while also attending to more evidence-based interventions on body image and its effects (Cash & Pruzinsky, 2004).

A current major empirical analysis of body image is neurologic, particularly those studies involving the brain and associated visual, vestibular, vascular, and proprioceptor stimuli. Most recently, impactful studies by Ramachandran and Rogers-Ramachandran (2007) indicate that body image can be shaped and changed by the brain. Using vision, and proprioceptor cues, they were able to map where in the brain (somatosensory, motor and parietal cortices) cues were received to fashion a virtual sense of body (2007) that did not correspond to actuality. The idea that body image can be so profoundly shaped by the brain has important implications for theory and for treatment. For example, Oliver Saks describes a patient whose loss of proprioception resulted in her inability to know her own bodily boundaries. She, therefore, could not control flailing her arms and legs about and could not sit or stand.

In a related set of studies, Ramachandran (2004) indicates that when motor signals are sent to muscles, duplicate signals are sent to the brain's parietal lobes, giving a sense of real limbs when there are actually amputations, leading to the phenomenon of phantom limb syndrome. Therefore, as is known in the field of prosthetics, amputees who are unable to incorporate a change in body image that genuinely indicate a lost limb were shown to be unable to use prosthetics effectively.

Of particular importance to healthcare professionals in chronic illness is the empirically derived idea that the perceptual elements of body image are complex. Fisher (1986) found that people not only compartmentalized their body image, but also differed in how they did so. Some localized their body image, whereas others had a more global view of their body. For instance, people with serious body defects might approach their bodies as separate regions, specifically isolating the defective region so that it will not influence their overall evaluation of self. Fisher believed that this ability suggests "important defensive and maturational significance in how differentiated one's approach to one's body is" (p. 635). He also argued that the rubric of body image itself is vague, representing a number of dimensions of the same and different constructs. New neurologic data indicate that certain brain regions governing specific body parts play a part in whether body images can be sustained or demarcated as separate. For example, clients with left-sided hemiplegia caused by a stroke often experience a disassociation from their paralyzed limbs.

Factors in the Definition of Body Image

Definitions of body image, although varied, share similarities. Common to many of the definitions is the belief that body image develops in response to multiple sensory inputs (visual, tactile, proprioceptive, and kinesthetic). Therefore, although physicality is included in one's body image, body image is subjective and dynamic because it is influenced by multiple factors (Cash, 2002; Pruzinsky, 2004). Body image is brought into the immediate focus of the individual by pain, physical or psychological illness, age, or weight (Krueger, 2002). Kinesthetic perceptions of function, sensation, and mobility are also part of our image. For example, children without sensation of body parts (e.g., spina bifida) often do not include in their art those body parts where they lack sensation.

Body image also includes feelings and thoughts. How one thinks and feels about one's body will influence social relationships and other psychological characteristics. Furthermore, how we feel and think about our bodies influences the way we perceive the world (Cash & Fleming, 2002).

Nezlek (1999) found three factors were included in the definition of body image. These included body attractiveness, social attractiveness (how attractive people believed others found them to be), and general attractiveness. For both men and women, self-perceptions of body attractiveness and social attractiveness were positively related to intimacy. Because body attractiveness is an important function of body image, this concept frequently is confused with body image itself, but body image encompasses more than attractiveness.

Many definitions of body image today involve the notions of the real and the ideal. Theorists would argue that the ideal image of one's self and the real image must be compatible, or dissonance results. A discrepancy between the real and the ideal body image may lead to conflicts that adversely affect personality, interactions, and health. For example, "normative discontent" refers to the pervasive negative feelings women and girls experience when they negatively distort their appearance, experience body image dissatisfaction, or overevaluate the appearance in defining a sense of self (Striegel-Moore & Franko, 2002).

For the healthcare professional, definitions of body image indicate the complexity of the concept, but more importantly, emphasize how significantly the client's cultural, social, historical, and biological factors affect body image. Perhaps even more important to healthcare professionals and their professionally derived norms is that body image and the factors affecting it are not merely cosmetic. A client's perceptions and attitudes about his or her body can affect health, social adjustment, interpersonal relationships, and general well-being. These perceptions are profoundly affected by chronic illness, as can be seen in this and other chapters.

Perhaps because body image is so vital to issues of ordinary health as well as chronic illness, it has come to be associated with, or even confused with, several other terms. The terms body image, self-concept, and self-esteem are frequently used interchangeably. Body image is not the same as body attractiveness but is related to both attractiveness and to self-esteem. Body image is a mental image of one's physical self, moderated by one's psychology and the social environment, and as is being discovered, by certain physiologic parameters of the brain. Body image, thus, is an integral component of self-concept. Self-concept is the total perception an individual holds of self—who one believes one is, how one believes one looks, and how one feels about one's self (Mock, 1993). Research extends self-concept to include not only ongoing perceptions of one's self, but also the idea that self-concept so mediates and regulates behavior that it is one of the most significant regulators of behavior (Markus & Wurf, 1987). Self-concept also is used to describe roles in which one casts the self, which can further stretch, and perhaps muddy, the concept. Finally, self-esteem is related to "the evaluative component of an individual's self-concept" (Corwyn, 2000, p. 357).

Factors Influencing Adjustment to Body Image

Meaning and Significance

As critical as each influence may be to the individual's adaptation, it is most important that the meaning of the event to the individual be understood.

Knowing that clients may compartmentalize both the meaning and the body part, the healthcare professional must recognize and accept how each client assesses the changes occurring in his or her body, their importance, and the way that the client chooses to incorporate (or not) change and image into their body image. Then, treatment of chronic illness, and by association, body image, functionality, or appearance cannot be far removed from the meaning attributed to such by the client or significant other.

In most cultures, body parts carry emotional attribution quite aside from functionality or appearance. The hands, for instance, are critical portrayals of the meanings and metaphysics of religions, whether shown invitingly open, in clasped position, or thumbs and forefingers together. Similarly, the mind is associated with the brain, with all the significance attached to that in a knowledge society, whereas the heart is universally seen as a major font of emotions. The heart is, to many, the symbol of love, courage, and life, and the seat of joy, hate, and sorrow. Indeed, in some cultures, the heart is seen as the location of the soul. Consider the emotional significance, then, that damage to the heart would engender in the body image of the affected client. Most nurses have been taught about clients who, after sustaining a myocardial infarction, are so anxious that they become a "cardiac cripple," owing to their fear of death from exercise or normal activity. Clearly, the self-image of such clients has sustained a serious insult. Clients with dementia create issues of self-images not only to the person undergoing the change, but also in the interactions and subsequent reappraisals of significant others. How many times have nurses heard families say that they "no longer know their loved one" as the disease progresses?

To counter the insult to body image and functionality, and knowing likely prognoses, the healthcare professional must reassure the client and family about their perceptions of body image, and help them reconcile to the present and future realities of the situation. That is, the healthcare professional will make efforts to reconcile the ideal body image of the client with the current attributes of the person, and encourage the client to move toward a more realistic body image, while recognizing that, for the client, losing their desired body image can create a grieving process that must also be managed.

Body image and the insults to functionality from chronic illness cannot be isolated from the meaning and significance the client gives to them. Furthermore, the meaning and significance to family members or significant others can also play an important role in the client's response. These are crucial factors to consider in offering and performing effective and sensitive care. Of all the aspects of body image in chronic illness, the appreciation and understanding of the meaning and significance to the client are areas that nursing can most contribute. The client's meaning and significance of the change in body image must not be overlooked or downplayed. Nursing's empathic and holistic approach can be of great value in this arena of health care.

The cause of the person's chronic illness and associated insult to one's body image can be an important coping factor. If the change is caused by an accident, healthcare mismanagement, or personal negligence, the person may harbor unresolved anger, blame, and shame. The person may also be guarded about sharing and discussing such matters, which confounds recovery and makes it more difficult. On the other hand, if the cause is recommended or life-saving interventions, the person perceives body image insult as an unavoidable consequence and a relatively small price to pay (Rybarczyk & Behel, 2002).

Another important factor the nurse must not forget is the "fifth vital sign," or pain. If pain is associated with the cause of the body image change, the meaning and significance of the altered body image can be negatively influenced. Pain may also nourish a persisting and even worsening negative body image and impair recovery in functionability (Rybarczyk & Behel, 2002). Hence, it is essential to assess the person for pain and discomfort, and to treat accordingly.

Influence of Time

The length of time during which body changes occur may influence one's body image and subsequent psychological adjustment (White, 2002). Changes in body image may occur slowly, over a lifetime, or quickly, within hours or days. Although some might argue that more time gives individuals greater opportunity to reformulate a body image, the fact remains that some individuals will never adapt their body image to the ideal they hold or their current attributes. A person with type 2 diabetes may have a slow progression of changes and ample time for denial and grief resolution, whereas trauma and sudden illness, such as head trauma, stroke, or certain surgeries, may lead to abrupt changes in the body and in body image. Individuals who experience sudden traumatic illnesses have no warning, and thus little opportunity to adjust to the changes (Bello & McIntire, 1995). A classic example is the lag between limb amputations and phantom pain, where clients are confused about whether they still have the appendage. To adjust to rapid change, the client must grieve the loss as well as physically adjust to the changes. Otherwise, the client who cannot cope with the dysfunction is at high risk for infection, noncompliance with therapeutic care, depression, social isolation, and obsession with or denial of the changes in body image (Dropkin, 1989).

The permanence of the change in appearance also affects adjustment to changes in body image. A person may better cope with changes in appearance that are temporary (i.e., temporary ileostomy) more so than those that are permanent (i.e., limb amputation). However, adjusting to body image changes depends partly on the meaning the individual ascribes to the changes and, in some cases, the length of time during which the change occurs (White, 2002).

Social Influences

Each sociocultural group establishes its own norms governing the acceptable, especially in terms of physical appearance and personality attributes (Jackson, 2002). Societies can hold a persistent, pervasive view using standards dictating ideal physical appearance and role performance. These standards, although some with caveats, serve all members of that social group, including those who have chronic illness and those who do not.

Groups target their social influence and affect the self-images of individuals. Family relationships are often important to the person with a chronic illness and their initial perception of their own body image. Negative family reactions about appearance, behavior, performance, and body image have been linked with recurrent poor body image consequences (Byely et al., 1999; Kearney-Cooke, 2002). Peer relationships are important mediating groups, particularly for those who are uncertain how to structure their life styles (e.g., adolescents). On one hand, peers can help shape conformance to a model. An example is the currently popular view of the muscle-bound, minimal-body-fat male model that is popular among young people (Olivardia, Pope, & Hudson, 2000). On the other hand, peer groups can call into question the appropriateness of such modeling for their own age group (e.g., older adults' perception of the aforementioned male model).

Persons with disfigurements are often, with little choice in the matter, forced to deal with their body image and the prevailing societal view. Depending on the visibility of the disfigurement and the coping of the disfigured person, sanctions such as staring, whispering, or shunning can negatively affect body image and personal value (Pruzinsky, 2002; Rumsey, 2002).

Untoward issues of body image often begin early in life. There is evidence now that in the United States and Britain, both girls and boys as young as 6 years old are overly conscious of their body weight and would begin dieting in an attempt to meet social norms of idealized thin and handsome young men and women. These young children, especially girls, are reported to be influenced by parental models and fashion magazines toward a desired thinness (Fornari & Dancyge,

2006; McCabe, Marita, Ricciaedelli, & Lina, 2005; Lowes & Tiggemann, 2003). The body image issues that begin in early years often persist throughout adolescence and into adulthood (Striegel-Moore & Franko, 2002).

The effect of society and environment on body image is reciprocal. Just as societal reactions can affect body image, the individual is not entirely passive, and so can react to such standards. Nevertheless, societal influences weigh heavily on behavior and body image, frequently leading to stereotypical assignments that affect individual body image adjustments. For example, persons with craniofacial disfigurement, or those who are chronically obese, have been subjected to societal reactions and expectations of ideal beauty throughout their lives. Over the years, having been constantly compared with the "ideal" beautiful or thin person, the individual with chronic illness has had to manage their own responses as well as those of others in the obvious discrepancy between an ideal body and their own real bodies.

Cultural Influences

Many aspects of culture affect body image. A cultural map has been suggested by Helman (1995) in which a view of the body is shared by the members growing up within a particular cultural or social group. This cultural map tells individuals how their body is structured and how it functions, includes ideal body definitions, and identifies "private" and "public" body parts as well as differentiating between a "healthy" and an "unhealthy" body (Helman, 1995).

The perceptions of health and illness and their effects on body image vary from culture to culture. In Altabe's study (1998) on ideal physical traits and body image, ethnic groups were similar in their identification of ideal body traits but different in assigning values to the body traits (e.g., valuing skin color or breast size). Findings indicated that African Americans had the most positive self-view and body image, whereas Asian Americans placed the least importance on physical appearance. Some non-caucasians had a more positive body image than did caucasians.

African Americans view health as a feeling of well-being, the ability to fulfill role expectations, and experiencing an environment free of pain and excessive stress. In the United States, the Hispanic culture perceives health as being and looking clean, feeling happy, getting adequate rest, and being able to function in expected roles. An imbalance in the emotional, physical, and social arenas may produce illness. Hispanic individuals often do not seek health care until they are very sick, and those with chronic illness may view themselves as victims of malevolent forces, attributed to God or punishment (Rhode Island Department of Health, 1998).

Native Americans view health as a balancing of mind, body, spirit, and nature. The practice of medicine is viewed as cooperative and offers choice and individual involvement in the pursuit of health. The Southeast Asian culture's health beliefs focus on the concept of Yin and Yang (balance) and maintaining this balance to achieve wellness. Obesity is viewed as a sign of contentment and socioeconomic status (Rhode Island Department of Health, 1998).

Influence of Healthcare Team Members

The care given to persons with a chronic disease or disability has a direct influence on their ability to adapt to societal pressures. Members of the healthcare team, although subject to the norms of the larger society, also have perceptions of illness and certain disabilities shaped by such professional norms as objectivity, compassion, or moral judgment. When caring for an individual with chronic illness, reactions from the healthcare team are important in the clients' adjustment and acceptance of body image.

Healthcare team members must understand that they are often the first person to see the changes engendered by the chronic illness or treatment. Their reactions often set the stage for body image expectations of clients. Seeing their caregiver's reactions may reinforce a body image for clients that continues for a long period of time, whether that image is positive or negative. Healthcare team members, therefore, must learn to manage their demeanor, voice, tone, and body reactions, avoiding any obvious rejections or trivialization of clients with chronic illness. One of the goals of the healthcare team should be to assist clients in having and/or maintaining a positive image and acceptance of self. For example, the client who has recently undergone breast reconstructive surgery following a mastectomy may have problematic issues of body image. The support and guidance by healthcare team members in helping the client with information about surgery, pain relief, self-care, positive reinforcement, family relationships, and emotional support are important to positive body image building (Van Deusen, 1993). Assessing concerns related to appearance and allowing clients to express fears, beliefs, thoughts, and life experiences also contributes to adjustment to body image changes (White, 2002).

Age

Erik Erikson's classic developmental theory is useful in examining phases of psychosocial development, particularly as this theory examines various stages throughout the life span that encourage or inhibit body image and personal feelings of value (Erikson, 1963). In younger age groups, conflicts about industry versus inferiority are changed into feelings of worth and competence (Cash & Pruzinsky, 1990). If there were negative effects during early developmental stages, altered or poor body image may result.

It is thought that younger children may be able to adapt more easily to changing body images because they have not fully come to recognize or appreciate their body image, unlike an adolescent or adult. Because their bodies are constantly changing, and because they are attending to their peers, adolescents can have an especially difficult time adapting to body image changes brought on by chronic illness. Patients with juvenile diabetes or adolescents with visible physical disfigurements, such as skin or neurologic diseases, frequently act out their frustrations via risky behaviors, depression, or withdrawal.

Body image in an adult has likely been well established and serves as an identity base. Adaptation to changes in body image can be more difficult to accept in an older group of individuals because illness challenges their fundamental identity. The older adults' acceptance of body image changes tends to be related more to the ability to be useful in society, loss of independence and health status, and, possibly, attractiveness to others (Krauss-Whitbourne & Skultety, 2002). Older adults may still feel young at heart but as their bodies age, they are subject to changes in skin, hair, posture, strength, or speed of action, which are compounded by various chronic illnesses such as cardiac, respiratory, orthopedic, visual, or hearing problems. They may feel young, but their outer appearances demonstrate their age and associated conditions in a culture that values the young. The elderly often want to maintain an accepted social body image, so it is important to consider these issues when possible body image disturbances arise.

Gender

The gender of a person may influence his or her response to a change in body image. Although both genders are subject to norms of beauty, women and girls are reported to be more affected by breaches of the norms of beauty than boys and men are (Emslie, Hunt, & McIntyre 2001). Women with burns, for example, generally have a more negative body image than do men with burns, although the effect of burns on body image depends on the locus of the burn and the percentage of body surface involved (Orr, Reznikoff, & Smith, 1989; Thombs, Notes, Lawrence, Magyar-Russell, Bresnick, & Faurerbach, 2008). It is important to note, however, that females tend to have negative body image perceptions more often than males across age and cultures; therefore, women

may experience more disturbances in body images than males when faced with chronic illnesses (Striegel-Moore & Franko, 2002).

Typically, the male gender is associated with a "masculine, strong" appearance, and the female gender is associated with a "feminine, softer" appearance. Role behaviors are less strictly segregated now than in the 1950s, 1960s, and 1970s, yet, many older clients were socialized to gender roles during those years and have strong expectations of clear role behaviors. Men were expected to be strong, active, rational, and silent, whereas women were expected to be indirect, passive, capable, and emotional. These views have an impact on their self-image and the differences engendered by chronic illness. Older chronically ill men or widowers who need assistance in learning to cook, or women learning to be more assertive even as their bodies are less conducive to these activities, often must change their body image. Often they do so gracefully, as we hear in the admonition, "Growing old is not for sissies." However, it behooves healthcare professionals, many of whom were not born in the times generating the social norms governing the body images of the older adults, to learn about the histories of those individuals whose chronic illnesses they treat. In that way, the healthcare professional can become more empathetic and understand the possible sources of body images of their clients. This is particularly important for chronically ill women with diabetes, whose diets are strictly managed but yet needs to be a good cook to accommodate their self-image as competent women. Another example is the hypertensive man whose medication limits his libido or sexual performance.

Prior Experience and Coping Mechanisms

Body image is thought to be individually developed through each person's concept of his or her "ideal" perception and based on his or her previous experiences within society as well (Cash & Pruzinsky, 2002). Because past experiences, positive or negative, can substantially affect present circumstances, understanding how a client is likely to perceive an event, and cope with it, is one of the more important assessments performed by the healthcare professional. This awareness is particularly beneficial to the individual who has not had much exposure to the healthcare system and may require advocacy by the healthcare professional.

Coping mechanisms already developed by the individual through support from family, the healthcare team, or the client's social group, are helpful in promoting adaptation to changes in body image during chronic illness. Understanding the individual's perception of body image before and during a diagnosis of chronic illness can be helpful to the healthcare professional in easing the client's adjustment to body image changes. Knowing that body image is an inferential diagnosis, it is helpful for the healthcare professional to estimate which stage of body image is most likely to reflect the client's situation, whether persevering, reformulating, or rejecting one's body image.

Most clients have an exacerbation of their typical coping mechanisms during illness. Therefore, under the stress of chronic illness and depending on its familiarity to the client, the healthcare professional is most likely to initially observe an exaggerated coping style, however inadequate it may be. Using that information as a first step in assessing a client, and moving from there to infer body image changes on the continuum presented in this chapter, is a good beginning for the healthcare professional and client.

Assessment of Body Image

Evidenced-based practice guidelines are not yet available for the assessment or treatment of impaired body image. Yet, there are many skilled assessment techniques from which the sensitive or skilled healthcare professional may derive interventions. Practice in psychological assessment is useful. The focus here is, therefore, on assessment.

Assessing the behaviors of individuals who have experienced an alteration in function or change leading to a disruption in body image is vital in planning appropriate interventions. This assessment leads to a determination of perceptions and meanings associated with the change that is unique to the client, and allows recognition of barriers to health. Such an assessment requires the observation and interviewing of the client to determine the nature and meaning of the threat. Only after such an assessment and validation of its correctness may the healthcare professional provide interventions.

A key to a successful assessment is a therapeutic relationship with the client. Trust, sensitivity to the client's thoughts and feelings, and provision of accurate and realistic support all help to build and strengthen the therapeutic relationship between the client and provider (Hayslip et al.,1997).

A complete assessment of a client's experience and meaning of change is facilitated by asking questions related to the client's perception of the experience, knowledge of the illness and its effects, and others' perceptions of the client's illness. Accounting for these factors in the assessment process creates a client-centered knowledge base for choosing appropriate interventions. In addition, assessing the client's psychosocial history and support systems allows the provider to elicit greater support for the client in areas already known to the client.

Assessing a client's unique influencing factors is essential in planning interventions. Knowing how much value is placed on the appearance or functioning of the body helps the healthcare professional to determine the impact of the image disruption. Assessing self-esteem and the client's perceived attitudes of others is also important in discovering the meaning and impact of the disruption to the client. Ascertaining the phase of recovery of the client is essential, and is particularly important in planning specific client-centered interventions. Knowing when to implement educational, supportive, or rehabilitative interventions makes these interventions most useful. Questions that might help the healthcare professional assess whether a client has a poor body image, particularly because of illness or injury,

CASE STUDY

Amy, a 13-year-old girl, was rather overweight, and came from a family with overweight parents and an overweight brother, Jack, who was 15 years old. Amy was in her bedroom, confiding in her best friend, Sara, who was also slightly overweight. "Like, I don't know, Sara, we had gym today, and I just hate having to undress in front of the other girls. They all seem to look me over and, I don't know, I don't think anyone likes me. They don't ask me over to their tables at the cafeteria, and anyhow, they're all like skinny sticks. Act like it, too."

"I'm not like Jack. Like, he doesn't seem to mind how he looks, and even makes jokes about his weight. I mean, I know I should lose weight and stuff, but like, I just can't seem to do it. Like, look at my thighs . . . thunder thighs! And even when I do try to lose some pounds, they just keep coming back, worse than ever. But Jack, he makes fun of himself and that seems to take the sting out of it . . . none of the other kids can poke fun at him because he does it first. He's the class clown and they all love him.

"I don't know. I think I'm always going to be fat. And anyhow, there's those actresses on TV who are overweight and they seem to make money on it, so maybe it's not so bad. And look at my mom, she got married and all. But, like, I think she was skinnier when she got married. It seems everybody wants to be super thin, but then, we're not. So I don't know . . . is it bad to be this way? What do you think?"

Discussion Questions

1. If you could infer body images from the case study, what might you think is Amy's body image? Jack's?
2. What opportunities do you see for a nurse in the case study as described? What would you do?
3. What would you, as a nurse, have said to Amy as she wondered about her weight? As a friend? Are there differences from what you might have said in either case? If so, what are these differences, and why?

might focus on hiding or denial. Denial of one's self, self-effacement, or denial of the injury's severity is one hint at a poor self-image. A more typical indication of poor self-image or self-esteem is hiding, physically or mentally, from others. Actions such as avoiding others, avoiding close contact (such as undressing in front of others or sexual intimacy), avoiding displays of the injury or scars, or feelings of shame or embarrassment when discussing the injury or illness, are important clues to self-image.

In some instances, it may be necessary to use a standardized assessment tool to measure body disturbances and number and types of support systems. Many tools are available for this use (Cash & Pruzinsky, 2002). Tools about body disturbances

generally have questions on general appearance, body competence, others' reaction to appearance, value of appearance, and so forth. These tools have incorporated related concepts to body image, such as self-esteem and self-concept, and are able to measure affective, cognitive, and behavioral components of body image (Thompson & Van Den Berg, 2002).

Incorporating families into assessment is encouraged. This can be done by interviewing, observing, and taking note of both verbal and nonverbal interactions within the family system (Wright & Leahey, 2000). Assessing family meanings of the chronic illness, perceived losses, and stresses placed on the family because of the illness are important in planning interventions.

BODY IMAGE ISSUES IMPORTANT TO CHRONIC ILLNESS

Chronic illness has many challenges, one of which includes the adaptation to changes in body image. The process of adaptation depends on many factors, but primary among those are the external changes to the person, functional limitations, the changes' significance and importance to the person, the time over which the change (and losses) occurred, social influences, and the impact of culture.

External Changes

Important external factors that influence body image are the visibility and functional significance of the body part involved, the importance of physical appearance to the individual, and the rate at which the change occurred (Rybarczyk & Behel, 2002). For example, epilepsy is a chronic disease that illustrates all of these factors. Epileptic seizures, such as a tonic–clonic seizure, can affect the entire body; the seizures are easily observed and happen suddenly. Epilepsy may also prevent the client from maintaining a job, driving a car, or engaging in sports or popular activities such as swimming. Typically epilepsy's onset is acute. The person does not have time to prepare for accepting this chronic disease. A seizure occurs and the person's life is changed from that moment onward. This can make it more challenging to accept and live "normally" with the image of "being an epileptic," and potentially having a very visible, sudden, and dysfunctional (possibly dangerous) experience. The severity of insult to appearance and functional significance, and the degree of importance to the person, must be considered on an individual basis. For example, some persons may find epilepsy a minor nuisance but mild psoriasis traumatizing, because the latter is visible and mildly dysfunctional. It is essential to assess the meaning and significance of the change to the person.

Another common example is the obese client. Obesity is now listed as one of the leading health indicators that are problematic in the United States (*Healthy People 2010*). Obesity is typically a nonacute, slowly progressing condition, which has come to be viewed as a major risk factor in several chronic illnesses, such as diabetes, heart disease, and osteoarthritis. Obesity is also considered déclassé in Western culture, often viewed as an indicator of overindulgence and sloth, and frequently associated with lower classes. Although the obesity risk has been challenged (Campos, 2005; Flegal, Graubard, Williamson, & Gail, 2007), most healthcare professionals still believe obesity must be medically managed. Today there are public health campaigns to reduce obesity, beginning in childhood. Obese persons are reacting to the medicalization of obesity, and a movement is underway denying obesity's current importance and stigmatization. The movement, however, is implicitly acknowledging that a person's body image can be negatively and powerfully influenced by obesity and others' reactions to it.

Mental illnesses can also influence body image, and yet, many healthcare professionals overlook this aspect of chronic mental illness. For instance, a person with schizophrenia may have a negatively altered body image as part of the disturbed thinking of the illness and/or from the perceived change the illness has on the behavior and presentation of the person. Furthermore, the medication used to treat schizophrenia can affect body image because of its side effects of palsy or weight gain. Therefore, ignoring the possible side effects in treating the mentally ill is likely to affect not only medication compliance, but, also, related possible physical self-image.

External changes and their rapidity of change are important in assessing body image. Healthcare professionals should not assume, but verify with the client, what the current body image is, and what it means to the client. Each person is unique, and, therefore, each experience with chronic illness and its impact on body image is unique.

Appearance

The physical appearance of a disease is frequently a change for which clients are unprepared. Given the possibility of perseverance, reformulation, or rejection of changes, further studies are needed of the ways in which body image and its accompanying variables affect acceptance by others. Empirical evidence and anecdotal data exist to guide us in considering suitable interventions. For example, when the appearance also draws attention to its underlying cause, clients and their significant others are often ostracized, particularly when the disease is one that carries a stigma (see Chapter 3). Many clients with AIDS develop Kaposi's sarcoma (KS), a common and sometimes disfiguring tumor related to HIV. Because the skin is a common site for KS, the characteristic purple hue of KS is easily visible, and is considered by many patients as a "public signature" of HIV (deMoore et al., 2000). In more severe cases of illness, in which the body is catastrophically debilitated, as in amyotrophic lateral sclerosis (ALS), Helman (1995) notes that the entire body image may accommodate the body as separated from the sense of self—that is, "It is my body that is diseased, but not me."

Visibility and Invisibility

Chronic illness and its treatment provide visible, outward changes in appearance and invisible, internal changes. Both types of change can significantly affect individuals' perceptions of themselves. In an adult, it is suggested that the more visible or extensive the body alteration, the more likely it is to be perceived as a threat to one's body image. Loss of hair, scarring, edema, amputations, and disfigurement are common examples in the body image literature. In reading the life accounts of severely disfigured persons, many choose to work at unusual times (nights) and in jobs in which they have little contact with others (see Chapter 5). In a meta-analysis of 12 articles that met their inclusion criteria, Bessel and Moss (2007) report that truly efficacious interventions are lacking for adults with visible differences. In an related study, Thompson and Kent (2001) report that persons with disfigurements shape their self-image by interactions with others in social contexts, and that interventions are available. Like Bessel and Moss, they note that

reports and interventions were not methodologically rigorous or informed by theory.

In another study of patients with severe burns and their adjustment to their disfigurement, Thombs and colleagues (2008) found that over time, women, more than men, suffered dissatisfaction with body image, particularly with larger burns, and that their dissatisfaction interfered with psychological functioning over time. The findings of these studies argue a need for more research of a longitudinal and qualitative nature, toward a better understanding of the processes and outcomes of visible differences and their impact on body image.

The matter of body image and incorporation of changes seems to be more ambiguous in children. Children are strongly subject to the norms imposed by their peers, with their self-image being readily influenced. A visible change or disfigurement in a child could ostracize the child from his or her peer group. Of particular strength and importance to children, especially for those with "stigmatized" body images, is the family member or healthcare professional who can support the child's acceptance of the body image changes. Puberty is one time of life in normal development in which personal identity and body image are affected. It is during this time then, that parents and adults who work with children should support healthy body images and intervene when a child begins to develop poor body images (see, for example, Fornari & Dancyge, 2006).

When a change is not markedly visible, as when an ostomy is created, or its treatment (e.g., colostomy appliances) is introduced, persons with chronic illness must take previously "invisible" body parts and make them "visible" (Helman, 1995). This dynamic is further compounded when the new intervention is preferentially hidden from others. Such procedures and the management of visible and hidden change likely lead to dramatic changes in an individual's lifestyle and self-image. For example, clients with a stoma must periodically empty the appliance bag, learn to change it, irrigate the stoma when needed, cope with social matters such as dressing to fit the appliance, and manage social etiquette with problems of leaking, odors, and the noises resulting from involuntary discharge into the appliance. The person dealing with such challenges may keep this hidden, and limit social functioning to avoid possible embarrassment (Kirkpatrick, 1986). Since the late 1980s, in a movement begun by former First Lady Betty Ford when she announced her decision to manage alcoholism and breast cancer, many are now openly announcing illnesses and treatments that were usually hidden. Nonetheless, the visibility or invisibility of an illness, injury, or treatment regimen, must be managed, and in that management exists the potential to enhance or diminish body images held by the individual.

Functional Limitations

Functionality is something that is conceptualized as "external," in that functionality is usually a visible part of enactment of one's role. It may be that the function is carried out privately, as in a sexual function, but function is the ability of a body part to be able to be used to conduct its usual purpose. The ability to function in a meaningful way is essential to a sense of well-being; consequently, any limitation of functional ability may alter one's concept of body image. Most clients and their significant others are not prepared for the appearance and functional limitations associated with chronic illness.

The function of a body part and its importance and visibility are critical to one's body image. The leg, because of its functional importance in mobility and a person's life, is more likely to be a more important part of body image than, say, a toe (Brown, 1977). Loss of a toe, for example, is likely to be viewed as less problematic than loss of a leg, because much function can be retained by compensatory body parts and because a toe is less visible. Therefore, one might expect different accommodations in body image to such amputations, even as it is recognized that perception of loss and its impact vary from person to person and culture to culture. Indeed, the oldest prosthesis found has been that of a wooden large toe that

was found attached by leather thongs to the foot of an ancient Egyptian female mummy. This well-carved prosthesis, unhidden by a sandal, aided the woman in walking and maintaining balance (Pittsburgh Post Gazette, 2007).

The roles of worker, gendered persona, and sexual being are three important facets of body image. Chronic illness or treatment can threaten the client's ability to perform each of these roles. Furthermore, the stage of one's life can make a major difference in the perception of the strength of the threat or its incorporation into one's body image. A teenager, perhaps, is likely to regard work or sexual function and their concomitant body image differently than would a seasoned elder who has had different experiences and usually, changed body appearance and function.

Loss of sexual function for most persons, particularly those who are sexually active, is often perceived as a profound loss. Women with breast removal from cancer, or men and women with genital cancers, frequently avoid sexual situations after treatments (Golden & Golden, 1986). The male client may feel especially vulnerable if he feels his sexuality or provider role is compromised by chronic illness. Testicular cancer is the most common cancer in young men ages 18 to 35 and typically results in the removal of the diseased testicle. Older men with prostate cancer may require the removal of both testicles, with a resultant loss of libido and virility and compromised perception of "manhood." Although implants can be used, the perception of functional loss can strongly persist. The nurse can be, and may often be, the main source of professional support and education, and thus assists clients with the sensitive issues involved with body image.

INTERVENTIONS

Interventions, particularly those of assessment, have been described throughout this chapter. Healthcare professionals and their interventions are used to help clients manage their own reactions and the reactions of others to changes in body structure, function, or appearance as the result of chronic illness. These changes are frequently interpreted as setting one apart and as different from one's peers (see Chapter 3), leading to self-doubt, inhibited participation in social activities, and a disruption of perceptions of self. Finding appropriate interventions for clients experiencing an altered body image can aid the client in healing and adapting to changes in body image (Norris, Connell, & Spelic, 1998).

Adapting to changes in body image resulting from chronic illness is a dynamic process. On a daily basis, clients are faced with thoughts and reminders of their illness and changes to their bodies. During periods of exacerbation, remission, and rehabilitation, clients are grieving the loss of their former selves, living with the uncertainty of their chronic illness, and learning to create new images of self (Cohen, Kahn, & Steeves, 1998). Knowing that the process is continually changing, with steps forward and backward, helps the nurse to support clients as they adapt to changes in body image.

Specific Interventions

Interventions are chosen after careful assessment of the client. As mentioned previously, a therapeutic relationship with the client is an essential beginning to the process. Before successful intervention can occur the following must be addressed: acknowledging of barriers to communication, feelings about the illness, changes the illness caused, and personal biases on the part of the healthcare professional. Accurate knowledge about the disease process and the client's response are also necessary if the healthcare professional is to assist the client. In addition, the healthcare professional must be able to recognize that body image changes will require a supportive, accepting, and consistent relationship that can withstand setbacks and emotional tension. It is important to be aware of the client's attitude and participation in the recovery process. This may involve professional rehabilitation, including physical and occupational therapy, or it may involve informal self- or family-directed interventions. The healthcare professional who is both knowledgeable about evidence-based practice, guidelines, and treatment regimens can be influential in acknowledging subtle progress that the client may or may not be aware of, and supporting the benefit of rehabilitation as part of the overall recovery process. By evidence-based practice, the knowledgeable healthcare professional can provide not only quality care in the chronic illness, but also begin helping the client toward forming a more balanced and realistic body image.

Communication

Providing opportunities for clients to express feelings and thoughts about the changes they are experiencing can be beneficial to both clients and healthcare professionals. It allows clients to speak and be heard, and also allows careful assessment of the clients' thoughts and feelings directly. Assumptions should not be made about the meaning of experiences relating to changes in body image (Cohen, Kahn, & Steeves, 1998). In addition, ensuring client comfort in expressing both positive and negative feelings and emotions helps strengthen the therapeutic relationship and facilitate the journey to wholeness. Allowing family members to express their thoughts, feelings, and concerns is also beneficial and should be incorporated into the recovery process.

Talk therapy, either individual or group, can be of much benefit in the recovery process. Cognitive-behavioral therapy has a proven record—that is, it is evidence-based practice—in helping clients change their dysfunctional thinking and related behaviors associated with chronic illness and negative body image (Peterson et al., 2004; Rumsey & Harcourt, 2004; Rybarczyk & Behel, 2002; Veale, 2004).

Self-Help Groups

Self-help groups for clients experiencing body image changes may help to buffer the stressors

EVIDENCE-BASED PRACTICE BOX

In one of the few studies reporting successful psychotherapeutic treatment of phantom pain, nurse authors Rebecca Zuckweiler and Merrie J. Kaas report that they had success treating phantom pain in 14 amputees with a guided-imagery intervention developed by Zuckweiler. Zuckweiler's Image Imprinting (ZIPS) is a multistep approach combining cognitive behaviors and the synthesis of several psychotheories, based on an overall systems framework. Symptoms are viewed as understandable when related to the whole (systems theory), and are only a part of the complete balance of body and mind. In the ZIPS approach, the experience of pain is alterable by manipulating both thought and areas of the body, particularly those areas where pain seems to be situated.

In their pre- and post-study, 14 clients, mostly men older than 50 years of age who had leg amputations because of illness and accidents and who had phantom pain or sensation post amputation, were given the therapy. Several aims guided the study: (1) the determination of changes in frequency of pain from pre- to post-intervention and at 3 and 6 months after the intervention; (2) changes in perceived control over life and disability pre- and post-intervention, (3) association of age, time since amputation, and cause of amputation with phantom pain/sensation pre-intervention and at 6 months post-intervention; (4) the association of number of treatments, daily practice of ZIPS, and the duration of ZIPS and phantom pain/sensation at 6 months post-intervention, and, finally, (5) the determination of the association of pre- and post-intervention control over life and disability with the phantom pain/sensation at pre-intervention and 6 months post-intervention.

Each intervention session was taped and later analyzed by the therapist, who also kept confidential progress notes. The clients were given recording logs to summarize their experiences and frequency of ZIPS practice outside their therapy sessions. ZIPS is a several-step imagery process of identifying and matching sensation to an accurate body image (see Zuckweiler & Kaas, 2005, for details). In their study, the intervention consisted of two, 1 hour sessions, followed by half-hour sessions thereafter, individualized to patient need. A telephone follow-up assessment 3 and 6 months after the ZIPS intervention assessed frequency and distress of phantom pain or sensation. Spearman's correlations, analysis of variance (ANOVA), Wilcoxon signed ranks tests, and the Mann-Whitney U tests were used in the data analyses. Tests of significance were two-tailed and confidence levels set at 95%.

Findings indicated that phantom pain was quickly treated but lessening phantom sensation was more difficult. The client's rating of his disability influenced pain reduction, but not phantom sensation. Conversely, level of control influenced the reduction of sensation, but not pain. The number of treatments was not a factor in reducing pain or sensation, although practice sessions did make a difference.

The *rate* at which clients proceeded through their sessions, redefining their body image seemed to be important to their success. The clients used sessions to try on body image and make the mind accept that there was no longer a body part to associate with phantom pain or sensation. The authors pointed out that the mirror box, another major intervention, does not seem to sustain relief of phantom pain or sensation when the box is removed. They attribute this to the mind's lack of connection of sensation to the individualized body part. The clients shifted

(Continued)

EVIDENCE-BASED PRACTICE BOX (*Continued*)

the use of the ZIPS technique from a structured three to four times a day to an as-needed basis, as their phantom pain or sensation lessened. Pain compounded by prosthetic fittings inhibited results from ZIPS treatments, suggesting that ZIPS should be employed at times when patients are not experiencing another form of severe pain. During treatments, many of the clients, despite reporting acceptance of their amputation and disability, showed signs of further grief processing. The management of grief had to occur before treatment began for the phantom pain or phantom sensation. Similarly, management of phantom pain or sensation helped some of those with post-traumatic stress syndrome make progress in managing their stress syndrome.

According to the nurse authors, the ZIPS approach can be effective and economical, as well as self-empowering, and can be used by a variety of mental health workers on an inpatient or out-patient basis.

Source: Zuckweiler, R. & Kaas, M. (2005). Treating phantom pain and sensation with Zuckweiler's image imprinting. *Journal of Prosthetics and Orthotics, 17*(4), 103–112.

experienced by the changes. Providing clients with opportunities to share experiences with others in similar situations can be therapeutic for some individuals. Self-help or support groups offer important emotional, social, and spiritual fellowship, as well as education about the focus of the support group. Before urging support groups as an intervention, it is important to assess the willingness of individuals to participate in a group setting. Support groups that are most helpful are those where the members are encouraged, but not forced, to share information, and where the leader can lead the discussions to bring out salient points intelligently, empathetically, and fairly. Groups should be avoided that are unstable, promote products or purchases, or that charge inordinate fees. Groups that encourage gripe sessions, allow individuals to dominate a discussion, or that demand cult-like allegiances or sharing of information clients don't wish to share should be avoided (Centers for Disease Control, 2008).

Some individuals are not comfortable in a group setting, especially when they are dealing with a body image disruption. For those who find it helpful, the benefits are many. Seeing others on the road to recovery, helping those who are struggling, developing friendships, or finding

where they themselves are in the journey can help with the healing process (Corey & Corey, 1997). Furthermore, these groups provide an opportunity for clients to begin socializing with others in a safe and nonthreatening environment.

Support groups became popular during the late 1970s, particularly after Spiegel's research (2008) indicated that breast cancer patients who participated in a support group lived, on average, 18 months longer than those who did not belong to a support group. Subsequent research could not duplicate those earlier findings, but women who have joined support groups showed other benefits, primarily experiencing less depression, distress, anxiety, and pain, and importantly, obtaining information about their disease and its treatment. In fact, in another survey of 367 women with advanced breast cancer, almost as many got their information from the internet (39%) as from their doctors (42%) (Y-Me National Breast Cancer Organization, 2007). These data as well as other data from that survey indicate that health-care professionals must find more meaningful ways to convey needed information to this group of patients. Since the early findings on support groups and breast cancer needs, support groups have found a place in the therapeutic regimens.

Almost all oncology centers can direct patients into such groups, as patients increasingly find them a useful adjunct and information site as they manage work, family, sexuality, and uncertain cancer prognoses.

Nurses and other healthcare professionals can locate a variety of support groups, or even begin one themselves as a therapeutic intervention. At this writing, the Internet is an excellent source of support groups and the resources needed to begin or maintain support groups. One site alone included almost 500 different support groups listed alphabetically, all relating to various illnesses or states of life (e.g., divorce, parenting). Nurses, by virtue of their place in the healthcare delivery system, are poised to address both physical and psychosocial needs of patients, and are able to deliver information in helpful ways: support groups are one intervention that nurses can develop to help patients meet their needs for information and emotional support.

Self-Care

Encouraging clients to participate in the activities of daily living that are meaningful to them helps restore feelings of normalcy. Whether engaging in personal grooming activities, such as applying cosmetics, jewelry, or hair accessories, caring for one's self can be an effective intervention. Self-care will help the client incorporate the change into the normal functioning of daily living. This intervention may also help the client become less sensitive to physical appearances and learn to manage everyday activities (Norris, Connell, & Spelic, 1998). Regular exercise can be helpful improve body-image, along with supporting physical health and function (Wetterhahn, Hanson, & Levy, 2002) (see Chapter 13).

Prostheses

Prostheses have been used for centuries, helping to modify functionality, external appearances, and, most likely, body image. Because so much of chronic illness is visible or involves body parts with need for additional support, prostheses have varied in sophistication and availability. Most healthcare professionals are familiar with prosthetic eyes, hearing aids, various "limbs" (e.g., hand, foot, leg, arm), or breast, penile, or testicular implants. In chronic disease involving amputations, the age of the client presents unusual concerns. The prosthetic hand, foot, or knee of a child, for example, may require, for the child's adequate social development, that the prosthetic stand up to repeated use in play, such as in swimming, with the effects of water, sand, and chlorine. Adults may wish to maintain a physically normal appearance and avoid the functional "hook" hand prosthesis. In older adults whose gait problems may be exacerbated by joint problems, the "fit" of a prosthesis, as in a hip replacement, is a special concern. The rehabilitation required after hip replacement is particularly necessary, and its success has much to do with subsequent body image improvement related to increased mobility.

Spinal cord injury has sparked research that focuses on current knowledge of spinal cord treatment, electrical stimulation, mechanisms of secondary damage, and possibilities for regeneration of nerves. Bioengineering, electric-powered prostheses, invasive and noninvasive sensors to control prostheses, or use of brain waves or pupillary contraction to power computers for communication are currently being used or being tested. Their success is a huge event for the affected person, and this specialized area of knowledge typically requires focus and specialization by healthcare professionals.

The use of prostheses and the unique technologies to power these prostheses will continue to expand in the future. It is important to understand that the field of prosthetics requires knowledge about the illness as well as the care with which clients implement and maintain their prosthetics and the impact of prosthetics on body image.

Education and Anticipatory Guidance

This intervention is effective only when the client has indicated a readiness to learn. Knowledge of disease processes, information about symptoms, and methods of treatment are important educational topics for the client. It is also helpful to consider the preferred learning style (e.g., visual, auditory, and/or practice) of the client, such as a visual or auditory learning style preference (Cohen, Kahn, & Steeves, 1998). The benefits of client education and anticipatory guidance should be stressed to stimulate and support the client's readiness to learn. (see Chapter 14).

OUTCOMES

Body image, the physical aspect of self-concept, is closely linked with the concept of self-esteem in the Nursing Outcomes Classification (NOC) (Moorhead, Johnson, & Maas, 2004). Disturbances of these along with personal identity disturbance, chronic low self-esteem, and situational low self-esteem are considered part of what Carpenito (2000) globally calls self-concept disturbance. These alterations can be a result of an immediate problem, such as sudden disfiguration from surgery or burns, or can be related to long-term changes from chronic illnesses such as cancer and its treatment effects, arthritis, Parkinson's disease, or a cerebrovascular accident.

Defining characteristics of this nursing classification can be multiple: denial, withdrawal of the individual, refusal to be part of the care required, refusal to look at the body part involved or let immediate family look at it, refusal to discuss rehabilitation efforts, signs and symptoms of grieving, self-destructive behavior such as alcohol or drug abuse, and hostility toward healthy individuals. One's sense of femininity or masculinity may also be threatened, which can lead to difficulty in sexual functioning, and, combined, these changes can lead to social anxiety, self-consciousness, and depression (Carpenito, 2000; Otto, 1991; White, 2002).

The 14 indicators for this outcome listed in the NOC include: internal picture of self; congruence between body reality, body ideal, and body presentation; description of affected body part; willingness to touch the affected body part; satisfaction with body appearance; satisfaction with body function; adjustment to changes in physical appearance; adjustment to changes in body function; adjustment to changes in health status; willingness to use strategies to enhance appearance; willingness to use strategies to enhance function; adjustment to body changes resulting from injury; adjustment to body changes resulting from surgery; and adjustment to body changes resulting from aging (Moorhead et al., 2004). However, the ultimate goal or outcome for individuals is adaptation to the change, a "positive perception of own appearance and body functions" (p. 161).

STUDY QUESTIONS

1. Name three concepts related to body image and explain their relationship.
2. Describe how you would assess a client with a changed body image.
3. Discuss how age, gender, and culture can affect body image.
4. How often in your own friendships do issues of body image come up in conversation?

What are the general themes of such discourse? Did this chapter help you in furthering the discussion or in understanding everyday concerns about body image?

5. What elements would you include in an educational intervention for a patient group with body image issues? Justify your choices.

INTERNET RESOURCES

Albert Einstein Sociedade Beneficente Israelita Brasileira Mental Help page (in Portugese): www.mentalhelp.com
American Heart Association on Obesity: www.americanheart.org/presenter.jhtml?identifier=4639
Daily Strength Support Group Resource: www.dailystrength.com
Kids Health: kidshealth.org/kid/exercise/weight/overweight.html
US Department of Health and Human Services Body Image Web page: http://www.womenshealth.gov/bodyimage/
US Department of Health and Human Services Women's Health: womenshealth.gov/
Weight-control Information Network: www.win.niddk.nih.gov/publications/health_risks.htm

REFERENCES

Altabe, M. (1998). Ethnicity and body image: Quantitative and qualitative analysis. *International Journal of Eating Disorders, 23*, 153–159.

Bello, L., & McIntire, S. (1995). Body image disturbance in young adults with cancer. *Cancer Nursing, 18*(2), 138–143.

Bessell, A. & Moss, T.P. (2007). Evaluating the effectiveness of psychosocial interventions for individuals with visible differences: A systematic review of the empirical literature. *Body Image, 4*(3), 227–238.

Blanke, O. (2007). I and me: Self-portraiture in brain damage. *Frontiers of Neurology and Neuroscience, 22*, 14–29.

Brown, M.S. (1977). The nursing process and distortions or changes in body image. In F.L. Bower (Ed.), *Distortions in body image in illness and disability* (pp. 1–19). New York: Wiley.

Byely, L., Archibald, A., Graber, J., & Brooks-Gunn, J. (1999). A prospective study of familial and social influences on girls' body image and dieting. *International Journal of Eating Disorders, 28*, 155–164.

Campos, Paul. (2005). *The Diet Myth* (2004), New York: Gotham.

Carpenito, L. (2000). *Nursing diagnosis: Application to clinical practice* (8th ed.). Philadelphia: Lippincott.

Cash, T., & Pruzinsky, T. (2004). *Body Image: A handbook of theory, research, and clinical practice.* New York: Guilford Press.

Cash, T.F. (2002). Cognitive behavioral perspectives on body image. In T. Cash & T. Pruzinsky (Eds.), *Body image: A handbook of theory, research, and clinical progress* (pp. 38–46). New York: Guilford Press.

Cash, T.F., & Fleming, E.C. (2002). The impact of body image experiences: Development of the body image quality of life inventory. *International Journal of Eating Disorders, 31*, 455–460.

Cash, T.F., & Pruzinsky, T. (1990). *Body images: Development, deviance, and change.* New York: Guilford Press.

Cash, T. F., & Pruzinsky, T. (2002). Understanding body image: Historical and contemporary perspectives. In T. Cash & T. Pruzinsky (Eds.), *Body image: A handbook of theory, research, and clinical progress* (pp. 30–37). New York: Guilford Press.

Centers for Disease Control and Prevention. (2008). Chronic fatigue syndrome: Support groups. Retrieved March, 2008, from www.cdc.gov/cfs www.cdc.gov/CFS/cfssupport.htm

Cohen, M.Z., Kahn, D.L., & Steeves, R.H. (1998). Beyond body image: The experience of breast cancer. *Oncology Nursing Forum, 25*(5), 835–841.

Corey, M., & Corey, G. (1997). *Groups: Process and practice* (5th ed.). Boston: Brooks/Cole.

Corwyn, R.F. (2000). The factor structure of global self-esteem among adolescents and adults. *Journal of Research and Personality, 34*, 357–379.

deMoore, G.M., Franzcp, N., Hennessey, P., Kunz, N. M., Ferrando, S.J., Rabkin, et al. (2000). Kaposi's sarcoma: The scarlet letter of AIDS. The psychological effects of a skin disease. *Psychosomatics, 41*(4), 360–363.

Dropkin, M.J. (1989). Coping with disfigurement and dysfunction after head and neck cancer surgery: A conceptual framework. *Seminars in Oncology Nursing, 5*(3), 213–219.

Emslie, C., Hunt, K., & Macintyre, S. (2001). Perceptions of body image among working men and women. *Epidemiology and Community Health, 55,* 406–407.

Erikson, E. (1963). *Childhood and society* (2nd ed.). New York: Norton.

Fisher, S. (1986). *Development and structure of the body image* (vol. 2). Hillsdale, NJ: Lawrence Erlbaum Associates.

Flegal, K.M., Graubard, B.I., Williamson, D.F., & Gail, M.H. (Nov 7, 2007). Cause-specific excess deaths associated with underweight, overweight, and obesity. *Journal of the American Medical Association, 298*(17), 2028–2037.

Fornari, V. & Dancyge, I.F. (2006). Physical and cognitive changes associated with puberty. In T. Jaffa & B. McDermott (Eds.), *Eating Disorders in Children and Adolescents,* (pp. 57–69). Cambridge: Cambridge University Press.

Frederick, D.A, Lever, J., & Peplau, L.A. (2007). Interest in cosmetic surgery and body image: Views of men and women across the lifespan. *Plastic & Reconstructive Surgery, 120*(5), 1407–1415.

Golden, J.S., & Golden, M. (1986). Cancer and sex. In J. M. Vaeth (Ed.), *Body image, self-esteem, and sexuality in cancer patients* (2nd ed.) (pp. 68–76). Basil: Karger.

Hayslip, B., Cooper, C.C., Dougherty, L.M., & Cook, D.D. (1997). Body image in adulthood: A projective approach. *Journal of Personality Assessment, 68*(3), 628–649.

Helman, C. G. (1995). The body image in health and disease: Exploring patients' maps of body and self. *Patient Education and Counseling, 26,* 169–175.

Jackson, L. A. (2002). Physical attractiveness: A sociocultural perspective. In T. Cash & T. Pruzinsky (Eds.), *Body image: A handbook of theory, research, and clinical progress* (pp. 13–21). New York: Guilford Press.

Kearney-Cooke, A. (2002). Familial influences on body image development. In T. Cash & T. Pruzinsky (Eds.), *Body image: A handbook of theory, research, and clinical progress* (pp. 99–107). New York: Guilford Press.

Kirkpatrick, J. R. (1986). The stoma patient and his return to society. In J. M. Vaeth (Ed.), *Body image, self-esteem, and sexuality in cancer patients* (2nd ed.) (pp. 24–27). Basil: Karger.

Krauss-Whitbourne, S. & Skultety, K. (2002). Body image development: adulthood and aging. In T. Cash & T. Pruzinsky (Eds.), *Body image: A handbook of theory, research, and clinical progress* (pp. 83–90). New York: Guilford Press.

Krueger, D. W. (2002). Psychodynamic perspectives on body image. In T. Cash & T. Pruzinsky (Eds.), *Body image: A handbook of theory, research, and clinical progress* (pp. 30–37). New York: Guilford Press.

Lewis, J. (1983). *Something Hidden: A Biography of Wilder Penfield.* Halifax, Nova Scotia: Goodread Biographies.

Lowes, J. & Tiggemann, M. (2003). Body dissatisfaction, dieting awareness, and the impact of parental influence in young children. *British Journal of Health Psychology, 8,* 135.

Markus, H., & Wurf, E. (1987). The dynamic self-concept: A social psychological perspective. *Annual Review of Psychology, 38,* 299–337.

McCabe, M., & Ricciardelli, P., & Lina A. (2005). A prospective study of pressures from parents, peers, and the media on extreme weight change behaviours among adolescent boys and girls. *Behaviour Research and Therapy, 43,* 653–668.

Mock, V. (1993). Body image in women treated for breast cancer. *Nursing Research, 42*(3), 153–157.

Moorhead, S., Johnson, M., & Maas, M. (Eds.), (2004). *Nursing outcomes classification (NOC)* (3rd ed.). St. Louis: Mosby.

Mueller, S. (December 2007-January 2008). Amputee envy. *Scientific American Mind, 18*(6), 60–65.

Nezlek, J.B. (1999). Body image and day-to-day social interaction. *Journal of Personality, 67*(5), 793–817.

Norris, J., Connell, M.K., & Spelic, S.S. (1998). A grounded theory of reimaging. *Advances in Nursing Science, 20*(3), 1–12.

Olivardia, R., Pope, H.J., & Hudson, J.I. (2000). Muscle dysmorphia in male weightlifters: A case control study. *American Journal of Psychiatry, 157,* 1291–1296.

Orr, D. A., Reznikoff, M., & Smith, G. M. (1989). Body image, self-esteem, and depression in burn-injured adolescents and young adults. *Journal of Burn Care and Rehabilitation, 10*(5), 454–461.

Otto, S. E. (1991). *Oncology nursing.* St. Louis, MO: Mosby.

Peelen, M.. & Downing, P.E. (2007). The neural basis of visual body perception. *Nature reviews neuroscience, 8*(8), 636–648.

Peterson, C.B, Wimmer, S., Ackard, D.M., Crosby, R., Cavanagh, L.C., Engbloom, S. et al. (2004). Changes in body image during cognitive-behavioral treatment in women with bulimia nervosa. *Body Image,* *1*(2), 139–153.

Pittsburgh Post Gazette. (July 28, 2007). A Ticklish Matter: Photograph and caption. No author.

Pruzinsky, T. (2002). Body image adaptation to reconstructive surgery for acquired disfigurement. In T. Cash & T. Pruzinsky (Eds.), *Body image: A handbook of theory, research, and clinical progress* (pp. 440–449). New York: Guilford Press.

Pruzinsky, T. (2004). Enhancing quality of life in medical populations: A vision for body image assessment and rehabilitation as standards of care. *Body Image, 1,* 71–81.

Ramachandran, V.S. (2004). *A Brief Tour of Human Consciousness.* New York: Pearson Education.

Ramachandran, V.S. & Rogers-Ramachandran, D. (August, 2007). It's all done with mirrors. *Scientific American Mind, 18*(4), 16–18.

Rhode Island Department of Health Office of Minority Health. (1998). Minority health fact sheets. Retrieved from http://www.health.state.ri.us/chic/minority/publications.php

Rumsey, N. (2002). Body image and congenital conditions with visible differences. In T. Cash & T. Pruzinsky (Eds.), *Body image: A handbook of theory, research, and clinical progress* (pp. 226–233). New York: Guilford Press.

Rumsey, N., & Harcourt, D. (2004). Body image and disfigurement: Issues and interventions. *Body Image 1,* 83–97.

Rybarczyk, B., & Behel, J. (2002). Rehabilitation medicine and body image. In T. Cash & T. Pruzinsky (Eds.), *Body image: A handbook of theory, research, and clinical progress* (pp. 387–394). New York: Guilford Press.

Schilder, P. (1950). *The image and appearance of the human body.* New York: International Universities Press.

Spiegel D., Butler L.D., Giese-Davis J., Koopman C., Miller E., Dimiceli S., Classen C., Fobair P., Carlson R.W. (2008). Reply to effects of supportive-expressive group therapy on survival of patients with metastatic breast cancer: A randomized prospective trial. *Cancer 112*(2): 444.

Striegel-Moore, R., & Franko, D. (2002). Body image issues among girls and women. In T. Cash &

T. Pruzinsky (Eds.), *Body image: A handbook of theory, research, and clinical progress* (pp. 183–191). New York: Guilford Press.

Thombs, B.D., Notes, L.D., Lawrence, John W., Magyar-Russell, G., Bresnick, M.G., Faurerbach, J.A., et al. (2008). From survival to socialization: A longitudinal study of body image in survivors of severe burn injury. *Journal of PsychosomaticResearch, 64*(2), 205–212.

Thompson, J., & Gardner, R. (2002). Measuring perceptual body image in adolescents and adults. In T. Cash & T. Pruzinsky (Eds.), *Body image: A handbook of theory, research, and clinical progress* (pp. 142–154). New York: Guilford Press.

Thompson, A., & Kent, G. (2001). Adjusting to disfigurement: Process involved in dealing with being visibly different. *Clinical Psychology Review, 21*(5), 663–682.

Thompson, J., & Van Den Berg, P. (2002). Measuring body image attitudes among adolescents and adults. In T. Cash & T. Pruzinsky (Eds.), *Body image: A handbook of theory, research, and clinical progress* (pp. 155–162). New York: Guilford Press.

Van Deusen, J. (1993). *Body image and perceptual dysfunction in adults.* Philadelphia: WB Saunders.

Veale, D. (2004). Advances in cognitive behavioural model of body dysmorphic disorder. *Body Image, 1*(1), 113–125.

Wetterhahn, K., Hanson, C., & Levy, C. (2002). Effect of participation in physical activity on body image of amputees. *American Journal of Physical Medicine and Rehabilitation, 81*(3), 194–201.

White, C. A. (2002). Body image issues in oncology. In T. Cash & T. Pruzinsky (Eds.), *Body image: A handbook of theory, research, and clinical progress* (pp. 379–386). New York: Guilford Press.

Wright, L. & Leahey, M. (2000). *Nurses and families: A guide to family assessment and intervention* (3rd ed.). Philadelphia: F.A. Davis.

Y-Me National Breast Cancer Organization (2007). Survey underscores importance of emotional, educational needs among women with advanced breast cancer. *Science Daily.* Retrieved from www.sciencedaily.com.

7

Quality of Life

Victoria Schirm

INTRODUCTION

This chapter focuses on quality of life for the 90 million Americans and their families who live with a chronic illness. Emphasis is on nursing practice issues related to the conditions of heart disease and cancer—the leading causes of death in the United States—and on arthritis, hypertension, and diabetes (Chronic Disease Overview, 2005). This approach aligns with the strategic focus of the National Institute of Nursing Research (NINR, 2006) on improving quality of life in persons with chronic, disabling, and life-threatening illnesses. NINR is leading the way in the development of nursing interventions for clients and families, many of whom face significant challenges as they now live with a chronic illness. This chapter includes theoretical conceptualizations and clinical research findings that demonstrate the unique contribution of nursing in assessment, intervention, and outcomes evaluation of quality of life in chronic illness.

Nursing practice and nursing research are well positioned to meet the challenge of identifying, testing, and applying interventions that promote quality of life for survivors of acute illness who are now disabled or otherwise living with a chronic condition. Application of research findings to an

individual's quality of life enables nurses in clinical practice to plan and deliver evidence-based care. Nursing interventions guided by the best available evidence can then be individualized to the values and preferences of the client, thereby assuring better adherence to a plan that must be a lifelong commitment. Client participation in clinical decision-making about the effect that treatments may have on quality of life can be used to monitor therapy over the long term.

Quality of life evaluations can also be used to scrutinize the appropriateness of treatments and show progress toward attainment of treatment goals and responses to therapy. Objective knowledge about desired treatment outcomes for chronic illness that incorporate quality of life domains (improved health and function, pain and symptom control, or prolonged life) can be considered against expected, negative treatment effects such as financial burdens, anxiety, and disrupted lives.

Quality of life assessments provide a way to evaluate the impact of chronic illness on clients and their families. The complex interrelationships of the associated burdens of chronic illness are appreciated more fully when the client's overall quality of life is known. In chronic illness research, quality of life is studied to identify and evaluate specific problems and needs of clients with illness or disability. In the larger arena of the healthcare system, quality of life evaluations are used to monitor the extent to which delivered services address client needs. Outcomes that promote quality of life are valued, particularly when positive results are achieved with efficiency and cost savings. This chapter demonstrates that managing the effects of chronic illness and enhancing quality of life is a multifaceted, complex endeavor.

Defining Quality of Life

Defining quality of life has never been easy. Each individual's unique circumstances and experiences shape quality of life, and this subjective component is an important defining element in quality of life. At the same time, objective indicators of what constitutes quality of life are needed to assess outcomes. The general or global meaning of quality of life and an overall sense of well-being may be anchored to an individual's social and economic conditions, living arrangements, and community environment as well as culture, personal values, happiness, life satisfaction, and spiritual well-being.

The more specific health-related quality of life is usually defined in relationship to physical health, emotional and mental well-being, and functional status. Evaluation of health-related quality of life has become an important indicator for outcomes evaluation and resource needs in chronic illness, and is used as a gauge to monitor progress in achievement of *Healthy People 2010* goals (Centers for Disease Control and Prevention, 2000).

Regardless of whether one is referring to global quality of life or health-related quality of life, the subjective or individual perspective is important to the definition. Rene Dubos' (1959) definition addresses the subjective nature and the multidimensionality of quality of life by saying, "Men naturally desire health and happiness . . . The kind of health that men desire most is not necessarily a state in which they experience physical vigor and a sense of well-being, not even one giving them a long life. It is, instead, the condition

best suited to reach goals that each individual formulates for himself" (p. 228). The World Health Organization (WHO) (1948) definition of health as "a state of complete physical, mental and social well-being and not merely the absence of disease or infirmity" recognizes the multidimensionality of health that is inclusive of a personal evaluation of one's circumstances. Nurses involved in chronic illness care have a stake in understanding distinctions and overlaps in quality of life, health-related quality of life, and self-perceived health.

CONCEPTUALIZING AND MEASURING QUALITY OF LIFE

Theoretical Frameworks

Theories, frameworks, or models in chronic illness explain the complex interrelationships among factors that influence the illness trajectory on quality of life. Such conceptualizations are important not only to generate new evidence for best nursing practice, but also to test and evaluate existing interventions that may affect quality of life in chronic illness. This section presents the literature on quality of life as a theoretical framework or conceptualization, and quality of life as an outcome influenced by various factors depicted in an explanatory model. Examples from the nursing literature are given that use quality of life as a specific outcome of nursing interventions for persons with chronic illness.

Understanding the theoretical underpinnings of quality of life in the context of chronic illness informs nursing research and nursing practice. For example, Moons, Budts, and DeGeest (2006) emphasize that achieving a better conceptual understanding of quality of life is important in conducting clear and meaningful research. They present a critique of various conceptualizations that include: quality of life focused on disease or impairment as a limitation to leading a normal life; quality of life as social utility or ability to lead a productive life; quality of life exemplified in feelings of happiness; quality of life as defined by personal achievement and self-actualization; and quality of life synonymous with life satisfaction and subjective well-being. They conclude that life satisfaction or appraisal of one's life as a whole is the best determinant of quality of life.

Whittemore's (2005) concept analysis of integration considered prior definitions of the term that included qualitative well-being and quality of life. Results of an integrative review produced a definition of integration that encompasses one's self, the environment, and activities of daily living that result in balance and harmony, outcomes that are congruent with quality of life in chronic illness. This perspective provides an understanding of the link between the process and circumstances of chronic illness with quality of life as an outcome measure. As a model for nursing research or practice, the concept of integration can be used to develop and evaluate appropriate nursing interventions that enhance quality of life in chronic illness, as measured by psychosocial adjustment and physical health.

Some quality of life theoretical frameworks have been posited from an ethical perspective. Allmark (2005) suggests that ethical theories are relevant to answering moral questions, especially regarding issues of quality of life versus quantity of life. An ethical framework is useful in clinical nursing practice because it gives guidance to ways that individuals' voices can be discerned; enhances development of decision-making in routine clinical practice; and considers the client's beliefs, values, and preferences in the context of complex questions (Allmark, 2005).

Hirskyj (2007) considers ethical ramifications of resource allocations associated with the Quality-Adjusted Life Years (QALY) concept. QALY is an outcome measure that can be used to determine the efficacy of nursing care as measured by not only the quantity of life but also the quality of life. The QALY framework provides a means to estimate and reveal client's values, beliefs, and preferences in relation to care outcomes. Although nurses may be hesitant to use formulas in providing holistic care, especially in the context of

resource allocation, the QALY concept is supported by evidence that suggests better clinical outcomes are achieved with cost-effective care. Consequently, QALY offers a systematic evidence-based model to practice nursing care and meet the individual needs of clients (Hirskyj). These frameworks provide a context in which to consider the ethical issues that surround quality of life outcomes in chronic illness.

Other researchers have expanded the knowledge base and theory development in understanding quality of life in chronic illness by investigating clients' priorities and perceptions. The work of Sullivan, Weinert, and Cudney (2003) offers guidance for theory development and for nursing interventions in rural women experiencing chronic illness. Women's lived experiences provided rich descriptions of adaptation strategies and the physical and emotional responses to chronic illness that can be used to promote and evaluate quality of life. At the same time, concepts of isolation and distance, common in rural settings, emerged as important components of nursing in chronic illness care for this vulnerable population.

Carter, MacLeod, Brander, and McPherson (2004) also found that clients' perspectives with regard to quality of life in terminal illness are important components. A framework that considers quality of life outcomes from clients' perspectives, as opposed to models developed by experts emphasizing a good death, can lead to interventions that are more client centered. For example, knowing that "being in charge" is more important to a dying person's quality of life than "having a good death" can support development of appropriate interventions that facilitate client control within the context of the illness.

Theoretical models have also been constructed to elicit variables that can significantly influence and predict quality of life for the many older adults who live with chronic illness (Low & Molzahn, 2007). Such models are helpful in understanding the complex interrelationships among physical functioning, perceived health, and emotional and mental well-being to quality of life as an outcome of nursing care. Low and Molzahn found that good health, financial stability, and meaning and purpose in life have substantial positive effects on the quality of life of older adults. This model provides conceptual links among several variables—financial resources, health, physical function, meaning and purpose in life, emotional support, and environment—to quality life. The underpinnings of this model provide direction for improving the quality of life of older adults through development of nursing interventions that promote activities of daily living, provide emotional support, or enhance the environment.

Theoretical models have been used to design specific nursing interventions for chronic illness care that can positively impact quality of life. The Watson Caring Model was used to evaluate quality of life in clients with hypertension (Erci et al., 2003). Components of the model with the nurse offering comfort, compassion, and empathy with an understanding of the individual's strengths and limitations were used to guide nursing interventions for community-residing clients with hypertension. Results demonstrated improved quality of life scores as measured by a 42-item scale and reduction in blood pressure. The structure, process, and outcome framework, originally developed by Donabedian (1988) to assess quality of healthcare delivery, guided a randomized clinical trial of a discharge intervention for hospitalized older adults with hip fractures (Huang & Liang, 2005). A structured discharge plan that was systematically implemented by an advanced-practice nurse was used to evaluate several outcomes, including quality of life, post-hospital discharge for elders who had sustained a hip fractures resulting from a fall.

In another study (Suhonen, Välimäki, Katajisto, & Leino-Kilpi, 2005), a model of individualized nursing care was used to evaluate outcomes of satisfaction, autonomy, and health-related quality of life in hospitalized clients. This model testing demonstrated a positive association between clients' perceptions of care given by nurses and their ratings of satisfaction with care, ability to

make decisions about care, and health-related quality of life. This affirmation of individualized nursing care as explicated in the model, provides supporting data for evidence-based nursing practice.

Saunders and Cookman (2005) explored the theoretical underpinnings of depression related to hepatitis C virus infection to gain a better understanding of quality of life in this client population where the illness is often chronic. The symptom experience, stigma associated with the illness, and uncertain illness trajectory were described as multidimensional components of hepatitis C–related depression. Saunders and Cookman proposed that the conceptualization provides a model for developing nursing interventions that are likely to be effective for maximizing quality of life outcomes in this special population.

Theoretical frameworks also have been advanced to explain the changing dimensions of cancer care. Once viewed as an acute, life-limiting illness, cancer in most instances is now managed as a chronic illness. Cancer nursing with children is one area where the science of nursing is embedded within the art of nursing practice (Cantrell, 2007). This conceptualization views quality of life as foundational to the experiences of children and adolescents with cancer. For quality of life to be an outcome, the values, beliefs, and wishes of children and their families as well as the values and expertise of the oncology nurse must be acknowledged and applied with the best available scientific evidence. One without the other is not sufficient to produce health-related quality of life in pediatric oncology.

Clark (2004) used quality of life as the conceptual basis to determine how psychiatric nurses assess and provide care to seriously mentally ill clients residing in community settings. Three themes emerged as ways in which quality of life influenced psychiatric nursing practice. One was that quality of life defined the goal of care in that it permeated everything nurses did. Second, was that the nurse's concern for quality of life focused interventions on the person and away from the mental illness. The third theme was that quality of life formed the foundation of the nurse–client relationship, where the focus is the individual client's perspective as opposed to management of a disease or symptoms.

Measuring Quality of Life

As described in the previous section, theoretical frameworks provide a systematic approach to study quality of life. Regardless of whether quality of life is conceptualized as a complex set of relationships that influence the chronic illness trajectory, or viewed as an outcome of the illness itself, an appropriate measure of quality of life is crucial. Valid and reliable measures are needed to capture accurately the elements or concepts that characterize quality of life. Quality of life has a subjective component as defined by the individual's unique situation that reflects happiness and life satisfaction (*Healthy People 2010*). This general quality of life includes health as well as culture, values, beliefs, and environment. The more specific health-related quality of life is usually defined in relationship to health and physical function, and emotional and mental well-being. Elements that contribute to the more general or global quality of life may not be considered in assessments about health-related quality of life. At the same time, reference to health-related quality of life may suggest illness or disease.

Nurses, in particular, have a stake in understanding the distinctions and the overlaps in the quality of life dimensions. When used as a framework, the dimensions of quality of life provide a context for assessing nursing's contribution to improved care outcomes for clients with chronic illness. In clinical practice, nurses can use standardized quality of life assessments to plan, implement, and evaluate evidence-based care for clients with chronic illnesses. Measurement is a first step in the process because accurate and appropriate assessment of symptom status has the potential for better care management and evaluation of nursing intervention effectiveness. To this end, Sousa, Ryu,

Kwok, Cook, & West (2007) created a model and validated a measure to assess the impact of rheumatoid arthritis on quality of life. They found two factors, arthritic pain and general symptoms, to be confirmatory and predictive of quality of life evaluations. They surmised that nursing interventions aimed at assessing pain and managing overall symptoms have the most potential to enhance quality of life and function for individuals with rheumatoid arthritis.

Quality of life measurement, especially assessment of health-related quality of life in populations, is important in monitoring progress in achievement of *Healthy People 2010* goals. One major goal is to improve quality of life and increase life expectancy for individuals of all ages.

The Centers for Disease Control and Prevention (CDC) (2000) is, likewise, concerned with quality of life as a health outcome. Traditional illness outcome measures of morbidity and mortality are limiting, in that they do not speak to risks, burdens, resource needs, or declines associated with illness, particularly as they relate to chronic conditions. To this end, the CDC created the "Healthy Days" measure that evaluates one's perception of well-being via four items: self-rated health, number of days of illness or injury, number of days of emotional distress, and days unable to do self-care or to work. The four-item measure was expanded to include 10 additional questions eliciting responses on individuals' days of activity limitations, pain, depression, anxiety, sleeplessness, and feeling energized.

The WHO (2004) has also developed a standardized tool to measure quality of life and health from the individual's perspective. In contrast to the CDC measure, the WHO Quality of Life measure has 26 items that assess an individual's feelings of satisfaction and enjoyment with life, limitations due to pain, capacity for work, ability to perform activities of daily living and to get around, access to health care, and satisfaction with relationships. Both the CDC and the WHO tools have the common objective to quantify and standardize measurement of quality of life. These tools are intended to measure health and well-being in healthy populations as well as to detect illness conditions that could benefit from early intervention and treatment.

Increasingly, nursing as a discipline has recognized that it too needs to focus on measurable outcomes related to interventions. The measurement of quality of life, including health-related quality of life, has become one such standardized assessment as an indicator for outcomes of nursing care. Quality of life determinations that use consistent measures provide an objective assessment of clients' care needs. Measures that include appropriate determinants that contribute to or influence quality of life can be used by nurses to give care based on the best available evidence.

As mentioned briefly in the introduction, the need for systematic measurement of quality of life outcomes in chronic illness has been recognized by the National Institute of Nursing Research (NINR). Specifically noted is the need for quality of life outcomes measurement associated with functional decline in older adults; assessments of how quality of life changes over time in chronic illness; quality of life evaluations for transplant recipients and those at end-of-life; and reasonable expectations for quality of life related to technology-based interventions (Reeve et al., 2007). NINR-funded intervention studies aimed at improving quality of life in chronic illness include investigations of problem solving, skill development for self management, appropriate resource use, application of self efficacy, and coping skills training. In addition, NINR supports research centers to enhance quality of life in chronic illness and to study the impact of chronic diseases on vulnerable populations (NINR, 2006).

Context of Quality of Life in Chronic Illness

Quality of life in chronic illness can be viewed within the context of health and functioning, psychological and spiritual well-being, societal roles, and economic status. These multiple dimensions provide a practical way to discuss the background that contributes to quality of life for individuals living with chronic illness. Considerable overlap exists among these components. For example, health and function is multifaceted and may include perceived health, energy level, pain experiences, stress levels, independence, capacity to meet responsibilities, access to and use of health care, and usefulness to others. This view of health and function as a quality of life component shows that reliance on any one clinical parameter may not capture the client's overall picture of health and well-being. People with chronic illness may report a good perceived quality of life, but clinically they have objective symptoms. Thus knowledge of how symptoms affect clients' health and function can lead to a better understanding of their quality of life in chronic illness. Typically, the presence of symptoms prompts an individual to seek health care—for example, weakness and poor coordination in the individual with multiple sclerosis. In addition, people with chronic illness are subjected to symptoms from the iatrogenic effects of their treatments. Regardless of the origin, physically distressing symptoms affect health and function and, ultimately, one's quality of life. Moreover, symptoms and the distress they cause result in varying reports about health and function as perceived by clients. Healthcare professionals and family members sometimes report conflicting views about a person's health and function, thereby producing quality of life ratings that may differ. Treatment decisions may be impacted by such ratings, demonstrating the importance of using quality of life assessments that consider clients' perspectives of their health and function.

The complexity of health and function in chronic illness suggests that neither good health nor optimal function is a necessary or sufficient condition for quality of life. Psychological and spiritual components are part of quality of life, and include intangibles such as happiness, peace of mind, and a belief system. Considerable overlap exists between psychological and spiritual well-being. Psychological well-being may be thought of as an essential component of quality of life that influences overall adjustment to chronic illness. More directly, spirituality has been advanced as an important element in quality of life measurement across different cultures (Moreira-Almedia & Koenig, 2006). At the same time, caution is urged that spirituality is different than religiosity as well as different from meaning in life, hope, and peace. In the nursing literature, spirituality is defined broadly as embracing "love, compassion, caring, transcendence, relationship with God, and connection of body, mind, and spirit" (O'Brien, 2003, p. 6). Most definitions take into consideration that spirituality affects all aspects of a person's well-being. Persons living with a chronic illness sometimes must make significant life changes in order to maintain quality of life. For many individuals with chronic illness, there may be an increased reliance on psychological and spiritual resources and on the social and emotional support offered by friends and confidantes.

Supportive care or the lack of it influences how individuals manage and cope with stress. Indeed, most people know the positive effect of having "moral support" and companionship at times of difficulty. Family health and relationships are a large part of this aspect of quality of life. Any illness affecting a family member inevitably affects other family members, resulting in a changed quality of life for them as well. For example, when family members become primary caregivers of a chronically ill member, there are role changes, additional responsibilities, and increased stressors that have varying effects on quality of life. Without a doubt, the overwhelming nature of chronic illness affects the quality of life not only for the client, but also for family members. Therefore, nursing interventions to promote quality of life in chronic illness are frequently aimed at caregivers. It is reasonable to expect that when caregivers are helped to manage their stress and anxiety, both the caregiver and the client realize better quality of life.

The social and cultural context of quality of life are far-reaching components, as is evidenced by the manner in which organizations such as WHO and the CDC define and measure quality of life. Unique cultural interpretations can influence perceived quality of life. Social conditions, expectations of individual behaviors, and cultural regulations affect and contribute to quality of life. Social support and cultural influences are intertwined frequently with economic aspects. Chronic illness affects the financial resources of individuals and their families. The negative impact causes psychological and emotional burdens, and drains financial assets. The reasons for financial strain and its effects vary. Frequently, a chronic illness requires individuals to decrease, suspend, or end their work, leading to a reduction or loss of income. Furthermore, if the care recipient requires much assistance or supervision, the primary family caregiver may also have to terminate employment. Therefore, a family with a member who is chronically ill now faces an increased financial burden resulting from the unemployment of two members. These situations contribute to an adverse quality of life through decreased workforce participation, and ultimately cause lost productivity, which further increases the overall cost of chronic illness.

Individuals with chronic illness also suffer financially because of the additional expenses incurred with medical insurance rates or out-of-pocket expenses for items not covered by insurance. Transportation to medical or treatment appointments, for example, or the extra cost of special dietary foods or supplements can add up quickly. The desperately ill person who has found little benefit from traditional therapies may spend large amounts of money on alternative forms of treatment to improve their health. The combined effect on quality of life associated with decreased income and increased expenses may not always be obvious. Therefore, nurses must be aware of how this financial burden may contribute to decreased quality of life. For example, clients may take fewer medications because they cannot afford to take the prescribed amount, or the family caregiver may be overtaxed by the caregiving burden because the family cannot afford assistance.

At the same time, caution is warranted in assuming that a positive relationship exists

CASE STUDY

Healthy Aging and Quality of Life

This case study illustrates many aspects of quality of life in chronic illness, including health and function, psychosocial elements of aging, the meaning of family, and death and dying. The story begins in 1989 when Mr. and Mrs. H made the decision to enter a continuing care retirement community. At the time Mrs. H was 70 years old and Mr. H was 68 years old and recently diagnosed with Parkinson's disease. Mr. H had a productive career as an educator and Mrs. H worked for a short time at a service agency and had been a longtime active volunteer with various organizations. They were the parents of four adult children who lived in various parts of the country.

It became clear to this couple that Mr. H would eventually need more attention and care, and that it would be difficult for Mrs. H to care for her husband as the disease progressed. The retirement community would allow them to be in an environment where both could receive health care that would be needed as they grew older, especially Mr. H. Moreover, the community was within walking distance from their former home, so the area was familiar to them. They felt they would not need to make many additional changes such as finding a new church, losing the friendships they had made in the area, or locating different places to shop. The children were supportive of this move, and they were pleased that their parents made these plans in the early stages of Mr. H's chronic illness.

Mr. and Mrs. H lived together at the retirement community for more than 10 years. Mrs. H, as she recalled the latter years of her husband's life, commented that "Those years were the hardest; it was difficult to see him gradually become completely disabled. He could not move or communicate at the end." After some time following the death of her spouse, Mrs. H made the decision to enter assisted living at the retirement community. This change and the fact that other health related services are readily available has been helpful to Mrs. H. She has experienced several falls, and the reassurance that assistance is nearby has given her comfort. These falls have been attributed to poor balance and neuropathy in her feet and legs. She wears glasses and uses hearing aids for "special occasions" such as a lecture or Sunday "sermons." She reports that her hearing aides are not useful in noisy situations such as in restaurants or public gatherings. She is independent in activities of daily living, and uses a walker or cane most of the time because of her poor balance. She no longer drives, so needs the community van or transportation for the elderly to do errands at the grocery or drug store.

In terms of her social and leisure activities, Mrs. H is an avid painter using watercolors, and she has taken advantage of further honing her skills by attending workshops. Mrs. H loves the weekly movies that are shown at the retirement community, but prefers viewing the television in her own room where she can hear and see better and choose what she likes. She uses the computer extensively for Internet access to shopping, information, and playing Scrabble online. She has an extensive social network and takes advantage of the many programs that are offered at the retirement community.

In summary, Mrs. H views her situation as one where she has maintained and enjoyed a good quality of life, despite losses: her husband's chronic illness and death, and her own frailty. She reports that she is content with her situation, remains interested in many things, and enjoys learning more. She recognizes her frailty and ailments, but admits that they do not disturb her greatly. Mrs. H is quick to say that her faith has been a big influence in her life; and that family with the special love of her children sustains her.

(Continued)

CASE STUDY (*Continued*)

Discussion Questions

1. How has Mrs. H's quality of life been influenced by her environment? By her past experiences? By her family?
2. Mr. and Mrs. H made the decision to change their living environment when Mr. H was diagnosed with Parkinson's

disease. What additional nursing assessments would be helpful in determining the level of care that would best maintain quality of life?

3. What nursing interventions to promote quality of life might Mrs. H need in the future?

Source: Marsha Haack, MS, RN, Coordinator, Nursing Research, Penn State Milton S. Hershey Medical Center, Hershey, Pennsylvania.

between a good quality of life and an adequate income. The high degree of subjectivity in quality of life and the existence of many interrelated components suggest that other aspects may influence one's quality of life. The interrelatedness of these various quality of life aspects is evident in literature that report results of interventions in chronic illness conditions.

EVIDENCE-BASED INTERVENTIONS TO PROMOTE QUALITY OF LIFE

Evidence-based nursing practice has the most potential to enhance quality of life in chronic illness. The best available research evidence combined with nursing expertise and consideration of individual values and preferences enables effectiveness and efficiency in nursing care. Nurses cannot afford to base practice solely on tradition or experience, or even from knowledge of experts or highly rated textbooks. Increasingly, nursing interventions are seen as having a direct impact on patient outcomes. In chronic illness care, this pivotal nursing role raises the bar to practice nursing that is systematic, produces outcomes that contribute to cost effectiveness, and enhances quality care. As a result of the efforts of nurse researchers and the NINR initiatives, interventions with known efficacy are being implemented to promote quality of life in chronic illness.

This section reviews nursing interventions in chronic illness that promote and evaluate quality of

life as an outcome. Overall, a reasonable outcome of any nursing intervention is improved quality of life for clients. In chronic illness, this goal is even more salient. Nurses as essential health care professionals to clients with chronic illness can be instrumental in planning, carrying out, and evaluating care that promotes quality of life. For clients, enhancing their quality of life amid the debilitating effects of a long-term illness becomes an especially relevant outcome. Moreover, quality of life from the client's context is a reasonable outcome measure of the effectiveness of clinical interventions. The review includes nursing and related investigations on quality of life outcomes for clients and families who have conditions that are the leading causes of death such as heart disease and cancer. Also included are studies that address quality of life as an outcome in chronic conditions such as arthritis, mental illness, and functional decline associated with aging. Review of the quality of life research for those at end-of-life is presented as well. These investigations provide examples of ways that nurses can intervene effectively to promote quality of life for clients and their families living with a chronic illness, disability, or condition.

Evidence-Based Guidelines

Clinical practice guidelines provide easily accessed and current, evidence-based information about recommendations, strategies, or information for care and decision-making in specific clinical conditions (Coopey, Nix, & Clancy, 2006). Guidelines about interventions specific to promoting quality of life are embedded in some guidelines; and many guidelines include nurses as the intended users. Four guidelines are presented in Table 7-1: (1) self-management in chronic care, (2) heart failure medication management, (3) radiation-oncology nursing, and (4) persistent pain in older adults. These and other evidence-based guidelines are readily available at the National Guideline Clearinghouse (2007). Guidelines can be used by nurses to evaluate quality of life as it is influenced by clinical decision-making and intervening in chronic illness situations. For example, the evidence-based guideline for chronic care self-management was developed for counseling, evaluation, and management of families who have children with chronic illnesses. This guideline, created by an expert panel at a major children's hospital, specifically targets families of children with chronic illness. Intended users include advanced practice nurses, among others. Clinical areas where chronically ill children and their families are cared for are the practice arenas in which these guidelines are most likely to be used. As an outcome, health-related quality of life, is one measure that healthcare professionals can use to evaluate the effect of their interventions on client outcomes.

The accessibility and ease of use related to evidence-based guidelines provide an efficient and effective manner for nurses to intervene and evaluate quality of life for clients and their families with chronic illness. At the same time, it is important that the user evaluate the relevance, currency, and validity of guidelines for measurement of intended outcomes. Consequently, along with guideline use, nurses must be aware of the recent quality of life research and measurement to apply the best available evidence at the client care level. Therefore, it is important to consider specific practice characteristics that may influence guideline effectiveness and the time and effort that might be required to implement recommendations (Coopey et al., 2006). The guideline should reflect the nurses'

clinical knowledge and experience as well as the clients' values and preferences (Clark, Donovan, & Schoettker, 2006).

Using guidelines from the National Guideline Clearinghouse offers assurances that the recommendations, strategies, and information are based on systematic literature reviews and scientific evidence. Guidelines offer recommendations for practice that are based on a specified level of evidence. For example, the table comparing evidence-based guidelines shows that expert consensus was the primary means to formulate the recommendations put forth in the guideline for pharmacologic management of heart failure. The evidence rating from the US Preventive Services Task Force was used to evaluate the quality of the recommendations for medication use in heart failure patients, with quality of life and cost-effective drug prescribing being outcomes. For application in clinical practice, nurses could review the guidelines and assess the methods and rating scheme that were used in development. A determination can be made that if a recommendation is strong, the intervention is always indicated and acceptable, and, therefore, likely to positively influence quality of life for clients. On the other hand, the nurse would need to use additional information and decision-making if the recommendation has a lower rating, such as useful, should be considered, or not useful.

Interventions from the Research Literature to Promote Quality of Life

A review of nursing and health-related literature that report the effects of various interventions on quality of life as one outcome in chronic illness conditions are presented in this section. Much of the research is descriptive in nature; therefore, cause-and-effect relationships between nursing interventions and quality of life as an outcome are not well established. It is also difficult to collect data on outcomes that are sensitive and unique to nursing care interventions. Individuals with chronic illness are seen by a variety of healthcare professionals who may potentially impact their

(*Text continues on page 151*)

TABLE 7-1			
Comparison of Guidelines That Measure Quality of Life Outcomes			
Guideline Title	Evidence-based care guideline for chronic care: self-management (2007)	The pharmacologic management of chronic heart failure (2001; Revised 2003)	Radiation-oncology nursing practice and education (1998; Revised 2005)	The management of persistent pain in older persons (1998; Revised 2002)
Guideline Developer(s)	Cincinnati Children's Hospital Medical Center	US Department of Veterans Affairs	Oncology Nursing Society	American Geriatrics Society
Disease/ Condition(s)	Chronic illness/ condition of more than 3 months and/ or persistent function limitations; and/or use of healthcare services beyond usual care.	Chronic heart failure	Cancer	Persistent pain
Clinical Specialty	Family practice, internal medicine, nursing, nutrition, pediatrics, physical medicine, rehabilitation psychology	Cardiology, family practice, internal medicine, nursing	Nursing, oncology, pediatrics, radiation-oncology	Family practice, geriatrics, internal medicine
Intended Users	Advanced practice nurses, allied health personnel, dietitians, healthcare providers, nurses, patients, pharmacists, physicians, psychologists/non-physician behavioral health clinicians, social workers	Advanced practice nurses, nurses, physician assistants, physicians	Advanced practice nurses, nurses	Advanced practice nurses, allied health personnel, healthcare providers, health plans, managed care organizations, nurses, patients, physician assistants, physicians, public health departments
Guideline Objective(s)	To provide evidence-based recommendations for self-management by families of children with chronic conditions in order to improve health outcomes and quality of life	To present updated evidence-based pharmacologic guidelines on the management of chronic heart failure	To provide specific recommendations for the education of nurses new to radiation-oncology and for the practice of quality radiation oncology nursing care	To update and revise previous recommendations from the clinical practice guideline titled "The Management of Chronic Pain in Older Persons," using the latest information in elderly persons

(Continued)

TABLE 7-1

Comparison of Guidelines That Measure Quality of Life Outcomes (*Continued*)

Guideline Objective(s)		To assist practitioners in clinical decision-making, to standardize and improve the quality of patient care, and to promote cost-effective drug prescribing To present guidelines to serve as a basis for monitoring local, regional, and national patterns of pharmacologic care	To assist with the articulation of the role of the radiation-oncology nurse, justification of nursing staff positions in the department of radiation-oncology, and the evaluation of radiation-oncology nurses' performance	To provide the reader with an overview of the principles of pain management as they apply specifically to older people and specific recommendations to aid in decision-making about pain management for this population
Client Population	Children with chronic conditions and their families	Veterans with chronic heart failure	Adult and pediatric patients undergoing radiation therapy	Older persons with persistent pain
Major Outcomes Considered	Self efficacy Health-related quality of life Healthcare utilization Parent/patient satisfaction Missed days from usual activities Cost Specific disease measures	Symptoms Functional capacity Quality of life Disease progression Need for hospitalization Survival rates	Quality of life Morbidity associated with radiation therapy	Patient-reported pain intensity recorded with standard pain scales Validity and acceptability of pain scales Safety and adverse effects of pain medications Pain relief, quality of life, and functional capacity
Methods Used to Access the Quality and Strength of the Evidence	Not stated	Weighting according to a rating scheme	Expert consensus; weighting according to a rating scheme	Weighting according to a rating scheme
Methods Used to Formulate the Recommendations	Expert consensus (Delphi Expert consensus and nominal group techniques)		Not stated	Not stated

Source: National Guidelines Clearinghouse. (2007). Retrieved November 21, 2007, from www.guidelines.gov

quality of life. Nevertheless, findings from many of the studies suggest that quality of life has usefulness as a nurse-sensitive quality indicator and as a measure of intervention effectiveness in chronic conditions. Doran and colleagues (2006) noted that linking outcomes to nursing interventions is necessary to determine and identify specific nursing interventions that improve health outcomes and provide the evidence base to improve nursing care in chronic illness.

Most of the reports view the quality of life of a client as an important outcome measure across several domains, and specific interventions have focused on outcomes such as stage of the disease, disability, and mortality rates. The view of outcomes in terms of morbidity and death discounts other aspects of health and function in chronic illness, such as the client's perceived health, pain experiences, stress levels, independence, capacity to meet responsibilities, access to and use of health care, and usefulness to others. These outcomes are important to clients who want to know how interventions are going to influence health and function. Clients also want guidance in choosing options that will produce the best outcomes. In addition, regulatory bodies and manufacturers of pharmaceuticals and technologic devices want guidance about product effectiveness on client outcomes, and in particular how an individual's quality of life is affected. The results of the research and of the other literature reviewed here show the many facets of client quality of life outcomes in chronic illness care.

Overview of Nursing Interventions

Nursing interventions can empower clients to practice healthy behaviors and enable them to be self-directed in their care and thereby contribute appreciably to quality of life. Feldman, Murtaugh, Pezzin, McDonald, and Peng (2005) found that use of an email reminder improved self-care management and health-related quality of life for heart failure clients. The email reminders were evidence-based, condition-specific information that

was provided to nurses as they cared for heart failure clients. These reminders were integrated into the assessment and routine teaching interventions that nurses carried out for clients. When compared with routine care, the basic email reminder to nurses that they should teach to the specific areas of medication knowledge, diet and weight monitoring produced positive results in clients' quality of life. Moreover, they found that this basic teaching for heart failure generated results similar to that of a more intensive intervention that included more reminders and additional nursing time. The study is limited in so far as the sample was from one urban home care agency. However, the results are useful in linking a nursing practice intervention to clients' quality of life, and thereby add to a better understanding of nursing interventions that are appropriate as well as cost-effective.

Nursing-led management and intervention in chronic disease care has been investigated and evaluated in relation to client quality of life outcomes. These investigations are hampered frequently by an inability to produce conclusive results regarding a nursing impact on quality of life. Results of one study provide evidence that nurse mediated interventions have the potential to yield positive quality of life outcomes for clients with implantable cardioverter–defibrillators (Dickerson, Wu, & Kennedy, 2006). However, establishing a link via statistically significant results is more complicated. This situation frequently occurs as the result of multiple factors that affect quality of life, inability to isolate a single nursing intervention, or failure in the adequacy of the measurement (Dickerson et al.). At the same time, the imperative to promote quality of life in chronic illness care requires continued nursing research. Taylor and colleagues (2005) acknowledged the urgency of the need for ongoing research in their systematic review of evidence effectiveness related to nursing's role in chronic obstructive pulmonary disease (COPD). As a chronic illness, COPD is a prime example of an escalating public health burden in terms of number of persons affected and the resources used. Nurses have been recognized as playing a critical role in chronic illness care of COPD. Taylor and colleagues called for reprioritization of nurse-led models of chronic illness care. The equivocal results of this study and many others investigating quality of life as an end result suggest the need for more carefully designed nursing interventions as well as measurement of additional outcomes.

Health and Function

Health and function as determinants of quality of life are used frequently with traditional clinical and disease indicators to evaluate outcomes for older adults with chronic illness conditions. In clinical practice, these quality of life assessments can enhance understanding about treatment preferences and future care needs. For example, health-related quality of life was used as a predictor of potential need for future hospital care for older adults in a large primary care practice (Dorr et al., 2006). Dorr and colleagues found that consideration of quality of life may improve decision making about treatment preferences and intensity for care. Knowledge of an older person's capacity for self-care and functional abilities can maximize appropriate resources and need for care when critical situations arise. Many times the needed information about quality of life addressing psychosocial aspects of chronic illness is missing from assessments. The assessment data can be used to plan, carry out, and evaluate treatments. In situations in which treatments are known to cause extreme debility, changes should be considered for older clients based on quality of life outcomes.

Nursing care for elderly cancer survivors is one area where information about potential effects on quality of life can be used in clinical practice. Quality of life and related symptoms in elderly women with breast cancer are entangled frequently with other chronic health conditions or are attributed to aging. Heidrich, Egan, Hengudomsub, and Randolph (2006) found that poor social situations, a pessimistic outlook on life, and not knowing the reason for many distressing symptoms further contribute to decreased quality of life. In

these situations, interventions may be helpful that help older women better understand why they are experiencing symptoms and that depression, anxiety, or lack of energy may be caused by cancer and are not part of normal aging.

Clients need information about the reason for symptoms and to know that some symptoms are intertwined with chronic illness and compounded by the aging process. This knowledge can help older adults develop more effective coping strategies. Targeting intervention strategies also can be done more appropriately when quality of life outcomes are better identified. Awareness that women report worse quality of life compared to men because women tend to have a higher prevalence of chronic illness and related functional declines can lead to more proactive early detection and health-promotion interventions (Orfila et al., 2006).

Frequently, lack of awareness about available help and treatments is an obstacle to better quality of life. In a study of bowel function and associated fecal incontinence among those older than 75 years of age, researchers found that decreased quality of life was influenced by the amount of dependence that symptoms caused (Stenzelius, Westergren, & Hallberg, 2007). Appropriate assessment of bowel symptoms and the extent of dependency along with nurses' encouragement of clients to seek appropriate care are straightforward interventions that can have a positive impact on quality of life for older adults with bowel dysfunction.

Cancer Care

Nursing research related to care of cancer clients and their families provides an excellent illustration of the complexity of measuring, intervening, and evaluating quality of life in chronic illness. Cancer is increasingly recognized as a chronic illness because of better survival rates that have resulted from effective treatments. With the increased survival following a diagnosis of cancer, quality of life emerges as a predominant issue. Identification, prevention, and management of the long-term effects of cancer and related treatments have received attention by nurse researchers. Bender, Ergun, Rosenzweig, Cohen, and Sereika (2005) identified the prevalence of symptoms experienced by women across three phases of breast cancer treatment. They assessed global quality of life, and evaluated how vasomotor, physical, psychosocial, and sexual components were experienced by women in the various phases of breast cancer care and treatment. Fatigue, cognitive impairments, and mood disturbances emerged as common symptoms experienced by the women, regardless of the phase of illness or treatment. Fatigue associated with cancer and related treatments was an especially bothersome symptom, suggesting that nursing interventions focused on alleviating and managing fatigue may promote better quality of life for women with breast cancer.

Survival rates for some clients with ovarian cancer have also resulted in the focus being given to nursing care for these clients over a much longer period than previously experienced. Knowledge about how women move through the trajectory of diagnosis, treatment, and surviving ovarian cancer is important to intervening to promote quality of life (Ferrell et al., 2005).

The positive effect on quality of life produced by interventions that prevent or lessen fatigue associated with cancer has been given attention in the nursing literature. Cancer-related fatigue is frequently measured as a quality of life component, and various interventions have been proposed to reduce fatigue. Mitchell, Beck, Hood, Moore, and Tanner (2007) conducted a systematic review of the literature and used a rating scheme to support the efficacy of different interventions to reduce fatigue associated with cancer care and treatment. For many interventions, effectiveness was not well established, owing to insufficient or poor-quality data. These interventions included alternative therapies such as yoga, acupuncture, and nutritional supplements; drugs that may help alleviate fatigue; and psychotherapy. Strategies that teach clients to manage and balance activity, rest, and sleep were rated as likely to be effective, because the evidence is based on small, descriptive studies or expert consensus. Exercise was the one intervention that was recommended for practice because of the strength

of the evidence and because the benefits outweighed the harm. Other studies have also shown that exercise is a safe and effective intervention for reducing fatigue and promoting quality of life in cancer patients. Exercise combined with structured group sessions was effective, owing in part to the group cohesion and atmosphere, and the direct effects that exercise has on reducing fatigue (Losito, Murphy, & Thomas, 2006). This understanding and awareness of the evidence supporting nursing interventions for cancer care promotes best practices interventions for clients and their families. In particular, the growing body of evidence that cancer clients reap many benefits from exercise provides substantial rationale for nurses to promote and use physical activity as a means of improving health and quality of life for many clients with cancer (Kirshbaum, 2006).

Quality of Life in Terminal Illness

Nursing's involvement as researchers and clinicians in end-of-life care has created heightened interest in measuring, promoting, and maintaining quality of life as a nursing care outcome for clients at the end-of-life. Indeed, the primary objective of palliative and hospice care is to optimize quality of life for individuals and their families. In their review of the literature, Jocham, Dassen, Widdershoven, and Halfens (2006) found that research on nursing interventions in quality of life in palliative cancer care creates special challenges. A primary challenge is the methodological issues related to measurement of quality of life. Most often the aim of end-stage treatment is to control physical symptoms and promote psychological, social, and spiritual comfort. Hence, an individual's quality of life becomes anchored in other aspects of life, and traditional measures may not be accurate or appropriate. Despite the presence of a terminal illness, clients may continue to give rather favorable ratings to their situation, suggesting that other values, goals, and preferences are important to quality of life. In older adults, quality of life at end-of-life, likewise, is beset by methodological issues and evaluating the experiences of clients and families. The aging process alters responses to illness, and disease and symptoms may not manifest in ways that nurses are familiar with in younger adults. Evidence-based activities that promote and maintain quality of life for terminally ill older adults include attention to age-related changes and the impact on sensory function and physiologic responses. Particular consideration should be given to pain assessment, medication management, and assessments of depression and cognitive status (Amella, 2003). Others have shown that by asking seriously ill clients what they view as quality of life is instructive in helping decide on treatment plans, making advance directives, or prioritizing activities (Vig & Pearlman, 2003).

Psychosocial and Other Supportive Interventions

Nursing studies have focused on interventions to promote quality of life when technology and other well-established treatments fail or when these tools and machinery are insufficient to maintain health and function. Facing suffering on a daily basis and the need to find meaning and purpose in living with a chronic disability challenges healthcare professionals to address a client's needs in other than physical ways. Psychosocial well-being like health and function contributes immensely to one's quality of life in chronic illness. This type of well-being can be characterized as the capacity to view oneself in a positive manner as well as see the world as meaningful, manageable, and logical. The capacity to view self in a positive manner, despite serious physical symptoms that accompany chronic illness, has been shown to be moderated by a strong sense of coherence (Delgado, 2007). In some situations, the simple act of listening to a client's burdens and feelings promotes quality of life. This response comes about through the contentment, respect, and nurturance that are shown by the nurse who listens without judgment (Jonas-Simpson et al., 2006). Interventions that enable better understanding and use of coping skills can be supportive of quality of life for clients and families experiencing chronic illness. Clients who

were post myocardial infarction and who reported quality of life improvements used optimistic, self-reliant, and confrontational coping strategies most frequently over a 1-year period (Kristofferzon, Lofmark, & Carlsson, 2005).

In addition to psychosocial-related activities that augment chronic illness care, evidence-based alternative interventions can likewise be part of the client's care routine. Interventions such as guided imagery and relaxation therapy have the potential to supplement traditional medical and health care that chronically ill clients need. The combination of guided imagery and relaxation techniques improved health-related quality of life for women with osteoarthritis by alleviating pain intensity and increasing mobility. Moreover, this intervention is easily taught and readily available to clients (Baird & Sands, 2006).

Chronically mentally ill clients are another group that can benefit from interventions that augment prescribed medication and counseling therapies. Crone (2007) reported that physical activity programs enabled mentally ill individuals to have positive emotional experiences, increased social interaction, and enhanced well-being. Nurses can be instrumental in facilitating development and referral to programs that help increase physical activity for clients with mental illnesses, and thereby promote quality of life. Individuals with other chronic conditions also have benefited from exercise programs. Knowing the stage of a client's readiness to engage in exercise is an additional factor that can give nurses information to tailor education more specifically (Lee, Change, Liou, & Chang, 2006).

Interventions for Family Quality of Life

Nursing interventions to promote quality of life are, likewise, important to family members and others who are caregivers to clients living with a chronic illness. Consequently, it is important to know how caregivers experience quality of life. In general, chronic illness affects quality of life for the entire family. Therefore, family assessment and intervention is necessary. The level of the nurse's involvement with the family will determine the extent of the interventions. Most nurses can meet the basic need that families of clients with chronic illness have for factual information. This information may include education about the disease, treatments, and prognosis. Being available to answer questions and to give practical advice is important. Intervening at this fundamental level establishes trust with families that helps foster continued support. Nurses can invite family members to participate in care activities as appropriate. Families with complex problems may need referral to a specialist. Appropriate use of support groups can create an added network for clients and relieve some of the family burden that may be present (Sutton & Erlen, 2006). The nurse is often in a position to evaluate how such supportive interventions may affect quality of life. A safe and supportive environment can facilitate family sharing of feelings about the illness. Support groups can be suggested that would be appropriate for clients and their family caregivers. The nurse is one of the members of a collaborative health care team that is needed to maintain and promote optimum quality of life for clients with a chronic illness and their families.

The complex trajectory of chronic illness poses difficulties in making a strict separation of interventions for quality of life for both clients and family members. It is reasonable, therefore, to expect that nursing interventions with families can be as helpful as interventions that directly promote health and function in the individual with chronic illness. Moreover, inclusion of the family may strengthen the adjustments that chronically ill clients must make during the course of illness. As family members increasingly are relied on to provide time-consuming health care, their health and well-being directly affects care outcomes for chronically ill members. As a result, defining and assessing quality of life is not limited to the client, but should include specific measures that enable nurses to assess and meet the needs of family caregivers (Kitrungrote & Cohen, 2006).

A study of the effects of mental illness on families offers insights into strategies that nurses can use to promote quality of life for the caregivers (Walton-Moss, Gerson, & Rose, 2005). An important finding of the research is that nurses need to recognize the variability among families in how they respond to mental illness. All families, regardless of where the mentally ill relative is within the illness trajectory, need to be listened to as they tell their story and want help to communicate with their loved one. This nursing care is supportive of a families' quality of life when they are coping reasonably well or when they are overwhelmed by numerous challenges. Ultimately, the social and emotional support and financial resources of families impact quality of life. Knowledge about resources, services, and organizations for chronic illness conditions can help in making appropriate and timely referrals that will better maintain quality of life and well-being of clients and families.

Individuals and families shift perspectives on their quality of life as they progress through the illness trajectory. At various points, the illness may be primary; at other times, wellness may predominate. When illness is at the center, a situation that occurs most often with a new diagnosis, the focus is on suffering, loss, and burden. Families may become overwhelmed. When the focus is on wellness, this may provide an opportunity to refocus on aspects that engage the family and client to promote quality of life. The nurse who is aware of these shifts in chronic illness behavior is better equipped to support clients through appropriate interventions.

Quality of Life and Technologic Interventions

Nurses are becoming increasingly involved either directly as researchers or indirectly as research coordinators in clinical trials that evaluate quality of life as one outcome for clients receiving new products, devices, and drugs. Attention to and awareness of the effects that technologic advances have on clients' quality of life, therefore, becomes important in nursing care. Federal agencies and regulatory bodies offer extensive guidance and recommendations for evaluating device and treatment effectiveness on client care (US Department of Health & Human Services et al., 2006).

Measurement of client-related outcomes is a particularly important evaluation component in these clinical trials, with quality of life being one such aspect. This approach provides insight regarding treatment effectiveness that can be determined only by clients. An individual's perspective about a drug or treatment effect provides corroboration with observable clinical data. This confirmation is important, because enhanced clinical outcomes such as better glucose control or decreased blood pressure may not necessarily correspond to improvements in function or well-being if the individual is experiencing side effects of the new treatment or drug. In addition, many clinical trials are investigating therapies that are expensive and carry with them uncertain outcomes with regard to quality of life (Grusenmeyer & Wong, 2007). In these instances it is important for clinicians to understand that extraordinary economic costs may be at issue with minimal impact on an individual's quality of life. Clients with life-threatening chronic illnesses also are confronted with choosing life-extending treatments at the expense of quality of life, as these treatments may cause debilitating side effects. Periodic quality of life assessments throughout the course of treatment may offer a better discrimination between improvements versus deterioration in quality of life; and allow client preferences to be included in the decision to continue or forego the specific treatment (Bozcuk et al., 2006).

Another issue with technologic interventions that extend life is deciding when to forego continued treatment. For example, implantable cardioverter–defibrillators have become a well-accepted evidence-based practice for high-risk life-threatening arrhythmias. Individuals with these devices are not only experiencing a better quality of life, they are also living longer. These issues bring to the forefront nurses' role in assessing and managing physical and psychological responses to the devices, and what to do when an individual needs end-of-life care. Care of clients and families in these situations requires nursing knowledge about the efficacy and cost effectiveness of interventions to promote quality of life (Dunbar, 2005).

Similar issues confront those receiving hemodialysis for end-stage renal disease. Hemodialysis frequently impacts quality of life throughout the course of the disease, such that physical and mental well-being are negatively affected. The concern at hand becomes identification of indicators that offer realistic appraisals of outcomes associated with the quality as well as the quantity of life (Cleary & Drennan, 2005).

OUTCOMES

Quality of life as an outcome of care is being increasingly addressed by all healthcare entities, including providers, payers, and consumers. In addition, the increased attention globally to chronic illness care makes it imperative that nurses address quality of life as a nurse-sensitive quality indicator. Clearly as an outcome of nursing care, quality of life can be influenced by appropriately designed care interventions. Nurses are in a position, through research and clinical application of interventions, to make a difference in the lives of clients and families. They can apply evidence-based practices that relieve symptoms and provide comfort; these are actions that promote quality of life. Decision-making to initiate, continue, modify, or withdraw treatments can be made by evaluating quality of life as an outcome. The efficacy of clinical nursing interventions and practice behaviors, likewise, can be evaluated based on their contribution to clients' quality of life. By evaluating the extent to which nursing interventions improve quality of life for clients and families, nurses are in a position to show the efficacy of what they do. That nurses can carry out interventions to promote quality of life becomes meaningful to cost-effective care as well.

Throughout this discussion, repeated emphasis has been given to interrelatedness and overlap of interventions that promote and maintain quality of life in a variety of chronic illness conditions. Physical, functional, and psychosocial components are related, especially in the context of chronic illness. As such they are significant determinants of one's quality of life. In many instances, these characteristics and the social and environmental context of the individual can influence quality of life negatively or positively, depending on the particular set of circumstances. The presence of resources, family support, and access to social and health services can have a powerful and affirming influence on quality of life, despite serious chronic illness disability.

Assessing outcomes of nursing interventions using quality of life as a measure contributes to a fuller description of the accountability nurses have in promoting quality care and outcomes. Knowledge of the individual circumstances that influence quality of life in chronic illness enables better care planning. This targeting of interventions to the specific quality of life for individuals can lead to successful preventive and therapeutic approaches in caring for people with chronic illness. With an ever-present awareness of the many components that influence quality of life in chronic illness, nurses can intervene more effectively.

STUDY QUESTIONS

1. What elements are a part of quality of life evaluations in chronic illness? Discuss how the perceptions of individual clients and healthcare professionals contribute to quality of life evaluations.
2. Identify a theoretical or conceptual framework that addresses quality of life as an outcome for clients and families with a chronic illness. Describe an intervention using that framework that demonstrates how nursing can make a difference in quality of life.
3. Describe the importance of quality of life as a nurse-sensitive quality indicator?
4. As an outcome of care, how is quality of life viewed by healthcare providers,

consumers, agencies, and third party payers?
5. Describe how nurses can use guidelines to promote evidence-based quality of life care to clients and families with chronic illness.
6. What interventions can nurses use to promote client and family quality of life at end-of-life?
7. Describe outcomes that indicate a good quality of life. How might quality of life outcomes change over time?
8. What potential ethical dilemmas arise when evaluating quality of life in chronic illness?

REFERENCES

Allmark, P. (2005). Can the study of ethics enhance nursing practice? *Journal of Advanced Nursing, 51*(6), 618–624.

Amella, E.J. (2003). Geriatrics and palliative care: Collaboration for quality of life until death. *Journal of Hospice and Palliative Nursing, 5*(1), 40–48.

Baird, C.L., & Sands, L.P. (2006). Effect of guided imagery with relaxation on health-related quality of life in older women with osteoarthritis. *Research in Nursing & Health, 29,* 442–451.

Bender, C.M., Ergün, F.Ş., Rosenzweig, M.Q., Cohen, S.M. & Sereika, S.M. (2005). Symptom clusters in breast cancer across 3 phases of the disease *Cancer Nursing, 28*(3), 219–225.

Bozcuk, H., Dalmis, B., Samur, M., Ozdogan, M., Artac, M., & Savas, B. (2006). Quality of life in patients with advanced non-small cell lung cancer. *Cancer Nursing, 29*(2), 104–110.

Cantrell, M.A. (2007). The art of pediatric oncology nursing practice. *Journal of Pediatric Oncology Nursing, 24*(3), 132–138.

Carter, H., Macleod, R., Brander, P., & McPherson, K. (2004). Living with a terminal illness: Patients' priorities. *Journal of Advanced Nursing, 45*(6), 611–620.

Centers for Disease Control & Prevention. (2000). Measuring healthy days: Population assessment of health-related quality of life. Atlanta, GA: CDC.

Chronic Disease Overview. (2005). Retrieved October 3, 2007, from Centers for Disease Control and Prevention website: http://www.cdc.gov/nccdphp/overview.htm

Clark, E., Donovan, E.F., & Schoettker, P. (2006). From outdated to updated, keeping clinical guidelines valid. *International Journal for Quality in Health Care, 18*(3), 165–166.

Clark, E.H. (2004). Quality of life: A basis for clinical decision-making in community psychiatric care. *Journal of Psychiatric and Mental Health Nursing, 11*, 725–730.

Cleary, J., & Drennan, J. (2005). Quality of life of patients on haemodialysis for end-stage renal disease. *Journal of Advanced Nursing, 51*(6), 577–586.

Coopey, M., Nix, M.P., & Clancy, C.M. (2006). Translating research into evidence-based nursing practice and evaluating effectiveness. *Journal of Nursing Care Quality, 21*(3), 195–202.

Crone, D. (2007). Walking back to health: A qualitative investigation into service users' experiences of a walking project. *Issues in Mental Health Nursing, 28*, 167–183.

Delgado, C. (2007). Sense of coherence, spirituality, stress and quality of life in chronic illness. *Journal of Nursing Scholarship, 39*(3), 229–234.

Dickerson, S.S., Wu, Y.B., & Kennedy, M.C. (2006). A CNS-facilitated ICD support group: A clinical project evaluation. *Clinical Nurse Specialist 20*(3), 146–153.

Donabedian, A. (1988). Quality assessment and assurance: Unity of purpose diversity and means. *Inquiry, 25*, 173–192.

Doran, D.M., Harrison, M.B., Laschinger, H.S., Hirdes, J.P., Rukholm, E., Sidani, S., et al. (2006). Nursing-sensitive outcomes data collection in acute care and long-term-care settings. *Nursing Research, 55*(2S), S75–S81.

Dorr, D.A., Jones, S.S., Burns, L., Donnelly, S.M., Brunker, C.P., Wilcox, A., et al. (2006). Use of health-related, quality-of-life metrics to predict mortality and hospitalizations in community-dwelling seniors. *Journal of the American Geriatrics Society, 54*(4), 667–673.

Dubos, R. (1959). *Mirage of health: Utopias, progress, and biological change.* Garden City, NY: Doubleday.

Dunbar, S.B. (2005). Psychosocial issues of patients with implantable cardioverter defibrillators. *American Journal of Critical Care, 14*(4), 294–303.

Erci, B., Sayan, A., Tortumluoğlu, G., Kiliç, D., Şahin, O., & Güngörmüş, Z. (2003). The effectiveness of Watson's caring model on the quality of life and blood pressure of patients with hypertension. *Journal of Advanced Nursing, 41*(2), 130–139.

Feldman, P.H., Murtaugh, C.M., Pezzin, L.E., McDonald, M.V., & Peng, T.R. (2005, June). Just-in-time evidence-based e-mail "reminders" in home health care: Impact on patient outcomes. *HSR: Health Services Research, 40*(3), 865–885.

Ferrell, B., Cullinane, C.A., Ervin, K., Melancon, C., Uman, G.C., & Juarez, G. (2005). Perspectives on the impact of ovarian cancer: Women's view of quality of life. *Oncology Nursing Forum, 32*(6), 1143–1149.

Grusenmeyer, P.A., & Wong, Y. (2007). Interpreting the economic literature in oncology. *Journal of Clinical Oncology, 25*(2), 196–202.

Healthy People 2010. *A systematic approach to health improvement* (n.d.). Retrieved October 11, 2007, from www.healthypeople.gov/Document/Word/uih/uih_bw.doc

Heidrich, S.M., Egan, J.J., Hengudomsub, P., & Randolph, S.M. (2006). Symptoms, symptom beliefs, and quality of life of older breast cancer survivors: A comparative study. *Oncology Nursing Forum, 33*(2), 315–322.

Hirskyj, P. (2007). QALY: An ethical issue that dare not speak its name. *Nursing Ethics, 14*(1), 72–82.

Huang, T., & Liang, S. (2005). Care of older people: A randomized clinical trial of the effectiveness of a discharge planning intervention in hospitalized elders with hip fracture due to falling. *Journal of Clinical Nursing, 14,* 1193–1201.

Jocham, H.R., Dassen, T., Widdershoven, G., & Halfens, R. (2006). Quality of life in palliative care cancer patients: A literature review. *Journal of Clinical Nursing, 15,* 1188–1195.

Jonas-Simpson, C.M., Mitchell, G.J., Fisher, A., Jones, G., & Linscott, J. (2006). The experience of being listened to: A qualitative study of older adults in long-term care settings. *Journal of Gerontological Nursing, 32*(1), 46–53.

Kirshbaum, M.N. (2006). A review of the benefits of whole body exercise during and after treatment for breast cancer. *Journal of Clinical Nursing, 16,* 104–121.

Kitrungrote, L., & Cohen, M.Z. (2006). Quality of life of family caregivers of patients with cancer: A literature review. *Oncology Nursing Forum, 33*(3), 625–632.

Kristofferzon, M., Löfmark, R., & Carlsson, M. (2005). Issues and innovations in nursing practice: Coping, social support, and quality of life over time after myocardial infarction. *Journal of Advanced Nursing, 52*(2), 113–124.

Lee, P., Chang, W., Liou, T., & Chang, P. (2006). Issues and innovations in nursing practice: Stage of exercise and health-related quality of life among overweight and obese adults. *Journal of Advanced Nursing, 53*(3), 295–303.

Losito, J.M., Murphy, S.O., & Thomas, M.L. (2006). The effects of group exercise on fatigue and quality of life during cancer treatment. *Oncology Nursing Forum, 33*(4), 821–825.

Low, G., & Molzahn, A.E. (2007). Predictors of quality of life in old age: A cross-validation study. *Research in Nursing & Health, 30,* 141–150.

Mitchell, S.A., Beck, S.L., Hood, L.E., Moore, K., & Tanner, E.R. (2007). Putting evidence into practice: Evidence-based interventions for fatigue during and following cancer and its treatment. *Clinical Journal of Oncology Nursing, 11*(1), 99–113.

Moons, P., Budts, W., & DeGeest, S. (2006). Critique on the conceptualization of quality of life: A review and evaluation of different conceptual approaches. *International Journal of Nursing Studies, 43,* 891–901.

Moreira-Almeida, A., & Koenig, H.G. (2006). Retaining the meaning of the words religiousness and spirituality: A commentary on the WHOQOL-SRPB group's "A cross-cultural study of spirituality, reli-gion, and personal beliefs as components of quality of life." *Social Science & Medicine, 63,* 843–845.

National Guideline Clearinghouse. (2007). Retrieved November 21, 2007, from www.guidelines.gov

National Institute of Nursing Research. (2006). Changing practice, changing lives: NINR strategic plan (2006–2010). *Journal of the American Academy of Nurse Practitioners, 20*(5):281–287.

O'Brien, M.E. (2003). *Spirituality in nursing: Standing on holy ground* (2nd ed.), Sudbury, MA: Jones & Bartlett.

Orfila, F., Ferrer, M., Lamarca, R., Tebe, C., Domingo-Salvany, A., & Alonso, J. (2006). Gender differences in health-related quality of life among the elderly: The role of objective functional capacity and chronic conditions. *Social Science & Medicine, 63,* 2367–2380.

Reeve, B.B., Burke, L.B., Chiang, Y., Clauser, S.B., Colpe, L.J., Elias, J.W., et al. (2007). Enhancing measurement in health outcomes research supported by agencies within the U.S. Department of Health and Human Services. *Quality of Life Research, 16,* 175–186.

Saunders, J.C., & Cookman, C.A. (2005). A clarified conceptual meaning of hepatitis C-related depression. *Gastroenterology Nursing, 16*(46), 123–130.

Sousa, K.H., Ryu, E., Kwok, O., Cook, S.W., & West, S.G. (2007). Development of a model to measure symptom status in persons living with rheumatoid arthritis. *Nursing Research, 56*(6), 434–440.

Stenzelius, K., Westergren, A., & Hallberg, I.R. (2007). Bowel function among people over 75 years reporting faecal incontinence in relation to help seeking, dependency and quality of life. *Journal of Clinical Nursing, 16,* 458–468.

Suhonen, R., Välimäki, M., Katajisto, J., & Leino-Kilpi, H. (2005). Provision of individualized care improves hospital patient outcomes: An explanatory model using LISREL. *International Journal of Nursing Studies, 44,* 197–207.

Sullivan, T., Weinert, C., & Cudney, S. (2003). Management of chronic illness: Voices of rural women. *Journal of Advanced Nursing, 44*(6), 566–574.

Sutton, L.B., & Erlen, J.A. (2006). Effects of mutual dyad support on quality of life in women with breast cancer. *Cancer Nursing, 29*(6), 488–498.

Taylor, S.J.C., Candy, B., Bryar, R.M., Ramsay, J., Vrijhoef, H.J.M., Esmond, G., et al. (2005). Effectiveness of innovations in nurse led chronic disease management for patients with chronic obstructive pulmonary disease: Systematic review of evidence. *British Medical Journal.* Retrieved July 30, 2007, from http://www.bmj.com/

U.S. Department of Health and Human Services, FDA Center for Drug Evaluation and Research, FDA Center for Biologics Evaluation and Research, and FDA Center for Devices and Radiological Health. (2006). Guidance for industry: Patient-reported outcome measures: Use in medical product development to support labeling claims: Draft guidance. *Health quality of life outcomes.* Retrieved on October 11, 2007, from http://www.fda.gov/cder/guidance/5460dft.htm

Vig, E.K., & Pearlman, R.A. (2003). Quality of life while dying: A qualitative study of terminally ill older men. *Journal of the American Geriatrics Society, 51*(11), 1595–1601.

Walton-Moss, B., Gerson, L., & Rose, L. (2005). Effects of mental illness on family quality of life. *Issues in Mental Health Nursing, 26,* 627–642.

Whittemore, R. (2005). Clinical scholarship: Analysis of integration in nursing science and practice. *Journal of Nursing Scholarship, 37*(3), 261–267.

World Health Organization. (1948). What is the WHO definition of health? Retrieved on October 11, 2007, from http://www.who.int/suggestions/faq/en/print.html

World Health Organization (2004). The World Health Organization quality of life (WHOQOL)–BREF. Retrieved on October 11, 2007, from http://www.who.int/substance_abuse/research_tools/en/english_whoqol.pdf

8

Adherence

Jill Berg, Lorraine S. Evangelista, Donna Carruthers, and Jacqueline M. Dunbar-Jacob

INTRODUCTION

Adherence of patients to prescribed treatment by their healthcare professionals has been discussed in the medical literature since the 1950s (Greene, 2004). The lack of agreement between healthcare recommendations and patient behavior has been defined as an issue of adherence or nonadherence [Haynes, 1979; Rand, 1993; World Health Organization (WHO), 2003]. Early research identified this problem of discrepancy between an ordered treatment and the actual implementation of the treatment by the patient as a factor that affected patient outcomes (Sackett & Snow, 1979).

In 2001, the World Health Organization (WHO) convened a meeting on treatment adherence. Poor adherence to treatment of chronic diseases was identified to be 50% in developed counties, with lower rates of adherence in developing countries (WHO, 2003). Adherence with medical recommendations is poor across all chronic disease regimens. This nonadherence increases healthcare expenditures and prevents patients from achieving the full benefit of any intervention. In addition, most chronic disorders are treated with a plan of care that encompasses a variety of components that may include medication, diet,

and exercise. Therefore, patients are often asked to manage a complex treatment regimen.

Goals for *Healthy People 2010*

Overall goals for Healthy People (US Department of Health and Human Services, 2000) are to help Americans lead healthy and long lives and to reduce health disparities. There are 467 objectives to be met by 2010, and many of these objectives in this document relate to behavior change strategies. For example, for diabetes, many of the goals in *Healthy People 2010* refer to lifestyle changes and education in order to better manage the disease and avoid complications such as end-stage renal disease and death. Goals for *Healthy People 2010* include health behavior change such as adherence to chronic illness regimens and preventive behaviors such as screenings to detect risk factors for disease.

Adherence and Chronic Illness

The predominant pattern of illness has changed from acute to chronic as science and technology have advanced. With that technology, treatment regimens have become more complex. However, because of changes in managed health care, these complex regimens are implemented with limited or no supervision as the patient and/or family caregivers carry out these prescribed regimens at home. Therefore, practitioners must be concerned with the extent to which patients can implement the treatment plans they design, as well as the evaluation of the patient's responses.

Patient responsibility for managing chronic conditions has increased, but there is concern about adherence as it relates to medical outcomes and economic costs. For example, an individual who has insulin-dependent diabetes mellitus (IDDM) may have a computerized insulin pump and a blood-testing device. This individual may, at some point, be a candidate for hemodialysis or renal transplantation because of complications. All of these treatment modalities require adherence behaviors to ensure maximal benefit and minimal harm to the patient. According to DiMatteo (2004), the average rate of nonadherence to treatment across all diseases is 24.8%. If this rate was extrapolated to physician visits by individuals with diabetes, as many as 7.6 million visits would result in nonadherence.

The managed care environment has also had an impact on patient burden in chronic illness. Managed care's influence on health care has been demonstrated by earlier hospital discharges, shortened office visits, and decreasing home health referrals. In addition, recent literature indicates that as many as 46% of healthcare professionals do not prescribe adequate therapy for their patients (McGlynn et al., 2003). Therefore, patients and family members have had to shoulder more of the responsibility for the treatment regimen, often in isolation. Although disease management programs have been developed by health maintenance organizations (HMOs), few programs have been implemented and critically evaluated to date. Healthcare professionals working within a managed care system often have little time to address the management of chronic illness and adherence with the recommended regimen (Miller, Hill, Kottke, & Ockene, 1997). Other findings suggest that healthcare professionals and agencies can make a difference in medical outcomes by means of integrating multidisciplinary interventions specifically aimed at assisting the patient to manage their chronic disease through education, self-management instruction, prevention, and outreach strategies (Feachem, Sekhri, & White, 2002).

Literally hundreds of studies have examined adherence behavior, but unfortunately that research has not effected significant changes in behavior (Dunbar-Jacob & Schlenk, 2001; McDonald, Garg, & Haynes, 2002). Even in the 1980s, health behavior researchers such as Conrad (1985) asserted that it was reasonable to assume that a patient with chronic illness attempts to self-regulate in order to gain some control over something that is not always controllable. Rosenstock (1988) also noted that healthcare professionals should "encourage people to make informed decisions, but decisions of their own choice . . ." (p. 72). He added that healthcare professionals are not always right, and there is always the potential for untoward side effects from ordered treatment. These assertions have not changed over the years, and, in fact, we have made little progress even in our understanding of adherence behavior. Furthermore, we have not successfully implemented interventions to ensure continuing adherence with chronic regimens.

Chronic illness regimens can be exceedingly complex, and resources to assist individuals with chronic illness are often limited. Therefore, it is important that the healthcare professional understands the variables that affect the ability of the person to adhere to a regimen. To facilitate understanding, this chapter addresses factors that have an impact on adherence behavior. A discussion of the theories and a description of techniques are also presented to provide a context for the behavioral changes that are required in treatment regimens. We will also present information on goals related to *Healthy People 2010*, as well as evidence-based guidelines and their relationship to adherence behaviors. Finally, interventions to improve adherence are presented, along with case studies to illustrate key strategies.

Ms. C is a 25-year-old Latina with a history of asthma. As a child, Ms. C had severe asthma, which was very difficult to control. Once she was in high school, her asthma improved. She had not had an asthma attack since she was 16 until this last weekend when she had to go the emergency room because she had difficulty breathing. She reports to you that she had a cold recently, and still has a frequent cough. She works at a local copy shop and this past week she was coughing so much at work she had to go home. She is also dating a young man who smokes. She needs help in restarting an asthma trigger reduction program, starting on some anti-inflammatory medications and speaking to her boyfriend about his smoking.

Discussion Questions

1. How can you, a healthcare provider, help Ms. C to develop a course of action to which she is likely to adhere?
2. How would you suggest that Ms. C's boyfriend help Ms. C with her recent health problems and new treatment regimens (other than by quitting smoking)?
3. Suggest possible measures of adherence behaviors that you might use to assess Ms. C's adherence.

Definition of Terms and Historical Perspectives

Greene (2004) addresses the first use of terms related to patients following recommended treatment regimens. He credits medical sociology and further describes the evolution of terms as well as the development of a discipline concerned with health behavior. There were a variety of labels associated with these behaviors, and patients were labeled as "uncooperative, non-compliant, poorly-controlled, resistant, devious, incorrigible, irresponsible and careless" (Greene, 2004, p. 330). Early descriptions of patients having difficulty following treatment regimens reflected societal attitudes related to tuberculosis in patients who were poor and foreign-born. Eventually, the terms used to describe behavior included compliance, adherence and concordance.

In 1974 a group of scientists gathered in Canada to discuss compliance with therapeutic regimens (Greene, 2004). The term compliance was chosen after some careful debate (well described in the Greene essay). Compliance was used as an umbrella term for all behavior related to healthcare recommendations, particularly in light of the shift from acute to chronic disease seen in the last half of the 20th century.

Adherence and nonadherence are generally used as synonyms for the original terms compliance and noncompliance. The term adherence has eventually been adopted instead of the term compliance on the global stage of healthcare delivery. An example of an interesting classic presentation in the meaning and use of these words was presented by Barofsky (1978), who proposed a continuum of self-care with three levels of patient response to healthcare recommendations: compliance, adherence, and therapeutic alliance. In his model, compliance is linked with coercion; adherence, to conformity; and self-care, to a therapeutic alliance with provider–patient interactions. Misselbrook (1998) used the term concordance to indicate the partnership between practitioner and patient in achieving health outcomes.

The literature reveals different schools of thought related to adherence presented in the literature. One school supports the notion that it is impossible to ever have patients completely adhere to medical regimens. A contradictory school of thought suggests that it is possible, through education or other means, to have patients adhere to their regimen requirements. These contrary schools of thought may be dependent on how the health plan was formulated (Dunbar, 1980). If the plan is formulated by a partnership between the patient and the healthcare professional, the possibility of the patient "adhering" to the plan increases. Should the patient be expected to follow a plan created exclusively by the healthcare professional, without input by the patient, then the patient may or may not "comply." The WHO has adopted "adherence" as the term of choice and suggests that it is necessary to incorporate the agreement of the patient with the prescribed treatment plan (WHO, 2003).

Creer and Levstek (1996) as well as Dunbar-Jacob (1993) questioned the extent to which we "blame the patient" for their adherence behavior. Part of the responsibility, they assert, belongs to healthcare professionals, and there are instances when nonadherence is wise, given the regimen. Trostle (1997) argued that there is too much emphasis placed on the authority physicians have in recommending healthcare regimens. He further asserted that nonadherence is viewed as "nonconformity with medical advice" (p. 116) and suggested that we look broadly at the behaviors that are being engaged in by patients within the context of their illness. He also cautioned that attempts to motivate patients to comply could be considered coercive and manipulative. In any event, healthcare professionals often make decisions about the effectiveness of treatments without knowing whether the patient is actually following the treatment or in agreement with their healthcare professional (Rand, 2004).

In order to provide efficacious treatment of chronic disease, healthcare professionals face two challenges. First, we must ascertain whether patients are following the regimen, and secondly we must find effective ways of helping patients to overcome barriers in carrying out complex regimens.

Components of Adherence

The relevance of adherence to the total wellness–illness continuum was first described by Marston, a nurse, in 1970. Marston considered adherence to be self-care behaviors that individuals undertake to promote health, to prevent illness, or to follow recommendations for treatment and rehabilitation in diagnosed illnesses. She is notable in the history of treatment adherence as the first reviewer of literature in the field (Greene, 2004).

It may be helpful, however, to consider adherence as more than self-care behaviors; rather, it is behavior that is often shared, because patients cannot always implement their medical regimens without the participation of others, even though the delineation of responsibilities is not always clear. Sackett and Haynes (1976) outlined three necessary ingredients before labeling a patient "non-compliant." These include (1) a correct diagnosis must be made, (2) the recommended treatment must be determined to be efficacious, (3) and the patient must be informed and willing. For example, Greenley, Josie, and Drotar (2006) note that there are misunderstandings about the responsibility for an asthma treatment regimen in inner-city children, and that this misunderstanding often leads to nonadherence. This is especially true when there is a change in the dependence/independence status of the patient, as with the teenager who assumes greater responsibility for management of his or her healthcare regimen or the older adult who now requires more supervision and assistance by family members.

In the classic book *Chronic Illness and the Quality of Life*, Strauss and associates (1984) noted that family members often take on assisting or controlling roles in influencing patients to adhere to medical regimens. A follow-up study of how couples managed chronic disease revealed that coordination and collaboration between the couple were necessary to carry out the work of the medical regimen (Corbin & Strauss, 1985). More recent work in the field of HIV, describes the role that family caregivers provide in the complex regimen (Beals, Wight, Aneshensel, Murphy, & Miller-Martinez, 2006). A review by Knafl and Gilliss

(2002) concludes that nursing needs to be more involved with family interventions for chronic illness management. Given that shared responsibility exists, it seems reasonable to conclude that adherence-increasing strategies should be directed toward all those involved in the regimen, and that there may be a need for discussing the division of responsibility among family members.

Theoretical Underpinnings for Adherence Behavior

Theoretical frameworks and conceptual models provide direction for healthcare professionals by guiding the assessment and providing structure for the interaction of patient and provider. At this point in time, the emphasis is on translation of theories and models to effective practice interventions. Although an extensive library devoted to adherence behavior exists, few studies support strategies to improve adherence (DiMatteo & Haskard, 2006). Models for understanding individual health behavior can only be useful if they are based on empirical research and can then be used to create effective interventions. This relates to the current mandate for translational research and evidence-based practice. Brief reviews of behavioral models that are currently used are presented in the following.

Health Belief Model

The health belief model (HBM), developed by Hochman et al. (as cited in Rosenstock, 1974) was devised to explain health-related behaviors, especially preventive health behaviors, and contains a cluster of pertinent beliefs and attitudes (Becker & Maiman, 1975). The model was modified to include general health motivation (Becker, 1976) and was again modified to include sick-role behaviors. The HBM's major proposition is that the likelihood of an individual taking recommended health actions is based on (1) the illness's perceived severity, (2) the individual's estimate of the likelihood that a specific action will reduce the threat, and (3) perceived barriers to following recommendations. The

HBM is still used frequently to explain the relationships of attitudes and behaviors to adherence behavior, specifically in relation to perceived susceptibility, perceived severity, and perceived barriers (McCall & Ginis, 2004; Rodriquez-Reimann, Nicassio, Reimann, Gallegos, & Olmedo, 2004; and Wutoh et al., 2005).

Health Promotion Model

A nursing model that evolved from the HBM is the health promotion model (HPM) (Pender, 1996; Pender, Murdaugh, & Parsons, 2001). Pender conceptualizes health as a goal and believes that only the desire to be healthy leads to engagement of health promotion activities. Pender organized the concepts under the framework of individual characteristics and experiences, behavior-specific cognitions and affect, and behavioral outcomes. The Health Promoting Lifestyle Profile is an instrument that assesses health promotion behaviors, and has been translated and validated in Spanish as well as English (Walker, Sechrist, & Pender, 1987). Recent studies using this model have supported that income and education negatively impact the use of health promotion activities (Chilton, Hu, & Wallace, 2006; Lee, Santacroce, & Sadler, 2007).

Common Sense Model of Self-Regulation

The Common Sense Model of Self-Regulation was developed from two prior models. One of them, the Common Sense model, was developed by Leventhal, Meyer, & Nerenz, in 1980 to explain how individuals process illness-related events and how this shapes coping and adherence. Early studies using this model were conducted primarily on individuals with asymptomatic illnesses (Baumann, Cameron, Zimmerman, & Leventhal, 1989; Meyer, Leventhal, & Gutmann, 1985).

In brief, an individual's processing of illness-related events is dependent on four dimensions: cause (what was responsible for the illness), consequences (how things will change because of the illness), identity (being able to identify the illness), and timeline (the course of the illness). In 1987,

CASE STUDY

Mr. W. is a 58-year-old African American college history professor with type 2 diabetes. He was diagnosed with diabetes 3 years ago and lost weight and started an exercise program. During the last year, he has gained weight and is no longer exercising daily. He admits to you that with some changes at work, he is extremely stressed. He starts every evening with a martini, relaxes after his long day, and then has a big dinner. His blood sugars are out of control and you are concerned that he will have to start insulin injections.

Discussion Questions

1. Would you, the health provider, label Mr. W as nonadherent? Why or why not?
2. Suggest several lifestyle modifications that may benefit Mr. W.
3. How might Mr. W's perspective of his illness differ from that of his provider?

Leventhal and colleagues identified a feedback mechanism to a behavioral model and called it the Self-Regulation Theory. The dimension of control–cure was examined as part of the illness representation. These two models are now combined into one model known as the Common Sense Model of Self-Regulation (Leventhal, Brisette, & Leventhal, 2003). Recent studies using this model have shown that beliefs about illness affect coping (Kelly, Sereika, Battista, & Brown, 2007; Ohm & Aaronson, 2006; Quinn, 2005; Searle, Norman, Thompson, & Vedhara, 2007).

The Theory of Reasoned Action and the Theories of Planned Behavior

The theory of reasoned action (Fishbein & Ajzen, 1975) and the theory of planned behavior (Ajzen, 1985) have intention as a main component. Individuals engage in health behaviors, intentionally, based on attitudes toward a behavior and social influence. The theory of planned behavior adds a component to the model, called "perceived behavioral control," which captures the extent to which a person has control over any given behavior. Both of these theories have been useful in the examination of preventive behaviors, such as engaging in exercise programs (Martin, Oliver, & McCaughtry, 2007; Norman & Connor, 2005), condom use (Gredig, Nideroest, & Parpan-Blaser, 2006), and binge drinking (Norman, Armitage, & Quigley, 2007), where intention has been found to be an important component of engaging in the desired behavior. Such theories have proven to be valuable in comprehending physical activity in chronic illness regimens (Eng & Martin-Guiness, 2007).

Cognitive Social Learning Theory

Cognitive social learning theory attempts to predict behavior that is dictated by outcome and efficacy expectancies. This theory combines environment, cognition, and emotion in the understanding of health behavior change (Bandura, 2004). Three necessary prerequisites to altering health behavior are the recognition that a lifestyle component can be harmful, the recognition that a change in behavior would be beneficial, and the recognition that one has the ability to adopt a new behavior (self-efficacy) (Schwarzer, 1992). To effect any change then, each individual must be able to self-monitor and self-regulate health behavior. This aspect of self-regulation has led to a variety of self-management strategies with which to cope with illness. The additional component of self-efficacy, defined as the patient's expectations or confidence in his or her ability to perform a recommended action, has also promoted research to test efficacy-enhancing strategies important in health behavior change. Self-efficacy has been found to be an important predictor of self-management behaviors useful in the treatment of AIDS (Johnson et al., 2006) cancer (Eiser, Hill, & Blacklay, 2000), cardiac disease (Hiltunen et al., 2005), depression (Harrington et al., 2000), and diabetes (Ott, Greening, Palardy, Holderby, & DeBell, 2000).

Transtheoretical Model of Change (Stages of Change)

The stages of change, or transtheoretical model, was developed by Prochaska and DiClemente (1983), and it is an eclectic model that aims to examine and predict the process of change. This model contains three constructs: the stages of change; processes of change; and levels of change. The model's underlying premise proposes that people are at different stages in their intentional desire to adopt certain health behaviors with or without assistance. It also proposes that interventions should be matched to each categorical stage of change. Although presented hierarchically, the process of change is considered to be spiral with relapse from a healthy behavior placing an individual in a position to move backward toward contemplation of the healthy behavior. The model also incorporates self-efficacy and decision-making as key factors in the process of change, but these factors have an impact at different stages of change. The stages include the following:

1. Pre-contemplation: no intention of changing behavior
2. Contemplation: considering future action
3. Pre-action: have a timetable for action
4. Action: involved in behavior change
5. Maintenance: after change is adopted; relapse is a possibility

The stage model of health behavior was initially applied to the treatment of addictive behaviors. Currently other research on behavioral change for chronic illness has embraced this model. Clinical interventions have been proposed at each stage. The use of motivational interviewing has been examined for use in moving patients to an action phase of readiness (Jackson, Asimakopoulou, & Scammell, 2007; Johnson et al., 2007), although critics warn that there is no theoretical link between motivational interviewing and the transtheoretical model.

In summary, there are many models that have been used to study adherence behavior in chronic illness. It is important to have a theoretical basis for proposed interventions; however, more work needs to be accomplished to evaluate the effectiveness of theory-based strategies.

Prevalence of Nonadherence

Individuals with chronic medical conditions face a variety of stressful life circumstances involving a range of adaptation demands. Individuals with chronic illness must deal with a loss of independence, the threat of disease progression, and the challenge of modifying their behavior to meet the demands of a prescribed regimen. Lifestyle modifications may become necessary and include, but are not limited to, dietary changes, use of medications, and change in physical activity. Adherence with these modifications has substantial implications for treatment success and decreased disease progression.

For the patient with chronic illness, failure to adhere can result in increased disease complications, increased hospitalizations, greater treatment costs, as well as disruptions in lifestyle, family dynamics, and coping skills. Although ascertaining the true picture of nonadherence in chronic illness is difficult, the consistency with which poor adherence rates are reported indicates that nonadherence is a major problem in health care. Recent studies indicate that adherence rates in chronic illness are approximately 50% (Dunbar-Jacob et al., 2000; Haynes, McDonald, Garg, & Montague, 2002; WHO, 2003). For example: in the United States, medication adherence to antihypertensive medications is 51% (Graves, 2000). However, this problem is not limited to the United States. In developing countries, it is estimated that adherence to antihypertensive medications rates is less than 50% (van der Sande et al., 2000).

Different definitions of adherence have contributed to difficulties in comparing studies of particular disease groups, and make it impossible to generalize to studies highlighting other diseases. Adherence studies are typically disease-specific; that is, the study population is defined by the presence of a specific disease. However, more recent reviews of adherence behaviors in persons with chronic illness indicate that the nature and extent of adherence problems are similar across diseases, across regimens, and across age groups (Vermeire, Hearnshaw, Van Royen, & Denekens, 2001). A review of studies examining medication adherence reported rates as low as 50%, with some differences in rates seen between settings and measurement methods (Dunbar-Jacob et al., 2000).

Medication adherence is one category of research that spans a variety of diseases. Unfortunately there is no gold standard to measure medication adherence, and current evidence suggests the use of several strategies besides disease outcomes to capture treatment adherence to medication (Krapek et al., 2004; Wagner & Rabkin, 2000; Wendel et al., 2001). Furthermore, polypharmacy in chronic disorders adds an additional variable in observing and measuring medication adherence (Vik, Maxwell, & Hogan, 2004).

Electronic monitors have been used to assess medication adherence in many recent studies. Studies of treatment adherence in HIV populations have used both self-report, diaries, and medication event monitors (MEMs). Not specific to HIV populations, electronic monitoring typically provides lower estimates of adherence than self-report data (Wagner & Rabkin, 2000). In a study of individuals with ankylosing spondylitis, only 22%

adhered strictly to prescribed medication (de Klerk & van der Linden, 1996). Although nonadherence rates were not as low among patients with epilepsy (34%) (Cramer, Vachon, Desforges, & Sussman, 1995); major depression (37–55%) (Demyttenaere, Van Ganse, Gregoire, Gaens, & Mesters, 1998; Carney, Freedland, Eisen, Rich, & Jaffe, 1995); schizophrenia (55%) (Duncan & Rogers, 1998), diabetes mellitus (47%) (Mason, Matsayuma, & Jue, 1995); hypertension (30–47%) (Mounier-Vehier et al., 1998; Lee et al., 1996); and ischemic heart disease (38–45%) (Carney et al., 1998; Straka, Fish, Benson, & Suh, 1997), these nonadherence behaviors were nonetheless significantly associated with poor control of symptoms.

Other methods for measuring medication adherence (drug-dosing recall, pill counts, self-report surveys, and pharmacy refills) have been used and have yielded similar rates of adherence (DiMatteo, 2004; Dunbar-Jacob, Schlenk, & Caruthers, 2002). In a study using subjects with chronic pain, paper diaries and electronic diaries were compared. The electronic diaries offered a time-stamped variation on the paper diary and outperformed the latter with regard to adherence of use by the subject (Stone, Shiffman, Schwartz, Broderick, & Hufford, 2003).

Forty-eight percent of patients with tuberculosis were reported as having defaulted on their recommended medication prescriptions (Pablos-Mendez, Knirsch, Barr, Lerner, & Frieden, 1997). Treatment adherence following renal transplantation is associated with loss of the graft. In addition, a history of poor adherence prior to transplantation has also been associated with graft loss (Butler, Roderick, Mullee, Mason, & Peveler, 2004). Self-reported medication nonadherence among renal transplant recipients ranged between 13 and 36% (Greenstein & Siegal, 1998; Hilbrands, Hoitsma, & Koene, 1995), whereas heart transplant recipients showed nonadherence rates of up to 37% (Grady et al., 1996). Although persons with life-threatening disorders may adhere somewhat better than other patients, researchers suggest that even moderate alterations in their treatment have a significant clinical impact (de Geest, Abraham, & Dunbar-Jacob, 1996; Dew et al., 2007).

Dunbar-Jacob and colleagues (2000) have summarized other behaviors that should be considered when assessing adherence:

- Nonadherence with low-fat, low-cholesterol diets (15–88%)
- Nonadherence with weight-reducing diets (greater than 50%)
- Nonadherence with therapeutic exercise (50% dropping out of exercise during the first 3 to 6 months; leveling to a drop-out rate between 55% and 75% at 12 months)
- Nonadherence with appointment keeping (8.5–63.4%)

ISSUES RELATED TO EXAMINING ADHERENCE BEHAVIOR

Studies have demonstrated that large numbers of individuals do not follow healthcare recommendations completely. Although nonadherence is increasingly recognized as a problem, there is no consensus about appropriate or effective methods to increase adherence. Some of the difficulty lies in the inadequacies of research on adherence, some lies in differing role expectations of patients and providers, and some relates to conflict in values. As healthcare professionals prescribe, teach, and counsel patients about medical regimens, they must be cautious in making assumptions about adherence behaviors in a given situation before imposing any specific strategy on the patient.

Individual Characteristics

Several patient characteristics that influence adherence have been examined. These include demographic factors, psychological factors, social support, past health behavior, somatic factors, and health beliefs (Dunbar-Jacob et al., 2002). Ethnicity was addressed in a review by Schlenk and Dunbar-Jacob (1996) and Joshi (1998), indicating that more

research is needed in this area. More recent literature has examined ethnicity as an influence in adherence with diagnostic testing (Strzelczyk & Dignan, 2002). Strzelczyk and Dignan (2002) reported that African American women were more likely to be nonadherent with mammography screening. With respect to retention in clinical trials, African American subjects were more likely to drop out of participation in a rheumatoid arthritis treatment adherence study than caucasians (Dunbar-Jacob et al., 2004). An interesting study by Taira et al. (2007) examined predictors of medication adherence among Asian-American subgroups in Hawaii and found that Filipino, Korean, and Hawaiian patients were less likely to adhere than Japanese patients. More research is needed to examine strategies among various ethnic groups to increase adherence behavior.

Because of the many inconsistencies in studies that examine age and adherence behavior, no overall statement can be made. According to Park and Skurnik, (2004), there may be a variety of factors that interfere with the ability of the older adult to adhere to medical instruction. It is important to rule out cognitive changes, which may occur with aging, versus the busy lifestyle barriers that pertain to the middle-aged adult. In a study by Hinkin et al. (2004), HIV patients who were middle aged were less adherent than older patients. For children, there are specific issues of adherence related to age that are associated with developmental stages rather than chronologic age. However, in general, developmental issues have not been well addressed in the adherence literature (Dunbar-Jacob et al., 2000).

Psychological Factors

Intuitively, healthcare professionals believe that psychological factors may affect adherence behavior. In the case of depression, many studies support the premise that depression is related to poor adherence. DiMatteo, Lepper, and Croghan (2000) completed a meta-analysis examining the relationship between depression and adherence and found that depressed patients were at a threefold risk for nonadherence. Depression has also been linked to mortality in patients not following medical recommendations in acute coronary syndromes (Kronish et al., 2006), and HIV (Lima et al., 2007). It may be helpful to treat depression in patients at risk for nonadherence (Berg, Nyamathi, Christiani, Morisky, & Leake, 2005). Other psychological factors, such as ambiguity, hostility, and general emotional distress, as single factors, are not predictive of adherence behavior but may, in fact, be components of motivation (Dunbar-Jacob, Schlenk, Burke, & Mathews, 1997).

Social Support

Social support is a variable that has frequently been explored in adherence studies. However, social support has not demonstrated to consistently have an impact on adherence behavior. In some cases social support increases adherence behavior, such as in pediatric patients with asthma who received social support from family and friends (Sin, Kang, & Weaver, 2005) or patients with HIV patients (Gonzalez et al., 2004). In contrast, other studies have found that social support has no impact on adherence (Sunil & McGehee, 2007).

Prior Health Behavior

It has been suggested that adherence to a particular healthcare regimen at a single point in time may predict subsequent adherence (Dunbar-Jacob, Schlenk, Burke, & Mathews, 1997). In the 10-year study of the Lipid Research Clinics Coronary Primary Prevention Trial, initial medication adherence accurately predicted adherence throughout the study; however, this did not extend to other health behaviors. In general, it was found that the more similar the initial behaviors were to the behaviors that need to be predicated, the greater the likelihood of accuracy (Dunbar-Jacob, Schlenk, Burke, & Mathews, 1997). In a recent study examining HIV treatment adherence, attending clinic appointments was associated with medication treatment adherence (Wagner, 2003).

Somatic Factors

It has been postulated that the presence of symptoms may lead to greater adherence with medical recommendations. For example, hypertensive individuals who are asymptomatic indicated that they could tell when their blood pressure was high and adhered with treatment at these times because of their belief that adherence relieved the symptoms (Meyer, Leventhal, & Guttman, 1985). In another study, of individuals with lung disease, increased dyspnea predicted greater adherence with nebulizer therapy (Turner, Wright, Mendella, Anthonisen, & IPPB Study Group, 1995). A more recent study found that lack of symptoms was a barrier to adherence with inhaled corticosteroids (Ulrik et al., 2006). Illness-related symptoms may be an important cue to following treatment recommendations.

Regimen Characteristics

Regimen type and regimen complexity have been linked to adherence behavior, with complexity being a more important factor (Dunbar-Jacob, Burke, & Puczynski, 1995). Complexity includes multiple medications, frequent treatments, a variety of treatments (e.g., diet, exercise, and medications), duration of the regimen, a complicated treatment delivery systems, as well as annoying side effects (Lemanek, 1990; Chesney, 2003). An early review of the literature (Wing, Epstein, Nowal, & Lamparski, 1986) substantiated that complicated regimens lead to low adherence rates. This effect has also been well documented in the HIV literature where patients have extremely complex medication regimens (Chesney, 2003; Hinkin et al., 2002).

Economic and Sociocultural Factors

Economic Factors

Poverty, poor English-language proficiency, and limited access to health care are predictors of nonadherence (Gonzalez, 1990). The burdens of financial costs alone may serve as a barrier to obtaining healthcare services, supplies, or medications needed to manage chronic illness. Another major economic barrier to adherence is a lack of resources, including inadequate or difficult transportation, inadequate availability of child care, loss of time from low-paying jobs, and little job security. Socioeconomic status has recently been associated with poor adherence in individuals using hormone-replacement therapy. This needs to be examined further with other studies of adherence (Finley, Gregg, Solomon, & Gay, 2001). Health literacy may also contribute to problems in managing chronic illness regimens. In some studies, limited health literacy has been associated with poor adherence to antiretroviral medications (Wolf et al., 2007) and with better adherence to other HIV medications (Paasche-Orlow et al., 2006).

Some barriers to adherence are clearly related to an ineffective healthcare system for chronic disease management. For example, some individuals with chronic disease who come to emergency departments for nonurgent care have limited access to primary care services that are more appropriate for chronic disease management (Mansour, Lanphear, & DeWitt, 2000). Well known is the decreased availability of primary care services, particularly in inner cities and rural areas, to groups such as migrant workers, new immigrants, the homeless, and those with AIDS. In addition, the maze of governmental and third-party payers' policies and regulations often deny provider reimbursement for preventive or educational services, making these services less available to patients.

Cultural Factors

More attention is being given to the ways in which culture influences health behaviors and the interactions of patients with healthcare providers. Cultural influences affect the way adults and children experience, interpret, and respond to illness and its treatment.

Because of the changing demographics and the influx of immigrants into the United States, studies examining the behaviors of different cultural groups have begun to appear in the literature.

Some of these studies explore the dimension of being a minority group with a health problem. For example, minority status has been associated with lower asthma medication adherence. Minorities were found to have lower adherence and a higher prevalence of negative asthma medication beliefs than caucasians. Tests of mediation suggested that such negative medication beliefs partially mediated the relationship between minority status and adherence (Le et al., 2008). Language issues affect the utilization of health care and the ability to form relationships with healthcare professionals. Different cultural norms may also interfere with adherence behaviors. For example, in Latino families, the stigma of having tuberculosis may be a factor in poor adherence with medication taking (Cabrera, Morisky, & Chin, 2002; Hovell et al., 2003). Latinos have also been described as seeking health care late, if at all, and then using folk healers and medications for illness (Talamantes, Lawler, & Espino, 1995; Zuckerman Guerra, Dorssman, Foland, & Gregory, 1996). Some of the delay in healthcare utilization relates to insurance issues, language barriers, and immigration status.

Asian immigrants may have difficulty accepting and actively engaging in regimen demands. Chinese immigrants were found to have ineffective self-care and coping strategies with diabetes in a study by Jaynes and Rankin (2001). Similarly, in a study by Im and Meleis (1999), Korean women ignored the symptoms of menopause until symptoms became intolerable.

It will become increasingly important for healthcare professionals to interpret the effect of culture and ethnicity on adherence behavior. One of the issues that confounds the link between health behavior and culture is socioeconomic status. There is a need to distinguish if poor adherence is related to ethnicity, cultural, or socioeconomic factors, as opposed to the interaction of these factors.

Patient–Provider Interactions

Of all of the variables associated with nonadherence, patient–provider interactions have been highlighted as being extremely important during the last decade. In 1993, in an editorial in the journal *Health Psychology*, Dunbar-Jacob asks if it is time to share the blame. Previously, the focus of adherence research and practice only examined patient characteristics. In the results from the Medical Outcomes Study, DiMatteo et al. (1993) found that patient satisfaction in an encounter with a healthcare provider may impact health behavior. A few years later, the American Heart Association addressed the "multilevel compliance challenge" (Miller et al., 1997), referring to the contributions of the patient, provider, and the healthcare system. More recent studies have focused on the relationship between provider and patient as a way of encouraging health behavior change (Beach, Keruly, & Moore, 2006; O'Malley, Sheppard, Schwartz, & Mandelblatt, 2004). Strategies such as motivational interviewing have been used successfully by healthcare professionals who are advocating health behavior change (Carels et al., 2007; Cook, Emiliozzi, & McCabe, 2007). Ockene, Hayman, Pasternak, Schron, and Dunbar-Jacob (2002) detail specific strategies that healthcare providers should use in counseling patients. These include:

- Simplify the regimen
- Tailor the regimen to each individual patient
- Ask about adherence behavior at every encounter
- Review patient's medication containers, noting renewal dates
- Involve the patient in designing the treatment plan
- Provide clear instructions (written and verbal)
- Use behavioral strategies (reminder systems, cues, self-monitoring, feedback, and reinforcement)

Perspectives of Patient and Healthcare Professional

Patients and providers are likely to have different perspectives of chronic illness, its treatment, and the relative merits of adherence behavior. The patient lives with the disease, and treatment is only one aspect of that individual's life. Living with treatment consequences is vastly different from offering advice, counsel, education, or exhortation about healthcare recommendations. Patients ask for help from healthcare professionals because they feel ill, they are worried, they are responding to others' recommendations, they need evidence to validate claims for entitlement benefits, and so forth. Providers, on the other hand, are concerned about adherence, which may be seen as the desired outcome of the patient–provider interaction (Anderson, 1985).

Anderson identifies two ways in which the patient's perspectives of chronic illness—in this case, diabetes mellitus—differs from those of healthcare providers. First, there is a relative difference in understanding the treatment regimen, not just on the level of specificity, rationale, and consequences, but also with respect to the sources of problems. Patients may see treatment as part of the problem of having diabetes, whereas providers see treatment as a solution. Second, patients are more concerned about the "here and now" experience, in contrast to providers' concern over a problem that places future health at risk. For example, patients express more concerns about preventing hypoglycemic reactions than about managing higher than normal blood glucose levels. Providers, on the other hand, express more concern about the importance of achieving close to normal blood glucose levels because of their perceptions of serious long-term consequences if control of blood glucose levels is not achieved (Anderson, 1985).

Ethics and Adherence Behavior

Adherence with recommendations for health behavior is an increasingly important ethical issue in healthcare cost containment, because conflicts arise when healthcare resources are limited and decisions about the best use of time, money, and the energy of providers must be made. However, economic and ethical issues in adherence differ.

Whereas economic issues are concerned with the most efficient distribution of resources, ethical issues are concerned with the most equitable distribution (Barry, 1982). Connelly (1984) believes that strategies that promote and improve a patient's active and effective self-care are both ethically and economically significant.

There is also concern about providing resources to help those with chronic disorders in developing countries, where treatment nonadherence is so high (WHO, 2003). Ethical issues center on reciprocal rights and responsibilities of caregivers and patients, use of paternalism and coercion by caregivers, autonomy of the patient, relative risks and benefits of proposed regimens, and the costs to society of nonadherence. Again, the focus upon the patients' active participation with their healthcare providers appears to also raise ethical concerns (Bernardini, 2004; Rand & Sevick, 2000). This questions whether healthcare directed solely by the practitioner without input by the patient is ethical and whether nonadherence should rest upon the shoulders of only the patient.

INTERVENTIONS TO ENHANCE ADHERENCE BEHAVIOR

The complexity of the variables associated with nonadherence should not deter the healthcare professional from working with the patient to achieve maximum possible integration of optimal health recommendations. To accomplish maximum adherence, those who use adherence-increasing strategies have a responsibility to ensure the patient's safety and comprehension. For the nurse, often working as liaison between patient and physician, communicating with either or both is often necessary before matters are sufficiently clear to select and begin specific adherence-increasing strategies. The WHO (2003) has suggested adopting the use of the five "A's" in an effort to assist patients with self-management aspects to their chronic disease, such as treatment adherence. The five "A's" include: assess, advise, agree, assist, and arrange (Locke & Latham, 2002). The

interventions suggested in this chapter are adaptable within this framework. However, advising the patient of the importance of treatment adherence, establishing agreement with a treatment plan, and arranging adequate follow-up are also necessary steps for healthcare professionals interested in providing treatment adherence interventions to their patients.

Assessment

If we are to assume that any measurement of patient adherence is an assessment of behaviors, then we must decide how to analyze those behaviors. Adherence behaviors can be assessed in many ways. Unfortunately, each measurement is prone to some error, usually consisting of a bias toward an overestimation of adherence (Burke & Dunbar-Jacob, 1995; Dunbar-Jacob et al., 2002). Unfortunately, there is no "gold standard" for measuring adherence. However, using a combination of methods to measure a specific adherence behavior is recommended to increase accuracy and reliability of the results, compared with a single method of measurement (WHO, 2003). An assessment of the patient's overall well-being and psychological structure is also essential to a better understanding of his or her adherence behaviors.

A systematic assessment of the patient should include the patient's family, sociocultural and economic factors, knowledge level, beliefs, attitudes, and current understanding of the proposed regimen. Attention should also be given to the patient's perceptions of the illness threat, the efficacy of recommendations, and the patient's ability to carry these out.

Enhancing adherence behaviors is not as simple as telling patients what to do and then telling them again when the desired effect is not achieved. In studying adherence, it is necessary to understand that it is not the length of their life that is of concern to many people with chronic illness, but their perception that the recommended behavior change will be worth the effort (Rapley, 1997). Understanding and respecting the social, cultural, and psychological factors that influence adherence behaviors may enhance efforts to manage the problem of nonadherence.

There should be a determination of the "rightness" of the prescriptions for the particular patient, including an estimation of the relative harm or benefit that is expected. The assessment will allow the nurse to determine which aspects of the regimen management (1) are most unlikely to achieve adherent behavior, (2) are most important in attaining therapeutic goals, and (3) require the most learning to attain the desired behavioral change. The following questions should be asked in an adherence-oriented history (Hingson, Scotch, Sorenson, & Swazey, 1981):

- Have you been taking anything for this problem already?
- Does anything worry you about the illness?
- What can happen if the recommended regimen is not followed?
- How likely is that to occur?
- How effective do you feel the regimen will be in treating the disorder?
- Can you think of any problems you might have in following the regimen?
- Do you have any questions about the regimen or how to follow it?

Healthcare professionals are not infallible, and errors can occur in prescribing, in dispensing, in communicating with the patient and family caregiver, and in maintaining updated written records, especially in settings in which multiple care providers are present. A second consideration is that the patient or caregiver simply may not understand, or remember, instructions. If patients lack the knowledge or skills to undertake a recommended behavior or treatment, it is unlikely that they will do so. Instructions related to treatment regimens need to be reinforced continually over time to enhance adherence behaviors.

Enhancing a patient's motivation requires careful assessment of his or her readiness to make and maintain behavioral changes. Building skills

requires that he or she be ready to learn tasks such as reading food labels, selecting appropriate foods in restaurants, and incorporating the taking of medications into his or her daily routine. In other words, patients must learn new strategies to help them adopt and maintain new behaviors, especially when daily routines are interrupted (Bandura, 1997; Miller et al., 1997).

It is also important to be aware of a tendency among care providers to see adherence behavior as positive, admirable, and wise (being the "good patient") and nonadherence behavior as being negative, deplorable, and unintelligible (being the "problem patient"). It seems probable that healthcare professionals who have this view would be less likely to search out barriers to nonadherence.

Assessment should also lead to a determination of the proper focus of adherence-increasing strategies. It was mentioned earlier that the notion of adherence as self-care may be too restrictive in situations where adherence with medical regimens cannot be achieved without the assistance of others. For instance, the combination of marked disability and chronic illness makes the conceptualization of adherence as self-care ability inappropriate. In such instances, social support networks may be the most important agents of adherence and, therefore, should become the focus of adherence-increasing strategies. However, the nurse should carefully assess the impact of social support on adherence. Although social support—by significant others or support networks—may help patients cope with chronic illness and reinforce adherence behavior in some populations (Burke & Dunbar-Jacob, 1995), this may not be true for all, because there are patients who do not always want tangible help from others.

Measuring Adherence Behaviors

There are several common methodological approaches that focus on adherence. Primary ones include self-report, practitioner report, observation, physiologic measures, medication monitoring, and electronic monitors.

Self-Report

Patient self-reports of adherence behaviors are the simplest and least expensive method of gathering nonadherence information and are feasible in virtually all care settings. Self-reports also allow the collection of more detailed information on the circumstances surrounding poor adherence than any other types of measures (Burke & Dunbar-Jacob, 1995). They may be elicited through simple questions or through a more complex, structured interview schedule. Common self-report measures include medication and symptom diaries, structured questionnaires, and interviews.

Self-reported adherence behavior has come under scrutiny because it is widely believed to be invalid and unreliable (Berg & Arnstein, 2006; Liu et al., 2006; Smith et al., 2007). There are many reasons that a patient's self-reported adherence may be inaccurate. Patients may honestly not remember whether they took their medications, or may have misconceptions about their dosing schedule (Barfod, Hecht, Rubow, & Gerstoft, 2006; Sankar, Nevedal, Neufeld, & Luborsky, 2007). There may also be other reasons for nonadherence such as economic factors, or lack of resources, or the patient's discomfort with being honest with healthcare providers. In any event, it is incumbent on the part of the provider to be able to assess whether a patient can and is willing to follow a recommendation. Toward this end, there are studies that recommend asking questions in a nonjudgmental way to get a valid answer about regimen adherence (Berg & Arnstein, 2006).

Several studies have attempted to evaluate and define the accuracy of self-reported adherence. Many of these have compared patient reports with pill counts, drug levels, or biological markers in body fluids. Most have found that individuals overestimate their adherence (Bender, Milgrom, Rand, & Ackerson, 1998; Dunbar-Jacob et al., 2000; Liu et al., 2006). Despite inherent problems, self-report is still the most common measure used in adherence behavior assessment.

Practitioner Report

Reports by healthcare professionals are an indirect method of adherence assessment. However, studies indicate that this method is not accurate. Because there are no readily observable characteristics of the patient who has trouble following a regimen, clinicians rely on intuition and presumption to gauge the adherence of a patient (Miller et al., 2002; Steele, Jackson, & Gutman, 1990). However, given that practitioner reports are fast, free, noninteractive, and consistent with the medical model, they are still used to assess adherence behavior.

Observation

Direct observation of the patient is not always possible. Therefore, observation is not a practical method of assessing adherence. Theoretically, this method would be an ideal way to provide evidence of adherence behavior; however, individuals often "play to an audience," and the knowledge that someone is watching affects behavior. An example of this behavior for the individual with asthma is the demonstration/return demonstration of the correct method of using metered-dose inhalers (MDIs). Patients with asthma are assessed on their ability to carry out the instructed regimen and adherence with teaching. Although nurses assess a patient's behavior in carrying out tasks related to healthcare management, the assumption cannot be made that this activity continues at home.

Physiologic Measures

Physiologic measures of adherence include serum drug levels, heart rate monitoring, muscle strength, urine sample analysis, cholesterol levels, and glycosylated hemoglobin levels. The advantage of physiologic methods is that these measures are not dependent on the patient's memory or veracity.

Of all of the physiologic measures, measurement of drug levels is most commonly used. Although drug-level measurements reflect a greater degree of accuracy than self-reports and practitioner reports, there are some difficulties with this type of assessment. First, these measures do not reflect the level of adherence (Dunbar-Jacob, Burke, & Puczynski, 1995). They merely classify a person as having followed or not followed some of the regimen (Burke & Dunbar-Jacob, 1995). Second, although assays offer a direct and objective approach to the measurement of nonadherence, this method is neither affordable nor available for every drug, is only applicable to medications with a long half-life, and may vary from individual to individual (de Geest, Abraham, & Dunbar-Jacob, 1996). Third, physiologic technologies are often unable to detect dosage levels. For example, many asthma medications are so rapidly absorbed systemically that it is not possible to detect them by biochemical assay (Rand & Wise, 1994). Finally, accurate detection of nonadherence through drug-level testing offers no explanation or insight into the reasons for nonadherence (Besch, 1995).

Medication Monitors

Pill counts, pharmacy-refill monitoring, and MDI canister weighing can all be used to measure medication adherence. In studies that use pill counts, the subject is given a vial each month that has a certain number of tablets, and this vial is exchanged for a new one each month. The medication left in the vial can be compared with the number that was supposed to be left if the medication were taken. Similarly, when a patient requests a refill from the pharmacy, the time of the request is compared with the expected date of refill if the medication were taken as prescribed. This does not take into account whether patients are sharing medications with others or "dumping" pills prior to refill.

Metered-dose inhaler canister weighing is used with patients who have respiratory illnesses. The canister is weighed before it is given to the patient and then at specific times during treatment. Although medication-monitoring methods appear highly accurate, they may overestimate adherence behavior (Rand & Wise, 1994; Rudd, Ahmed, Zachary, Barton, & Bonduelle, 1990). Berg & Arnstein (2006) suggest that asking a patient to

bring in the medications for a check of pill count may, in fact, be offensive and be counterproductive to the rapport building between patient and provider.

Electronic Monitoring

Electronic monitors are the newest technology for the assessment of adherence behaviors. The most common electronic monitoring device is the electronic medication monitor. Electronic monitors may also be used to capture heart rate and muscle movement with exercise adherence (Iyriboz, Powers, Morrow, Ayers, & Landry, 1991) or to document nasal continuous positive airway pressure adherence for patients with sleep apnea (Kribbs et al., 1993).

Electronic monitors that assess medication adherence are used with tablets, eye drops, and MDIs (Berg & Arnstein, 2006). These monitors function with the use of microprocessors placed in special bottle caps or blister packs and can monitor the date and time of day for each manipulation of the drug container and provide information on drug-taking behavior for days or weeks. Knowing the pattern of pill taking (or not taking) can be useful in evaluating clinical responses (or lack thereof) or side effects, and provide guidance for interventions specifically tailored for each patient (Quittner, Modi, Lemanek, Ievers-Landis, & Rapoff, 2007).

Strategies to Enhance Adherence

There is universal agreement that it is important for patients with chronic illness to follow evidence-based provider recommendations (WHO, 2003). In order to enhance adherence to treatment, there are a variety of strategies that healthcare providers can employ. Some of these strategies are educational, some are behavioral, and some are organizational.

Education

Educational interventions should include an assessment of the patient's level of knowledge, cultural background, and particular goals. Educational information should be presented in manageable segments, with additional information and reinforcement at subsequent meetings. The nurse should focus on the key issues in the management of the regimen and should select the most important aspects necessary for health maintenance. Difficult skills should be demonstrated, and then the patient should be allowed to practice and do a return demonstration. Difficult skills should also be reviewed each time the patient visits.

Written material should be geared to the patient's reading level and language. Glazer and colleagues (1996) evaluated printed materials to teach breast self-examination and found that, although the reading level of the materials being provided was at the ninth-grade level, the average reading level of the target population was at the sixth-grade level. Another study on health literacy found that 24% of patients could not understand even the most basic written medication instructions and that an additional 12% had very limited literacy (Gazmararian, Williams, Peel, & Baker, 2003). These findings underscore the need to prepare materials that can be used by the maximum number of patients. Other educational materials can be provided, such as videotapes, audiotapes, and computer-assisted instruction.

Often patients rely on family members to interpret regimen details at home and may feel embarrassed about their issues with health literacy (Williams et al., 2007). Therefore, when educating those with chronic illnesses, family members or significant others should be involved in the teaching session. Emphasis in teaching needs to be directed toward not only knowledge of the disease, but also the skills needed for the regimen (Burke & Dunbar-Jacob, 1995). In addition, the regimen should be simplified as much as possible.

Beyond Knowledge and Comprehension

Abilities beyond knowledge and comprehension are required. Therefore, educational goals must be broader than solely the acquisition of knowledge if adherence is to result. The outcome of adherence depends on participation of the learner beyond that of listening, reading, or assimilating information. Clinicians should also encourage patients' participation in their own care. Flexible self-care regimens enable people to exercise a degree of autonomy that is not an option in standard regimens, even when these are adapted to some extent for individuals. The flexibility of instructions, such as "If you have this sign or this symptom, then try this activity," allows people some freedom to make informed choices, and having choices fosters independence and a better quality of life (Rapley, 1997).

Behavioral Strategies to Enhance Adherence

Behavioral strategies attempt to influence specific adherence behaviors directly through the use of various techniques. These strategies may be used as a single intervention, or in combination, to achieve desired results.

It is generally believed that adherence is increased when patients actively participate in learning and deciding how to implement prescribed regimens. However, insistence by the healthcare provider on a preconceived or stereotyped notion of the most desirable level of participation may be inappropriate. A mismatch between an authoritarian provider and an assertive, active learner may influence adherence adversely. On the other hand, the provider who expects an active involvement process can overwhelm a passive and nonactive learner.

Tailoring

The minimal outcome of patient participation with the nurse in developing an adherence strategy should be tailoring the treatment to the patient's daily behaviors, because this process may help cue adherence (Burke & Dunbar-Jacob, 1995). Integrating treatment activities so that they coincide with routine activities, called rituals, is an important way of individualizing and enhancing the treatment plan. The daily schedule of eating, arising and retiring, hygiene, favorite television program, and so on, identifies rituals that may be used to incorporate health behaviors into daily life.

Simplifying the Regimen

As a result of discussions between patient and nurse, it may become apparent that the patient is unable to manage the complexity of the prescribed regimen. Negotiation with the prescribing source may result in better adherence if this barrier is cleared and the regimen is simplified. As a general rule, the number of times medications are taken and the number of doses should be held to a minimum.

Providing Reminders

Reminders or memory aids are useful when the problem is a failure of the behavior to occur because patients have forgotten to perform one or more aspects of the desired behavior. Calendars, clocks, and individually prepared posters with medication and food reminders can be very helpful. Separating a day's supply of medications can also help the person who has difficulty remembering if a particular dose was taken.

The healthcare professional can reinforce the importance of adherence at episodic visits. Such reinforcement may involve pill counting, attention to patient diaries or to other reports of behavior, and self-monitoring; these are all methods that remind the patient of the value of adherence and that elicit participation.

Telephone calls are also useful in reminding patients about healthcare recommendations, in encouraging adherence with medications in the elderly (Cargill, 1992), and as an effective intervention in enhancing adherence with making and keeping follow-up appointments after referral from emergency (Komoroski, Graham, & Kirby, 1996). Friedman and colleagues (1996) tested a variation of telephone follow-up, which demonstrated a 17.7% improvement in medication adherence

among those receiving automated telephone calls. Bosworth et al. (2008) used a telephone intervention for patients with hypertension and found a significant change in medication-taking behavior. Telephone reminders not only provide a personal touch, but also allow individuals who wish to reschedule an appointment the opportunity to do so at that time (Crespo-Fierro, 1997). A newer strategy, the use of text messaging to adolescents with diabetes, increased disease self-efficacy and adherence to medical regimen (Franklin, Waller, Pagliari, & Greene, 2006).

Enhancing Coping

The nurse should be sensitive to cues from individual patients suggesting emotional responses that interfere with learning optimal health behaviors. Situational anxiety, marked depression, and denial are associated with low levels of adherence. These three emotional responses should be interpreted as signals that a patient's coping skills are inadequate and that a modification in approach may be more effective.

Ethnocultural Interventions

Recognition that the patient and family's patterns of communication may differ from the provider's is important for effective interactions. In addition, cultural components need to be integrated into any strategies that are proposed. There are some basics to delivering culturally competent care to enhance treatment adherence. Most of the strategies have been addressed in other documents for example, *Healthy People 2010*. It has been acknowledged that one of our goals for the health of all is to ensure that we eliminate the disparities that currently exist in providing care. Flaskerud (2007) acknowledges that the provision of culturally competent care rests on the shoulders of the healthcare provider. Therefore, it is up to each individual healthcare provider to provide these key ingredients to our practices:

- Ask about health practices that may interfere with a treatment regimen
- Seek understanding when a patient says something that you do not understand
- Acknowledge to patients that there may be additions to recommendations that stem from culture and tradition, and inquire about these
- Listen carefully to verbal and nonverbal communication

For effective interaction with persons of a different culture, "cultural translation" may be needed. One requisite for a cultural translator is learning about the historical rituals and norms that relate to health of the particular group. Another requisite is evaluating health behaviors in the patient's cultural context to determine competing priorities, environmental obstacles, or degree of knowledge and skills (George, 2001).

Providers need to recognize that *their* belief system, values, and attitudes toward healthcare management also are culturally determined and may be responsible for ideologic or philosophic differences. The emphasis on self-care in Western medical systems is ideologically consistent with the value of individual enterprise in Western cultures (Anderson, Blue, & Lau, 1993). Persons of other cultures may find this value for self-care foreign.

EVIDENCE-BASED PRACTICE AND HEALTH OUTCOMES

There has been a slow explosion of interest in documenting the evidence of particular strategies to improve health outcomes. Evidence based

EVIDENCE-BASED PRACTICE BOX

Purpose: The purpose of this study was to evaluate the efficacy of the telephone as a tool to improve adherence to a cholesterol-lowering diet.

Method: Subjects were randomized to a control group and to a treatment group. Usual care for the control group consisted of follow-up physician visits and/or lipid measurements every 3–6 months. Subjects assigned to the treatment group received the intervention described in the following text.

Sample: The study enrolled 65 men and women diagnosed with hypercholesterolemia, who were considered nonadherent to a cholesterol-lowering diet.

Intervention: Members of the treatment group were required to participate in six intervention sessions delivered every 2 weeks via telephone. Telephone interventions were individually tailored and designed to focus on methods of managing eating behavior in difficult situations.

Results and Implications for Nursing Practice: There was a significant difference in total and saturated fat, dietary cholesterol adherence, and serum low-density lipoprotein cholesterol (LDL-C) between the control group and the intervention group. This behavioral intervention enhanced adherence to the recommended cholesterol-lowering diet. Implications are as follows: In light of the difficulties patients often face when attempting to follow a therapeutic eating plan, healthcare providers must rely on methods of improving adherence that have proved successful in similar situations.

Source: Burke, L.E., Dunbar-Jacob, J., Orchard, T.J., et al. (2005). Improving adherence to a cholesterol-lowering diet: A behavioral intervention study. *Patient Education and Counseling, 57*(1), 134–42.

practice guidelines for a variety of physiologic and behavioral interventions are now readily available to all healthcare practitioners (AHRQ, NGC). This means that what we recommend to patients is based on evidence of efficacy. We still, however, face the challenge of helping patients to follow recommendations. No matter the quality of our interventions, they are only beneficial if patients use them. And, it is up to healthcare professionals to better assess if patients can do what we suggest, and then to evaluate the outcomes.

This chapter has discussed hundreds of studies that have assessed adherence behavior. Ultimately, it is up to each of us to build rapport with our patients, and to simply ask the patient what they can and cannot do.

STUDY QUESTIONS

1. Why is trying to increase adherence behaviors important for clients with chronic illness?
2. What factors are involved in adhering to medical regimens? Discuss them.
3. How prevalent is nonadherence? Can you think of examples from your own practice?
4. How does adherence behavior affect evidence-based practice?
5. What ethical issues arise when a provider tries to increase a client's adherence behavior? Discuss an ethical approach.
6. Using your own or a client's culture, identify how norms, rituals, and practices affect adherence with healthcare recommendations.
7. What are the strengths and weaknesses of education as a means of increasing adherence?
8. What role does health literacy have on adherence behavior?
9. How can you encourage client participation to increase adherence? Discuss tailoring, simplifying the regimen, and reminders.
10. How can you enhance coping to increase adherence?
11. What are the advantages and disadvantages of support groups to aid adherence behavior?

REFERENCES

Ajzen, L. (1985). From intention to action: A theory of planned behavior. In J. Kuhl & J. Beckman (Eds.), *Action control: From cognition to behavior.* Heidelberg: Springer.

Anderson, J.M., Blue, C., & Lau, A. (1993). Women's perspectives on chronic illness: Ethnicity, ideology, and restructuring of life. *Diabetes Spectrum, 6*(2), 102–115.

Anderson, R.M. (1985). Is the problem of noncompliance all in our head? *Diabetes Educator, 11,* 31–34.

Bandura, A. (1997). *Self-efficacy: The exercise of control.* New York: W.H. Freeman and Company.

Bandura, A. (2004). Swimming against the mainstream: The early years from chilly tributary to transformative mainstream. *Behaviour Research and Therapy, 42*(6), 613–630.

Barfod, T.S., Hecht, F.M., Rubow, C., & Gerstoft, J. (2006). Physicians' communication with patients about adherence to HIV medication in San Francisco and Copenhagen: A qualitative study using grounded theory. *BMC Health Services Research, 6,* 154.

Barofsky, I. (1978). Compliance, adherence, and the therapeutic alliance: Steps in the development of self-care. *Social Science and Medicine, 12,* 369–376.

Barry, V. (1982). *Moral aspects of health care.* Belmont, CA: Wadsworth.

Baumann, L.J., Cameron, L.D., Zimmerman, R.S., & Leventhal, H. (1989). Illness representations and matching labels with symptoms. *Health Psychology, 8*(4), 449–469.

Beach, M.C., Keruly, J., & Moore, R.D. (2006). Is the quality of the patient-provider relationship associated with better adherence and health outcomes for patients with HIV? *Journal of General Internal Medicine, 21*(6), 661–665.

Becker, M.H. (1976). Socio-behavioral determinants of compliance. In D.L. Sackett & R. Haynes (Eds.), *Compliance with therapeutic regimens.* Baltimore: Johns Hopkins University Press.

Becker, M.H., & Maiman, L.A. (1975). Sociobehavioral determinants of compliance with health and medical care recommendations. *Medical Care, 13*, 10–24.

Bender, B., Milgrom, H., Rand, C., & Ackerson, L. (1998). Psychological factors associated with medication nonadherence in asthmatic children. *Journal of Asthma, 35*, 347–353.

Berg, J., Nyamathi, A., Christiani, A., Morisky, D., & Leake, B. (2005). Predictors of screening results for depressive symptoms among homeless adults in Los Angeles with latent tuberculosis. *Research in Nursing & Health, 28*(3), 220–229.

Berg, K.M., & Arnstein, J.H. (2006). Practical and conceptual challenges in measuring antiretroviral adherence. *Journal of Acquired Immune Deficiency Syndromes, 43*(Suppl 1), 79–87.

Bernardini, J. (2004). Ethical issues of compliance/adherence in the treatment of hypertension. *Advances in Chronic Kidney Disease, 11*(2), 222–227.

Besch, C.L. (1995). Compliance in clinical trials. *AIDS, 9*(1), 1–10.

Bosworth, H.B., Olsen, M.K., Neary, A., Orr, M., Grubber, J., Svetkey, L., et al. (2008). Take Control of Your Blood pressure (TCYB) study: A multifactorial tailored behavioral and educational intervention for achieving blood pressure control. *Patient Education and Counseling, 70*(3), 338–347.

Burke, L.E., & Dunbar-Jacob, J. (1995). Adherence to medication, diet and activity recommendations: From assessment to maintenance. *Journal of Cardiovascular Nursing, 9*(2), 62–79.

Butler, J.A., Roderick, P., Mullee, M., Mason, J.C., & Peveler, R.C. (2004). Frequency and impact of nonadherence to immunosuppressants after renal transplantation: A systematic review. *Transplantation, 77*(5), 769–776.

Cabrera, D.M., Morisky, D.E., & Chin, S. (2002). Development of a tuberculosis education booklet for Latino immigrant patients. *Patient Education and Counseling, 46*(2), 117–124.

Carels, R.A., Darby, L., Cacciapaglia, H.M., Konrad, K., Coit, C., Harper, J., et al. (2007). Using motivational interviewing as a supplement to obesity treatment: A stepped-care approach. *Health Psychology, 26*(3), 369–374.

Cargill, J.M. (1992). Medication compliance in elderly people: Influencing variables and interventions. *Journal of Advanced Nursing, 17*(4), 422–426.

Carney, R.M., Freedland, K.E., Eisen, S.A., Rich, M.W., & Jaffe, A.S. (1995). Major depression and medication adherence in elderly patients with coronary artery disease. *Health Psychology, 14*(1), 88–90.

Carney, R.M., Freedland, K.E., Eisen, S.A., Rich, M.W., Skala, J.A., & Jaffe, A.S. (1998). Adherence to a prophylactic medication regimen in patients with symptomatic versus asymptomatic ischemic heart disease. *Behavioral Medicine, 24*(1), 35–39.

Chesney, M. (2003). Adherence to HAART regimens. *AIDS Patient Care and STDs, 17*(4), 169–177.

Chilton, L., Hu, J., & Wallace, D.C. (2006). Health-promoting lifestyle and diabetes knowledge in Hispanic American adults. *Home Health Care Management Practice, 18*, 378–385.

Connelly, C.E. (1984). Economic and ethical issues in patient compliance. *Nursing Economics, 2*, 342–347.

Conrad, P. (1985). The meaning of medications: Another look at compliance. *Social Science and Medicine, 20*, 29–37.

Cook, P.F., Emiliozzi, S., & McCabe, M.M. (2007). Telephone counseling to improve osteoporosis treatment adherence: An effectiveness study in community practice settings. *American Journal of Medical Quality, 22*(6), 445–456.

Corbin, J.A., & Strauss, A.L. (1985). Managing chronic illness at home: Three lines of work. *Qualitative Sociology, 8*(3), 224–247.

Cramer, J., Vachon, L., Desforges, C., & Sussman, N. (1995). Dose frequency and dose interval compliance with multiple antiepileptic medication during a controlled clinical trial? *Epilepsia, 36*, 1111–1117.

Creer, T.L., & Levstek, D. (1996). Medication compliance and asthma: Overlooking the trees because of the forest. *Journal of Asthma, 33*, 203–211.

Crespo-Fierro, M. (1997). Compliance/adherence and care management in HIV disease. *Journal of the Association of Nurses in AIDS Care, 8,* 43–54.

de Geest, S., Abraham, I., & Dunbar-Jacob, J. (1996). Measuring transplant patients' compliance with immunosuppressive therapy. *Western Journal of Nursing Research, 18*(5), 595–605.

deKlerk, E., & van der Linden, S. (1996). Compliance monitoring of NSAID drug therapy in ankylosing spondylitis, experiences with an electronic monitoring device. *British Journal of Rheumatology, 35,* 60–65.

Demyttenaere, K., Van Ganse, E., Gregoire, J., Gaens, E., & Mesters, P. (1998). Compliance with depressed patients treated with fluoxetine or amitriptyline. *International Clinical Psychopharmacology, 13*(1), 11–17.

Dew, M.A, DiMartini, A.F., De Vito Dabbs, A., Myaskovsky, L., Steel, J., Unruh, M., et al. (2007). Rates and risk factors for nonadherence to the medical regimen after adult solid organ transplantation. *Transplantation, 83*(7), 858–873.

DiMatteo, M.R. (2004). Variations in patients' adherence to medical recommendations: A quantitative review of 50 years of research. *Medical Care, 42*(3), 200–209.

DiMatteo, M.R., & Haskard, K.B. (2006). Further challenges in adherence research: Measurements, methodologies, and mental health care. *Medical Care, 44*(4), 300–303.

DiMatteo, M.R., Lepper, H.S., & Croghan, T.W. (2000). Depression is a risk factor for noncompliance with medical treatment. *Archives of Internal Medicine, 160,* 2101–2107.

DiMatteo, M.R., Sherbourne, C.D., Hays, R.D., Ordway, L., Kravitz, R.L., McGlynn, E.A., et al. (1993). Physicians' characteristics influence patients' adherence to medical treatment: Results from the Medical Outcomes Study. *Health Psychology, 12*(2), 93–102.

Dunbar, J. (1980). Adhering to medical advice: A review. *International Journal of Mental Health, 9*(1–2), 70–78.

Dunbar-Jacob, J. (1993). Contributions to patient adherence: Is it time to share the blame? *Health Psychology, 12,* 91.

Dunbar-Jacob, J., Burke, L.E., & Puczynski, S. (1995). Clinical assessment and management of adherence to medical regimens. In P.M. Nicassio &

T.W. Smith (Eds.), *Managing chronic illness: A biopsychosocial perspective.* Washington, DC: APA.

Dunbar-Jacob, J., Erlen, J.A., Schlenk, E.A., Ryan, C.M., Sereika, S.M., & Doswell, W.M. (2000). Adherence in chronic disease. *Annual Review of Nursing Research, 18,* 48–90.

Dunbar-Jacob, J., Holmes, J.L., Sereika, S., Kwoh, C.K., Burke, L.E., Starz, T.W., et al. (2004). Factors associated with attrition of African Americans during the recruitment phase of a clinical trial examining adherence among individuals with rheumatoid arthritis. *Arthritis Rheumatology, 51*(3), 422–428.

Dunbar-Jacob, J. & Schenk, E. (2001). Patient adherence to treatment regimen. In A. Baum & T. Revenson (Eds.), *Handbook of health psychology* (pp. 321–657). Mahwah, NJ: Lawrence Erlbaum Associates Publishers.

Dunbar-Jacob, J., Schenk, E.A., Burke, L.E., & Mathews, J.T. (1997). Predictors of patient adherence: Patient characteristics. In S.A. Schumaker, E.B. Schron, J.K. Ockene (Eds.), *The handbook of health behavior change* (2nd ed.). New York: Springer.

Dunbar-Jacob, J., Schenk, E., & Caruthers, D. (2002). Adherence in the management of chronic disorders. In A. Christensen & M. Antoni (Eds.), *Chronic physical disorders: Behavioral medicine's perspective.* (pp. 69–82). Malden, MA: Blackwell Publishers.

Duncan, J., & Rogers, R. (1998). Medication compliance in patients with chronic schizophrenia: Implications for the community management of mentally disordered offenders. *Journal of Forensic Sciences, 43,* 1133–1137.

Eiser, C., Hill, J.J., & Blacklay, A. (2000). Surviving cancer: What does it mean for you? An evaluation of a clinic based intervention for survivors of childhood cancer. *Psycho-Oncology, 9,* 214–220.

Eng, J.J., & Maeatin-Guiness, K. (2007). Using the theory of planned behavior to predict leisure time physical activity among people with chronic kidney disease. *Rehabilitation Psychology, 52*(4), 435–442.

Feachem, R.G., Sekhri, N.K., & White, K.L. (2002). Getting more for their dollar: A comparison of the NHS with California's Kaiser Permanente. *British Medical Journal, 324*(7330), 135–141.

Finley, C., Gregg, E.W., Solomon, L.J., & Gay, E. (2001). Disparities in hormone replacement therapy use by socioeconomic status in a primary care population. *Journal of Community Health, 26*(1), 39–50.

Fishbein, M., & Ajzen, I. (1975). *Belief, attitude and intention: An introduction to theory and research.* Reading, MA: Addison-Wesley.

Flaskerud, J.H. (2007) Can we achieve it? *Issues in Mental Health Nursing, 28*(3), 309–311.

Franklin, V.L., Waller, A., Pagliari, C., & Greene, S.A. (2006). A randomized controlled trial of Sweet Talk, a text-messaging system to support young people with diabetes. *Diabetic Medicine, 23*(12), 1332–1338.

Friedman, R., Kazis, L.E., Jette, A., Smith, M.B., Stollerman, J., Torgeson, J., et al. (1996). A telecommunication system for monitoring and counseling patients with hypertension: Impact on medication adherence and blood pressure. *American Journal of Hypertension, 9*(1), 285–292.

Gazmararian, J.A., Williams, M.V., Peel, J., & Baker, D.W. (2003). Health literacy and knowledge of chronic disease. *Patient Education and Counseling, 51*(3), 267–275.

George, M. (2001). The challenge of culturally competent health care: Applications for asthma. *Heart and Lung, 30*(5), 392–400.

Glazer, H., Kirk, L., & Bosler, F. (1996). Patient education pamphlets about prevention, detection, and treatment of breast cancer in low literacy women. *Patient Education and Counseling, 27*, 185–189.

Gonzalez, J. (1990). Factors relating to frequency among low-income Mexican American women: Implications for nursing practice. *Cancer Nursing, 13*, 134–142.

Gonzalez, J.S., Penedo, F.J., Antoni, M.H., Durán, R.E., McPherson-Baker, S., Ironson, G., et al. (2004). Social support, positive states of mind, and HIV treatment adherence in men and women living with HIV/AIDS. *Health Psychology, 23*(4), 413–418.

Grady, K.E., Lemkau, J.P., McVay, J.M., Carlson, S., Lee, N., Minchella, M., et al. (1996). Clinical decision-making and mammography referral. *Preventive Medicine, 25*(3), 327–338.

Graves, J.W. (2000). Management of difficult-to-control hypertension. *Mayo Clin Proceedings, 75*, 539–542

Gredig, D., Niderost S., & Parpan-Blaser, A. (2006). HIV-protection through condom use: Testing the theory of planned behaviour in a community sample of heterosexual men in a high-income country. *Psychology & Health, 21*(5), 541–555.

Greene, J.A. (2004)."Noncompliance" enters the medical literature, 1955–1975. 2002 Roy Porter Memorial Prize Essay Therapeutic Infidelities. *Social History of Medicine, 17*(3), 327–343.

Greenley, R.N., Josie, K.L., & Drotar, D. (2006). Perceived involvement in condition management among inner-city youth with asthma and their primary caregivers. *Journal of Asthma, 43*(9), 687–693.

Greenstein, S., & Siegal, B. (1998). Compliance and non-compliance in patients with a functioning renal transplant: A multicenter study. *Transplantation, 66*(12), 1718–1726.

Harrington, R., Kerfoot, M., Dyer, E., McNiven, F., Gill, J., Harrington, V., et al. (2000). Deliberate self-poisoning in adolescence: Why does a brief family intervention work in some cases and not others? *Journal of Adolescence, 23*, 13–20.

Haynes, R. B. (1979). Determinants of compliance: The disease and the mechanics of treatment. In R.B. Haynes (Ed.), *Compliance in healthcare.* Baltimore, MD: Johns Hopkins University Press.

Haynes, R.B., McDonald, H., Garg, A.X., & Montague, P. (2002). Interventions for helping patients to follow prescriptions for medications. [Update of Cochrane Database Syst Rev. 2000;(2):CD000011; PMID: 10796686]. Cochrane Database of Systematic Reviews (2), CD000011.

Hilbrands, L., Hoitsma, A., & Koene, R. (1995). Medication compliance after renal transplantation. *Transplantation, 60*, 914–920.

Hiltunen, E.F, Winder, P.A., Rait, M.A., Buselli, E.F., Carroll, D.L., & Rankin, S.H. (2005). Implementation of efficacy enhancement nursing interventions with cardiac elders. *Rehabilitation Nursing, 30*(6), 221–229.

Hingson, R., Scotch, N., Sorenson, J., & Swazey, J. (1981). *In sickness and in health.* St. Louis: Mosby.

Hinkin, C.H., Castellon, S.A., Durvasula, R.S., Hardy, D.J., Lam, M.N., Mason, K.I., et al. (2002). Medication adherence among HIV positive adults: Effects of cognitive dysfunction and regimen complexity. *Neurology, 59*(12), 1944–1950.

Hinkin, C.H., Hardy, D.J., Mason, K.I., Castellon, S.A., Durvasula, R.S., Lam, M.N., et al. (2004). Medication adherence in HIV-infected adults: Effect of patient age, cognitive status, and substance abuse. *AIDS, 18*(1), 19–25.

Hovell, M.F., Sipan, C.L., Blumberg, E.J., Hofstetter, C.R., Slymen, D., Friedman, L., et al. (2003). Increasing Latino adolescents' adherence to treatment for latent tuberculosis infection: A controlled trial. *American Journal of Public Health, 93*(11), 1871–1877.

Im, E., & Meleis, A. (1999). A situation-specific theory of Korean immigrant women's menopausal transition. *Journal of Nursing Scholarship, 31,* 333–338.

Iyriboz, Y., Powers, S., Morrow, J., Ayers, D., & Landry, G. (1991). Accuracy of the pulse oximeters in estimating heart rate at rest and during exercise. *British Journal of Sports Medicine, 25*(3), 162–164.

Jackson, R., Asimakopoulou, K., & Scammell, A. (2007). Assessment of the transtheoretical model as used by dietitians in promoting physical activity in people with type 2 diabetes. *Journal of Human Nutrition & Dietetics, 20*(1), 27–36.

Jaynes, R., & Rankin, S. (2001). Application of Leventhal's self-regulation model to Chinese immigrants with type 2 diabetes. *Journal of Nursing Scholarship, 31,* 333–338.

Johnson, S.S., Paiva, A.L., Cummins, C.O., Johnson, J.L., Dyment, S.J., Wright, J.A., et al. (2007). Transtheoretical model-based multiple behavior intervention for weight management: Effectiveness on a population basis. *Preventive Medicine, 46*(3), 238–246.

Johnson, M.O., Chesney, M.A., Goldstein, R.B., Remien, R.H., Catz, S., Gore-Felton, C., et al. (2006). Positive provider interactions, adherence self-efficacy, and adherence to antiretroviral medications among HIV-infected adults: A mediation model. *AIDS Patient Care and STDs, 20*(4), 258–268.

Joshi, M.S. (1998). Adherence in ethnic minorities: The case of South Asians in Britain. In L. Myers & K. Midence (Eds.), *Adherence to treatment in medical conditions.* Amsterdam: Harwood.

Kelly, M.A., Sereika, S.M., Battista, D.R., & Brown, C. (2007). The relationship between beliefs about depression and coping strategies: Gender differences. *The British Journal of Clinical Psychology, 46*(3), 315–332.

Knafl, K.A., & Gilliss, C.L. (2002). Families and chronic illness: A synthesis of current research. *Journal of Family Nursing, 8*(3), 178–198.

Komoroski, E., Graham, C., & Kirby, R. (1996). A comparison of interventions to improve clinic follow-up compliance after a pediatric emergency department visit. *Pediatric Emergency Care, 12,* 87–90.

Krapek, K., King, K., Warren, S.S., George, K.G., Caputo, D.A., Mihelich, K., et al. (2004). Medication adherence and associated hemoglobin A1c in type 2 diabetes. *Annals of Pharmacotherapy, 38*(9), 1357–1362.

Kribbs, N., Pack, A., Kline, L., Smith, P., Schwartz, A.R., Schubert, N.M., et al. (1993). Objective measurement of patterns of nasal CPAP use by patients with obstructive sleep apnea. *American Review of Respiratory Disease, 147*(4), 887–895.

Kronish, I.M., Rieckmann, N., Halm, E.A., Shimbo, D., Vorchheimer, D., Haas, D.C., et al. (2006). Persistent depression affects adherence to secondary prevention behaviors after acute coronary syndromes. *Journal of General Internal Medicine, 21*(11), 1178–1183.

Le, J.Y., Kusek, J.W., Greene, P.G., Bernhard, C., Norris, K., Smith, D., et al. (1996). Assessing medication adherence by pill count and electronic monitor in the African American Study of Kidney Disease and Hypertension. *American Journal of Hypertension, 9*(8), 719–725.

Le, T.T., Bilderback, A., Bender, B., Wamboldt, F.S., Turner, C.F., Rand, C.S., et al. (2008). Do asthma medication beliefs mediate the relationship between minority status and adherence to therapy? *Journal of Asthma, 45*(1), 33–37.

Lemanek, K. (1990). Adherence issues in the medical management of asthma. *Journal of Pediatric Psychology, 15*(4), 437–458.

Leventhal, H., Brisette, I., & Leventhal, E. (2003). The common-sense model of self-regulation of health and illness. In Cameron, L., *The self-regulation of health and illness behaviour* (pp. 42–65). New York: Routledge.

Lima, V.D., Geller, J., Bangsberg , D.R., Patterson, T.L., Daniel, M., Kerr, T., et al. (2007). The effect of adherence on the association between depressive symptoms and mortality among HIV-infected individuals first initiating HAART. *AIDS, 21*(9), 1175–1183.

Liu, H., Miller, L.G., Hays, R.D., Wagner, G., Golin, C., & Hu, W. (2006). A practical method to calibrate self-reported adherence to antiretroviral therapy. *Journal of Acquired Immune Deficiency Syndromes, 43*(Suppl. 1), 104–112.

Locke, E.A., & Latham, G.P. (2002). Building a practically useful theory of goal setting and task motivation. A 35-year odyssey. *American Psychologist, 57*(9), 705–717.

Mansour, M.E., Lanphear, B.P., & DeWitt, T.G. (2000). Barriers to asthma care in urban children: Parent perspectives. *Pediatrics, 106,* 512–519.

Marston, M. (1970). Compliance with medical regimens: A review of the literature. *Nursing Research, 19,* 312–323.

Martin, J., Oliver, K., & McCaughtry, N. (2007). The theory of planned behavior: Predicting physical activity in Mexican American children. *Journal of Sport & Exercise Psychology, 29*(2), 225–232.

Mason, B., Matsayuma, J., & Jue, S. (1995). Assessment of sulfonylurea adherence and metabolic control. *Diabetes Educator, 21,* 52–57.

McCall, L.A., & Ginis, K.A. (2004). The effects of message framing on exercise adherence and health beliefs among patients in a cardiac rehabilitation program. *Journal of Applied Biobehavioral Research, 9*(2), 122–135.

McDonald, H.P., Garg, A.X., & Haynes, R.B. (2002). Interventions to enhance patient adherence to medication prescriptions: Scientific review. *The Journal of the American Medical Association, 288*(22), 2868–2879.

McGlynn, E., Asch, S., Adams, J., Keesey, J., Hicks, J., & DeCristofaro, A. (2003). The quality of health care delivered to adults in the United States. *New England Journal of Medicine, 348*(26), 2635–2645.

Meyer, D., Leventhal, H., & Gutmann, M. (1985). Common-sense models of illness: The example of hypertension. *Health Psychology, 4*(2), 115–135.

Miller, N.H., Hill, M., Kottke, T., & Ockene, I. (1997). The multilevel compliance challenge: Recommendations for a call to action. A statement for healthcare professionals. *Circulation, 95,* 1085–1090.

Miller, L.G., Liu, H., Hays, R.D., Golin, C.E., Beck, C.K., Asch, S.M., et al. (2002). How well do clinicians estimate patients' adherence to combination antiretroviral therapy? *Journal of General Internal Medicine, 17*(1), 1–11.

Misselbrook, D. (1998). Managing the change from compliance to concordance. *Prescriber, 19,* 23–33.

Mounier-Vehier, C., Bernaud, C., Carre, A., Lequeuche, B., Hotton, J.M., & Charpentier, J.C. (1998). Compliance and antihypertensive efficacy of amlodipine compared with nifedipine slow-release. *American Journal of Hypertension, 11,* 478–486.

Norman, P., Armitage, C.J., & Quigley, C. (2007). The theory of planned behavior and binge drinking: Assessing the impact of binge drinker prototypes. *Addictive Behaviors, 32*(9), 1753–1768.

Norman, P., & Conner, M. (2005). The theory of planned behavior and exercise: Evidence for the mediating and moderating roles of planning on intention-behavior relations. *Journal of Sport and Exercise Psychology, 27,* 488–504.

Ockene, I.S., Hayman, L.L., Pasternak, R.C., Schron, E., & Dunbar-Jacob, J. (2002). Task force No.4: Adherence issues and behavior changes: Achieving a long-term solution. 33rd Bethesda Conference. *Journal of the American College of Cardiology, 40*(4), 630–640.

Ohm, R, & Aaronson, L.S. (2006). Symptom perception and adherence to asthma controller medications. *Journal of Nursing Scholarship, 38*(3), 292–297.

O'Malley, A.S., Sheppard, V.B., Schwartz, M., & Mandelblatt, J. (2004). The role of trust in use of preventive services among low-income African-American women. *Preventive Medicine, 38*(6), 777–785.

Ott, J., Greening, L., Palardy, N., Holderby, A., & DeBell, W.K. (2000). Self efficacy as a mediator variable for adolescents' adherence to treatment for insulin dependent diabetes mellitus. *Children's Health Care, 29,* 47–63.

Paasche-Orlow, M.K., Cheng, D.M., Palepu, A., Meli, S., Faber, V., & Samet, J.H. (2006). Health literacy, antiretroviral adherence, and HIV-RNA suppression: A longitudinal perspective. *Journal of General Internal Medicine, 21*(8), 835–840.

Pablos-Mendez, A., Knirsch, C.A., Barr, R.G., Lerner, B.H., & Frieden, T.R. (1997). Nonadherence in tuberculosis treatment: Predictors and consequences in New York City. *American Journal of Medicine, 102*(2), 164–170.

Park, D.C., & Skurnik, I. (2004). Aging, cognition, and patient errors in following medical instructions. In M.S. Bogner (Ed.), *Misadventures in health care: Inside stories* (pp. 165–181). Mahwah, NJ.: Lawrence Erlbaum.

Pender, N.J. (1996). *Health promotion in nursing practice* (2nd ed.). Norwalk, CT: Appleton-Century-Crofts.

Pender, N.J., Murdaugh, C.L., & Parsons, M.A. (2001). *Health promotion in nursing practice.* Upper Saddle River, NJ: Prentice Hall.

Prochaska, J., & DiClemente, C. (1983). Stages and processes of self-change of smoking: Toward an integrative model of change. *Journal of Consulting & Clinical Psychology, 51,* 390–395.

Quinn, J. R. (2005). Delay in seeking care for symptoms of acute myocardial infarction: Applying a theoretical model. *Research in Nursing & Health, 28*(4), 283–294.

Quittner, A.L., Modi, A.C., Lemanek, K.L., Ievers-Landis, C.E., & Rapoff, M.A. (2007). Evidence-based assessment of adherence to medical treatments in pediatric psychology. *Journal of Pediatric Psychology.* Retrieved October 1, 2007, from http://jpepsy.oxfordjournals.org/cgi/content/abstract/jsm064v1

Rand, C.S. (1993). Measuring adherence with therapy for chronic diseases: Implications for the treatment of heterozygous familial hypercholesterolemia. *American Journal of Cardiology, 72*(10), 68D–74D.

Rand C. (2004). Non-adherence with asthma therapy: More than just forgetting. *The Journal of Pediatrics, 146,* 157–159.

Rand, C.S., & Sevick, M.A. (2000). Ethics in adherence promotion and monitoring. *Controlled Clinical Trials, 21*(Suppl. 5), 241–247.

Rand, C.S., & Wise, R.A. (1994). Measuring adherence to asthma medication regimens. *American Review of Respiratory and Critical Care Medicine, 149,* 289–290.

Rapley, P. (1997). Self-care: Re-thinking the role of compliance. *Australian Journal of Advanced Nursing, 15,* 20–25.

Rodríguez-Reimann, D.I., Nicassio, P., Reimann, J.O., Gallegos, P.I., & Olmedo, E.L. (2004). Acculturation and health beliefs of Mexican Americans regarding tuberculosis prevention. *Journal of Immigrant Health, 6*(2), 51–62.

Rosenstock, I.M. (1974). Historical origins of the health belief model. *Health Education Monographs, 2,* 354–386.

Rosenstock, I.M. (1988). Enhancing patient compliance with health recommendations. *Journal of Pediatric Health Care,* 2(2), 67–72.

Rudd, P., Ahmed, S., Zachary, V., Barton, C., & Bonduelle, D. (1990). Improved compliance measures: Applications in an ambulatory hypertensive drug trial. *Clinical Pharmacology and Therapeutics, 48*(6), 676–685.

Sackett, D.L., & Haynes, R.B. (Eds.) (1976). *Compliance with therapeutic regimens.* Baltimore: Johns Hopkins University Press.

Sackett, D.L., & Snow, J.C. (1979). The magnitude of compliance and noncompliance. In R.B. Haynes, D.W. Taylor, & D.L. Sackett (Eds.), *Compliance in health care* (pp. 11–22). Baltimore: Johns Hopkins University Press.

Sankar, A.P., Nevedal, D.C., Neufeld, S., & Luborsky, M.R. (2007). What is a missed dose? Implications for construct validity and patient adherence. *AIDS Care, 19*(6), 775–780.

Schlenk E., & Dunbar-Jacob, J. (1996). *Ethnic variations in adherence: A review.* Unpublished manuscript.

Schwarzer, R. (1992). Self-efficacy in the adoption and maintenance of health behaviors: Theoretical approaches and a new model. In R. Schwarzer (Ed.), *Self-efficacy: Thought control of action* (pp. 217–243). Washington, DC: Hemisphere.

Searle, A., Norman, P., Thompson, R., & Vedhara, K. (2007). A prospective examination of illness beliefs and coping in patients with type 2 diabetes. *British Journal of Health Psychology, 12*(4), 621–638.

Smith, S.R., Wahed, A.S., Kelley, S.S., Conjeevaram, H.S., Robuck, P.R., & Fried, M.W. (2007). Assessing the validity of self-reported medication adherence in hepatitis C treatment. *The Annals of Pharmacotherapy, 41*(7), 1116–1123.

Sin, M.K., Kang, D.H., & Weaver, M. (2005). Relationships of asthma knowledge, self-management, and social support in African American adolescents with asthma. *International Journal of Nursing Studies, 42*(3), 307–313.

Steele, D.J., Jackson, T.C., & Gutmann, M.C. (1990). Have you been taking your pills? *The Journal of Family Practice, 30*(3), 294–299.

Stone, A., Shiffman, S., Schwartz, J., Broderick, J., & Hufford. (2003). Patient compliance with paper and electronic diaries. *Controlled Clinical Trials, 24*(2), 182–199.

Straka, R., Fish, J., Benson, S., & Suh, J. (1997). Patient self-reporting of compliance does not correspond with electronic monitoring: An evaluation using isosorbide dinitrate as a model drug. *Pharmacotherapy, 17,* 126–132.

Strauss, A. L.(1984). *Chronic illness and the quality of life* (2nd ed.). St. Louis: Mosby.

Strelczyk, J.J., & Dignan, M.B. (2002). Disparities in adherence to recommended followup on screening mammography: Interaction of sociodemographic factors. *Ethnic Disparities, 12*(1), 77–86.

Sunil, T.S., & McGehee, M.A. (2007). Social and religious support on treatment adherence among HIV/

AIDS patients by race/ethnicity. *Journal of HIV/AIDS & Social Services, 6*(1–2), 83–99.

Taira, D.A., Gelber, R.P., Davis, J., Gronley, K., Chung, R.S., & Seto, T.B. (2007). Antihypertensive adherence and drug class among Asian Pacific Americans. *Ethnicity & Health, 12*(3), 265–281.

Talamantes, M., Lawler, W., & Espino, D. (1995). Hispanic American elders: Caregiving norms surrounding dying and the use of hospice services. *The Hospice Journal, 19*, 35–49.

Trostle, J.A. (1997). The history and meaning of patient compliance as an ideology. In David S. Gochman et al. (Eds.), *Handbook of health behavior research II: Provider determinants.* New York: Plenum Press.

Turner, J., Wright, E., Mendella, L., Anthonisen, N., & IPPB Study Group. (1995). Predictors of patient adherence to long term home nebulizer therapy for COPD. *Chest, 108*, 394–400.

Ulrik, C.S., Backer, V., Soes-Petersen, U., Lange, P., Harving, H., & Plaschke, P. (2006). The patient's perspective: Adherence or non-adherence to asthma controller therapy. *Journal of Asthma, 43*(9), 701–704.

U.S. Department of Health and Human Services. (2000). Office of Disease Prevention and Health Promotion. (n.d.). *Healthy People 2010.* Retrieved January 22, 2001, from http://www.health.gov/healthypeople/

van der Sande, M.A., Milligan, P.J., Nyan, O.A., Rowley, J.T., Banya, W.A., Ceesay, S.M., et al. (2000). Blood pressure patterns and cardiovascular risk factors in rural and urban gambian communities. *Journal of Human Hypertension, 14*(8), 489–496.

Vermeire, E., Hearnshaw, H., Van Royen, P., & Denekens, J. (2001). Patient adherence to treatment: Three decades of research. A comprehensive review. *Journal of Clinical Pharmacological Therapy, 26*(5), 331–342.

Vik, S.A., Maxwell, C.J., & Hogan, D.B. (2004). Measurement, correlates, and health outcomes of medication adherence among seniors. *Annals of Pharmacotherapy, 38*(2), 303–312.

Wagner, G. (2003). Placebo practice trials: The best predictor of adherence readiness for HAART among drug users? *HIV Clinical Trials, 4*(4), 269–281.

Wagner, G., & Rabkin, J.G. (2000). Measuring medication adherence: Are missed doses reported more accurately then perfect adherence? *AIDS Care, 12*(4), 405–408.

Walker, S.N., Sechrist, K.R., & Pender, N.J. (1987). The health-promoting lifestyle profile: Development and psychometric characteristics. *Nursing Research, 36*, 76–80.

Wendel, C.S., Mohler, M.J., Kroesen, K., Ampel, N.M., Gifford, A.L., & Coons, S.J. (2001). Barriers to use of electronic adherence monitoring in an HIV clinic. *Annals of Pharmacotherapy, 35*(9), 1010–1015.

Williams, L.K., Joseph, C.L., Peterson, E.L., Wells, K., Wang, M., Chowdhry, V.K., et al. (2007). Patients with asthma who do not fill their inhaled corticosteroids: A study of primary nonadherence. *The Journal of Allergy & Clinical Immunology, 120*(5), 1153–1159.

Wing, R.R., Epstein, L.H., Nowal, M.P., & Lamparski, D. (1986). Behavioral self-regulation in the treatment of patients with diabetes mellitus. *Psychological Bulletin, 99*(1), 78–89.

Wolf, M.S., Williams, M.V., Parker, R.M., Parikh, N.S., Nowlan, A.W., & Baker, D.W. (2007). Patients' shame and attitudes toward discussing the results of literacy screening. *Journal of Health Communication, 12*(8), 721–732.

World Health Organization.(2003). *Adherence to long-term therapies: Evidence for action.* Geneva, Switzerland: World Health Organization.

Wutoh, A.K., Brown, C.M., Dutta, A.P., Kumoji, E.K., Clarke-Tasker, V., & Xue, Z. (2005). Treatment perceptions and attitudes of older human immunodeficiency virus-infected adults. *Research in Social and Administrative Pharmacy, 1*(1), 60–76.

Zuckerman, M., Guerra, L., Dorssman, D., Foland, J., & Gregory, G.G. (1996). Health-care-seeking behaviors related to bowel complaints: Hispanics versus non-Hispanic Whites. *Digestive Diseases and Sciences, 41*(1), 77–82.

II

Impact on the Client and Family

9

Family Caregiving

Linda L. Pierce and Barbara J. Lutz

INTRODUCTION

Few adults receive paid homecare services. Outside support is not always welcome. Caregivers often refuse help and resources, as they may feel that professionals are prying into their private lives (Pierce, 2001).

Many adults who are in need of help receive unpaid care (Johnson & Wiener, 2006). The term *unpaid caregiver* refers to a range of kin and non-kin individuals who provide both functional (task-oriented) and affective (emotional) unpaid assistance to a dependent person with whom a long-term or life-long commitment usually exists (Shirey & Summer, 2000). Family members, friends, and neighbors who provide unpaid care may also be referred to as *informal caregivers* (Pierce, Steiner, Govoni, Thompson, & Friedemann, 2007). These individuals care for spouses, other relatives, friends, and disabled children (Scott, 2006). The most common informal caregiving relationship is between an adult child and an aging parent (Scott, 2006). However, in a study financed by the US Administration of Aging, over 900,000 households include a child caregiver between the ages of 8 and 18 years who care for ill or disabled family members (Hunt, Levine, & Naiditch, 2005). The value of

this total care is estimated at $257 billion annually (Pandya, 2005).

The decisions about caring for a person with chronic illness are complex and multifaceted for caregivers. Each choice an individual makes has advantages and disadvantages for the person with chronic illness, the caregiver, and the family. Health-care professionals generally find that no two situations are alike. Each and every situation needs to be individualized to best meet the needs of everyone involved. This chapter focuses on the multiple aspects of coping and decision making that caregivers face, often on a daily basis.

Current Family Caregiving

The incidence of chronic disease in the United States is increasing. More than 90 million Americans live with chronic conditions such as diabetes, heart disease, and cancer (The Dartmouth Atlas Project, 2006). Nearly one third of young adults aged 18 to 44 years suffer from a chronic condition (Shapiro, 2002). Most important, the number of adults older than 65 years (37.3 million in 2006) will continue to rise by more than 19 million by 2020; by 2030 there will be about 71.5 million of these individuals (DHHS, 2007; Moore, 2006). Almost 75% of older persons have at least one chronic condition and many have multiple conditions (AHRQ, 2002). With advances in health care, the number of older adults living with debilitating and/or chronic conditions will grow (Williams, Dilworth-Anderson, & Goodwin, 2003).

At the other end of the age spectrum is the growing number of children with chronic illness, disabilities, or both. Advances in neonatal care can now save increasing numbers of preterm and low birth weight infants. According to a 2003 report from the National Center for Health Statistics, the percentage of low birth weight infants (born weighing less than 2500 grams) increased to the highest level in more than 30 years. In addition, the percentage of preterm births (infants born at less than 37 weeks of gestation) increased to 12% of live births. Low birth weight and prematurity both lead to an increased incidence of chronic health problems in the pediatric population. About 15 to 18% of children have a chronic disease (University of Michigan Health System, 2006) that continues into adulthood.

A 2004 study by the National Alliance for Caregiving and the American Association of Retired Persons estimated that 21% of the American population provides unpaid care to family and friends aged 18 years and older. This translates into 44.4 million caregivers in the United States (Pandya, 2005). The duration of caregiving can last from a few months to decades. Although time spent in caregiving varies depending on the type of condition, caregivers of cognitively impaired adults spend 13 hours each day providing care (Bohse & Associates, 2001), while others report an average of 20 hours per week in caring for a person with a chronic condition (DHHS, 2003a).

Preferences for Family Care

It is important to clarify that some dependent individuals will always need the level of care provided in institutional settings and that not all families are willing or able to provide care over the long term. However, for all but the most severely impaired

individuals, most chronically ill, dependent persons have their long-term care needs met in the home or with community-based care arrangements. Approximately two thirds of dependent persons in the community rely solely on informal caregivers (Mittelman, 2003). For these arrangements to work, family members, friends, or neighbors must play central roles in long-term plans of care.

The decision about where and how to provide care for family members with chronic conditions is emotionally charged and multifaceted. Home-based care is financially cost-effective for the healthcare system. However, the reliance on family members as care providers creates multiple stressors for the family (Hunt, 2003). When formal assistance is required, married persons prefer help in the home regardless of the level of disability of the care recipient; however, financial difficulty and the strain of extended caregiving, especially on the caregiver's health, often lead family caregivers to decisions that favor institutionalized care (Family Caregiver Alliance, 2006).

Characteristics of Family Caregivers

Today, the term *family caregiver* extends beyond the traditional family boundaries. *Caregiver* is defined as anyone who provides assistance to another in need. The *informal caregiver* is anyone who provides care without pay and who usually has personal ties to the care recipient. *Family caregiver* is a term used interchangeably with informal caregiver and can include family, friends, or neighbors (DHHS Administration on Aging, n.d.c). *Caregiver coalition* is a term used to describe the addition of a support person or persons in traditional relationships when the caregiver–recipient arrangement is no longer sufficient (Haigler, Bauer, & Travis, 2004).

Motivations for caregiving, such as love, duty, or obligation (often based on ethnicity and culture), strongly influence a caregiver's willingness to accept primary caregiving status (Geister, 2005). Additional reasons given by family caregivers for accepting their role are their expectations of themselves and others, religious training and spiritual experiences, and role modeling (Piercy & Chapman, 2001).

Caregiver Dyads and Caregiver Systems

Early caregiving research identified a care recipient and a caregiver as separate entities; the caregiver had primary responsibility for the care and well-being of the care recipient. These studies often did not recognize that caregiving usually occurs within the context of larger, more complex family systems (Palmer & Glass, 2003) or other social networks (Weitzner, Haley, & Chen, 2000). Furthermore, the helping networks used by widowed and never-married individuals may be larger than those of married people (Barrett & Lynch, 1999).

In recent years, caregiving research has placed more emphasis on the dynamics of the family relationships (Palmer & Glass, 2003) and the dyadic relationship (Badr & Actielli, 2005; Lyons, Zarit, Sayer, & Whitlach, 2002). As would be expected, these studies indicate that the dynamics of the family or other close personal relationships that exist before the illness experience can influence caregiving relationships post illness. The increasing number of stepfamilies also adds to the complexity of caregiving. Today, people of both genders and of all ages, ethnicities, and economic classes occupy positions as caregivers with varying levels and types of responsibilities, especially in long-term care arrangements. Because caregivers have varying degrees of responsibility for providing or arranging for care, the terms *care provider* and *care manager* may be used to differentiate two types of caregivers (Stoller & Culter, 1993). This designation helps clarify the previously invisible contributions of all family caregivers. If a son is close to his dependent parents, especially if he is not married, he is likely to be accountable for seeing that things get done, even if he does not provide all of the direct care that is required (Allen, Goldscheider, & Ciambrone, 1999; Keith, 1995;

Thompson, Tudiver, & Manson, 2000). Similarly, an adult grandchild may help a grandparent in the absence of a nearby adult child, or children-in-law may find their relationships to relatives with chronic illness make them better suited to caregiving roles than the biological children (Peters-Davis, Moss, & Pruchno, 1999; Pruchno, Burant, & Peters, 1997; Travis & Bethea, 2001).

Changes in the modern family social structure have resulted in more families where both parents work outside the home. This so-called sandwich generation is often not available to provide care for aging family members, which creates a new level of caregivers—children and adolescents. These young caregivers assist with or even assume care of adults with chronic illness in their homes (Hunt et al., 2005; Lackey & Gates, 2001).

Racial and Ethnic Diversity

The family caregiving experience is also shaped by race and ethnicity. These two factors influence one's life experiences in terms of socioeconomic status, education, marital status, health, living arrangements, and general lifestyle (Binstock, 1999). In chronic illness, access to programs and services and preferences for certain types of assistance are often sharply divided along racial and ethnic lines. The number of minority older adults is increasing at a faster rate than that of non-Hispanic whites, with the largest proportionate increases projected in the over-75-years group. While the number of African-American older adults will increase slightly in the next 50 years, proportionately larger and more rapid increases will occur among Hispanic and Asian elders (He, Sengupta, Velkoff, & DeBarros, 2005).

Comparative research indicates that patterns of family response to a family member with a chronic illness may be significantly different across ethnic groups (Chesla & Rungreangkulkij, 2001). Gerontologic researchers are building a substantial body of literature on African American, Asian American, Native American, and Hispanic older adults and their family caregiving experiences and preferences for support. Because this literature is extensive, only one example of diversity is provided to illustrate ethnic influences.

Cultural precedence, historical events, and the needs of extended kin and family structure shape African-American caregiving. Documented barriers to formal programs and services include poverty and economic disparity, lower educational levels, ageism, and racial discrimination (Jones, 1999). As a result, persistent underutilization of formal assistance programs and a reliance on family and friends are typical patterns of long-term care for dependent African-American older adults (Cox, 1999).

While it is known that African-American families have a strong sense of respect, duty, and obligation to elderly members of their communities, it may also be the case that generations have learned to be self- and family-reliant in the face of both overt and covert forms of racial discrimination (Binstock, 1999; Edmonds, 1999). As a result of this self-reliance, African-American family caregivers, especially women, may be perceived to have a lower level of role strain than their white counterparts. Research demonstrates a large variation in the female African-American caregiver's perception of role strain (Williams et al., 2003).

Gender Differences

The choice of who becomes the primary caregiver and what the family caregiving system looks like depends on many factors. In a spousal relationship, the unaffected spouse usually assumes the caregiving role. Often, both spouses are forced to cope with role renegotiation in addition to their new roles as the giver and receiver of care (Gordon & Perrone, 2004).

Among married adult children, daughters or daughters-in-law are most often the primary caregivers for aging parents (Shirey & Summer, 2000). Daughters are more likely to offer assistance to their father who is serving in a caregiving role than their mother. This may be because they are more comfortable with their mother in that role

and feel that their father needs additional assistance performing the tasks required of a caregiver (Mittelman, 2003). Sarkisian and Gerstel (2004) found that much of the relationship between gender and helping parents is explained by gender differences in employment patterns. They suggest that gender differences in adult care may be fading as women's and men's work lives become more similar (Sarkisian & Gerstel). National studies in the 1980s suggested that though women predominate as caregivers, somewhere between one in five and one in three caregivers are men (Chang & White-Means, 1991; Stone, Cafferata, & Sangl, 1987). Other studies in the 1990s estimated that men constituted nearly half of in-home caregivers and of caregivers to the elderly, chronically ill, and disabled (Kramer & Thompson, 2001).

Although men are just as likely as women to be involved in caring for and helping seniors, women, wives, mothers, and adult daughters spend more time as the designated primary caregiver (Stobert & Cranswick, 2004). The gendered nature of caregiving is certainly one important characteristic of long-term caregiving that is likely to continue in the future. All things being equal, the person who is closest to and the most involved in the daily life of the dependent person is usually the person most accountable for either doing or seeing that care is done.

Types of Care Provided by Family Caregivers

Over the long term, a dependent person requires two types of care: social care and health-related care. Social care includes both functional and affective assistance in daily living while health-related care refers to specialized care by professionals and daily treatments performed by family caregivers, such as the administration of medication.

Functional assistance is determined by the care recipient's ability to perform various tasks of daily existence, which are categorized as either instrumental or basic activities of daily living. Instrumental activities of daily living (IADLs) are the functions an adult would be expected to perform in the process of everyday life, including cooking, cleaning, buying groceries, doing yard work, and paying bills. For a child, these tasks might include getting to school, playing, or cleaning his or her room. Basic activities of daily living (ADLs) are the tasks required for personal care and basic survival. These tasks include eating, bathing, dressing, going to the bathroom, maintaining personal hygiene, and getting around (mobility).

Affective assistance, also called emotional support, includes behaviors that convey caring and concern to the care recipient. Affective assistance is most often linked with enhanced feelings of self-esteem, contentment, life satisfaction, hope of recovery, dignity, and general well-being (Brody & Schoonover, 1986; Horowitz, 1985).

In the past, there was a somewhat clearer division between the formal and informal care network. The informal network—family caregivers or significant others—provided both emotional and functional aspects of care and monitored the care provided by formal providers. The formal network provided specialized care that was highly task-oriented and goal-directed. Today the roles of the formal and informal network reveal a more blended approach to caregiving. Family caregivers perform highly skilled tasks formerly reserved for the professional. Professional caregivers function as a team with the family in care decisions for the client (Haigler, Bauer, & Travis, 2004).

Caregiving Histories and Maturation over Time

Longitudinal studies of family caregiving have documented the many changes that occur in the role of family caregiver and note that family caregiving is not a static event. Pearlin (1992) equated caregiving to career development. There are two factors that contribute to this notion of a caregiving career or caregiving history: maturation of the caregiver over time, and ongoing role development associated with the inevitable transitions in care over the long term.

The expectations of the family caregiver are many. They often begin their roles with little or no training or support. In addition to the psychological aspects of caregiving, they are expected to provide competent, skilled health care for their loved ones (Elliot & Shewchuk, 2003). Most caregivers begin their experiences as novices with little or no experience or knowledge of how to navigate the healthcare system (McAuley, Travis, & Safewright, 1997; Skaff, Pearlin & Mullan, 1996). Over time, mature caregivers master a new language system of entitlements (Medicare, Medicaid) and treatments (medication administration, illness symptomatology), and learn how to incorporate the needs of a dependent person into their daily lives (Leavitt et al., 1999). Some caregivers mature more quickly and with greater ease than others, and some caregivers are never able to achieve adequate skill and/or confidence in the caregiver role. Thus, tremendous variability can be found in the levels, lengths, and forms of care provided by family caregivers, which are at least partially attributed to successful mastery of their roles (Seltzer & Wailing, 2000).

Transitions in care occur at three points: entry into a caregiving relationship, institutionalization (or transitions into other formal care arrangements), and bereavement (Seltzer & Wailing, 2000). Unlike acute or episodic care that has an end point, the only natural end to long-term caregiving is the death of the care recipient. Even families that ultimately opt for institutional placement of their dependent family members do not abandon their relatives over the long term. Most caregivers stay engaged as care managers following the institutional placement decision (Seltzer & Wailing).

Montgomery and Kosloski (n.d.) have identified a similar concept called a caregiving trajectory. Their seven markers of caregiving are (1) performance of initial caregiving task; (2) self-definition as a caregiver; (3) provision of personal care; (4) seeking out or using assistive services; (5) consideration of institutionalization; (6) actual nursing home placement; and (7) termination of the caregiver role. In this trajectory, Montgomery and Kosloski believe that the order and timing of the markers are indicative of the individual, their culture, and the relationship of the caregiver to the care recipient.

One of the reasons that family caregiving precipitated by acute hospitalization is so stressful for new caregivers is that they have not had a period of maturation and development before the intense caregiving demands and the decision-making requirements that follow (Kane, Reinardy, & Penrod, 1999). In addition, the transitions in care occur rapidly and over a highly compressed period. In a matter of days the caregiver may transition from having no care responsibilities to being fully engaged in rehabilitation after hospitalization, or home or institutional long-term care (Kane et al., 1999).

Positive Aspects of Caregiving

In the past, research on stress, strain, burden, and burnout has overshadowed the positive aspects of providing care to a dependent family member. As a result, less is understood about how and why caregivers provide care even under difficult circumstances. While not much has been published on satisfaction with caregiving, Kramer's (1997) review of research on positive aspects of caregiving noted that some caregivers gain experience when assisting others. Gain was conceptualized as "the extent to which the caregiving role is appraised to enhance an individual's life space and be enriching" (p. 219). Caregivers do report satisfaction with their role. Adults who functioned as caregivers during their childhood have reported that their participation taught them responsibility, allowed them to be "part of the family," provided opportunities to be "appreciated" and to be "useful." They also reported pride at learning skills at an early age (Lackey & Gates, 2001). Many couples feel that caring for their partner strengthened their relationship (Gordon & Perrone, 2004). Coherence, a sense of togetherness in caring for others, was discovered by Pierce (2001) to be important for maintaining stability within the family. Through coherence, family caregivers felt connected and

this helped them survive in stressful times related to caring situations (Pierce, 2001).

A number of factors have been reported over the past three decades as contributors to caregivers' satisfaction. These factors include the care recipient's levels of physical, cognitive, and social impairment (Blake & Lincoln, 2000; Deimling, & Bass, 1986; Williams, 1993); the types of care provided by the caregiver (Draper, Poulos, Cole, Poulos, & Ehrlich, 1992; Montgomery, Stull, & Borgatta, 1985); the caregiver's gender and marital status (Zarit, Todd, & Zarit, 1986); the extent to which the caregiver's personal and social life are disrupted by the demands of caregiving (George & Gwyther, 1986; Poulshock, & Deimling, 1984); the quality of the relationship between caregiver and care recipient as perceived by the caregiver (Bowdoin, 1994; Caron & Bowers, 2003); and the satisfactory assistance with caregiving perceived by the caregiver (Bowdoin, 1994; George & Gwyther). For instance, caregivers and their families may experience less satisfaction if the care recipient is severely disabled and if they perceive that needed assistance in caring is unavailable. Other caregivers may report more satisfaction if the care recipient is only mildly disabled and if relatives, or friends, or both are able to help provide the needed assistance (Pierce, 2001). Family style, including receptivity, has been suggested as an area for future study (Gilliss, 2002). Longitudinal research and research with caregivers in diverse arrangements are needed to provide a more comprehensive view of what contributes to a positive caregiving experience.

The Future of Caregiving

Looking to the future, it is likely that the next cohort of older adult baby boomers will be very different from their parents and grandparents and will further confound the current reliance on family caregivers. Declining family sizes, increasing childlessness, and rising divorce rates will limit the number of family caregivers (Johnson, Toohey, & Wiener, 2007) during the lifetimes of adult baby boomers. Parents of the baby boom generation have several children from whom to seek assistance, while older baby boomers with smaller families will not be so fortunate. It remains to be seen what this societal trend will mean to this cohort.

In the future, racial caregiving trends are likely to escalate. In particular, African-American and Hispanic caregivers will be more available for long-term caregiving than will Caucasian caregivers. Furthermore, Caucasian caregivers are expected to purchase more services for dependent family members (Shirey & Summer, 2000). Most researchers agree, however, that any predictions about family caregiving in the future are tenuous because public policy is difficult to predict from one generation to the next. That policy will need to change to accommodate the caregiving needs of the aging baby boom cohort is the only certainty.

PROBLEMS AND ISSUES

Family caregivers face multiple problems, issues, and concerns throughout their caregiving experiences. The case study of the H. family is typical of the effort most family caregivers put into fulfilling their responsibilities, attending to the wants and needs of the care recipient, and continuously adjusting their lives to the physical and emotional requirements of the caregiving situation.

Family caregiving experiences incorporate societal values and are shaped by governmental policy. Policies that affect family caregiving in the United States have been created with the presumption that families are responsible for caring for their disabled members and will provide the majority of the care that is needed (Montgomery, 1999). For many years, these expectations were consistent with caregivers' resources and abilities.

Over the past two decades, however, there has been a blurring of the lines of responsibility for long-term caregiving. Increased technology, greater acuity of those in need of assistance, and competing demands on available caregivers have created an imbalance between the demand for family care and the ability of family

caregivers to provide care. Family caregivers are being asked to provide highly technical treatments; administer complex medication regimens; provide labor-intensive, hands-on care; and monitor the medical conditions of very ill family members.

The one responsibility that has remained constant over time, whether the family caregiver is a direct care provider or arranges care as a care manager, is the extensive decision-making demands placed on family caregivers. When the dependent family member cannot make decisions or has difficulty communicating choices, the responsibility for countless decisions associated with managing daily life falls to the caregiver. These decisions include the initiation, timing, and provision of assistance from informal and formal sources; integration of caregiving demands into work and family life; and planning for future long-term care needs (McAuley, Travis, & Safewright, 1997; Travis & Bethea, 2001).

The Influence of Public Policy on Family Caregiving

Containing the rising costs of healthcare services has become a national policy imperative. This goal is demonstrated through policies that promote prevention of premature or unwanted institutionalization of disabled elders in nursing homes, limit publicly funded home care services to individuals with the lowest incomes, and curtail the Medicare home health benefit. Such policies limit the amount and scope of services that are provided to persons who need ongoing assistance by formal caregivers as well as their family caregivers. Recent cost-containment measures are occurring precisely when the demand for help in providing long-term care at home is increasing (Riggs, 2004). These changes in government-sponsored services mean that many families, particularly low- and middle-income families, are faced with difficult choices about providing assistance while receiving minimal help from professional healthcare providers.

CASE STUDY

The H. Family

Mrs. H. had coronary artery disease and congestive heart failure that caused increasing fatigue, dyspnea, and angina over a 5-year period. Frequent upper respiratory infections exacerbated her dyspnea.

Home Setting: Mrs. H. lived at home with her husband in a small rural town, in a home they had owned since their children were small. Mr. H. was 4 years younger than his wife.

Role Issues: Mr. H. assumed cooking tasks in the home and was the primary caregiver for his wife, assisting her to ambulate to the bathroom for toileting and bathing, making sure her clothes were clean and accessible, and making sure she took her medicine as prescribed.

Support: The couple's married daughter and married son lived within a 10-minute drive of their parents' house. Both had children of their own but assisted their parents at least once a week. The daughter did the major housecleaning for her parents and drove them regularly to the grocery store, the frequent doctor's visits, and the pharmacy. The son assisted his father with lawn work and household repairs; he was also called on in cases of medical emergency to be the decision maker.

Transitions: Over several years, Mrs. H.'s health declined. Her upstairs bedroom became inaccessible because stair climbing became exhausting. The living room was converted to a bedroom. She was hospitalized for a series of short-term stays for complaints of chest pain and/or difficulty breathing over this time span. Whenever she was hospitalized, the daughter and son took turns driving their father to the hospital because he visited their mother daily.

During the next 5 years, these hospitalizations increased in frequency to several times yearly. She used portable oxygen at home.

Initially it was only used for brief intervals during the night, and she was able to accompany her daughter for brief shopping trips or drives "to get out of the house." As her health declined, Mrs. H. used the oxygen continuously, remaining in her room. The family got a "medi-alert" call button that Mrs. H. always wore in case she needed emergency help.

With each hospitalization, Mrs. H. returned home weaker. Mr. H. began to worry that he could no longer care for his wife at home because of her increasing weakness. He moved her commode adjacent to her wheelchair; even so, Mrs. H. had difficulty transferring from her chair to the commode. Mrs. H. was heavier than her husband; he worried about her safety, fearing that she might fall and injure herself and he would be unable to assist her. The daughter had a part-time job but visited her parents more frequently, twice weekly. She began to express concerns about both parents' health to her brother, her friends, and her husband.

Decisions: When Mrs. H. was hospitalized at the age of 78 for chest pain and difficulty breathing, the physician approached Mr. H. and his son and daughter with a request that they sign a Do Not Resuscitate (DNR) agreement. Mrs. H. had vehemently expressed, "I don't want them damn machines," so the family readily agreed to the DNR order. They were concerned for Mrs. H. because the DNR had never been brought up by the doctor before.

Mr. H. told his children that Mrs. H. would have to go to a nursing home when she was discharged from the hospital, as he could no longer care for her with her severely diminished abilities. Although the family discussed this problem, they did not resolve it. After visiting Mrs. H. one evening at the hospital, during which time she was alert and talkative, the family returned to their homes. That evening Mrs. H. died. The family expressed relief that

(Continued)

■ CASE STUDY (*Continued*)

her suffering was over, that she died the way she wanted to, without machines. They were also relieved that the whole family did not have to struggle with the nursing home decision.

Discussion Questions

1. What are the advantages and disadvantages of the client being cared for at home? For the family? For the caregiver?
2. What factors influence the cost-effectiveness of home care versus institutionalization?
3. Who are the primary providers of home care? What are some of the providers' competing demands?
4. What are some of the emotional responses to family caregiving?
5. What is the financial impact of caregiving on the caregiver?
6. How does public policy affect caregiving?
7. How can health professionals assist family caregivers?
8. Where can family caregivers go for assistance and information?

Several government initiatives have attempted to address the needs of family caregivers. In 1993, the Family and Medical Leave Act (FMLA) became law. This act gives qualified caregivers the option of taking up to 12 weeks of unpaid leave from their jobs to care for a family member (US Department of Labor, 1993). In 2000, approximately 24 million or 16.5% of eligible employees used family and medical leave. Of these, approximately 30% used the leave to care for an ill child, spouse, or parent. Approximately 3% of the surveyed qualified employees who needed family and medical leave did not take it. The top barriers were not being able to afford unpaid leave (54%), being worried about losing their job (32%), or feeling that job advancement would be hurt (43%) (Workplace Flexibility 2010, 2004).

In addition to these barriers, many caregiving situations require that the caregiver be available for a longer period of time than the 12 weeks afforded by the FMLA. These barriers present difficult choices for family members of individuals in need of caregiving assistance—many are faced with leaving or reducing gainful employment to provide the necessary care because they have no other options. The Older Americans Act Amendments of 2000 established the National Family Caregiver Support Program (NFCSP) (DHHS Administration on Aging, n.d.a). Federal funds are given to states based upon their proportionate share of the 70-plus population. States, working in partnership with local agencies on aging and faith and community-service providers and tribes, offer five direct services to best meet the range of caregiver needs. The services include provision of the following:

- Information to caregivers about available services
- Assistance to caregivers in gaining access to supportive services
- Individual counseling, organization of support groups, and caregiver training to assist caregivers in making decisions and solving problems relating to their roles
- Respite care to enable caregivers to be temporarily relieved from their caregiving responsibilities
- Supplemental services, on a limited basis, to complement the care provided by caregivers

Family caregivers eligible for the NFCSP are those who care for adults aged 60 years or more and grandparents and relatives of children not more than 18 years of age, including grandparents who are sole caregivers of grandchildren and those individuals who are affected by mental retardation or have developmental disabilities. Priority is given to caregivers with social and economic need, particularly low-income and minority individuals, or older individuals providing care and support to persons with mental retardation and related developmental disabilities (DHHS Administration on Aging, n.d.a). While the NFCSP has been lauded as an important step in recognizing the needs of family caregivers, it lacks the appropriate funding to support the needs of caregivers at any meaningful level. Furthermore, each state decides how the funds are used, resulting in inconsistencies of services across states. In addition, with the aging of the baby boomers over the next several decades, the reliance on family members and friends for the long-term care needs of those with chronic conditions is expected to increase significantly (Montgomery & Feinberg, 2003; Riggs, 2004).

The lack of adequate monetary assistance for the family unit is a complex problem. Currently, public financing of long-term care in a home setting is minimal. Medicare offers a hospice benefit with a time-limited period at the end of life and some states have limited home and community-based waiver programs that provide some home-based services for low-income residents. Oftentimes the waiting lists for these services are long, with residents never receiving the services for which they are qualified. Many private insurers offer long-term care policies through employers, fraternal organizations, retirement communities, and health management organizations. Unfortunately, in the past, most of these policies did not cover many aspects of the personal care provided by family caregivers, leaving this in-home care as out-of-pocket expenses. Long-term care policies now on the market are more comprehensive, but are expensive to purchase.

Recently, individual states were authorized to craft their own programs to provide paid leave to workers who need to care for family members. In 2001, the Clinton administration proposed relief to families in the form of a $1,000 annual tax credit for those receiving or providing long-term care in the home, but the proposal generated controversy among legislators. Many believed that government intervention would discourage people from purchasing long-term care insurance to cover nursing home care and healthcare services in the home (DuPont, 1999). The issue of the government's role in assisting caregivers remains a strongly debated one.

Emotional Effects of Being a Caregiver

Although not all persons experience stress when providing care, many do. There are a number of factors that influence caregiving and the stress it may cause. Factors include the intensity of the care provided; types of care tasks performed; gender; personal characteristics of the caregiver; the relationship between the caregiver and the person receiving care; support from other family members; and competing obligations of the caregiver. Research on caregiver stress spans more than two decades, and researchers have labeled caregiver stress as either strain or burden.

Strain or Burden

Caregiver strain and burden are multidimensional, closely related concepts that include both subjective perceptions of caregivers, such as role overload, and objective factors, such as physical care needs of the care recipient. Caregiver strain is usually related to the stress, hardship, or conflicting feelings one has when performing the caregiving role (Hunt, 2003). For example, a caregiver may feel a high level of role strain when trying to decide between caring for an ailing parent and maintaining gainful employment.

One area of caregiver research that has focused heavily on caregiver strain is dementia care. In particular, caregiving is more stressful and produces more emotional and physical strain when the caregiver is caring for a person with dementia or Alzheimer's disease. Caregivers of persons with dementia are more likely than nondementia caregivers to say that they suffer mental or physical problems as a result of caregiving (Ory, Hoffman,

Yee, Tennstedt, & Schulz, 1999). Caregivers also report higher levels of strain when they perceive the patient to be manipulative, unappreciative, or unreasonable (Nerenberg, 2002).

Caregiver burden is defined as "the oppressive or worrisome load borne by people providing direct care for the chronically ill" (Hunt, 2003, p. 28). Burden is relative to the level of the care recipient's disability, including behavioral and cognitive issues; the extent of care required; and the caregiver's level of worry or feelings of being overwhelmed (Nerenberg, 2002). Financial strain also contributes to the level of caregiver burden (Evercare & National Alliance of Caregiving [NAC], 2007). Caregiver burden has been associated with increased depressive symptoms in caregivers of patients with stroke (Chumbler, Rittman, Van Puymbroeck, Vogel, & Qin, 2004), coronary artery bypass (Halm & Bakas, 2007), and Alzheimer's disease (Mausbach et al., 2007), among others. The Family Caregiver Alliance (FCA) estimates that between 40 and 70% of caregivers have "clinically significant" depressive symptoms (FCA, 2006). Higher levels of depression have been found among dementia caregivers who cared for persons with moderate to severe functional impairment and greater amounts of behavioral disturbance (wandering and aggression) than among non-dementia caregivers (Meshefedjian, McCusker, Bellavance, & Baumgarten, 1998).

In another study of caregivers and patients with dementia (N = 5627), 32% of the caregivers were classified as clinically depressed on the basis of elevated scores on the Geriatric Depression Scale (Covinsky et al., 2003) When caregivers' appraisals of the burden of caregiving are high, there is greater likelihood of caregiver depression and depressive symptoms (Clyburn, Stones, Hadjistavropoulos, & Tuokko, 2000).

Caregiving is also a risk factor for poorer health and increased mortality in some caregivers (FCA, 2006). One study reported that among spousal caregivers experiencing strain, there was a 63% higher mortality risk for family caregivers

during a 4-year period than that among non-caregivers (Schulz & Beach, 1999).

There also appears to be a gender component associated with caregiver burden. Female caregivers experience more psychiatric disorders than do male caregivers (Yee & Schulz, 2000) and are much more likely than men to report being depressed or anxious and to experience lower levels of life satisfaction. The irony is that, while they report more caregiver burden, role conflict, or strain, women are more likely than male caregivers to continue caregiving responsibilities over the long term. Women are less likely than men to obtain assistance from others with caregiving. Finally, women are less likely than men to engage in preventative health behaviors, such as rest, exercise, and taking medications as prescribed, while caregiving (Burton, Newsom, Schulz, Hirsch, & German, 1997).

Caregivers for spouses have reported a higher incidence of depression and stress than those caring for a disabled parent. The caregiving roles and responsibilities may have a major impact on the relationship itself. Health-care professionals must realize that the relationship between the caregiver and the spouse receiving the care needs to be supported and nurtured in terms of love, affection, and intimacy (Gordon & Perrone, 2004).

Children and adolescents who have functioned in the role of caregiver report difficulty watching their loved one progress with a chronic problem. They have memories of unpleasant smells and sights. They also report feeling helpless because of their lack of knowledge and fear that they would not be able to deal with a crisis (Lackey & Gates, 2001).

Recent research has found that caregivers who have a higher sense of self-efficacy and control over their life situations (i.e. personal mastery) have less burden and fewer depressive symptoms (Chumbler et al. 2004; Chumbler, Rittman, & Wu, 2007; Mausbach et al., 2007). These studies suggest that interventions that enhance self-efficacy or personal mastery will decrease health risks and improve health-related outcomes for caregivers (Chumbler et al., 2007; Rabinowitz, Mausbach, Thompson, Gallagher-Thompson, 2007; Halm & Bakas, 2007)

Burned Out and Giving Up

Burnout has been defined as a "state of physical, emotional, and mental exhaustion caused by long-term involvement in emotionally demanding situations" (Pines & Aronson, 1988, p. 9). For the caregiver, the term burnout can be used to describe this type of physical, mental, and/or emotional exhaustion (Nerenberg, 2002).

Figley (1998) developed a model of burnout for professional caregivers (e.g., nurses and social workers) that has implications for caregiver and caregiver family situations as well. In this model, burnout begins with a caregiver's stress response, that is, compassion stress, which refers to "the stress connected with exposure to a sufferer" (Figley, 1998, p. 21). In this case, the sufferer is the care recipient. When compassion stress is accompanied by prolonged exposure to the suffering and/or unresolved trauma, compassion fatigue sets in. Compassion fatigue can also be exacerbated by a substantial degree of life disruption. These factors lead to caregiver burnout, which may be dealt with by placing the care recipient in an institution, by having another family member assume primary caregiver duties, or, in some cases, by neglecting or abusing the care recipient. Parents caring for children with severe developmental disabilities or others caring for individuals with Alzheimer's disease are especially at risk for burnout due to prolonged exposure and high levels of life disruption. However, to date, little research has been done on the incidence of compassion fatigue in informal caregivers.

Family Relationships and Shifting Roles

Providing care to others, especially spouses and parents, often requires changes in the ways that family members interact with each other. For the care provider, this decision may be a life-long commitment to another family member (Elliot & Shewchuk, 2003). These changes in family interactions have been labeled role reversal, role renegotiation, or role reconstruction. Although most family caregivers handle these role changes over time, some caregivers struggle with changes in their family relationships (Lutz, Chumbler, & Roland, 2007).

In role reversal, for example, wives providing care to husbands are often required to make financial decisions or perform tasks to maintain their homes that have always been their husbands' responsibility. Adult children often speak of becoming "parents" to their frail parents (Plowfield, Raymond, & Blevins, 2000). Some researchers view the term role reversal as being inadequate for describing family relationships in late life (Brody, 1990; Seltzer, 1990). They view the use of the term role reversal as a simplistic way of viewing a complex phenomenon and express concern that it reinforces negative stereotypes of dependency in general and old age in particular. If being a parent, child, or spouse is a social position in a family, these positions do not change during the lifetime of the family. A parent is always a parent. A spouse is always a spouse. Although behaviors toward each other may change as health or functioning decline, the roles remain stable. Therefore, the term role renegotiation or reconstruction may be more accurate to describe changes in familial relationships due to caregiving.

Support for this argument was offered in a study of adult child caregivers that found that adult child caregivers respected traditional parental autonomy for as long as possible (Piercy, 1998). The caregivers in this study described sensitivity to the parents' wishes, even when they disagreed with the parent, and well beyond the point at which the parent experienced significant cognitive or physical decline. This is particularly evident in studies of non-white cultures where familial roles are revered and respected (Evans, Coon, & Crogan, 2007). However, Lackey and Gates (2001) found that in some cases child caregivers who provide care to their parents at times perceived a reversal of roles. When caring for a parent, children reported serving as the person and confidant of the parent. In addition to the changed family dynamics, the child caregivers reported a pronounced effect on their school life and their friendships.

Elder Abuse and Neglect

The 2000 Survey of State Adult Protective Services stated that there were 472,813 reported cases of elder or vulnerable adult abuse. For substantiated reports, the most common environment for abuse was in domestic settings. The typical abuser was a man between the ages of 26 and 50 years. Almost 62% of the perpetrators were family members (spouse, parents, children, grandchildren, siblings, and other family members). The family member or perpetrator with the highest incidence of perpetration was the spouse or intimate partner, followed by an adult child (Teaster, 2003). Even with the impact of these statistics, one must realize that it is likely that the majority of elder or vulnerable adult abuses go unreported.

The DHHS Administration on Aging (n.d.d) defines the following types of abuse and neglect: physical, sexual, psychological, financial or material exploitation, and neglect. Physical abuse is defined as the willful infliction of physical pain or injury. Examples of this are slapping, bruising, sexually molesting, or restraining. Sexual abuse is the infliction of nonconsensual sexual contact of any kind. Psychological abuse is infliction of mental or emotional anguish. Examples of psychological abuse are humiliating, intimidating, or threatening. Neglect is the failure of a caretaker to provide goods or services necessary to avoid physical harm, mental anguish, or mental illness. Examples of neglect include abandonment, denial of food, or denial of health-related services.

It is important for health-care professionals to recognize the precipitating factors for caregiver abuse of an elder. There appears to be a strong link between the likelihood for abuse and the caregiver's perception of their situation. Caregivers who have had a positive relationship with care recipients are less likely to become abusive. In certain situations, the risk of abuse increased in direct relationship to the amount of care required. The personality characteristics and behaviors of the care recipient have also been indicated in relationship to the caregiver's stress level. Finally, an abusive incident may be triggered by the use of alcohol, substance abuse, or psychiatric illness (Nerenberg, 2002).

Although it is more common to think about the potential abuse of a dependent person by a family caregiver, it is also possible that a caregiver may be the victim of an abusive care recipient. Patterns of dysfunctional behavior in families can extend over decades. If a wife was abused by her husband before he became ill or dependent on her for assistance, there is no reason to believe that he would suddenly discontinue all forms of abusive behavior because of illness.

Family caregivers, especially women, who never know about the family finances and must always ask the care recipient or other family members for money or who rely solely on the care recipients' families for other types of assistance, may be very vulnerable to neglect. In addition, self-neglect, behavior that threatens a person's own health or safety can be an adverse consequence of profound caregiving stress and associated depression. Self-neglect usually manifests as refusal to provide oneself with adequate food, water, clothing, and shelter.

Excessive Caregiving

Although a very subjective notion, providing excessive care to an impaired adult occurs in some caregiving situations. One form of excessive care is assistance that puts the caregiver's physical or emotional health at risk. Excessive care may have deleterious effects on the health of spouse caregivers (Plowfield, Raymond, & Blevins, 2000; Schultz & Beach, 1999). In the Caregiver Health Effects Study, persons who felt burdened while providing long-term care for demented spouses had a high risk of mortality over a 4-year period (Schultz & Beach, 1999).

Given and colleagues (1990) found that spouse caregivers who experienced a combination of negative care recipient behaviors, such as cognitive impairment and antisocial behaviors, were more likely to feel higher levels of responsibility and react negatively to the caregiver role than did persons caring for spouses not exhibiting such behaviors. Despite negative responses to the caregiver role, the greater levels of responsibility felt by these spouses may contribute to the provision of excessive care and the caregivers' rejection of or failure to take advantage of respite care opportunities.

A second type of excessive care occurs when caregivers assume responsibilities or perform tasks for their care recipients that they are capable of performing themselves. For example, a caregiver recently informed of her parent's heart disease may react by taking over responsibilities, such as paying bills or cooking, that her parent can still perform adequately. Such excessive care can rob parents of feelings of autonomy that may be beneficial to their health and emotional well-being. Caregiving is a delicate balance of providing for the care recipient's safety while preserving their autonomy to the fullest extent possible (Piercy, 1998). Albert and Brody (1996) found that greater feelings of burden on the part of caregivers were associated with viewing parent care as childcare. These burdened caregivers were also less likely to encourage parental autonomy. Such findings suggest that promotion of care recipient autonomy to the greatest extent possible for as long as possible may be beneficial for both caregiver and care recipient.

Financial Impact of Caregiving

Caregiving has different degrees of financial impact on families, depending on their particular caregiving situations and financial resources. For elderly couples with a spouse as caregiver, the impact may range from minimal to considerable, depending on the extent to which other family help is available, formal services are used, and how they are financed. For families of frail elderly relatives, reduced employment is most likely to occur when the caregivers are of ethnic minorities and for patients with specific clinical characteristics (Covinsky, Eng, Lui, & Sands, 2001). When adult children are the caregivers, the picture becomes murky because it is the financial resources of the care recipient that are usually considered for public assistance.

The current public financing system for in-home and community-based services targets persons with the lowest incomes. Well-off family caregivers can afford to pay for home or community-based care out of pocket, regardless of the financial eligibility of the care recipient. However, families in the middle ranges of income may be unable to purchase in-home services or receive public financing for needed care. White-Means (1997) found that care recipients who were within 150 to 250% of established poverty levels and who were not receiving the Medicare home health benefit or state-financed programs were less likely to use in-home services than were individuals in other income ranges. In other words, these low-income care recipients were not financially eligible for assistance, nor were their family caregivers able to purchase services for them.

The cost of caregiving is associated with the level of need for the affected individual. According the Department of Health and Human Services Administration of Aging (2003b) caregivers spend an average of 11% out of pocket for services not covered by Medicare.

A study conducted by Evercare and the National Alliance for Caregiving (NAC, 2007) found that in a survey of 1000 caregivers the average annual costs of caregiving was $5531. However, in a smaller subsample of caregivers (N = 41), who maintained a 1-month diary of expenses, the annualized expenses were $12,348. The most common expenses were in the areas of "household goods, food, and meals (42%), travel and transportation costs (40%), and medical care co-pays and pharmaceuticals (31%)" (NAC, 2007, p. 7). Those in the lowest income categories provided the most number of hours of care per week. Caregivers whose income was less that $25,000 per year provided an average of 41 hours of care each week. Estimates of costs of care for these caregivers is more that $5,000 annually (or approximately 20% of their income). Forty-nine percent of the caregivers in this group also reported that their finances had gotten worse since they started providing care. Of the total sample, 43% reported that their financial worries had increased since taking on the role of caregiver.

Research shows that relatively few adult children contribute financially to parent care; only 5 to 10% of adult children transfer money to parents in a year's time (Boaz, Hu, & Ye, 1999). These "financial caregivers" tend to have higher levels of asset income and proportionally more women engaged in the paid labor force full time than those who do not offer any financial assistance to dependent parents. Furthermore, financial help almost always goes to single parents (usually widowed mothers) and for caregiving situations that require extensive personal assistance.

Employment

In the mid-1980s, the first national study of its kind revealed the shocking effects that being a caregiver had on the nation's workforce. About 14% of caregiver wives, 12% of daughters, 11% of husbands, and 5% of sons quit their jobs to care for elderly relatives. Of employed caregivers, 29% rearranged their work schedules, 21% reduced work hours, and 19% took time off without pay (Stone, Cafferata, & Sangl, 1987). A 2004 national survey estimated that 44 million Americans were providing care for a friend or family member older than 18 years. Of these, 7 million were providing between 12 and 87 hours of care per week, which included personal care and other tasks such as shopping and transportation; more than 26 million had to adjust their work schedules; and almost 8 million quit working to accommodate their caregiving responsibilities

(MetLife & NAC, 2004). In another survey of 1000 caregivers, of those who were employed or had been employed sometime during the caregiving experience, 37% cut back or quit working, 14% changed jobs, 48% used sick leave or vacation days, and 15% used unpaid leave (Evercare & NAC, 2007).

Employees most in need of support are those who function as primary caregivers and those who care for older adults with high care needs (Evercare & NAC, 2007; Stone & Short, 1990). Being female, Caucasian, and in fair to poor health increased the caregiver's likelihood of needing some assistance to accommodate work and caregiving demands. There is also evidence to suggest that caregivers who have lower amounts of education and those less likely to view their work as a career are more likely than others to decide to leave paid employment altogether. Dautzenberg (2000) found that the daughter living closest with the least competing demands was most vulnerable to being called upon for caregiving duties.

Clearly, there are hidden costs, both economic and noneconomic, of informal care to older adults receiving care, their caregivers, and to other family members (Evercare & NAC, 2007; Fast, Williamson, & Keating, 1999). Unfortunately, these costs are frequently ignored by policy makers focused primarily on cost containment of services. The emotional well-being of the care recipient, who struggles with conflicting issues of dependency and burden to the family, and the emotional well-being of the family caregiver, who struggles with loss of control and independence in his or her daily life, can become very tenuous in these situations (Pyke, 1999). The most dramatic economic costs to caregivers include giving up paid employment, lost income from unpaid leave or time off work, relinquishment of career advancement opportunities, and the prospect of out-of-pocket expenses to support home care. Those in the lowest income categories have the highest economic burden. Employers need to consider flexible options to help the caregiver/employee meet the demands of their multiple roles.

INTERVENTIONS

The Interface of Informal and Formal Caregiving Networks

The interface of a formal caregiving network with the family caregiver is important for the long-term emotional and physical health of the family caregiver. There are several diverse models currently in use to explain the ways in which informal and formal caregiving networks exist over the long term.

Dual Specialization Model

One model that is particularly useful for studying the shared care between formal and informal networks is the dual specialization or complementary model (Litwak, 1985). The model is based on the notion that formal and informal networks have certain kinds of caregiving responsibilities and abilities that are best suited to each particular network. Because of this specialized division of labor, there is the potential for friction and conflict among caregivers. Therefore, the networks work best when the amount of contact or level of involvement between them is minimized, and the groups perform only those tasks for which they are best suited.

This conceptualization of a clear division of labor worked well until the early 1990s when, as already described, highly technical aspects of care were expected of family caregivers. With a new emphasis on family caregivers receiving support and empowerment from formal providers to become competent caregivers, a somewhat less restrictive interpretation of the complementary model is required today. Still, the model is useful for thinking about potential stress and tension that family caregivers may feel toward formal caregivers.

Family Empowerment Model

A model that more appropriately reflects the current emphasis on support of the family caregivers

and the inclusion of those caregivers as members of the care-planning team is the Family Empowerment Model (see Figure 9-1). Families with members who have chronic health conditions, especially if those members are children, often feel a sense of powerlessness in satisfying the health-care needs of that family member and in sustaining family life (Hulme, 1999). The Family Empowerment Model depicts an interactive intervention process that consists of phases corresponding to the amount of trust and decision making that a family shares with health professionals: professional dominated, participatory, challenging, and collaborative (Hulme, 1999). Family members interact with each other, nurses and other health-care professionals, the health-care system, and their community as they participate in the family empowerment process.

In the professional-dominated phase there is a high level of trusting dependency on health

FIGURE 9-1

Family Empowerment Model.

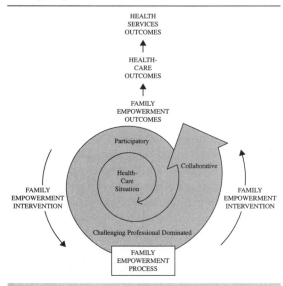

Source: Hulme, P.A. (1999). Family empowerment: A nursing intervention with suggested outcomes for families of children with a chronic health condition. *Journal of Family Nursing, 5*(1), 33–50. Thousand Oaks, CA: Sage.

professionals to direct health care while the family adjusts to the health-care situation. This phase occurs during an initial diagnosis of the chronic illness and during a life-threatening situation or relapse (Hulme, 1999).

The participatory phase occurs as the family responds to the continuing chronic illness and its disruptive effect on family life. "Critical consciousness and action" (Hulme, 1999) become apparent and family members begin to perceive themselves as important members in the decision-making process about health care for their family member. During this phase, family members focus on learning about the care of their chronically ill family member and the rules of the health-care system. They also seek support and try out changing roles and responsibilities to improve their family life (Hulme, 1999).

In the challenging phase the balance of power begins to shift from the health-care professional to the family. Family members question aspects of care, sometimes triggering conflict with the health-care professional over control of their family member's health care. Family frustration, uncertainty, disillusionment, and loss of trust in the health-care professionals are not uncommon during this phase (Hulme, 1999).

The collaborative phase is entered as the family becomes more self-confident and assertive and less reliant on the health-care professional. The family is now a full partner in the health-care team (Hulme, 1999).

When using the Family Empowerment Model, it is important to remember that the phases are interdependent and overlapping, and that a family's progress through the phases may be delayed or reversed because of a prolonged or extremely challenging phase, a disruption in family life, or changes in the health-care situation (Hulme, 1999). Health-care professionals can help prevent these events by implementing Family Empowerment Interventions, such as guiding the family in assessing its own strengths and in mobilizing the use of those strengths for problem solving. The goal of such interventions is to recognize, promote, and enhance a family's ability to meet the health-care needs of their family member

with chronic illness and to sustain their family life (Hulme, 1999). A valuable resource for nurses as well as family caregivers is the National Organization for Empowering Caregivers (www. nofec.org and www. care-givers.com).

Family Caregivers as Members of Care-Planning Teams

Although the two terms are sometimes used interchangeably, interdisciplinary teams are very different from multidisciplinary models of care. The older concept of teaming included multidisciplinary teams. These teams typically included members from different disciplines who shared common goals but worked independently from one another to propose and implement patient interventions. When a family caregiver interacts with a multidisciplinary team, he or she is more or less forced to compartmentalize caregiving needs, problems, or concerns into disciplines, such as a nursing problem, a therapy concern, or a social need.

In contrast, the more contemporary concept of teaming calls for interdisciplinary teams. These teams work together to identify and analyze problems, plan actions and interventions, and monitor results of the care plan. Team meetings are used to make or negotiate assignments, share information, and evaluate the team's effort toward achieving client and caregiver outcomes. Lines of communication among team members are highly visible, while disciplinary boundaries are connected on interdisciplinary teams (Travis & Duer, 2000). Family caregivers who participate as members of interdisciplinary teams need only to convey their problems, needs, issues, or concerns to activate a team effort for resolution.

Active inclusion as a member of the interdisciplinary team may help in overcoming a still common complaint of family caregivers: that of dissatisfaction with the level of their involvement in health-care decision making. Family caregivers have identified four markers of satisfactory involvement: feeling that information is shared; feeling included in decision making; feeling that there is someone you can contact when you need

CASE STUDY

The C. Family

Ms. L.C. is a 29-year-old white woman divorced from her husband. She lives with her 2-year-old son Andrew, who has central hypoventilation syndrome (he does not breathe unassisted when asleep) and prolonged expiratory apnea (he has frequent hypoxic episodes when awake). It was Andrew's illness that led to the couple separating. After birth, Andrew was hospitalized for approximately 3 months with his mother remaining near the hospital rather than returning home, 70 miles away. Her husband saw her absence as inattentiveness and neglect. After they learned that the baby had a poor prognosis, the parents disagreed about his treatment, resulting in much conflict, domestic violence, and eventual separation.

Home Setting. L. C. and Andrew live in a small, one-bedroom upstairs apartment on the outskirts of a small city. The living room is largely taken up with Andrew's crib and equipment: ventilator, apnea monitor, oxygen tanks, and suction equipment. Ms. C. keeps the apartment very clean to avoid respiratory irritants for her son. Toys are in every room.

Support System. Ms. C does not trust Mr. C. There is a restraining order to keep him out of the apartment, as he has stated he wishes to take Andrew off life support. Mr. C's mother and sister do not acknowledge Andrew as part of the family. They visited once in the hospital after Andrew was born, but tried to take out the baby's tracheostomy tube, for, in their culture only "normal" healthy babies are allowed to live.

L.C.'s mother comes to visit her daily. Her sister visits several times a week when she is off from work. Two nephews also visit once or twice weekly. Thus, there is extended family support for her from her family and much conflict from Mr. C.'s family. The consistent emotional support provided by her family keeps Ms. C. strong in her belief that her son deserves to live as normal a life as possible. She maintains a positive, almost stoic attitude about raising him at home.

Growth and Development Issues. The developmental task for this family is to incorporate the child into the family unit. The family unit itself changed after Andrew's birth, given the separation of the parents due to conflicts between their values of the child's right to live. Andrew is part of his mother's extended family system. L. C. has begun to date again, which has positive implications for her meeting her own needs as well as potential long-term implications for the family unit.

Andrew is played with in developmentally appropriate ways. He is frequently held and cuddled by his mother and her extended family. He is able to get around the apartment in his walker and is taken for age-appropriate excursions outside the home with his ventilator and the nurse.

Professional Assistance for the Child. Andrew has 24-hour-a-day nursing care. Importantly, Ms. C. refers to two of the nurses as part of the family, because they have cared for him for so long. In addition, he has a special education teacher once weekly, and a physical therapist and a speech therapist, who come every other week.

Assistance for the Parent Caregiver. The mother identified her need for support and counseling services. She was provided with the following information: The American Red Cross offers support groups for parents of children at home on high-technology care. The New York State Department of Health Council on Child and Adolescent Health

(Continued)

CASE STUDY (*Continued*)

offers a Directory of Self-Help/Mutual Support for Children with Special Health Needs and Their Families (1992). The National Organization of Rare Disorders is also a reference for self-help groups. The local county Mental Health Association is an additional resource for parent caregivers. L. C. is fortunate that her family allows her respite from her parenting and caregiving responsibilities. She can therefore participate in such self-help and support groups.

Discussion Questions

1. What challenging behaviors do you identify in this case study?
2. What do you think is causing these behaviors? Give some examples.
3. How would you handle these behaviors?
4. What are the worst ways to handle these behaviors? Please explain.
5. How might ethnicity/culture influence family caregiving?

Source: This case study was provided by Allison M. Goodell, R.N., B.S.N., staff nurse in the Pediatric Intensive Care Unit of the Children's Hospital at Albany Medical Center Hospital, Albany, New York.

to; and feeling that the service is responsive to your needs (Walker & Dewar, 2004). A goal of interdisciplinary teams should be to help family caregivers achieve these markers of involvement satisfaction. Use of the Family Empowerment Model (as previously discussed) can assist the interdisciplinary team in reaching that goal.

Interdisciplinary teaming works well in long-term care situations because it is virtually impossible to tease apart the ever-changing social and health-care needs of dependent individuals and their family caregivers. If an elderly diabetic client and his spousal caregiver cannot afford to purchase appropriate food and medications in the same week, the health care plan will fail until the social needs of the couple are met. Similarly, a wheelchair-bound adult in a potentially neglectful situation will not be able to remain in community-based care with only health-care support.

Transdisciplinary teams are the newest form of long-term care team. With shrinking health-care dollars and limited access to care, the trans-disciplinary team model seeks to "maximize the strengths of team members and minimize duplication in effort" (Lutz & Davis, 2008, p. 26). In this type of team, one member is selected to direct the care on the basis of the primary needs of the

family and patient. This team leader then coordinates the care with other members of the team and the family and patient. In this model, there is a blurring of disciplinary boundaries and team members may be cross-trained in the duties of other disciplines (without exceeding the standards of practice within their own discipline) to provide better continuity in care. For example, the nurse may also be cross-trained in some of the duties of the social worker or physical therapist (Lutz & Davis, 2008).

Life-Span Development and Developmentally Appropriate Care

Knowledge of growth and development helps caregivers separate normal changes from disease-related changes in the dependent family member, regardless of the client's age. This knowledge helps caregivers deal more effectively with decision-making issues, obtain appropriate available community resources, and secure emotional support for themselves. Numerous specialty organizations, such as the March of Dimes, provide this type of educational material for families of recipients of different ages (e.g., children and adolescents). The case study of Andrew, the ventilator-dependent child in the C. Family case study, demonstrates the importance of support and education for the parent.

For families of children with chronic illness, regardless of the type of chronic illness, certain developmental changes or times of transition trigger disequilibrium and stress in the family. Five principal periods of transition are at the initial diagnosis; when symptoms increase; when the child goes to a new setting (such as the hospital); during a parent's absence; and during periods of developmental change (Meleski, 2002). Of the developmental milestones, five specific times are associated with increased stress: periods when most children learn to walk, talk, and enter school; the onset of puberty, and the child's 21st birthday. Nurses need to recognize these times of transition and to teach families how to foster the healthy development of their children as well as the family. The literature reveals several types of adaptation that parents use during times of transition: support, assigning meaning to the illness, managing the condition, role reorganization, and normalization. Nursing interventions should consider the type of adaptation, the family, and its specific situation (Meleski, 2002).

Andrew's story illustrates some of the client and family needs that must be addressed. Andrew's growth, development, and social needs are addressed by his mother, her extended family, his nurses, and his therapists. As he grows older, his changing needs must be considered by individualizing the services he obtains and by treating him as normally as possible. His mother must learn about the changes he will undergo and how to interface effectively with institutions such as hospitals, clinics, and schools. To achieve this, she needs various supportive services. She also needs to have her own needs met so that she can more effectively deal with Andrew's chronic condition. Andrew's restructured family, without his father, has successfully incorporated him into a coherent unit and has not allowed his illness to be a major obstacle.

Helping Families Learn to Cope

Part of the maturation of individual family caregivers and caregiving systems involves the development of realistic expectations of the individual member's abilities and limitations, as well as an understanding of the anticipated trajectory of dependent care that lies ahead. To provide adequate care for a dependent relative and at the same time secure their own well-being, family caregivers need support, aid, and understanding from their families and friends and from the health-care system. To get that support, it is crucial that family caregivers learn to recognize when they need help, what kind of help to ask for, how to ask for the help they need, and whom to ask (Mittelman, 2003). Individual family caregivers and their caregiving systems may need assistance in learning how to cope with the positive and negative feelings and the emotional and social impacts of caregiving. Health-care professionals need to promote family caregivers' well-being, which is a complex, multidimensional concept that includes personal meanings (George & Gwyther, 1986). In doing so, caregivers may need assistance in acquiring the information, support, and services to meet those needs (Elliott & Shewshuk, 2003; Piercy & Chapman, 2001).

Family caregivers need formal providers who have time and the training necessary to help them learn effective interventions. Because nurses with clinical training also understand behavioral and counseling techniques, they are often considered the most appropriate member of the team to work with family caregivers and to oversee educational programs. Stress-Point Intervention by Nurses (SPIN) (Kauffmann & Harrison, 1998) has proved useful in assisting families whose children have a chronic condition and are repeatedly hospitalized. A nurse helps the family develop a unique set of coping strategies, based on the family's own concerns and resources and the nurse's expertise. The nurse helps the family explore issues together. This helps the family identify critical stress points and to design a customized family intervention. A central strategy that nurses use in the SPIN process is to express realistic confidence in the family's ability to cope (Kauffmann & Harrison, 1998). While SPIN was developed for families with children who have chronic conditions, the SPIN process could be adapted for families of adult members with chronic illness.

In general, programs that build family caregiver confidence and skill and a feeling of support are more effective than those that simply impart knowledge (Piercy & Chapman, 2001). Problem-solving interventions that target the specific concerns of family caregivers are especially effective and can reduce caregiver depression and distress (Elliott & Shewshuk, 2003). Kaye and colleagues (2003) found that an early intervention screening for family caregivers of older relatives resulted in caregivers accessing sources of community support before a crisis and impending burnout. In all cases, intervention programs must be developmentally appropriate and tailored to be culturally relevant and learner specific.

The types of intervention programs available range from individual or group caregiver counseling in the presence of a professional facilitator to self-paced, self-help computerized programs that can be completed in relative isolation from others. Software packages that provide caregivers with information and advice on promotion of personal psychological health, relaxation, and other coping strategies plus a caregiver self-assessment tool on coping with the caregiver role have proved useful to caregivers (Chambers & Connor, 2002). Caregivers report that the use of such software provides reassurance and emotional support and enables them to assess and enhance their own coping skills.

The time constraints of most contemporary family caregivers are now being addressed by such strategies as telephone conferencing, Internet chat rooms, and e-mail. Link$_2$Care and Caring~Web are examples of successful, innovative Internet-based programs that combine high technology with traditional service to increase caregiver well-being and coping skills (Pierce et al., 2004; Kelly, 2003–2004; Steiner & Pierce, 2002). Caregivers using both of these sites found features of updated news and research, information articles and fact sheets, online discussion groups, and ask an expert to be of value.

The Veteran's Administration (VA) is using home-telehealth technologies to link caregivers and veterans with chronic conditions to primary care providers at the VA (Lutz, Chumbler, Lyles, Hoffman, & Kobb, 2008; Lutz, Chumbler, & Roland, 2007). It is no longer the case that an intervention program is only effective with direct face-to-face contact. The key is to make the interventions relevant, multicomponent, tailored to caregivers' needs, and accessible when the caregiver needs it (Chambers & Connor, 2002; Elliott & Shewchuk, 2003; Gitlin et al., 2003; Mittelman, 2003). Many of the caregiving Internet site resources presented at the end of the chapter contain support interventions specific to caregivers.

Caregivers also need the opportunity for activities other than providing care to avoid a sense of entrapment and feelings of loss of self and burnout. Attention to self-help activities sustains one's sense of well-being and revitalizes energy that can later be used in providing care to the client, but many caregivers feel guilty about activities that focus on themselves (Medalie, 1994).

Spirituality and Caregiving

Spiritual beliefs and faith-based behaviors play multiple roles in caregivers' lives. Spirituality involves not only connectedness with a sacred other, but also with other people, perspectives, and sources of value and meaning beyond oneself (Faver, 2004). Such connectedness can produce happiness and energy to sustain a caregiver's ability to care for a chronically ill family member (Faver; Haley & Harrigan, 2004). Whether caregivers hold religious beliefs or not, they express needs for love, meaning, purpose, and, sometimes, transcendence in their lives (Murray et al., 2004). Caregivers draw strength from maintaining relationships with their families and value opportunities to give and receive love, to feel connected to their social world, and to feel useful (Murray et al., 2004).

Religious beliefs and formal religious practices are essential aspects of caregiving. Heavy reliance on prayer to cope with adversity is reported by many caregivers (Paun, 2004; Stuckey, 2001). African American women caregivers describe their prayer as an ongoing dialogue that keeps them connected with their God rather than as a formal religious ritual (Paun, 2004). Religiosity is also demonstrated by the belief that God has a plan; belief in a loving God; hope in an afterlife; and a sense of the evidence of God all around (Stuckey, 2004). Reading the Bible and other religious materials and listening to music are also aspects of formal religion used by caregivers (Theis, Biordi, Coeling, Nalepka, & Miller, 2003). Churches provide an important source of encouragement and social support for caregivers (Faver, 2004; Murray et al., 2004; Theis et al., 2003). A strong connection with a caring community is what caregivers value in their church relationships. Caregivers find that the consistent presence of fellow parishioners is a powerful sustaining force (Faver, 2004). Efforts to maintain chronically ill spouses' engagement in religious practices, such as church attendance, are important for caregivers. When church attendance is no longer possible, caregivers substitute televised or videotaped services and arrange for other formal religious practices like communion to be given at their home (Paun, 2004).

A spiritual or religious perspective seems to benefit caregivers in several ways. Caregivers report that attending religious services regularly is what keeps them going. Second to church attendance is prayer (Paun, 2004). Feelings of being supported and comforted by religious faith are associated with positive emotional experiences while caring for persons with Alzheimer's disease (Paun, 2004). A sense of sacred companionship

with God or a sacred other acts as a sustaining force for many caregivers (Faver, 2004). Thus, a spiritual approach to caregiving may help caregivers cope with stressful situations and benefit those for whom they care. Strong faith-based beliefs, such as moral living and being of service to others, can motivate persons to become caregivers as well as to continue caregiving (Stuckey, 2001).

Although caregivers report the importance of spirituality and religion in their lives, they are often reluctant to initiate raising such issues with healthcare professionals. Murray and colleagues (2004) found that caregivers (as well as the care recipients) did not broach the subject of spiritual care need because they perceived the healthcare professionals to be busy and/or did not see spiritual care as part of health-care professionals' role. Caregivers even actively tried to disguise their spiritual distress. Nurses need to be alert to caregivers' need for spiritual care and to create conditions where caregivers feel comfortable in discussing their spiritual needs. Giving caregivers this opportunity validates their concerns and needs and helps them feel connected and cared for. Spiritual support professionals, such as ministers and rabbis, should be included as an integral part of any interdisciplinary or transdisciplinary team.

Churches and Communities in Care Solutions

In addition to government-sponsored programs to help caregivers, churches have a potentially important role to play in caregivers' lives. Though little research has been conducted on the role of churches in eldercare, Stuckey (2001) found that churches supported caregivers by encouraging continued church participation whenever possible and by taking services to care recipient and caregiver when needed.

An example of a church collaboration is the Interfaith CarePartners (www.interfaithcarepartners.org) "Creating Caring Communities." An innovative aspect of this program is the Care

Team model of caregiving that was implemented nearly 25 years ago to provide in-home support to individuals with chronic health conditions and to offer respite support to their caregivers. Volunteers are recruited from Jewish and Christian congregations, and are trained to provide companionship, meal preparation, transportation, light household chores, shopping assistance, spiritual, emotional, and physical support, and personal care to adults and children with debilitating illnesses and disabilities. A Second Family Care Team serves chronically ill and frail adults. As the title suggests, the vision of this Care Team is to be a "second family" for frail adults and their caregivers. As well as providing types of support and assistance for the chronically ill adult, the team provides caregivers with encouragement, hope, respite, emotional support, and physical assistance. Collaboration efforts like Interfaith CarePartners are generally perceived as very helpful resources for caregivers. This care venture has consisted of over 9400 Care Team members who have donated 1.3 million hours of service since 1985.

Communities also have a role in providing assistance to those in need of care. An excellent example of a community partnership to accomplish this goal is the Gatekeeper Model developed in Spokane, Washington (Substance Abuse & Mental Health Administration, 2004). Employees of community businesses and corporations who work with the public are trained to identify and refer community-dwelling older adults who may be in need of aid. On referral by these gatekeepers, home-based assessments are conducted by interdisciplinary teams provided by the local mental health services, with referrals made for additional services as needed.

Another community example that benefits older adults and caregivers is the interfaith volunteer program organized by Faith in Action (www.fiavolunteers.org), which administers 1000 community programs across the United States. The program, funded by the Robert Wood Johnson Foundation and directed by Wake Forest University, aims to connect volunteers with older and disabled people who need help and to provide a source of respite for caregivers.

Programs, Services, and Resources for Family Caregivers

A Google Internet search was performed using the key words "family caregiving" and 169,000 matches were found. The sites included information and referral links, products and services, educational sites, and online caregiver support groups. Clearly, there is no shortage of programs, services, and resources for family caregivers. The problem is in finding affordable programs that are accessible and convenient for hassled family caregivers. In addition, a search for agencies and organizations to assist family caregivers resulted in 185,000 matches and that for books for caregivers and professionals in 158,000 matches. An easy-to-use comprehensive list of agencies and organizations with resources for family caregivers plus a list of books for caregivers and professionals can also be found in the Winter 2003–2004 volume of *Family Caregiving* (Kelly, 2003–2004).

Utilization of community services by family caregivers provides a range of benefits for caregivers. Unfortunately, barriers to the services continue to exist. Benefits reported by caregivers include renewal, sense of community, and knowledge and belief that their family member also benefited from the service. Barriers include care recipient resistance, reluctance of the caregiver, hassles for the caregiver, concerns about quality, and concerns about finances (Winslow, 2003). Nurses and other healthcare professionals involved in community services need to work to decrease or eliminate the barriers faced by family caregivers.

Respite Programs and Services

Respite is temporary relief from caregiving responsibilities that provides intervals of rest and relief for the caregiver. Family members may provide respite for the primary caregiver by taking over some tasks; for example, daughters may assist their caregiving mothers by shopping, cleaning, and so forth. There are also formal sources of respite, such as adult day care, in-home companions, and special weekend respite programs.

It is important for caregivers to recognize the warning signs that indicate that their coping skills are overwhelmed and they are in need of outside help. For many caregivers, the hardest step is acknowledging that help is needed; the next most difficult step is extending the effort to seek this help. Caregivers often feel guilty about seeking respite and delay using formal respite services until they are exhausted and debilitated. Ambivalence on the part of caregivers to make use of respite services is illustrated by a study of family caregivers' experiences with in-hospital respite care for family members with dementia (Gilmour, 2002). Caregivers' feelings varied from acceptance to qualified acceptance to marked ambivalence. Caregivers were torn between the need to have a break and the worry over the impact of the in-hospital respite care on their family member. Nurses have the interpersonal skills to help decrease tensions and anxieties that caregivers have over respite care. Caregivers need to see respite services as a reasonable and appropriate action, not as a sign of personal failure, if they plan to continue caregiving without being overwhelmed by the physical and social demands.

When caregiving becomes too physically demanding or emotionally draining, short-term institutional placement of the client may be a care alternative. Planned short-term hospital admission provides in-facility professional care with relief for the caregiver. These programs can prevent the threshold of family tolerance being exceeded. To enhance family caregivers' comfort with this type of respite, nurses need to put themselves in a secondary and supporting care provider role and acknowledge the family caregiver as the authority on the care required by their family member (Gilmour, 2002). Family members are more fully able to relinquish care when they are confident that their relative is receiving care comparable to what is provided at home and that the relative is not negatively affected by the hospital stay (Gilmour, 2002).

Both Medicare and many long-term care insurance policies provide a short-term nursing home placement for a dependent family member. Longer or more frequent temporary stays are also possible, if the family is able to pay the expenses out of pocket.

Adult Day Services

Adult day services (formerly known as adult day care) are congregate programs that provide opportunities for impaired adults to socialize and participate in organized activities, and for their families to receive respite time. Use of adult day care results in decreased caregiver worry and stress and improved psychological well-being (Ritchie, 2003). Caregivers appreciate the client socializing and improved health as well as the respite for themselves (Warren, Kerr, Smith, Godkin, & Schalm, 2003).

Great variation exists in the type and amount of services that these centers provide. In general, the centers are broadly classified as health or social models of care. Social models emphasize socialization and cognitive stimulation. Health models of care are often supported by a state's Medicaid program and include health-care monitoring in the day program. In general, the major difference between the two types of programs is the presence or absence of a registered nurse on site in a center commonly called adult day health care. Some day health programs with advanced rehabilitation or restorative programs are certified by Medicare as day treatment hospitals and include rehabilitation specialists on staff.

Work by Campbell and Travis (1999) highlights the interesting ways in which family caregivers integrate formal programs and services into their informal caregiving routines. In their study of spousal caregivers, these researchers concluded that weekends were a time when other caregivers were not at work and were more readily available to help. Thus, better support to the primary caregiver appeared to have contributed to low interest in paying for additional adult day services during the weekend.

Social day programs have a variety of funding options, but most reimbursement sources are limited to low-income families or those with long-term care insurance (DHHS Administration on Aging, n.d.b). Day health programs are primarily Medicaid programs or those skilled rehabilitation programs that are Medicare reimbursed. The out-of-pocket cost of day care to the family caregivers varies widely, depending on the region of the country and the type of program offered. In an analysis of cost implications of adult day services for persons with dementia, Gaugler (2003) found that the daily costs to reduce caregivers' role overload and depression decreased with adult day utilization over 1 year. Apparently, the adult day programs are most cost-effective for caregivers who use them consistently and for longer periods of time.

Home Care Programs

Home care has expanded in recent years as a result of earlier hospital discharge and the increase in technically more complex therapies. The home represents a different context for provision of care than the medical office or community clinic. Toth-Cohen and colleagues (2001) discuss four key factors that must be considered when providing care within the home setting: understand the personal meaning of the home for the family; view the caregiver as a "lay practitioner"; identify the caregiver's beliefs and values; and recognize the potential impact of the interventions on caregiver well-being.

Multiple benefits as well as challenges for the caregiver and the health-care professional are present in home care (Toth-Cohen et al., 2001). Benefits for the caregiver include (1) saving of time

and mental and physical energy; (2) remaining in control and guiding interaction with the provider; (3) being more comfortable and at ease in own surroundings; (4) practicing newly learned skills in the context in which they will be used.

Benefits for the health-care professional include (1) gaining an in-depth understanding of the client, the caregiver, and the home context; (2) designing interventions tailored to specific home situations; (3) identifying safety issues that caregivers may be unaware of, (4) observing performance in the context in which it occurs. Challenges and potential solutions are presented in Table 9-1. Nurses can work more effectively with families in their homes by being aware of the benefits, challenges, and possible solutions to those challenges. The nurse's ability to meet whatever challenges are encountered will influence a caregiver's response to interventions and recommendations.

Some home care programs provide respite services for families. Services can include homemaking, monitoring of both client and caregiver health status, and performing various skills, such as taking vital signs or changing catheters. Unfortunately, reimbursement for these programs is increasingly limited to those families with the greatest financial need. Paying out of pocket can be very expensive over the long term.

Psychotherapeutic Approaches

Individual, couple, group, or family counseling may be needed to help families respond to the demands of caregiving. Individual counseling is directed toward enhancing the caregiver's capacity to deal with the day-to-day rigors of caregiving. As described by Montcalm (1995), counseling for couples can be complex because of the multiple issues involved, such as dependency, grief over the losses in the relationship, and fear. When peer interaction and feedback seem appropriate, group therapy can be effective in steering a family caregiver toward more positive resolutions of internal conflict over the caregiving role.

TABLE 9-1

Summary of Challenges and Recommendations for Providing Services in the Home

Challenge	*Recommendations*
Building rapport	Identify caregiver's goals for intervention
	Use and respect caregiver's language
	Validate caregiver's existing strategies
	Involve and collaborate with family members and other supportive persons
Incorporating needs of both caregiver and person with dementia into interventions	Use holistic approach that addresses needs of both caregiver and person with dementia
	Involve person with dementia in meaningful activities
	Consider effects of education and home modification on both caregiver and person with dementia
Obtaining assessment data	Actively involve care receiver in intervention, when feasible
	Ask permission of care receiver to discuss ways of helping caregiver
	Schedule telephone contacts to discuss sensitive issues.
	Obtain assessment data when person with dementia is not present
Ensuring optimal fit between intervention and family	Reflect on possible differences between self and caregiver
	Review caregiver's management practices step by step
	Refocus on the caregiver's needs and priorities
	Discuss and try out possible strategies
Matching the intervention to caregiver expertise and knowledge of dementia	Recognize that caregiver may need more time to accept family member's condition and use provider's strategies
	Ensure that recommendations fit the caregiver's perspective and priorities
	Address quality-of-life issues in master caregivers
	Obtain information on specific strategies from master caregivers that may be helpful for other caregivers
	Follow up on how recommended strategies are working; if necessary, modify strategies
	Reinforce value of strategies
	Photograph physical adaptations or develop pre–post photos to reinforce positive changes
Working within the family system of roles	Role play using simple language and validation of care receiver's feelings
	Recognize roles of multiple caregivers and reflect on how they fit into the caregiving and relationships situation
	Facilitate communication and collaborative problem solving between caregivers
Helping caregivers access and use resources	Be aware of existing resources available to caregiver
	Educate caregiver about appropriate resources
	Help caregiver identify tasks that others could perform
	Role play with caregiver ways of asking for help

Source: Toth-Cohen, S., Gitlin, L.N., Corcoran, M.A., Eckhardt, S., Johns, P., & Lipsitt, R. (2001). Providing services to family caregivers at home: Challenges and recommendations for health and human service professions. *Alzheimer's Care Quarterly, 2*(1), 23–32. Reprinted with permission of Lippincott Williams & Wilkins.

Family treatment often includes a strategy called the "family meeting," at a time when all affected family members meet face to face. A family-based therapy, found effective for caregivers of family members with dementia, is the Structural Ecosystems Therapy (SET) (Mitrani & Czaja, 2000). The aim of SET is to address the entire family's needs within a "cojoint context" (p. 201). SET views the behavior of family members as interdependent and repetitive. Sometimes the repetitive patterns are maladaptive and cause symptoms such as caregiver stress. Other interaction patterns are adaptive and relieve caregiver burden. SET focuses on improving the caregiver's interactions within her whole social ecosystem, that is, family, community, health-care providers, and so on, thus increasing the extent to which the caregiver's emotional, social, and instrumental needs are met. SET is particularly appropriate for minority families because it acknowledges the importance of culture as a contextual variable that can have a marked influence on family interaction (Mitrani & Czaja, 2000).

Support Groups

Also called self-help groups, these forums focus on specific client populations and related caregivers' needs. Self-help groups for caregivers have been established in many communities throughout the United States. Some are self-directed or run by volunteers; others are led by health-care professionals who act as group facilitators. These groups provide information, emotional support, advocacy, or a combination of these services. They address such areas as skills in the care and maintenance of the disabled person and managing problems in the family; information regarding the aging process; emotional needs for recognition and support from caring people; and concrete service needs for referral and information regarding resources. Telephone support networks and Internet chat rooms are simply contemporary versions of the traditional face-to-face support group.

The Need for Culturally Sensitive Interventions

During the past century, the United States and Canada experienced massive waves of immigration, as well as a growing population of native-born minorities. Given the diversity of racial, ethnic, and religious groups in North America, there is a need for helping health-care professionals learn more about the many cultural groups with which they work so that they can provide interventions that are sensitive to the client's culture. To that end, there has been a rapid rise of multicultural consciousness in the United States. However, cultural awareness among healthcare professionals continues to be inadequate to serve those of other cultures.

Awareness that the definition of family differs from one cultural group to another is important. For example, the dominant Caucasian definition focuses on the intact nuclear family. However, African-Americans focus on a wider network of kin and community, and often include nonbiological family members in their family networks. The Chinese culture includes all of a person's ancestors and descendants in the definition of family and the needs of the family are valued more highly than the needs of the individual. However, these values may be changing because of globalization and the influence of Western values (Lee, 2007). Who the client considers to be family and who is providing care will influence who should be included in interventions.

Cultural groups vary greatly in how they respond to problems and their attitudes toward seeking help. For example, Hispanic families typically want to keep problems confidential and view caregiving as a responsibility of the female family members (Evans, Coon, & Crogan 2007; Rittman, Kuzmeskus, & Flum, 1998). To assist an Hispanic family, a helping professional will have to work on *personalismo*, knowing the older adult and her caregiver as total persons, before focusing on personal matters; *dignidad*, developing a working relationship that reflects dignity and self-worth;

TABLE 9-2

Examples of Systematic Reviews of Research on Caregiving Interventions

Authors (date)	Focus of Review and Number of Studies Rreviewed	Findings	Recommendations
Forster, Smith, Young, Knapp, House, & Wright (2001)	Effectiveness of information provision for patients with stroke and their CGs (N = 9 studies)	Providing information combined with educational sessions improves health of patients and CGs Variable quality of evidence Effectiveness of providing information alone is not demonstrated	Appropriate teaching strategies should focus on the needs identified by patients and CGs Limited evidence, more research needed
Lee & Cameron (2004)	Effectiveness of respite care for persons with dementia and their CGs (N = 3 RCTs)	No demonstrated evidence of the benefits of respite care Lack of high-quality evidence	Insufficient evidence to make a recommendation Limited evidence, more research needed
Selwood, Johnston, Katona, Lyketosos, & Livingston (2007)	Effectiveness of psychological interventions for family CGs of persons with dementia (N = 62 RCTs)	Individual behavioral management therapy with 6 or more sessions is effective in improving CG depression Group behavioral management therapy is not as effective Individual or group therapy focusing on coping strategies is also effective Education on dementia and supportive therapy are not effective	Individual behavioral management and individual and group coping strategy therapy improves CG mental health Educational sessions should be individualized to each CG More research is needed
Thompson, Spilsbury, Hall, Birks, Barnes, & Adamson (2007)	Effectiveness of technology-, individual-, and group-based information and support interventions for CGs of persons with dementia (N = 44 RCTs)	Group-based interventions improve depression in CGs No demonstrated effectiveness of any other type of intervention Clinical significance is uncertain Poor quality evidence	Insufficient evidence to make a recommendation Limited evidence, more research needed Specifically, more systematic reviews of qualitative findings are needed

CG, caregiver; RCT, randomized controlled trial.
Note: See individual citations for more details.

respeto, respect between the helping professional and Hispanic elder; and *confianza*, trust between the two parties (Evans, Coon, & Crogan, 2007; Gallagher-Thompson, Solano, Coon, & Arean, 2003).

Ethnic differences exist in attitudes toward caregiving and caregiving responsibilities. For example, Cuban Americans often have a hierarchical relational orientation and adhere to traditional family roles. Because of this, female caregivers may have difficulty in adopting the leadership role of caregiving (Mitrani & Czaja, 2000). Other cultural characteristics of Cubans are collectivism, giving precedence to the needs of the family over the individual, and the high degree of emotional and psychological closeness or enmeshment between caregiver and the care recipient. Enmeshment, observed more frequently in Cuban families than in Caucasian American families, can produce a lack of objectivity and an unwillingness to delegate care tasks, making it difficult for the caregiver to be an effective care manager (Mitrani & Czaja, 2000). To work effectively with families from varied ethnic and cultural heritages, the nurse must tailor family interventions to be culturally congruent.

Providing assistance to family caregivers of minority elders for any number of issues is most effective when the members of the targeted minority group are represented in the provider or intervention group. For this reason, neighborhood-centered services, in which minority caregivers can interact with bilingual professionals, tend to be highly effective. These programs are well suited to respecting the values and customs of families in need of help and to offering culturally relevant solutions to the caregivers (Spector, 2000).

Evidence-Based Practice

Evidence-based practice is based on the demonstrated effectiveness of interventions tested in multiple clinical trials. Systematic reviews of the research are considered to be the highest level of evidence. As described in the previous paragraphs,

there are numerous studies testing various interventions to help improve the health and well-being of caregivers. However, there are only a few systematic reviews of the literature that focus on these widely varying interventions. Furthermore, the reviews available cite the lack of high-quality evidence and poor consistency in the clinical trials testing these interventions (Forster et al. 2001; Lee & Cameron, 2004). Therefore, it is imperative that more intervention research is conducted with a focus on replicating previous clinical trials. Researchers also suggest the inclusion of qualitative findings in the systematic reviews to better determine the specific effects of the interventions from the perspectives of caregivers (Thompson et al. 2007). Table 9-2 includes examples of systematic reviews of the literature on caregiver interventions.

OUTCOMES

Care Recipient, Caregiver, and Caregiving System Outcomes

Providing care to another person has both positive and negative outcomes for the primary caregiver and the caregiver system. Because caregiving is a very personal journey, it is almost impossible to predict how each caregiver or care recipient will respond to the demands of dependency and caregiving support. Therefore, all of the interventions provided by an interdisciplinary or transdisciplinary team are ultimately directed toward supporting family caregivers when the situation is going well, and to helping caregivers correct practices that will lead to potentially negative outcomes.

Much of the caregiving literature reflects a focus on the negative aspects of caregiving. Less available are the positive aspects of the caregiver role. The literature continues to need studies that identify the potential benefits of caregiving (Hudson, 2004), for the purpose of increasing our understanding of the caregiving experience (Tarlow et al., 2004) as well as preventing the likelihood of viewing caregiving only from a pathologic perspective and thus socializing caregivers to expect burden (Gaugler, Kane, & Langlois, 2000). The study of caregiver benefits can also provide data for the development of evidence-based supportive care strategies for families and family caregivers (Harding & Higginson, 2003).

Despite the paucity of information regarding the benefits derived from the caregiver role, studies available indicate that most caregivers find some element of satisfaction in the caregiving experience (Nolan, 2001; Scott, 2001). Hudson (2004) reported that 60% of caregivers readily identified positive aspects of the caregiver role. Given what is known about long-term family caregiving, there are three outcomes that are commonly monitored. Together, these outcomes form a gold standard by which caregiving experiences can be measured. Outcomes for both the family caregivers and their care recipients include improved quality of life and meaning in life, enhanced autonomy and control, and reduced family stress and enhanced coping ability.

Quality of Life and Meaning in Life

It has been written that human beings "can be at their best when they are behaving with altruism and commitment to a person they love" (Lattanzi-Licht, Mahoney, & Miller, 1998, p. 31). Finding enhanced quality of life and meaning in life associated with the caregiving experience is one of the most positive outcomes of caregiving for the care recipient and the caregiver (Sheehan & Donorfio, 1999). Evidence of enhanced meaning of life can be seen in caregivers' comments about positive aspects of caregiving: "Love doing it—we've been given an opportunity we'd never thought we'd have" (Hudson, 2004, p. 62).

Until recently, systematic assessments of these positive outcomes of caregiving have been limited because of the difficulty clinicians have encountered in finding and accessing psychometrically sound measures of these abstract constructs (Farran, Miller, & Kaufman, 1999). The new generation of measurement tools allows interdisciplinary (or transdisciplinary) teams to tap into the day-to-day meaning and ultimate meaning of caregiving relationships so that these aspects of caregiving become a visible outcome of the experiences (Farran et al.). One such measurement tool is the Positive Aspects of Caregiving (Tarlow et al., 2004).

Perceived Autonomy and Control

Autonomy, as an outcome of family caregiving, means that the choices of long-term caregivers and their care recipients are self-determined. Consistent with the principles of self-determination is the need to have some control over events and decisions. In chronic care situations, autonomy and control are interrelated and both are affected by the ability of professional providers to support family caregivers in the choices they make and the care that they give. It follows that autonomy and control may need to be renegotiated with the formal network and within the informal caregiving system as the caregiving situation changes.

Those caregivers who are able to feel most relaxed and confident in managing their caregiving situations have reported that being successful does not mean being in total control (Karp & Tanarugsachock, 2000). Learning to "go with the flow" is how caregivers frequently describe their approach to control issues (Travis et al., 2000). If interdisciplinary teams respect the values and goals of the caregivers and their care recipients and help to translate these into real world plans of care, then perceived autonomy and control for both caregivers and care recipients are enhanced. Evidence of an enhanced sense of autonomy and control can be seen in caregivers' comments about positive aspects of caregiving: "Taking responsibility for things I had not previously been responsible for;" "I feel like I'm a stronger person now;" and "I've been able to undertake much more than I thought I could" (Hudson, 2004, p. 62).

Reduced Family Stress and Coping

As previously discussed, the many adverse effects of caregiving include an array of affective responses by caregivers to the demands of long-term caregiving. The goal of most care teams is to reduce this distress to a level that is perceived to be manageable for the caregivers. Caregivers are able to voice positive aspects in the role despite the negative aspects, such as stress and burden (Hudson 2004; Roff et al., 2004). Perhaps caregivers use positive emotions to augment and maintain their coping strategies when faced with an ongoing stressor like caregiving (Folkman, 1997). Because family stress and coping are global, multidimensional, and multifaceted, interventions are often designed to address a specific aspect of stress and coping, such as perceived burden, depression, or fatigue (Buckwalter et al., 1999).

Societal Outcomes

A number of studies have examined the cost-effectiveness of community-based home services to groups of individuals at risk for nursing home use. Even though the most consistent justification for delivering long-term care services in home- and community-based environments is cost containment, such claims have not been supported in the research (Weissert & Hedrick, 1999). Part of the problem is the way that costs of care are compared across settings. For example, while nursing home care appears to be more costly than community-based care, the calculations do not take into consideration the out-of-pocket expenses and subsidized programs and services that family caregivers must use to make community-based care a viable long-term care option for them and their dependent family members.

Delayed or Diverted Episodes of Institutional Care

Despite the fact that home- and community-based care may not be cost-effective, providing such care remains a goal for many families and a priority of policy makers. This is because institutional care is perceived as more expensive by most policy makers, and is less desirable than home care by older adults and policy makers alike, who clearly prefer noninstitutional solutions to long-term care.

In their study of the influence of service use on consequences for caregivers, Bass, Noelker, and Rechlin (1996) conceptualized services as a type of social support. They found that certain services, such as health care, personal care, and homemaker services, reduced the adverse effects of heavy or burdensome care on the family caregivers. These types of programs serve a clientele that may not be at imminent risk of nursing home placement, but their needs for assistance in the home or community are real (Weissert & Hedrick, 1994).

Instead of looking to home and community-based services as a cost-effective alternative to nursing home placement, a better outcome of success may be measures of diverted hospital stays (Weissert & Hedrick, 1994). Advanced death planning and decisions about when to institutionalize, as well as working with clinicians and families as dependent persons transition from active treatment to palliation, can reduce inappropriate and expensive care (Weissert & Hedrick, 1994). This outcome requires more discussions and decision making among care recipients and their family members regarding care decisions and increased communication with their physicians to ensure that the decisions are respected and carried out. Nurses can foster this decision making by encouraging families to talk openly with one another about care and by assisting families to put the plans into place in advance of the need to make decisions about hospitalizations or other unwanted aggressive measures.

ACKNOWLEDGMENT

The authors of the previous edition of the chapter, Tama L. Morris and Lienne D. Edwards, are recognized for their work.

STUDY QUESTIONS

1. Who are the primary providers of home care? What are some of the providers' competing demands?

2. What are the advantages and disadvantages of the person with chronic illness or disease being cared for at home? For the family? For the caregiver?

3. Are there differences for caregivers in caring for children with disability versus caring for older adults? Please be specific and discuss.

4. How does ethnicity influence family caregiving?

5. In what way(s) does culture affect family caregiving?

6. What factors influence the cost effectiveness of home care versus institutionalization?

7. What is the financial impact of caregiving on the caregiver?

8. How does public policy affect caregiving?

9. How can health professionals assist family caregivers?

10. As an advocate for family caregivers, what facts would you present to lawmakers related to supportive legislation?

11. What are some of the emotional responses to family caregiving? Discuss positive and negative consequences for family caregivers.

12. Choose a scenario that you are familiar with or use a case study from this chapter and apply the Family Empowerment Model.

13. How does spirituality or religious preference help family caregivers cope with their caring situation?

14. Where can family caregivers go for assistance and information?

15. What are some of the issues with implementing evidence-based practice when working with family caregivers? How can we address these issues?

16. What are some positive outcomes for family caregivers? What are some strategies that could be implemented to reinforce positive caregiving outcomes?

INTERNET RESOURCES

AssistGuide Information Services: www.agis.com/
CancerNet Support and Resources: www.cancer.gov/cancer_information/support/
Caregiver Resources. Because We Care: http://www.aoa.gov//eldfam/For_Caregivers/For_Caretgivers.aspx
Caregiving: www.acponline.org/public/h_care/2-caregv.htm
CarePages for your Patients: www.carepages.com/home_page.jsp
Caring for Someone with Alzheimer's: http://nihseniorhealth.gov/alzheimerscare/toc.html
Caring from a Distance: www.cfad.org/
Faith in Action: www.fiavolunteers.org
Family Caregiving Alliance: www.caregiver.org/caregiver/jsp/home.jsp
Heart of Caregiving: www.americanheart.org/presenter.jhtml?identifier=3039829
Interfaith CarePartners: www.interfaithcarepartners.org
National Alliance for Caregiving: www.caregiving.org/
National Family Caregivers' Association: www.nfcacares.org/
National Family Caregivers Association and National Alliance for Caregiving: www.familycaregiving101.org/
National Organization for Empowering Caregivers: www.nofec.org and www.care-givers.com

REFERENCES

Agency for Healthcare Research and Quality. (2002). *Preventing disability in the elderly with chronic disease.* AHRQ Publication No. 02–0018. Rockville, MD: Agency for Healthcare Research and Quality. Retrieved November 29, 2007 from www.ahrq.gov/research/elderdis.htm

Albert, S.M., & Brody, E.M. (1996). When elder care is viewed as child care. *American Journal of Geriatric Psychiatry, 4,* 121–130.

Allen, S.M., Goldscheider, F., & Ciambrone, D. (1999). Gender roles, marital intimacy, and nomination of spouses as primary caregivers. *The Gerontologist, 39,* 150–158.

Badr, H., & Acitelli, L.K. (2005). Dyadic adjustment in chronic illness: Does relationship talk matter? *Journal of Family Psychiatry, 19*(2), 465–469.

Barrett, A.E., & Lynch, S.M. (1999). Caregiving networks of elderly persons: Variation by marital status. *The Gerontologist, 39,* 695–704.

Bass, D.M., Noelker, L.S., & Rechlin, L.R. (1996). The moderating influence of service use on negative caregiving consequences. *Journal of Gerontology, Social Sciences, 51B,* S121–S131.

Binstock, R.H. (1999). Public policies and minority elders. In M. L. Wykle & A. B. Ford (Eds.), *Serving minority elders in the 21st century,* (pp. 5–24). New York: Springer.

Blake, H., & Lincoln, N. (2000). Factors associated with strain in co-resident spouses of patients following stroke. *Clinical Rehabilitation, 14*(3), 307–14.

Boaz, R.F., Hu, J., & Ye, Y. (1999). The transfer of resources from middle-aged children to functionally limited elderly parents: Providing time, giving money, sharing space. *The Gerontologist, 39,* 648–657.

Bohse and Associates. (2001). *Facts on aging.* Retrieved January 18, 2008, from http://www.bohse.com/html/facts_on_aging.html

Bowdoin, C. (1994). Commentary on new diagnosis: Caregiver role strain. *AACN Nursing Scan in Critical Care, 4*(1), 23.

Brody, E.M. (1990). Role reversal: An inaccurate and destructive concept. *Journal of Gerontological Social Work, 15,* 15–22.

Brody, E.M., & Schoonover, C. B. (1986). Patterns of parent-care when adult daughters work and when they do not. *The Gerontologist, 26,* 372–381.

Buckwalter, K.C., Gerdner, L., Kohout, F., Hall, G. R., et al. (1999). A nursing intervention to decrease depression in family caregivers of persons with dementia. *Archives of Psychiatric Nursing, 13,* 80–88.

Burton, L.C., Newsom, J.T., Schulz, R., Hirsch, C.H., German, P.S. (1997). Preventative health behaviors among spousal caregivers. *Preventative Medicine, 26,* 162–169.

Campbell, D.D., & Travis, S.S. (1999). Spousal caregiving when the adult day services center is closed. *Journal of Psychosocial Nursing, 37,* 20–25.

Caron, C.D., & Bowers, B.J. (2003). Deciding whether to continue, share, or relinquish caregiving: Caregiver views. *Qualitative Health Research, 13*(9), 1252–1271.

Chambers, M., & Connor, S.L. (2002). User-friendly technology to help family carers cope. *Journal of Advanced Nursing, 40*(5), 568–577.

Chang, C., & White-Means, S. (1991). The men who care: An analysis of male primary caregivers who care for frail elderly at home. *Journal of Applied Gerontology, 10,* 343–358.

Chesla, C.A., & Rungreangkulkij, S. (2001). Nursing research on family processes in chronic illness in ethnically diverse families: A decade review. *Journal of Family Nursing, 7*(3), 230–243.

Chumbler, N.R., Rittman, M., Van Puymbroeck, M., Vogel, W.B., & Qin, H. (2004). The sense of coherence, burden, and depressive symptoms in informal caregivers during the first month after stroke. *International Journal of Geriatric Psychiatry, 19*(10), 944–953.

Chumbler, N.R., Rittman, M.R., & Wu, S.S. (2007). Associations of sense of coherence and depression in caregivers of stroke survivors across 2 years [Electronic Version]. *The Journal of Behavioral Health Services Research, 2007, Sept 17.*

Clyburn, L.D., Stones, M.J., Hadjistavropoulos, T., & Tuokko, H. (2000). Predicting caregiver burden and depression in Alzheimer's disease. *Journal of Gerontology, Social Sciences, 55B,* S2–S13.

Covinsky, K.E., Eng, C., Lui, L., Sands, L.P., et al. (2001). Reduced employment in caregivers of frail elders. *The Journals of Gerontology Series A: Biological Sciences and Medical Sciences, 56*, M707–M713.

Covinsky, K.E., Newcomer, R., Fox, P., Wood, J., et al. (2003). Patient and caregiver characteristics associated with depression in caregiving of patients with dementia. *Journal of General Internal Medicine, 18*(12), 1006–1014.

Cox, C. (1999). Race and caregiving: Patterns of service use by African American and white caregivers of persons with Alzheimer's disease. *Journal of Gerontological Social Work, 32*, 5–19.

Dautzenberg, M.G.H. (2000). The competing demands of paid work and parent care. *Research on Aging, 22*, 165–188.

DHHS Administration on Aging (n.d.a). *About NFCSP.* Retrieved September 21, 2004, from http://www.aoa.gov/prof/aoaprog/caregiver/caregiver.aspx

DHHS Administration on Aging (n.d.b). *Because we care.* Retrieved September 21, 2004, from http://www.aoa.gov/prof/aoaprog/caregiver/carefam/taking_care_of_others/we-care.pdf

DHHS Administration on Aging (n.d.c). *Common caregiving terms.* Retrieved September 21, 2004, from http://www.aoa.gov/prof/aoaprog/caregiver/careprof/progguidance/resources/caregiving_terms.aspx

DHHS Administration of Aging (2003a). *Family caregivers: Our heroes on frontlines of long-term care.* Retrieved September 20, 2004, from http:///www.aoa.gov/prof/aoaprog/caregiver/careprof/TownHall/townhall_12_16_03.aspx

DHHS Administration of Aging. (2003b). *National family caregiver support program townhall meetings.* Retrieved September 20, 2004, from http://www.aoa.gov/prof/aoaprog/caregiver/careprof/TownHall/townhall_12_16_03.aspx

DHHS Administration on Aging. (2007). *Statistics on the aging population.* Retrieved November 30, 2007, from http://www.aoa.dhhs.gov/index.asp

Deimling, G., & Bass, D. (1986). Symptoms of mental impairment among elderly adults and their effects on family caregivers. *Journal of Gerontology, 41*(6), 778–84.

Draper, B., Poulos, C., Cole, A., Poulos, R., & Ehrlich, F. (1992). A comparison of caregivers for elderly stroke and dementia victims. *Journal of the American Geriatic Society, 40*(9), 896–901.

DuPont, P. (1999). *The short term problem facing long-term care. National Center for Policy Analysis.* Retrieved August 30, 2004, from http://www.ncpa.org/oped/dupont/dup010699.html.

Edmonds, M.M. (1999). Serving minority elders: Preventing chronic illness and disability in the African American elderly. In M.L. Wykle & A.B. Ford (Eds.), *Serving minority elders in the 21st century* (pp. 25–36). New York: Springer.

Elliot, T.R., & Shewchuk, R.M. (2003). Social problem-solving and distress among family members assuming a caregiving role. *British Journal of Health Psychology, 8*, 149–163.

Evans, B.C., Coon, D.W., & Crogan, N.L. (2007). Personalismo and breaking barriers: Accessing Hispanic populations for clinical services and research. *Geriatric Nursing 28*(5), 289–296.

Evercare° & National Alliance for Caregiving. (2007). *Evercare° study of family caregivers – What they spend, what they sacrifice.* Minnetonka, MN: Author. Retrieved January 3, 2008 from http://www.caregiving.org/data/Evercare_NAC_CaregiverCostStudyFINAL20111907.pdf

Family Caregiver Alliance. (2006). *Fact sheet: Caregiver health.* San Francisco, CA: Author. Retrieved November 30, 2007, from http://caregiver.org/caregiver/jsp/content_node.jsp?nodeid=1822

Farran, C.J., Miller, B.H., & Kaufman, J.E. (1999). Finding meaning through caregiving: Development of an instrument for family caregivers of persons with Alzheimer's disease. *Journal of Clinical Psychology, 55*(9), 1107–1125.

Fast, J.E., Williamson, D.L., & Keating, N.C. (1999). The hidden costs of informal elder care. *Journal of Family and Economic Issues, 20*, 301–326.

Faver, C.A. (2004). Relational spirituality and social caregiving. *Social Work, 49*(2), 241–249.

Figley, C.R. (1998). Burnout as systemic traumatic stress: A model for helping traumatized family members. In C. R. Figley (Ed.), *Burnout in families: The systemic costs of caring* (pp. 15–28). Boca Raton, FL: CRC Press.

Folkman, S. (1997). Positive psychological states and coping with severe stress. *Social Science & Medicine, 45*(8), 1207–1221.

Forster, A., Smith, J., Young, J., Knappp, P., House, A., & Wright J. (2001). Information provision for stroke patients and their caregivers. *The Cochrane Database Systematic Review, 2001*(3), Article CD001919.

Retrieved January 15, 2007, from The Cochrane Library Database.

Gallagher-Thompson, D., Solano, N., Coon, P., & Areán, P. (2003). Recruitment and retention of Latino dementia family caregivers in intervention research: Issues to face, lessons to learn. *The Gerontologist, 43*, 45–51.

Gaugler, J.E. (2003). Evaluating community-based programs for dementia caregivers: The cost implication of adult day services. *Journal of Applied Gerontology, 22*(1), 118–133.

Gaugler, J., Kane, R., & Langlois, J. (2000). Assessment of family caregivers of older adults. In R. Kane & R. Kane (Eds.), *Assessing older persons: Measures, meaning and practical applications* (pp. 321–359), New York: Oxford University Press.

Geister, C. (2005). The feeling of responsibility as core motivation for care giving – why daughters care for their mothers. *Pflege, 18*(1), 5–14.

George, L.K., & Gwyther, L.P. (1986). Caregiver well-being: A multidimensional examination of family caregivers of demented adults. *The Gerontologist, 26*(3), 253–259.

Gilliss, C.L. (2002).There is science, and there is life. *Families, Systems & Health, 20*(1), 49.

Gilmour, J.A. (2002). Disintegrated care: Family caregivers and in-hospital care. *Journal of Advanced Nursing, 39*(6), 546–553.

Gitlin, L., Burgio, L., Mahoney, D., Burns, R., et al. (2003). Effect of multicomponent interventions on caregiver burden and depression: The REACH Multisite Initiative at 6-month follow-up. *Psychology and Aging, 18*(3), 361–374.

Given, B., Strommel, M., Collins, C., King, S., et al. (1990). Responses of elderly spouse caregivers. *Research in Nursing and Health, 13*, 77–85.

Gordon, P.A., & Perrone, K.M. (2004). When spouses become caregivers: Counseling implications for younger couples. *Journal of Rehabilitation, 70*(2), 27–32.

Haigler, D.H., Bauer, L.J., & Travis, S.S. (2004). Finding the common ground of family and professional caregiving: The education agenda at the Rosalynn Carter Institute. *Educational Gerontology, 30*, 95–105.

Haley, J., & Harrigan, R.C. (2004). Voicing the strengths of Pacific Island parent caregivers of children who are medically fragile. *Journal of Transcultural Nursing, 15*(3), 184–194.

Halm, M.A., & Bakas, T. (2007). Factors associated with depressive symptoms, outcomes, and perceived physical health after coronary bypass surgery. *Journal of Cardiovascular Nursing, 22*(6), 508–515.

Harding, R., & Higginson, I. (2003). What is the best way to help caregivers in cancer and palliative care? A systematic literature review of interventions and their effectiveness. *Palliative Medicine, 17*, 63–74.

He, W., Sengupta, M., Velkoff, V., & DeBarros, K. (2005). *65+ in the United States: 2005.* Washington, D.C.: U.S. Government Printing Office.

Horowitz, A. (1985). Sons and daughters as caregivers to older parents: Differences in role performance and consequences. *The Gerontologist, 25*, 612–617.

Hudson, P. (2004). Positive aspects and challenges associated with caring for a dying relative at home. *International Journal of Palliative Nursing, 10*(2), 58–64.

Hulme, P.A. (1999). Family empowerment: A nursing intervention with suggested outcomes for families of children with a chronic health condition. *Journal of Family Nursing, 5*(1), 33–50. Thousand Oaks, CA: Sage.

Hunt, C.K. (2003). Concepts in caregiver research. *Journal of Nursing Scholarship, 35*(1), 27–32.

Hunt, G., Levine, C., & Naiditch, N. (2005). *Young caregivers in the U.S.* NY: National Alliance for Caregiving and the United Hospital Fund.

Interfaith care partners. (n.d.) Retrieved November 2007, from http://www.interfaithcarepartners.org

Johnson, R., Toohey, D., & Wiener, J. (2007). *Meeting the long-term care needs of the baby boomers.* Retrieved December 10, 2007, from http://www.urban.org/publications/311451.html

Johnson, R., & Wiener, J. (2006). *A profile of frail older Americans and their caregivers: The retirement project.* Washington, D.C.: The Urban Institute. Retrieved November 29, 2007, from http://www.urban.org/UploadedPDF/311284_older_americans.pdf

Jones, S. (1999). Bridging the gap: Community solutions for black-elderly health care in the 21st century. In M. L. Wykle & A. B. Ford (Eds.), *Serving minority elders in the 21st century,* (pp. 223–234). New York: Springer.

Kane, R.A., Reinardy, J., & Penrod, J.D. (1999). After the hospitalization is over: A different perspective on family care of older people. *Journal of Gerontological Social Work, 31*, 119–141.

Karp, D.A., & Tanarugsachock, V. (2000). Mental illness, caregiving, and emotion management. *Qualitative Health Research, 10,* 6–25.

Kauffmann, E. & Harrison, M.B. (1998). Stress-point intervention for parents of children hospitalized with chronic conditions. *Pediatric Nursing, 24* 4), 362–366.

Kaye, L.W., Turner, W., Butler, S.S., Downey, R., et al. (2003). Early intervention screening for family caregivers of older relatives in primary care practices. Establishing a community health service alliance in rural America. *Family Community Health, 26*(4), 319–328.

Keith, C. (1995). Family caregiving systems: Models, resources, and values. *Journal of Marriage and the Family, 57,* 179–190.

Kelly, K. (2003–2004). Link₂Care: Internet-based information and support for caregivers. *Family Caregiving,* Winter, 87–88.

Kramer, B. (1997). Gain in the caregiving experience: Where are we? What next? *The Gerontologist, 37,* 218–232.

Kramer, B., & Thompson, E. (2001). *Men as caregivers: Theory, research and service implications.* New York: Springer.

Lackey, N.R., & Gates, M.F. (2001). Adults' recollections of their experiences as young caregivers of family members with chronic physical illnesses. *Journal of Advanced Nursing, 34*(3), 320–328.

Lattanzi-Licht, M., Mahoney, J.J., & Miller, G.W. (1998). *The hospice choice: In pursuit of a peaceful death.* New York: Simon & Schuster.

Leavitt, M., Martinson, I.M., Liu, C.Y., Armstrong, V., et al. (1999). Common themes and ethnic differences in family caregiving the first year after diagnosis of childhood cancer: Part II. *Journal of Pediatric Nursing, 14,* 110–122.

Lee, H., & Cameron, M. (2004). Respite care for people with dementia and their carers. *The Cochrane Database Systematic Review, 2001*(3), Article CD004396. Retrieved January 15, 2007, from The Cochrane Library Database.

Lee, M.D. (2007). Correlates of consequences of intergenerational caregiving in Taiwan. *Journal of Advanced Nursing, 59*(1), 49–56.

Litwak, E. (1985). *Helping the elderly: The complementary roles of informal networks and formal systems.* New York: Guilford Press.

Lutz, B.J., Chumbler, N.R., Lyles, T., Hoffman, N, & Kobb, R. (2008). Testing a home-telehealth programme for US veterans recovering from stroke and their family caregiver. *Disability and Rehabilitation., 7,* 1–8.

Lutz, B.J., Chumbler, N.R., & Roland, K. (2007). Care coordination/home-telehealth for veterans with stroke and their caregivers: Addressing an unmet need. *Topics in Stroke Rehabilitation 14*(4), 32–42.

Lutz, B.J., & Davis, S.M. (2008). Theory and practice models for rehabilitation nursing. In S. Hoeman (Ed.) *Rehabilitation nursing: Prevention, intervention, and outcomes* (4th ed.) (pp. 14–29), St. Louis, MO: Mosby-Elsevier.

Lyons, K.S., Zarit, S.H., Sayer, A.G., & Whitlach, C.J. (2002). Caregiving as a dyadic process: Perspectives from caregiver and receiver. *Journal of Gerontology: Psychological Sciences, 57B*(3), P195–P204.

Mausbach, B.T., Patterson, T.L., Von Känel, R., Mills, P.J., et al. (2007). The attenuating effect of personal mastery on the relations between stress and Alzheimer caregiver health: A five-year longitudinal analysis. *Aging & Mental Health, 11*(6), 637–644.

McAuley, W.J., Travis, S.S., & Safewright, M.P. (1997). Personal accounts of the nursing home search and selection process. *Qualitative Health Research, 7,* 236–254.

Medalie, J.H. (1994). The caregiver as the hidden patient. In E. Kahana, D. E. Biegel, & M. L. Wykle (Eds.), *Family caregiving across the lifespan,* (pp. 312–330). Thousand Oaks, CA: Sage.

Meleski, D.D. (2002). Families with chronically ill children. *American Journal of Nursing, 102*(5), 47–54.

Meshefedjian, G., McCusker, J., Bellavance, F., & Baumgarten, M. (1998). Factors associated with symptoms of depression among informal caregivers of demented elders in the community. *The Gerontologist, 38,* 247–253.

MetLife® & NAC. (2004). *Caregiving in the U.S.* Retrieved January 18, 2008, from http://www.caregiving.org/data/04finalreport.pdf

Mitrani, V.B. & Czaja, S.J. (2000). Family-based therapy for dementia caregivers: Clinical observations. *Aging & Mental Health, 4*(3), 200–209.

Mittelman, J.S. (2003). Community Caregiving. *Alzheimer's Care Quarterly, 4*(4), 273–285.

Montcalm, D.M. (1995). Caregivers: Resources and services. In Z. Harel & R. E. Dunkle (Eds.), *Matching people with services in long term care,* (pp. 159–179). New York: Springer.

Montgomery, R.J.V. (1999). The family role in the context of long-term care. *Journal of Aging and Health, 11,* 383–416.

Montgomery, A., & Feinberg, L.F. (2003). *The road to recognition: International review of public policies to support family and informal caregiving.* San Francisco: National Center on Caregiving, Family Caregiver Alliance.

Montgomery, R.J.V. & Kosloski, K.D. (n.d.). *Change, continuity and diversity among caregivers.* Retrieved September 24, 2004 from http://www.aoa.gov/prof/aoaprog/caregiver/careprof/progguidance/background/program_issues/Fin-Montgomery.pdf

Montgomery, R., Stull, D., & Borgatta, E. (1985). Measurement and the analysis of burden. *Research in Aging, 7*(1), 137–52.

Moore, J. (2006). *The impact of the aging population on the health workforce in the United States.* Rensselaer, NY: University at Albany. Retrieved November 29, 2007, from http://www.albany.edu/news/pdf_files/impact_of_aging_full.pdf

Murray, S.A., Kendall, M., Boyd, K., Worth, A., Boyd K., Benton, T.F., et al. (2004). Exploring the spiritual needs of people dying of lung cancer or heart failure: A prospective qualitative interview study of patients and their carers. *Palliative Medicine, 18,* 39–45.

National Center for Health Statistics. (2003). *U.S. birth rate reaches record low.* Retrieved September 20, 2004, from http://www.cdc.gov/nchs/pressroom/03news/lowbirth.htm

Nerenberg, L. (2002). *Preventing elder abuse by family caregivers.* Washington, DC: National Center of Elder Abuse.

Nolan, M. (2001). Positive aspects of caring. In S. Payne & C. Ellis-Hill (Eds.), *Chronic and terminal illness: New perspectives on caring and carers,* (pp. 22–44). Oxford: Oxford University Press.

Ory, M.G., Hoffman, R.R. III, Yee, J.L., Tennstedt, S., & Schulz, R. (1999). Prevalence and impact of caregiving: A detailed comparison between dementia and nondementia caregivers. *The Gerontologist, 39,* 177–185.

Palmer, S., & Glass, T.A. (2003). Family function and stroke recovery: A review. *Rehabilitation Psychology, 48*(4), 255–265.

Pandya, S. (2005). *Caregiving in the United States.* Washington, D.C.: American Association of Retired Persons. Retrieved November 30, 2007, from http://www.aarp.org/research/housing-mobility/caregiving/fs111_caregiving.html

Paun, O. (2004). Female Alzheimer's patient caregivers share their strength. *Holistic Nursing Practice, 18*(1), 11–17.

Pearlin, L.I. (1992). The careers of caregivers. *The Gerontologist, 32,* 647.

Peters-Davis, N.D., Moss, M.S., & Pruchno, R.A. (1999). Children-in-law in caregiving families. *The Gerontologist, 39,* 66–75.

Pierce, L. (2001). Coherence in the urban family caregiver role with African American stroke survivors. *Topics in Stroke Rehabilitation, 8*(3), 64–72.

Pierce, L., Steiner, V., Govoni, A., Hicks, B., Thompson, T., & Friedemann, M. (2004). Caring~Webª: Internet-based support for rural caregivers of persons with stroke shows promise. *Rehabilitation Nursing, 29*(3), 95–99; 103.

Pierce, L., Steiner, V., Govoni, A., Thompson, T., & Friedemann, M. (2007). Two sides to the caregiving story. *Topics in Stroke Rehabilitation, 14*(2), 13–20.

Piercy, K. W. (1998). Theorizing about family caregiving: The role of responsibility. *Journal of Marriage and the Family, 60,* 109–118.

Piercy, K.W., & Chapman, J.G. (2001). Adopting the caregiver role: A family legacy. *Family Relations, 50,* 386–393.

Pines, A.M., & Aronson, E. (1988). *Career burnout: Causes and cures.* New York: The Free Press.

Plowfield, L.A., Raymond, J.E., & Blevins, C. (2000). Wholism for aging families: Meeting needs of caregivers. *Holistic Nursing Practice 14*(4), 51–59.

Poulshock, S., & Deimling, G. (1984). Families caring for elders in residence: Issues in the measurement of burden. *Journal of Gerontology, 39*(2), 230–239.

Pruchno, R.A., Burant, C.J., & Peters, N.D. (1997). Understanding the well-being of care receivers. *The Gerontologist, 37,* 102–109.

Pyke, K. (1999). The micropolitics of care in relationships between aging parents and adult children: Individualism, collectivism, and power. *The Journal of Marriage and the Family, 61,* 661–673.

Rabinowitz, Y.G., Mausbach, B.T., Thompson, L.W., & Gallagher-Thompson, D. (2007). The relationship between self-efficacy cumulative health risk associated with health behavior patterns in female caregivers of elderly relatives with Alzheimer's dementia. *Journal of Aging and Health, 19*(6), 946–964.

Riggs, J. (2004). A family caregiver policy agenda for the twenty-first century. *Generations, 27*(4), 68–73.

Ritchie, L. (2003). Adult day care: Northern perspectives. *Public Health Nursing, 20*(2), 120–131.

Rittman, M., Kuzmeskus, L.B., & Flum, M.A. (1998). A synthesis of current knowledge on minority elder abuse. In T. Tatara (Ed.), *Understanding elder abuse in minority populations,* (pp. 221–238). Philadelphia: Brunner/Mazel.

Roff, L., Burgio, L., Gitlin, L., Nichols, L., et al. (2004). Positive aspects of Alzheimer's caregiving: The role of race. *Journals of Gerontology Series B: Psychological Sciences and Social Sciences, 59B*(4), 185–190.

Sarkisian, N., & Gerstel, N. (2004). Explaining the gender gap in help to parents: The importance of employment. *Journal of Marriage and Family, 66,* 431–451.

Schulz, R., & Beach, S.R. (1999). Caregiving as a risk factor for mortality: The caregiver health effects study. *Journal of the American Medical Association, 282,* 2215–2219.

Scott, G. (2001). A study of family carers of people with a life-threatening illness 2: The implications of the needs assessment. *International Journal of Palliative Nursing, 7*(7), 323–330.

Scott, J. (2006). *Informal caregiving.* Orono, ME: University of Maine System. Retrieved November 30, 2007, from http://www.maine.gov/dhhs/beas/bhcoa/FinalReport-Caregiving_Family.pdf

Seltzer, M.M. (1990). Role reversal: You don't go home again. *Journal of Gerontological Social Work, 15,* 5–14.

Seltzer, M.M., & Wailing, L. (2000). The dynamics of caregiving: Transitions during a three-year prospective study. *The Gerontologist, 40,* 165–178.

Selwood, A., Johnston, K. Katona, C., Lyketsos, C., & Livingston, G. (2007). Systematic review of the effect of psychological interventions on family caregivers of people with dementia. *Journal of Affective Disorders, 101,* 75–89.

Shapiro, E.R. (2002). Chronic illness as a family process: A social-developmental approach to promoting resilience. *JCLP/in session: Psychotherapy in practice, 58*(11), 1375–1384.

Sheehan, N.W., & Donorfio, L.M. (1999). Efforts to create meaning in the relationship between aging mothers and their caregiving daughters: A qualitative study of caregiving. *Journal of Aging Studies, 13,* 161–176.

Shirey, L., & Summer, L. (2000). *Caregiving: Helping the elderly with activity limitations.* Washington, DC: National Academy on Aging Society.

Skaff, M.M., Pearlin, L.I., & Mullan, J.T. (1996). Transitions in the caregiving career: Effects on sense of mastery. *Psychology and Aging, 11,* 247–257.

Spector, R.E. (2000). *Cultural diversity in health and illness* (5th ed.). Upper Saddle River, NJ: Prentice Hall Health.

Steiner, V., & Pierce, L. (2002). Building a Web of support for caregivers of persons with stroke. *Topics in Stroke Rehabilitation, 9*(3), 102–111.

Stobert, S., & Cranswick, K. (2004). Looking after seniors: Who does what for whom? *Canadian Social Trends, 74,* 2–6.

Stoller, E.P., & Cutler, S.J. (1993). Predictors of use of paid help among older people living in the community. *The Gerontologist, 33*(1), 31–40.

Stone, R., Cafferata, G.L., & Sangl, J. (1987). Caregivers of the frail elderly: A national profile. *The Gerontologist, 27,* 616–626.

Stone, R.I., & Short, P.F. (1990). The competing demands of employment and informal caregiving to disabled elders. *Medical Care, 28,* 513–526.

Stuckey, J.C. (2001). Blessed assurance: The role of religion and spirituality in Alzheimer's disease caregiving and other significant life events. *Journal of Aging Studies, 15*(1), 69–84.

Substance Abuse and Mental Health Service Administration (2004). *SAMHSA model programs.* Retrieved September 20, 2004 from http://modelprograms.samhsa.gov

Tarlow, B., Wisniewski, S., Belle, S., Rubert, M., et al. (2004). Positive aspects of caregiving. *Research on Aging, 26*(4), 429–453.

Teaster, P.B. (2003). *A response to the abuse of vulnerable adults: The 2000 survey of state adult protective services.* Retrieved from http://www.ncea.aoa.gov/ncearoot/Main_Site/pdf/research/apsreport030703.pdf The Dartmouth Atlas Project. (2006). *The care of patients with chronic illness.* Hanover, NH: The Dartmouth Atlas of Healthcare.

Retrieved November 29, 2007, from http://www. rwjf.org/files/research/DartmouthSevereChronic-Medicare2006.pdf

Theis, S.L., Biordi, D.L., Coeling, H., Nalepka, C., & Miller, B. (2003). Spirituality in caregiving and care receiving. *Holistic Nursing Practice, 17*(1), 48–55.

Thompson, B., Tudiver, F., & Manson, J. (2000). Sons as sole caregivers for their elderly parents. How do they cope? *Canadian Family Physician, 46,* 360–365.

Thompson, C.A., Spilsbury, K., Hall, J., Birks, Y., Barnes, C., & Adamson, J. (2007). Systematic review of information and support interventions for caregivers of people with dementia. *BMC Geriatrics, 2007,* 7–18.

Toth-Cohen, S., Gitlin, L.N., Corcoran, M.A., Eckhardt, S., et al. (2001). Providing services to family caregivers at home: Challenges and recommendations for health and human service professions. *Alzheimer's Care Quarterly, 2*(1), 23–32.

Travis, S.S., & Bethea, L.S. (2001). Medication administration by family members of elders in shared care arrangements. *Journal of Clinical Geropsychology, 7,* 231–243.

Travis, S.S., Bethea, L.S., & Winn, P. (2000). Medication administration hassles reported by family caregivers of dependent elders. *Journal of Gerontology, Medical Sciences, 55A,* M412–M417.

Travis, S.S., & Duer, B. (2000). Interdisciplinary management of the older adult with cancer. In A.S. Luggen & S.E. Meiner (Eds.), *Handbook for the care of the older adult with cancer,* (pp. 25–34). Pittsburgh, PA: Oncology Nursing Press.

University of Michigan Health System. (2006). *Children with chronic conditions.* Ann Arbor, MI: Author. Retrieved November 29, 2007, from http://www. med.umich.edu/1libr/yourchild/chronic.htm

U.S. Department of Labor. (1993). *The family and medical leave act of 1993.* Washington, DC: U.S. Department of Labor, Wage and Hour Division.

Walker, E. & Dewar, B.J. (2004). How do we facilitate carers' involvement in decision making? *Journal of Advanced Nursing, 34*(3), 329–337.

Warren, S., Kerr, J., Smith, D., Godkin, D., & Schalm, C. (2003). The impact of adult day programs on fam-

ily caregivers of elderly relatives. *Journal of Community Health Nursing, 20*(4), 209–221.

Weissert, W.G., & Hedrick, S.C. (1994). Lessons learned from research on effects of community-based long-term care. *Journal of the American Geriatrics Society, 42,* 348–353.

Weissert, W.G., & Hedrick, S.C. (1999). Outcomes and costs of home and community-based long-term care: Implications for research-based practice. In E. Calkins, C. Boult, E. H. Wagner, & J.T. Pacala (Eds.), *New ways to care for older people,* (pp. 143–157). New York: Springer.

Weitzner, M.A., Haley, W.E., & Chen, H. (2000). The family caregiver of the older cancer patient. *Hematology and Oncology Clinics of North America, 14,* 269–281.

White-Means, S.L. (1997). The demands of persons with disabilities for home health care and the economic consequences for informal caregivers. *Social Science Quarterly, 78,* 955–972.

Williams, A. (1993). Caregivers of persons with stroke: Their physical and emotional well-being. *Quality of Life Researsh, 2*(3), 213–220.

Williams, S.W., Dilworth-Anderson, P. & Goodwin, P.Y. (2003). Caregiver role strain: The contribution of multiple roles and available resources in African-American women. *Aging and Mental Health, 7*(2), 103–112.

Winslow, B.W. (2003). Family caregivers' experiences with community services: A qualitative analysis. *Public Health Nursing, 20* (5), 341–348.

Workplace Flexibility 2010. (2004). *Family and medical leave: Selective background information.* Retrieved January 3, 2008, from http://www.law.georgetown .edu/workplaceflexibility2010/law/fmlaFiles/fmla_ DataPoints.pdf

Yee, J.L., & Schulz, R. (2000). Gender differences in psychiatric morbidity among family caregivers: A review and analysis. *The Gerontologist, 40,* 147–164.

Zarit, S., Todd, P., & Zarit, J. (1986). Subjective burden of husbands and wives as caregivers: A longitudinal study. *The Gerontologist, 26*(3), 260–66.

10

Sexuality

Margaret Chamberlain Wilmoth

INTRODUCTION

Humans are sexual beings from birth until death. Sexuality is an integral aspect of our personalities and is more than sexual contact and the ability to function to reach sexual satisfaction. Sexuality includes views of ourselves as male or female, feelings about our body, and the ways we communicate verbally and nonverbally our comfort about ourselves to others. It also includes the ability to engage in satisfying sexual behaviors alone or with another. Sexuality does not end when one reaches a certain age, nor does it end with the diagnosis of a chronic illness. In fact, sexuality and intimacy may become *more* important after such a diagnosis as a way of reaffirming human connection, aliveness, and continued desirability and caring. Sexuality is a critical aspect of quality of life that, unfortunately, is often ignored by healthcare professionals.

This chapter briefly reviews standards of nursing practice as they relate to sexuality, sexual physiologic functioning, and alterations in sexuality caused by common chronic illnesses and their treatments, and nursing interventions. This chapter also provides nurses with suggestions with ways to incorporate discussions of sexuality into their practice.

Definitions

Sexuality is a complex construct with terminology that has yet to be defined in a manner that is accepted by all. When discussing sexuality with other professionals or with clients, it is important to be sure that everyone has the same frame of reference for the many descriptors that are used for aspects of sexuality. Nurses also are encouraged to know the more "scientific" terms, yet remember that these are not the words used by most of their clients when they talk about their sexuality. Nurses need to find out what terms their clients use, clarify the meaning to ensure understanding, then use words the client knows and understands when discussing the impact of chronic illness on sexuality. Nurses should avoid using the term "sexual dysfunction," as this is a psychiatric diagnosis that most nurses are not qualified to make. The American Psychiatric Association (APA) has identified sexual dysfunctions that are a result of chronic medical condition and which have specific diagnostic criteria. Examples of psychiatrically diagnosed sexual dysfunctions include hypoactive sexual desire, dyspareunia, and erectile disorder (APA, 1994). The definitions used in discussing sexuality in this chapter are in Table 10-1.

TABLE 10-1	
Definitions	
Sexuality	Everything that makes us man or woman, including the need for touch, feelings about one's body, the need to connect with another human being in an intimate way, interest in engaging in sexual behaviors, communication of one's feelings and needs to one's partner, and the ability to engage in satisfying sexual behaviors
Sexual behaviors	Specific activities used to obtain release of sexual tension alone or with another in order to achieve sexual satisfaction; refers also to the multiple ways one verbally and nonverbally communicates sexual feelings and attitudes to others
Sexual functioning	The physiologic component of sexuality, including human sexual anatomy, the sexual response cycle, neuroendocrine functioning, and life cycle changes in sexual physiology
Sexual dysfunction	Characterized by disturbances in the processes of the sexual response cycle or by pain associated with sexual intercourse; is a *Diagnostic and Statistical Manual, version IV (DSM-IV)* diagnosis and should not be used by nurses unless they are specially trained in treating sexual dysfunctions

Sources: Wilmoth, M.C. (1998). Sexuality. In C. Burke (Ed.), *Psychosocial dimensions of oncology nursing care* (pp. 102–127). Pittsburgh: Oncology Nursing Press and American Psychiatric Association. (1994). *Diagnostic and statistical manual of mental disorders* (4th ed.).

Standards of Practice

Standards of practice infer both a legal standard of practice as well as an ethical responsibility that nurses adhere to in their practice of nursing (Andrews, Goldberg, & Kaplan, 1996). Standards of practice for the profession, published by the American Nurses Association (ANA) (2004), include six standards of care that encompass significant actions taken by nurses when providing care to their clients. These standards include the components of the nursing process. These standards also assume that all relevant healthcare needs of the client will be assessed and appropriate care provided, including needs surrounding sexuality.

Specialty organizations may have derived standards of nursing practice from those published by the ANA that are specific to their practice. For example, the Oncology Nursing Society (2004) published nursing practice standards that specifically identified sexuality as one potential area of client concern. These standards include both Assessment Criteria and Outcome Criteria. Nurses who care for cancer patients then are expected to follow each of these standards in the provision of patient care (Figure 10-1).

Nurses and physicians are legally obligated to ensure that clients have the necessary information to make decisions regarding treatment. The provision of informed consent also requires that all risks, benefits, and side effects of diseases and their treatments be provided to clients as they choose treatments for any illness. This includes information about potential sexual side effects of proposed treatments. Failure to provide this information could potentially lead to legal action by the client.

The Sexual Response Cycle and Sexual Physiology

There are two frameworks commonly used to describe what is called the "sexual response cycle." The first was proposed by Dr. William Masters and Virginia Johnson and is a four-stage model of sexual response of the male and female (1966). The four phases of the Masters and Johnson Model are

FIGURE 10-1

Oncology Nursing Society Statement on the Scope and Standards of Oncology Nursing Practice

Standard I Assessment	Standard III Outcome Identification
The oncology nurse systematically and continually collects data regarding the health status of the patient.	The oncology nurse identifies expected outcomes individualized to the patient.
Measurement Criteria	**Measurement Criteria**
The oncology nurse collects data in the following 14 high-incidence problem areas that may include but are not limited to:(j) sexuality.	The oncology nurse develops expected outcomes for each of the 14 high-incidence problem areas within a level consistent with the patient's physiology, psychosocial,spiritual capacities,cultural background, and value system.The expected outcomes include but are not limited to (j) sexuality. The patient and/or family:
1. Past and present sexual patterns and expression.	1. Identifies potential or actual changes in sexuality, sexual functioning or intimacy related to disease and treatment.
2. Effects of disease and treatment on body image.	2. Expresses feelings about alopecia, body image changes,and altered sexual functioning.
3. Effects of disease and treatment on sexual function.	3. Engages in open communication with his or her partner regarding changes in sexual functioning or desire, within cultural framework.
4. Psychological response of patient and partner to disease and treatment.	4. Describes appropriate interventions for actual or potential changes in sexual function.
	5. Identifies other satisfying methods of sexual expression that provide satisfaction to both partners, within cultural framework.
	6. Identifies personal and community resources to assist with changes in body image and sexual functioning.

Source: Oncology Nursing Society. (2004). Statement on the scope and standards of oncology nursing practice. Pittsburgh, PA: Author.

excitement, plateau, orgasm, and resolution (1966). The excitement stage causes an increase in the heart rate and vasocongestion to the penis. This is accompanied by lengthening and widening of the vagina, elevation of the cervix and uterus, and initial swelling of the labia minora (Guyton & Hall, 2006; Masters & Johnson, 1966). These changes are caused by vasocongestion and are secondary to a parasympathetic response mediated to S2 and S4 through the pudendal nerve and sacral plexus (Guyton & Hall, 2006).

The second stage is the plateau stage, which is an increased state of arousal causing the heart rate, and blood pressure to increase with a subsequent increase in respiratory rate (Katz, 2007). The third stage is the orgasm, the phase of maximal muscular contraction (men ejaculation, and women pelvic muscle contraction), with a peak of respirations and heart rate, and a subjective feeling of intense pleasure that radiates throughout the body (Katz, 2007). Impending orgasm is determined by the presence of an intense color change in the labia minora in women and full elevation of the scrotal sac to the perineal wall in men, all a result of intense vasocongestion (Masters & Johnson, 1966). Orgasm is mediated by the sympathetic nervous system and is the physical release and peak of pleasurable expression, followed by relaxation (Guyton & Hall, 2006). The sympathetic nerves between T12 and L2 control ejaculation (Koukouras et al., 1991). The intensity of orgasm in women is dependent upon the duration and intensity of sexual stimulation.

The final stage is resolution, when vasocongestion resolves and the body returns to its normal nonaroused state (Katz, 2007). Men also have what is referred to as a "refractory period," which is the period within which the male is unable to achieve an erection satisfactory for penetration. This period of time is age and health-status dependent (Masters & Johnson, 1966).

Physical changes that occur in both men and women as a result of sexual stimulation are vasocongestion and myotonia. Vasocongestion occurs in the penis in men and in the labia in women, and is an essential requirement for orgasm and subsequent sexual satisfaction. *Myotonia* refers to the involuntary muscular contractions that occur throughout the body during sexual response (Kolodny, Masters, Johnson, & Biggs, 1979).

The second framework is from Kaplan. Kaplan's (1979) modification of the sexual response cycle includes aspects of sexual physiology involving the prelude to sexual activity as well as the consequences of sexual activity. These three phases are desire, arousal, and orgasm. Desire is the prelude to engaging in satisfying sexual behaviors and is the most complex component of the sexual response cycle. Desire is often affected by factors such as anger, pain, and body image, as well as disease processes and medications (Kaplan, 1979). When sexual stimuli are perceived by women, they are processed physiologically and physically, leading to subjective feelings of arousal and a responsive feeling of desire (Katz, 2007). This may explain why psychogenic factors can be a determinant cause of male and female sexual dysfunction.

Arousal, manifested by erection in males, is mediated by the parasympathetic nervous system and is the result of either psychic or somatic sexual stimulation (Masters & Johnson, 1966). Alternately, activation of the sympathetic nervous system will lead to loss of an erection through vasoconstriction. It was previously thought that an analogous process of parasympathetic nervous system stimulation led to arousal in women. However, recent evidence suggests that it is stimulation of the sympathetic nervous system (SNS) that is responsible for female arousal (Meston, 2000). Data also suggest that stimulation of the SNS may enhance arousal in women with low sexual desire (Meston & Gorzalka, 1996) and that induction of relaxation may negatively affect arousal (Meston, 2000).

Although many women suggest that the Gräfenberg spot (G-spot) plays an important role in their sexuality, the existence of this sensitive area remains open for verification (Hines, 2001). The G-spot is purportedly located in the anterior wall of the vagina, about halfway between the back of the pubic bone and the cervix along the course of the urethra (Ladas, Whipple, & Perry, 1982). When stimulated, this tissue swells from the size of a bean to greater than a half dollar (Ladas et al., 1982). Stimulation of this area appears to cause a different orgasmic sensation, and it is hypothesized that this response is mediated by the pelvic nerve, causing the uterus to contract and descend against the vagina rather than elevate, as with stimulation mediated by the pudendal nerve (Ladas et al., 1982). Approximately 40% of women will experience expulsion of a fluid upon orgasm caused by G-spot stimulation (Darling, Davidson, & Conway-Welch, 1990). Research suggests that this is a prostatic-like fluid that is released during orgasm (Zaviacic &

Whipple, 1993; Zaviacic & Ablin, 2000). Belief that this is not urine but a normal release of fluid that occurs during sexual response may lead to a reduction in embarrassment for many women.

The neurohormonal system influences sexual functioning through its effect on hormone production. The hypothalamic–hypophysial portal system plays an important role in sexual functioning in both genders through production of gonadotropin-releasing hormone (GnRH) and subsequent stimulation of gonadotropin production by the anterior pituitary gland. The anterior pituitary gland secretes six hormones, two of which play an essential role in sexual functioning. Follicle-stimulating hormone (FSH) and luteinizing hormone (LH) control growth of the gonads and influence sexual functioning. In men, LH influences production of testosterone by the Leydig cells in the testes through a negative feedback loop (Guyton & Hall, 2006). Production of GnRH is reduced, once a satisfactory level of testosterone has been attained. A negative feedback loop also exists in the woman, although it is much more complex, given the concurrent production of estrogen and progesterone by the ovary and the production of androgens by the adrenal cortex.

Psychic factors appear to play a larger role in sexual functioning in woman than in that of men, particularly in relation to sexual desire. Multiple neuronal centers in the brain's limbic system transmit signals into the arcuate nuclei in the mediobasal hypothalamus. These signals modify the intensity of GnRH release and the frequency of the impulses (Guyton & Hall, 2006). This may explain why desire in women is more vulnerable to emotions and distractions than it is in men.

Aging affects the sexual response cycle in predictable ways, but it does not signal the end of sexuality. In fact, the old adage, "Use it or lose it," is applicable to continued sexual activity throughout life (Masters & Johnson, 1981). The general impact of aging on the sexual response cycle is a slower, less intense sexual response (Lindau, Schumm, Gaumann, Levinson, O'Muircheartaigh, & Waite, 2007). The frequency of sexual activity in earlier years is predictive of frequency as one ages. The quality of the sexual relationship appears to be the greatest influence on the frequency and satisfaction of sexual activity (Masters & Johnson, 1981). As in younger adults, the quality of communication in a relationship, degree of mutual intimacy, and level of commitment to the relationship are vital to a satisfying sexual relationship and to achieving sexual satisfaction.

In clients aged 60 or older, organic factors are the most important determinant of erectile dysfunction (Corona et al., 2007). The frequent comorbidity of multiple metabolic and hemodynamic abnormalities in the aging clients can increase substantially the incidence and progression of atherosclerotic lesions, leading to vascular forms of erectile dysfunction (Corona et al., 2007). Masters and Johnson (1966) found that in men between 51 and 90 years of age, the time to achieve erection was two to three times longer than in younger men. Achieving erection also required more tactile stimulation than in younger years. However, once achieved, older men can maintain a full erection for a longer period before ejaculation. Scrotal vasocongestion is reduced, with a subsequent decrease in testicular elevation. Basal and dynamic peak cavernosal velocity was reduced in older patients with Doppler ultrasound penile examination (Corona et al., 2007).The ability to attain orgasm is not impaired with aging, but there is an overall decrease in myotonia and fewer penile and rectal sphincter contractions. There is an increase in time from hours to days before older men can achieve another erection once they have ejaculated and achieved an orgasm (refractory period).

Women also experience sexual response cycle changes as they age, primarily after completing the menopausal transition. Common complaints include decreased desire, dry vagina, and difficulty attaining orgasm (Lindau et al., 2007). Vaginal changes include a thinning of the mucosa, with a decrease in vaginal lubrication. In women who abstain from sexual intercourse, narrowing and stenosis of the introitus and vaginal vault can occur (Leiblum & Segraves, 1989). Older women experience a decrease in the vasocongestion of the labia and other genitalia analogous to the decrease in penile tumescence experienced by men. Orgasm in sexually active women is not impaired; however, there is some decrease in the degree of myotonia experienced. Intense orgasm may lead to involuntary distension of the external meatus, leading to an increase in frequency of urinary tract infections in older women.

■ SEXUALITY AND CHRONIC ILLNESS

The presence of a chronic illness affects all aspects of an individual's life, including their sexuality. There are numerous chronic illnesses, and discussion of the impact of each on sexuality is beyond the scope of this chapter. Therefore, this chapter is limited to the provision of a brief discussion that the effects of coronary artery disease, diabetes mellitus, cancer, and multiple sclerosis have on sexuality.

Coronary Artery Disease

The heart is linked to romance and to the soul, so any threat to cardiac functioning is emotionally linked to matters of the self, sexuality, and intimacy. Cardiovascular disease, that includes coronary artery disease (CAD) and stroke, causes more death in both genders and all racial and ethnic groups in the United States than any other disease (Centers for Disease Control and Prevention, 2004). More men and women than ever before are living longer and continue to lead productive lives after experiencing a myocardial infarction (MI); however, recent data suggest that women experience a lower degree of quality of life than men (Agewall, Berglund, & Henareh, 2004; Svedlund & Danielson, 2004). Therefore, having adequate and accurate knowledge about sexuality post diagnosis may have a positive impact crucial to individuals' self-concept, to their sexuality, and to their sexual relationships.

The consensus study from the Second Princeton Consensus Conference collaborates and clarifies the risk stratification algorithm that was developed by the first Princeton Consensus Panel to evaluate the degree of cardiovascular risk associated with sexual activity for men with varying degrees of cardiovascular disease (Kostis et al., 2005). The algorithm emphasizes the importance of risk factor evaluation and management for all patients with erectile dysfunction (ED). The relative safety at which clients can engage in sexual activity is dependent on their degree of cardiac disease. This panel recommended a classification system that would stratify clients into a risk category based on the extent of their cardiac disease. These categories and management recommendations are found in Table 10-2. Patients with less than three major risk factors for cardiovascular disease (age, hypertension, diabetes mellitus, cigarette smoking, dyslipidemia, sedentary lifestyle, and family history of premature coronary artery disease) are generally at low risk for significant cardiac complications from sexual activity or the treatment of sexual dysfunction (Kostis et al., 2005). Clients whose cardiac conditions are uncertain, as well as those with multiple risk factors, require further testing or evaluation before resuming sexual activity (Kostis et al., 2005). Patients with a history of MI (>2 weeks and <6 weeks) may be at somewhat greater risk for coitus-induced ischemia and reinfarction, as well as malignant arrhythmias (Kostis et al., 2005). The level of risk associated within this time period post-MI can be assessed with an exercise stress test.

Counseling of all clients regarding lifestyle changes and activity restrictions should begin as soon as the client is stabilized. Discussions regarding sexual activity should be included in the counseling. Potential fear of cardiac arrest during sexual activity should be eradicated as soon as possible by assuring clients and their partners that this risk is only 1.2% and that sex accounts for only 0.5–1.0% of all acute coronary incidents (DeBusk, 2000).

Recent reports continue to validate the appropriateness of the stair-climbing tolerance test for successful return to sexual activity after 6 weeks post-MI. Sexual activity conceptualized simply as

TABLE 10-2		
Management Recommendations Based on Graded Cardiovascular (CV) Risk Assessment		
Grade of Risk	*Categories of CVD*	*Management*
Low risk	Asymptomatic, 6 weeks); mild valvular disease, LVD/CHF (NYHA class I); patients with pericarditis, mitral valve prolapse, or atrial fibrillation with controlled ventricular response should be managed on an individualized basis	Primary care management; consider all first-line therapies; reassess at regular intervals
Intermediate risk	Three major risk factors for CAD; moderate, stable angina; recent MI (>2, <6 weeks); LVD/CHF (NYHA class II); noncardiac sequelae of atherosclerotic disease (e.g., CVA, PVD)	Specialized CV testing; restratification into high or low risk based on results of CV testing
High risk	Unstable or refractory angina; uncontrolled hypertension; LVD/CHF (NYHA class III/IV); recent MI (<2 weeks), CVA; High-risk arrhythmias; obstructive hypertrophic and other cardiomyopathies; moderate–severe valvular disease	Priority referral for specialized CV management; treatment for sexual dysfunction deferred until cardiac condition stabilized and dependent on specialist recommendations; sexual activity should be deferred until a patient's cardiac condition has been stabilized by treatment or a decision has been made by a specialist

CAD, coronary artery disease; CHF, congestive heart failure; CVA, cerebrovascular accident (stroke); CVD, cardiovascular disease; LVD, left ventricular dysfunction; NYHA, New York Heart Association; PVD, peripheral vascular disease.
Sources: From DeBusk, R., Drory, Y., Goldstein, I., Jackson, G., Kaul, S., & Kimmel, S.E. (2000). Management of sexual dysfunction in patients with cardiovascular disease: Recommendations of the Princeton Consensus Panel. *The American Journal of Cardiology, 86* (2), 175–181, and Kostis, J.B., Jackson, G., Rosen, R., Barrett-Connor, E., Billups, K., Burnett, A.L. et al. (2005). Sexual Dysfunction and Cardiac Risk, The Second Princeton Consensus Conference. Retrieved November 3, 2007, from www.AJConline.org

arousal is unassociated with physical exertion. It is not until exertion is coupled with arousal that energy expenditure occurs. Data indicate that the man in the top position results in greater responses of heart rate and VO_2, and thus greater energy expenditure that may or may not reflect both heightened arousal and exertion. If sexual activity is conceptualized as exertion, then the capacity to climb two flights of stairs without limiting symptoms is a clinical benchmark of exercise tolerance

and subsequent ability to engage in sexual activity without symptoms (DeBusk, 2000).

Depression has been indicated as a psychological cause of sexual dysfunction and may increase the risk of cardiac mortality in both genders (Roose & Seidman, 2000). A discrepancy between male and female sexual desire, which could disturb relationships, can be observed in many aging couples (Corona et al., 2007). Roose and Seidman (2000) indicate that the male client with ischemic heart disease who is depressed is also likely to have erectile difficulties. This is also a predisposing factor for other adverse cardiac events. Therefore, it appears prudent that all post-MI clients be evaluated for depression and receive appropriate therapy. A wide body of evidence supports the hypothesis of a strong association between depression and ED (Corona et al., 2007). The age-dependent increased use of psychotropic drugs such as antidepressants and antipsychotics may play an important role in ED in older clients (Corona et al., 2007).

Clients should be counseled regarding the effects of medications on sexuality. Calcium channel inhibitors, nonselective β-blockers, angiotensin II antagonists, and diuretics may increase the risk of ED. Erectile dysfunction does not seem to be a problem in men using organic nitrates, angiotensin-converting enzyme inhibitors, selective β-blockers or serum lipid-lowering agents (Shril, Koskimaki, Hakkien, Auvinen, Tammela, & Hakama, 2007). Organic nitrates, including sublingual nitroglycerin, isosorbide mononitrate, isosorbide dinitrate, and other nitrate preparations used to treat angina, as well as amyl nitrite or amyl nitrate ("poppers" used for recreation), are absolutely contraindicated in patients taking PDE-5 inhibitors (Kostis et al., 2005).

Counseling and education about return to pre-infarct activities, including sexuality, should be a part of a comprehensive cardiac rehabilitation program. Age and marital status should not be a factor in determining who receives information about resuming sexual activity. If clients have a spouse or regular partner, they should be included in education and counseling sessions unless the clients request otherwise. Discussions about sexual activity should include talking about anxieties concerning resumption of sexual activities with one's partner, scheduling sexual encounters after periods of rest, avoiding sex after heavy meals or alcohol ingestion, and keeping nitroglycerin at the bedside as a form of reassurance (Steinke, 2000). An integral part of successful resumption of sexual activity is engaging in regular exercise based on physician recommendations. Partners of cardiac clients also experience distress because of the disease that may manifest as decreased intimacy and may require intervention to assist them in adjusting to disease-related stressors (O'Farrell, Murray, & Hotz, 2000).

Diabetes Mellitus

The incidence of diabetes mellitus in the United States is on the increase, with 1.5 million new cases of diabetes in people aged 20 years or older in 2005, according to the National Diabetes Information Clearing House (NDIC) (NDIC, 2007), and with this disease, the number of persons who have alterations in their sexuality will increase. Nurses must be prepared to assist these individuals with the multiple life changes they will experience because of this disease, including changes in sexual functioning.

It is well known that diabetes mellitus has serious effects on sexual functioning in men. Prevalence of ED in diabetic males range from 33–75% depending on age, glycemic control, and presence of other behaviors such as smoking (Jackson, 2004). There is great variability in reports on the effect of diabetes on the sexual response cycle in women (Sarkadi & Rosenquist, 2004).

Men with diabetes typically experience minimal changes in their desire for sexual activities. Any changes in desire may be attributable to difficulties in achieving satisfactory arousal. Arousal difficulties are manifested by the lack of adequate penile erection typically referred to as erectile ED. The term *impotence* has multiple negative psychological connotations and is no longer used by healthcare professionals (NIH, 1992). An estimated 50–75% of diabetic men have ED to some degree, a rate about fourfold higher than in non-diabetic men [Consortium for Improvement in Erectile Dysfunction (CIEF), 2007]. Acute onset of ED may reflect poor glycemic control of the disease; however, ED may be reversible if control is regained. Acute onset of ED reflects accumulation of sorbitol and water in autonomic nerve fibers and is generally a temporary condition. Erectile dysfunction can result from vasculogenic, neurogenic, hormonal, and/or psychogenic factors as well as alterations in the nitric oxide/cyclic guanosine monophosphate pathway or other regulatory mechanisms (Safarine & Hosseini, 2004).

Treatment options for ED in diabetic men include use of sildenafil or similar medications, intracavernosal injection therapy or placement of a penile prosthesis (Jackson, 2004). Men who experience ED should be referred to a urologist for work-up before making a decision about treatment options (see Table 10-3 for treatment options). In addition, because patients' responses to therapy vary according to risk factors, the more difficult-to-treat patients (e.g., those with conditions such as hypertension or diabetes) will most likely have a lower response rate and need more frequent follow-up visits than those with fewer risk factors (CIEF, 2007).

Men with diabetes are capable of experiencing orgasm and ejaculation even after developing ED, because the disease has lesser effects on the sympathetic autonomic nervous system. Men may experience a retrograde ejaculation due to autonomic system disruption of the internal vesical sphincter (Tilton, 1997). Fertility may also be impaired in diabetic men secondary to ED, low semen volume, and lowered sperm counts. Couples should be referred to a counselor to help them adjust to the relationship strains of chronic illness, and those desiring children should be referred to a fertility specialist.

Despite recent efforts in identifying and quantifying the prevalence of sexual problems in women with diabetes, data continue to be inadequate (Bhasin, Enzlin, Coviello, & Basson, 2007). Although less evidence exists on the relationship among patients with diabetes, the female genitourinary system, and sexual dysfunction in women, sexual dysfunction has been identified as a prevalent problem in women, and some evidence indicates that diabetes increases the risk for sexual dysfunction in this population (Grandjean & Moran, 2007). Other prevalence data suggest that all phases of the sexual response cycle are

negatively affected in women with insulin-dependent diabetes mellitus (IDDM), with diabetic women reporting 27% dysfunction as compared with 15% of those in a control group (Enzlin, Mathieu, Van den Bruel, Bosteels, Vanderschueren, & Demyttenaere, 2002). In addition, there appears to be a difference between diabetic women and healthy women regarding vaginal lubrication, with diabetic women reporting decreased lubrication (Enzlin et al., 2002). Data are scarce in comparing levels of desire between women with IDDM and non–insulin-dependent diabetes mellitus (NIDDM). Recent work suggests a correlation between sexual dysfunction and depression in women with diabetes (Bhasin et al., 2007).

Vaginal lubrication is a manifestation of sexual arousal and can be viewed as analogous to erection in men. As such, women would experience alterations in vaginal capillary dilation and loss of transudate formed in the vagina. The most common hormonally related problem associated with diminished sexual arousal is estrogen, because sexual arousal is influenced by levels of this chemical. Women experiencing estrogen deficiencies at menopause are often impacted by changes in vaginal structure and function (Grandjean & Moran, 2007). Diabetic women may be at higher risk for sexual dysfunction because of vaginal dryness, dyspareunia, decreased arousal or desire, and psychological factors. Treatment modalities are discussed for each of these specific problems (Grandjean & Moran, 2007). Women also reported that it took longer to reach a level of arousal necessary to be orgasmic, but that there were no discernible changes in their orgasms since the onset of diabetes. Other research reports varying frequencies of orgasmic difficulties. Kolodny (1971) found that 35% of his sample reported complete loss of orgasm, whereas Jensen (1981) had only 10% reported decreased or absent orgasm. Clearly much more research is needed in this area.

Although the data cannot pinpoint the exact percentage of diabetic women and men with sexual difficulties or identify exactly when in the course of the disease sexual problems occur,

TABLE 10-3

Treatments for Erectile Dysfunction

Treatment	Mechanism of Action	Side Effects	Pro/Con
Sildenafil citrate (Viagra), tadalafil (Cialis), vardenafil (Levitra)	Blocks enzyme phosphodiesterase type 5 and allows for persistent levels of cyclic GMP. This chemical is produced in the penis during sexual arousal and leads to smooth muscle relaxation in the penis and increases blood flow, leading to erection.	Headache, flushing of face, GI irritability, nasal congestion, muscle aches	Pro: Allows for some degree of spontaneity Con: Cannot be taken if the client also takes nitrates for cardiac disease
Intraurethral prostaglandin	Relaxes smooth muscle of ductus arteriosus. Produces vasodilation, inhibits platelet aggregation, and stimulates intestinal and uterine smooth muscle. Induces erection by relaxation of trabecular smooth muscle and by dilation of cavernosal arteries.	Flushing, bradycardia, diarrhea, urethral pain, hematoma, back pain, and pelvic pain.	Pro: Allows for some degree of spontaneity
Intracavernosal injections	Medications act on sinusoidal smooth muscle to induce relaxation and enhance corporal filling.	Penile pain during injection Priapism in 1% Hematoma in 8%	Pro: Allows for some degree of spontaneity Con: Requires office visits to ensure proper technique; can use only qod; expensive
Vacuum extraction device (VED)	Places negative pressure on corporal bodies of the penis to allow for blood flow into the penis and cause an erection. A constriction band is placed around the base of the penis to prevent loss of erection until the sex act is completed.	Penile hematoma; injury to erectile tissue or penile skin necrosis may lead to permanent penile deformity. Painful erections due to impairment of blood flow by the constriction band at the base of the penis.	Pro: Allows for penile–vaginal penetration Con: Loss of spontaneity; erection only involves a part of the penis
Malleable device	Straightens the penis for intercourse	Potential for postoperative infection; may place prolonged pressure on corporal bodies and cause tissue damage	Pro: May be used in patients with neurologic disease Con: Surgical procedure

(Continued)

TABLE 10-3

Treatments for Erectile Dysfunction (*Continued*)

Treatment	Mechanism of Action	Side Effects	Pro/Con
Inflatable penile prosthesis	Inflate erectile cylinders from reservoir. As fluid moves from the reservoir into corporal bodies, the penis becomes erect.	Infection in first few months after implanted; may have failure of device, requiring removal and replacement	Pro: Allows intercourse to continue Con: Reports of sexual dissatisfaction caused by loss of girth and length of erection Surgical procedure
External prosthetic penis	A strap-on dildo made of silicone rubber. Shaft of dildo is mounted at angle on flanged base, which holds it in the harness. Cleaning: soap/water	No physiologic implications; may require counseling with partner to overcome hesitancy	Pro: Allows intercourse to continue; enhances partner satisfaction Con: Personal inhibition may make this appear as a nonlegitimate option

nurses still have an obligation to address this aspect of care. Factors influencing sexual dysfunction in diabetic women include depression, marital dissatisfaction, difficulty adjusting to the diagnosis, and low satisfaction with diabetic treatment options. Sexual dysfunction in men also appears to be related to depression, as well as poor adjustment to the diagnosis and negative appraisal of the disease (Enzlin, Matieu, & Demytteanere, 2003). Nurses should assume that all clients with diabetes will experience a sexual difficulty at some point after diagnosis and *routinely* assess the sexual concerns of their clients. Women who report vaginal dryness can be encouraged to use over-the-counter water-soluble vaginal lubricants. Eating yogurt with active cultures may help in reducing the frequency of yeast infections. Maintaining close control over fluctuations in their blood glucose levels will also reduce the frequency of yeast infections. Couples should be referred to counseling as issues arise related to the strains of living with a chronic illness in order that better communication may occur about these issues.

Cancer

Cancer occurs in people of all ages. Cancer happens to an individual, a couple, and to a family. A complete discussion of the multiple ways cancer can have an impact on sexuality is beyond the scope of this chapter; for more detailed information, the reader is referred to any of the major cancer nursing textbooks and publications by the Oncology Nursing Society. This discussion is limited to the general ways that cancer and cancer treatments affect sexuality.

In general, surgical treatments for cancer have an impact on body image and the ability to function sexually. Surgical procedures for cancers of the gastrointestinal system can lead to sexual difficulties secondary to damage to nerves that enervate sexual organs or cause alterations in body image that affect sexuality. Other procedures may involve removal of or alterations in organs that directly impact the ability to function sexually. Radical hysterectomy renders a woman unable to bear children and will lead to a surgically induced menopause if oophorectomy is included in the procedure. Because of removal of the upper portion of the vagina, women and their partners may be concerned that having a shortened vagina may preclude satisfactory sexual intercourse. Postoperative discussions should include discussion of positions that might reduce dyspareunia.

Men also experience sexual side effects from surgical intervention. Characteristics associated with postoperative sexual recovery after radical prostatectomy include younger age, use of nerve-sparing techniques, smaller prostate at time of surgery, pretreatment erectile ability, presence of a sexually functional partner, and absence of androgen deprivation (Hollenbeck, Dunn, Wei, Sandler, & Sanda, 2004). Specific information regarding the effects of other surgical procedures on sexual functioning is found in Table 10-4.

Radiation therapy can cause alterations in organ functioning, primary organ failure resulting in either permanent or temporary alterations in fertility, as well as side effects that are not directly related to sexual functioning (Table 10-5). Fertility may be preserved by the use of modern radiation therapy techniques and the use of lead shields to protect the testes. Women diagnosed with invasive cervical cancer are frequently treated by a combination of external and internal radiation therapy. Side effects include fatigue, diarrhea, vaginal dryness, and vaginal stenosis (Maher, 2005). Vaginal dryness will definitely occur; however, vaginal stenosis can be prevented. A patent vagina is important in maintaining sexual function as well as allowing for adequate follow-up evaluations. Women must be educated about the need to either use a vaginal dilator or have vaginal intercourse on a regular basis (Wilmoth & Spinelli, 2000). In women older than 40 years, infertility may occur at lower doses of radiation. Women may undergo surgery to protect the ovaries by moving them out of the field of radiation (National Cancer Institute, 2007). Likewise, men who receive either external beam or brachytherapy for prostate cancer are at increased risk of sexual dysfunction (Hollenbeck et al., 2004). Current techniques such as conformal external-beam radiation therapy are reported

to lead to ED in as many as 40–60% of men with prostate cancer (Zelefky et al., 2006). These rates of ED are also reported in newer techniques of delivery of radiation therapy such as intensity-modulated radiation therapy (IMRT).

Chemotherapy treatments frequently cause temporary or permanent infertility. These side effects are related to a number of factors, including the client's gender, age at time of treatment, the specific type and dose of radiation therapy and/or chemotherapy, the use of single therapy or multiple therapies, and the length of time since treatment (National Cancer Institute, 2007). The extent of the impact on fertility varies according to the patient's gender, type of cancer, and the type and dosage of chemotherapy. Combination chemotherapy that includes alkylating agents and being a woman older than age 35 appear to be the primary factors related to altered fertility. In addition to altered fertility, chemotherapy can lead to altered ovarian function and subsequent menopause (McInnes & Schilsky, 1996). Menopausal symptoms such as hot flashes, vaginal dryness, and skin changes in addition to chemotherapy side effects can be traumatic for women, particularly if they are not aware of the potential for menopause (Wilmoth, unpublished data). The nurse could suggest use of vitamin E, use of water-soluble vaginal lubricants, and doing Kegel exercises to reduce symptoms (Wilmoth, 1996). In addition to the lubricating effect of the over-the-counter water-soluble lubricants, several products have demonstrated a positive effect against HIV infection with use. Astroglide, Vagisil, and ViAmor inhibited HIV production by 0.1000-fold when mixed with cells in seminal fluid, and 0.30-fold when layered on the cells in the two experiments shown in comparison with nonoxynol-9 (Baron, Poast, Nguyen, & Cloyd, 2004).

The use of alkylating agents in men has a major impact on their sexuality and fertility. Men who receive cumulative doses greater than 400 mg are always azoospermic, as are those treated with cisplatin (Krebs, 2005). Adult men, regardless of age, are likely to experience long-term side

TABLE 10-4

Effects of Cancer Surgery on Sexual Functioning

Type of Surgery	Effects on Sexual Functioning	Client Education
Colorectal surgery with colostomy	Varies; depends on type and extent of surgical procedure; major impact on body image and self-concept	Encourage expression of feelings and communication with partner.
Abdominoperineal resection	Females: shortening of vagina; vaginal scarring may cause dyspareunia; decreased lubrication if ovaries also are removed Males: erectile dysfunction; decrease in amount/force of ejaculate or retrograde ejaculation because of interruption of sympathetic and parasympathetic nerve supply. Amount of rectal tissue removed appears to determine degree of dysfunction. Capacity for orgasm not altered.	Use water-soluble lubricant prior to intercourse; allow more time for pleasuring before attempting penetration; with shortened vagina, use coital positions that decrease depth of penetration (e.g., side-to-side lying, man on top with legs outside the woman's, woman on top). Erectile dysfunction may be temporary or permanent; encourage use of touch, other means of communication.
Transurethral resection of bladder/partial cystectomy	Mild pain or dyspareunia	Encourage more time for pleasuring.
Radical cystectomy	Females: surgery usually includes removal of bladder, urethra, uterus, ovaries, fallopian tubes, and anterior portion of vagina. Males: surgery involves removal of bladder, prostate, seminal vesicles, pelvic lymph nodes, and possibly urethra. May cause retrograde or loss of ejaculation and decrease in or loss of erectile ability.	Vaginal reconstruction is possible; use water-soluble lubricant; encourage self-pleasuring and use of dilators; encourage use of touch and other means of sexual communication. Explore possibility for penile implant.
Radical prostatectomy	Involves removal of prostate, seminal vesicles, and vas deferens. Damage to autonomic nerves near prostate may cause loss of erectile ability; loss of emission and ejaculation.	Desire, penile sensations, and orgasmic abilities not altered. Explore possibility for penile prosthesis.
Transurethral resection of prostate	Causes retrograde ejaculation because of damage to internal bladder sphincter	Reassure that erection and orgasm will still occur but that ejaculate will be decreased or absent; urine may be cloudy.
Bilateral orchiectomy	Results in low levels of testosterone; causes sterility, decreased libido, impotence, gynecomastia, penile atrophy, and decreased growth of body hair and beard.	Discuss option of sperm banking prior to surgery; discuss optional ways of expressing sexuality with patient and partner.

(Continued)

TABLE 10-4		

Effects of Cancer Surgery on Sexual Functioning (*Continued*)

Type of Surgery	Effects on Sexual Functioning	Client Education
Retroperitoneal lymph node dissection	Damages sympathetic nerves necessary for ejaculation; results in temporary or permanent loss of ejaculation; patient maintains potency and orgasmic ability	Discuss option of sperm banking.
Total abdominal hysterectomy with bilateral salpingo-oophorectomy	Loss of circulating estrogens; decrease in vaginal elasticity, decrease in vaginal lubrication; some women report decreased desire, orgasm, and enjoyment.	Use water-soluble lubricants; intercourse may be resumed after 6-week post-op check; encourage discussion about meaning of loss of uterus to self-identity.
Mastectomy	Decrease in arousal associated with nipple stimulation; affects body image, self-concept	Encourage communication with partner.
Radical vulvectomy	Removal of labia majora, labia minora, clitoris, bilateral pelvic node dissection; loss of sexually responsive tissue with concomitant loss of vasocongestive neuromuscular response	Possibility of perineal reconstruction with split-thickness skin graft or gracilis muscle grafts. Intercourse is still possible; explore ways of achieving arousal other than genital stimulation. Preoperative and postoperative counseling are essential.
Penectomy	Degree of sexual limitation depends on length of remaining penile shaft. Glans will be removed; remainder of shaft of penile tissue will respond with tumescence and will allow ejaculation and orgasm.	Discuss possibility of artificial insemination if children are desired.

effects of chemotherapy. However, age, total dose, and time since therapy are essential to recovery of fertility. If fertility is to recover, normal sperm counts should return to normal within 3 years after completion of treatment. In women older than 40 years, infertility may occur at lower doses of radiation. Fertility may be preserved by the use of modern radiation therapy techniques and the use of lead shields to protect the testes. Men and their partners should be counseled about the effects of chemotherapy on fertility and sexuality and offered the option of semen cryopreservation (Krebs, 2005).

Multiple Sclerosis

Multiple sclerosis (MS) has the potential to have a profound impact on the sexual relationships of couples, owing to the resulting motor, sensory, and cognitive alterations. The prevalence of sexual difficulties ranges between 60–80% in males and 20–60% in women (McCabe, 2002). Sexual difficulties in persons with MS can be classified as being primary, secondary, or tertiary in origin (Lowden, O'Leary, & Stevenson, 2005). Primary sexual problems are those that are caused by the pathologic damage to the central nervous system and hormonal issues (Lowden et al., 2005).

TABLE 10-5

Site-Specific Effects of Radiation Therapy on Sexuality

Radiated site	Effect on Sexuality	Client Education
Testes	Reduction in sperm count begins in 6 to 8 weeks and continues for 1 year. Doses of 2 Gy will result in temporary sterility for about 12 months. Doses ≥5 Gy result in permanent sterility. Libido and potency will be maintained.	Discuss sperm banking prior to therapy and continued use of contraceptives.
Prostate	External beam: temporary or permanent erectile dysfunction because of fibrosis of pelvic vasculature or radiation damage of pelvic nerves. Interstitial: less incidence of impotency	Age is variable—men older than age 60 have higher incidence of impotence. Erectile dysfunction—may experience pain during ejaculation because of irritation of urethra. Potency preserved in 70–90% of men who were potent before treatment.
Cervix/vaginal canal	External beam: vaginal stenosis and fibrosis, fistula, cystitis Intracavitary: vaginal stenosis, dry, friable tissue, loss of lubrication. Both result in decreased vaginal sensation and dyspareunia.	Use of water-soluble lubricant; empty bladder before and after sex; encourage pleasuring prior to attempting penetration; use dilators or frequent intercourse to lessen amount of stenosis. Explore new positions for intercourse to allow woman control over depth of penile penetration.
Pelvic region	Women: temporary or permanent sterility dependent on dose of radiation, volume of tissue irradiated, and woman's age; the closer to menopause, the more likely permanent sterility will result. A single dose of 3.75 Gy will cause complete cessation of menses in women older than age 40. Men: temporary or permanent erectile dysfunction secondary to vascular or nerve damage	Oophoropexy and shielding may help to maintain fertility in women; continue use of contraceptives; use of water-soluble lubricant Both genders: encourage alternate means to express sexuality, such as touch.
Breast	Skin reactions, changes in breast sensations	Explore alternate pleasuring techniques and good communication techniques; breastfeeding should occur on nonradiated side.

Source: Wilmoth, M.C. (1998). Sexuality. In C. Burke (Ed.), *Psychosocial dimensions of oncology nursing care* (pp. 102–127). Pittsburgh: Oncology Nursing Press.

Secondary problems arise from symptoms including bladder dysfunction, fatigue, pain, cognitive dysfunction, and mobility issues (Lowden et al., 2005). Tertiary causes are psychological in nature, and are primarily related to attitudes and feelings about sexuality that are compounded by the interaction of the disease process and societal norms about sexuality (Lowden et al., 2005).

CASE STUDY

Jackson Smith is a 67-year-old African American man who has been living in the Willow Haven retirement center since June of 2006. Upon admission he had been diagnosed with chronic hypertension, depression, hyperthyroidism, and with one occurrence of being admitted to the emergency department with a reported medical diagnosis of pneumonia. Mr. Smith stayed at the hospital for treatment for 12 days and was then released.

Within the last 2 months Mr. Smith has become noticeably fatigued and has been having frequent headaches, which he has documented daily. Upon admission the client weight was 192 pounds. Mr. Smith has reported a loss of 24 lbs in a 2-month period. Mr. Smith's memory and attention span have been decreased, and when questioned about his memory he always replied either "It's probably due to my medications" or "I'm just getting old." From the given information the nurse reviewed Mr. Smith's current medications.

Current scheduled medications include: Inderal (propranolol), Prinivil (lisinopril)), Tapazole (methimazole), Viagra (sildenafil citrate), and Lexapro (escitalopram). PRN orders include: Ativan (lorazepam) and Tylenol (acetaminophen).

When questioned about his current medications he reported that he hadn't changed any medications, although he had been taking Viagra for the last couple of years in which he said it has been extremely effective in his social life, Mr. Smith states "I feel like a new man." In the course of completing a sexual assessment, Mr. Smith reported still having sex with multiple female partners weekly at the retirement home. He stated that he has always been sexually active, and that now he is able to assist his ED, which is caused primarily by his chronic hypertension with the simple easy use of Viagra

(sildenafil citrate). The nurse included assessment of Mr. Smith's knowledge and use of safe sex practices. The nurse also prepared Mr. Smith for having a complete physical examination, including having laboratory studies that would include complete blood count (CBC), HIV testing, and tests for sexually transmitted diseases.

Findings from the physical examination included finding that the patient had recently experienced finding blisters around his genitalia. A sample of the lesion was cultured and was diagnosed as herpes simplex type 2 (HSV-2). Blood work revealed that he was HIV-1- positive and CD4 count was 120 (fewer than 200 cells per mm3 may result in suppressed immune function).

During a counseling session with the nurse once all results were in, the nurse shared with Mr. Smith that he indeed had contracted the HIV virus, that he would have to begin a regular regimen of treatment, and that it was now critical for him to practice safe sex to prevent the spread to other partners. Mr. Smith was devastated with the results and exclaimed he didn't understand how he could have been affected with this illness, for when he was younger HIV/ AIDS wasn't around or heard of. He was educated on how this illness is a growing problem across the United States, and that anyone who is not using safe sex measures can contract the illness. In addition, he was instructed that he probably contracted the illness during unprotected sex with a female partner in which a blood to blood interaction could have occurred. He was informed that he now is a carrier of the disease, and that it is most important for him to understand how to prevent the spread to others. Mr. Smith shook his head, and then offered up any important information related to the other partners with whom he had a sexual relationship with at the retirement center.

(Continued)

CASE STUDY *(Continued)*

The occurrence of this HIV diagnosis was discussed with the nursing staff, and it was decided that all cognitively sound residents would receive a pamphlet concerning the increased risk of HIV/AIDS in the elderly population. In addition, included in the pamphlet would be ways to prevent the contracting of HIV virus by the use of safe sex practices, and by restating constantly throughout the pamphlet that there is no age limit on who can contract the HIV virus.

Discussion Questions

1. How would the nurse approach teaching safe sex practices in a senior living environment?
2. What signs or symptoms of early HIV would a geriatric patient most likely present with?
3. How would the nurse approach teaching senior citizens how to begin to use safe sex practices?

Neurologic changes caused by MS can affect sexual feelings as well as sexual response. There are common issues that affect both men and women in achieving sexual response; most prominently changes in sensation that lead to sexual stimuli and the ability to achieve orgasm (Lowden et al., 2005). Counseling for underlying emotional concerns as well as depression may affect treatment of desire problems as well. Changes in genital sensations can be troubling, because something that used to feel good may now be noxious. Teaching couples to communicate about these changes and to try new techniques may be helpful. Vaginal dryness can be improved with the use of water-soluble lubricants. Unfortunately, treatment of ED in men is not as easily remedied. Treatment options for ED in MS are the same as those for men with other chronic illnesses and can be found in Table 10-3.

Secondary sexual alterations caused by MS are a result of the physical symptoms that accompany the disease. Spasticity during sexual activity appears to affect women more than it does men and may be controlled by baclofen, chemical nerve blocks, and surgery. Bowel and bladder problems can cause significant alterations in sexuality and can severely impair spontaneity of sexual activity. Engaging in sexual activity successfully requires open communication as well as aggressive symptom management. Limiting fluid intake for several hours prior to sexual activity and urinating immediately before sexual activity can help with bladder control. Medications are available for incontinence; however, these medications may also increase vaginal dryness. Intermittent catheterization or taping a permanent catheter out of the way can allow successful activity. Bowel problems may be either ones of constipation, no control, or lack of predictability of function. A regular bowel regimen consisting of laxatives, enemas, or disimpaction can allow stress-free sexual interactions.

Fatigue is a pervasive symptom of MS as well as other chronic illnesses. In MS, fatigue can be managed with several pharmacologic agents and energy-conserving techniques. Medications include amantadine or pemoline. Use of wheelchairs or motorized carts or regular naps during the day can allow clients to conserve energy for activities they enjoy, including sexual activity. Cognitive impairment can also have a pervasive impact on a relationship. Memory loss, impaired judgment, and other problems can impair the interpersonal communication that is integral in any intimate relationship.

The psychosocial changes that accompany MS cause tertiary sexual dysfunction. Decreased self-concept, grieving for loss of self, and role changes affect both the client and the partner. Persons with MS report lower levels of sexual activity, sexual satisfaction, and relationship satisfaction than those without MS (McCabe, McKern, McDonald,

& Vowels, 2003). Ongoing counseling and participation in support groups can help couples deal with these sexual and relationship issues caused by MS (McCabe, 2002).

INTERVENTIONS

Sexual Assessment

Sexuality should be a routine part of every physician- or nurse-initiated assessment for nearly every client diagnosed with a chronic illness (Wilmoth, 2000, 2006). Assessing sexuality as routinely as other body systems serves two purposes. First, it decreases embarrassment on the part of the client and practitioner if it is accepted as a normal aspect of health care. Second, routine inclusion will give the client permission to mention sexual difficulties to the practitioner and give the practitioner permission to ask specific questions when it is suspected that the client might be experiencing a sexually related side effect of the disease or treatment.

The clinician should keep the same principles in mind when discussing sexuality, as any other topic, with a client and/or partner. The CIEF) suggests that many clients have unrealistic expectations about the efficacy of not only phosphodiesterase type 5 (PDE5) inhibitors but also other treatment options (CIEF, 2007). Clients need reassurance about the safety of treatments for issues with sexuality. These instances again reinforce the importance of the clinician as an educator, and emphasize the professional nature of these discussions: clarify the content component of communications, and reinforce permission to include sexuality in the plan of care. An example of a bridge question is, "has anyone talked with you about how your (injury/illness/treatments) can affect your ability to have sex?" "Unloading" a topic is another technique that is useful in discussing sexuality and can ease a client's concern once he or she learns that others have experienced this problem (Woods, 1984). An example of unloading is, "Many women who have received chemotherapy have had problems with vaginal dryness. What problems have you had with this?"

The inclusion of questions on sexuality in the admission assessment is an excellent way to legitimize the role of the nurse in addressing sexuality. Woods (1984) suggests that such questions should proceed from less intimate questions, such as role functioning, to more personal ones on sexual functioning. Closed (yes/no) questions should be avoided, as they eliminate opportunities for further discussion. Questions for an initial assessment include the following (Woods, 1984; Wilmoth, 1994a):

- How has (diagnosis/treatment) affected your role as wife/husband/partner?
- How has (diagnosis/treatment) affected the way you feel about yourself as woman/man?
- What aspects of your sexuality do you believe have been affected by your diagnosis/treatment?
- How has your (diagnosis/treatment) affected your ability to function sexually?

A more medically focused sexual evaluation might include determination of chief complaint, sexual status, medical status, psychiatric status, family and psychosexual history, relationship assessment, and summary with recommendations (Auchincloss, 1990; Krebs, 2007). A complete sexual history is not usually indicated unless initial assessment indicates the presence of a sexual problem. Most nurses are not adequately prepared to conduct a full sexual assessment; therefore, referral to a more appropriate practitioner is appropriate.

Including Sexuality in Practice

Four areas of competency must be achieved for nurses to successfully include sexuality into practice to attain the published standards of practice: comfort with one's own sexuality and comfort in discussing sexuality with others; excellent communication skills; a knowledge base about sexuality in health and illness; and role models to demonstrate integration of sexuality into practice (Woods, 1984; Wilmoth, 1994b).

Comfort with sexuality and enhancement of communication skills can be attained through reading, values clarification exercises, and participation in courses on sexuality. Some options include semester-long college courses related to sexuality or shorter weekend courses, often referred to as "SARs." Sexual attitude reassessment, or SAR, programs combine explicit films with small group discussions over a 2- or 3-day period to allow for analysis of one's personal values surrounding sexuality. Knowing one's own values and attitudes toward a variety of other sexual practices and sexual orientation is the first step in becoming comfortable with sexuality (Wilmoth, 1994a). Values clarification exercises can assist in this process. The outcome of clarifying one's values about sexuality is knowing what one believes is acceptable sexual behavior. It is important to remember that there is no right or wrong set of behaviors or values, just different ones.

Comfort in discussing sexuality and enhancing the ability to communicate clearly about sexuality can be achieved through a variety of methods. One option is to form a discussion group or journal club among colleagues. This group could engage in discussion of values clarification exercises or articles related to human sexuality in general or disease-focused articles on sexuality. Sharing with a peer group, particularly an interdisciplinary peer group, is a nonthreatening way in which to become comfortable talking about sexuality. This approach also assists with increasing knowledge about a variety of illnesses, their treatments, and their effects on sexuality.

Nurses are skilled communicators, but they initially may find initiating discussions with clients about sexuality anxiety provoking. Nurses should assume that their clients have some form of sexual experience rather than none at all, and should also assume that they have questions about the impact of their disease or its treatments on their sexuality. Experience has shown that patients are most appreciative when asked about this part of life in relation to their chronic illness. Nurses should use terminology, including slang that their clients understand, and should not hesitate to use appropriate humor in seeking clarification. For example, "that's a new one for me . . . What is that?" This can help diffuse a tense situation for both client and nurse.

Participation in each of the aforementioned processes will add to the nurse's knowledge base about normal sexual functioning. The professional nurse should also engage in independent study within their specialty regarding the effects that the illnesses, treatments, and medications have on sexuality. Engaging in discussions with other healthcare providers, such as physicians or pharmacists, or through participation in interdisciplinary journal clubs and research projects, can add depth to the nurses' knowledge. Such interdisciplinary efforts will have large payoffs for clients and their partners.

Nurses who are comfortable with their own sexuality, are proficient communicators, and have knowledge about sexuality possess the foundation necessary to include sexuality into their practice. However, many are still reluctant to do so. Peers who can role-model the incorporation of sexuality into nursing practice may be influential in helping others incorporate it into their practices. Role models can assist in this process by relating positive experiences with clients about discussions surrounding sexuality, by role-playing ways of initiating discussions about sexuality, and by acting as a resource for staff. However, there is little research documenting the effectiveness of role models in teaching others to incorporate sexuality into practice.

Grand rounds and presentations of individual cases that exemplify typical sexual concerns associated with a particular treatment, medication, or diagnosis are other strategies for enhancing comfort in including sexual discussions into practice. Physicians and pharmacists could discuss a particular disease process and treatment options, including medications and their effect on sexual functioning. A social worker or clinical nurse specialist skilled in assessing and educating about sexual issues could lead practitioners through the sexual assessment and educational process. Finally, a clinician or sex therapist could discuss interventions that the majority of practitioners could use in their counseling of persons with sexual issues.

Many health professionals use the PLISSIT model (Annon, 1976) to assist them in their sexual assessments. In this model, P stands for *permission;* LI, for *limited information,* SS, for *specific suggestions,* and IT, for *intensive therapy* (Figure 10-2). Mims and Swenson (1978) suggest that all nurses should be able to intervene at all levels except for provision of intensive therapy. If assessment suggests a problem beyond the level of needing specific suggestions, the client and partner should be referred to a sex therapist.

OUTCOMES

Desired client and partner outcomes that may be anticipated after nursing intervention include the following (American Nurses Association/Oncology Nursing Society, 2004):

- The ability to identify potential/actual changes in sexuality, sexual functioning, or intimacy related to disease and treatment.

- The ability to express feelings about alopecia, body image changes, and altered sexual functioning.
- The ability to engage in open communication with his or her partner regarding changes in sexual functioning or desire, within a cultural framework.
- The ability to describe appropriate interventions for actual or potential changes in sexual function.
- The ability to identify personal and community resources to assist with changes in body image and sexuality.

ACKNOWLEDGMENTS

The authors would like to acknowledge Vanessa LaLoggia, RN, BSN, MSN(c) and Devin High, BSN student for assistance in preparation of the evidence-based practice box, case study, and revisions.

FIGURE 10-2

PLISSIT Model

Permission (P):	(Assessment) Actions taken by the nurse to let the patient/partner know that sexual issues are a legitimate aspect in providing nursing care. This could include questions about sexuality that are incorporated into the general admission assessment or questions specifically related to their disease process or treatment.
Limited Information (LI):	(Education) Sharing of information regarding the effects of disease, treatments, and medications. Examples of limited information include discussing when sexual intercourse may be resumed after surgery, the possibility of menopause occurring in conjunction with chemotherapy, or medications leading to erectile dysfunction.
Specific Suggestions (SS):	(Counseling) This level of care requires specialized knowledge about specific conditions and their relationship to sexual functioning. Various techniques, positions, and alternate techniques useful in achieving sexual satisfaction are examples of counseling concerns.
Intensive Therapy (IT):	(Referral) Treatment of sexual dysfunction requires specialized training in psychotherapy, sex therapy techniques, crisis intervention, and behavior modification.

Source: Annon, J.S. (1976). *The behavioral treatment of sexual problems: Volume I: Brief therapy.* New York: Harper & Row.

EVIDENCE-BASED PRACTICE BOX

The Agency for Healthcare Research conducted a phase 1 feasibility study in November 2004, for the determination of *Quality Sexuality and Reproductive Health following Spinal Cord Injury (SCI)*. The reviewed evidence included published and unpublished studies along with any study involving randomized controlled trials (RCTs) that enrolled male, female, adult and adolescent populations with SCI. The study addressed two main inquiries related to sexuality post–spinal cord injury. The topics included the current fertility rate for men and women and how the availability of Viagra (sildenafil citrate) and other interventions have affected sexual function, frequency of activity, and adjustment post injury. The results concluded that in the arena of fertility, to achieve pregnancy and birth rates of 50% or greater, SCI couples needed to use an advanced fertility technique illustrated as Testicular Biopsy or Intracytoplasmic Sperm Injection. These techniques improved the chances of a live birth to greater than 50%, but were accompanied by a high level of expense and risks associated with an invasive procedure.

The second inquiry of the study explored how the availability of Viagra and other alternate interventions have affected sexual function, frequency of activity, and adjustment post spinal cord injury. The alternate interventions explored included biofeedback, perineal exercises, topical agents (e.g., nitroglycerin, minoxidil, prostaglandin, and papaverine), and intracavernous penile injections (e.g. papaverine, phentolamine, and prostaglandin E1) with an overall patient satisfactory erection response of 90%. In comparison, the use of vacuum tumescence devices, and penile implants demonstrated 20–50% effectiveness in erection response. The exclusive examination of the use of Viagra demonstrated an overall 79% success rate in treatment of erectile dysfunction, and an 84% overall patient satisfactory erection response. The frequency of activity, and adjustment post spinal cord injury correlated with the patient satisfactory response to each method. The analytic approach for this project was a combined qualitative and quantitative exploration on the data available for erectile dysfunction. It provides the strongest possible evidence-based interventions in the arena of sexuality post spinal cord injury available to date.

Source: US Department of Health and Human Services, Agency for Healthcare Research and Quality. (2004). *Sexuality and Reproductive Health Following Spinal Cord Injury*. AHRQ Publication No. 05-E003–2. November, 2004.

STUDY QUESTIONS

1. Why is it important for nurses and other healthcare professionals to include a sexual assessment and sexual education when providing care?
2. What are key changes in sexual response that should be expected to occur with healthy aging?
3. In general, what changes in sexuality are caused by chemotherapy in women? In men?
4. What do men and their partners need to know about the pathophysiology of diabetes mellitus on erectile ability and options to continue sexual intercourse?

5. What should be discussed about sexuality with a patient newly diagnosed with multiple sclerosis?

6. What are some methods that a nurse manager could implement with a nursing staff to increase comfort and knowledge regarding the impact of disease on sexuality?

REFERENCES

Agewall, S., Berglund, M. & Henareh, L. (2004). Reduced quality of life after myocardial infarction in women compared with men. *Clinical Cardiology, 27*(5), 271–274.

American Nurses Association. (2004). *Nursing: Scope and standards of practice.* Washington DC: Author.

American Psychiatric Association. (1994). *Diagnostic and statistical manual of mental disorders* (4th ed.). Washington DC: Author.

American Nurses Association/Oncology Nursing Society. (2004). *Statement on scope and standards of oncology nursing practice.* Washington DC: Author.

Andrews, M., Goldberg, K., & Kaplan, H. (Eds.). (1996). *Nurse's legal handbook* (3rd ed.). Springhouse, PA: Springhouse Corporation.

Annon, J.S. (1976). *The behavioral treatment of sexual problems: Volume I: Brief therapy.* New York: Harper & Row.

Auchincloss, S.S. (1990). Sexual dysfunction in cancer patients: Issues in evaluation and treatment. In J.C. Holland & J.H. Rowland (Eds.), *Handbook of psychooncology* (pp.383–413). New York: Oxford University Press.

Baron, S., Poast, J., Nguyen, D., & Cloyd, M. (2004). Practical prevention of vaginal and rectal transmission of HIV by adapting the oral defense: Use of commercial lubricants. *AIDS Research and Human Retrovirus, 17*(11), 978–1002.

Bhasin, S., Enzlin, P., Coviello, A., & Basson, R. (2007). Sexual dysfunction in men and women with endocrine disorders. *Lancet, 369*(9561), 597–611.

Centers for Disease Control, Office of Minority Health. (2004). Eliminate disparities in cardiovascular disease. Accessed November 3, 2004 from www.cdc.gov/omh/AMH/factsheets/cardio.htm

Consortium for Improvement in Erectile Dysfunction, (CIEF) (2007). *Collaborative for advancement of urological, sexual, and endocrine education.* Retrieved November 11, 2007 from erectilefunction.org/index.html

Corona, G., Mannucci, R., Mansani, R., Petrone, L., Bartolini, M., Glommi, R., et al. (2007). Aging and pathogenesis of erectile dysfunction. *International Journal of Impotence Research, 16*(5), 395–402.

Darling, C.A., Davidson, J.K., & Conway-Welch, C. (1990). Female ejaculation: Perceived origins, the Grafenberg spot/area, and sexual responsiveness. *Archives of Sexual Behavior, 19,* 29–47.

DeBusk, R. (2000). Evaluating the cardiovascular tolerance for sex. *The American Journal of Cardiology, 86*(2A), 51F–56F.

Enzlin, P., Mathieu, C., Van den Bruel, A., Bosteels, J., Vanderschueren, D., & Demyttenaere, K. (2002). Sexual dysfunction in women with Type 1 diabetes: A controlled study. *Diabetes Care, 25,* 672–677.

Enzlin, P., Matieu, C., & Demytteanere, K. (2003). Diabetes and female sexual functioning: A state-of-the-art. *Diabetes Spectrum,16,* 256–259.

Grandjean, C., & Moran, B., (2007). The impact of diabetes mellitus on female sexual well-being. Retrieved November 22, 2007 from www.nursing.theclinics.com

Guyton, A.C., & Hall, J.E. (2006). *Textbook of medical physiology* (11th ed.) Philadelphia: Elsevier Saunders.

Hines, T.M. (2001). The G-spot: A modern gynecologic myth. *American Journal of Obstetrics and Gynecology, 185*(2), 359–362.

Hollenbeck, B.K., Dunn, R.L., Wei, J.T., Sandler, H.M., & Sanda, M.G. (2004). Sexual health recovery after prostatectomy, external radiation or brachytherapy for early stage prostate cancer. *Current Urology Reports, 5,* 212–219.

Jackson, G. (2004). Sexual dysfunction and diabetes. *International Journal of Clinical Practice, 58*(4), 358–362.

Jensen, S. B. (1981). Diabetic sexual dysfunction: A comparative study of 160 insulin-treated diabetic men and women and an age-matched control group. *Archives of Sexual Behavior, 10,* 493–504.

Kaplan, H.S. (1979). *Disorders of sexual desire and other new concepts and techniques in sex therapy.* New York: Simon & Schuster.

Katz, A. (2007). *Breaking the silence on cancer and sexuality. A handbook for healthcare providers.* Pittsburgh: Oncology Nursing Society.

Kolodny, R.C. (1971). Sexual dysfunction in diabetic females. *Diabetes, 20,* 557–559.

Kolodny, R., Masters, W., Johnson, V., & Biggs, M. (1979). *The textbook for human sexuality for nurses.* Boston: Little, Brown.

Kostis, J.B., Jackson, G., Rosen, R., Barrett-Connor, E., Billups, K., Burnett, A.L., et al. (2005). Sexual dysfunction and cardiac risk, the second Princeton consensus conference. Retrieved November 3, 2007 from www.AJConline.org

Koukouras, D., Spiliotis, J., Scopa, C.D., Dragotis, K., Kalfarentzos, F., Tzoracoleftherakis, E., et al. (1991). Radical consequence in the sexuality of male patients operated for colorectal carcinoma. *European Journal of Surgical Oncology, 17,* 285–288.

Krebs, L.U. (2005). Sexual and reproductive dysfunction. In C.H. Yarbro, M.H. Frogge, M. Goodman, & S.L. Groenwald (Eds.), *Cancer nursing: Principles and practice* (6th ed.) (pp. 841–869). Sudbury, MA: Jones & Bartlett.

Krebs, L.U. (2007). Sexual assessment: Research and clinical. *Nursing Clinics of North America, 42*(4), 515–529.

Ladas, A.K., Whipple, B., and Perry, J.D. (1982). *The G-spot.* New York: Dell.

Leiblum, S.R., & Segraves, R.T. (1989). Sex therapy with aging adults. In S.R. Leiblum & R.C. Rosen (Eds.), *Principles and practice of sex therapy: Update for the 1990s* (2nd ed.) (pp. 352–381). New York: Guilford Press.

Masters, W.H., & Johnson, V.E. (1966). *Human sexual response.* Philadelphia: Lippincott-Raven.

Lindau, S.T., Schumm, L.P., Gaumann, E.O., Levinson, W., O'Muircheartaigh, C.A. & Waite, L.J. (2007). A study of sexuality and health among older adults in the United States. *New England Journal of Medicine, 357*(8), 820–822.

Lowden, D., O'Leary, M., Stevenson, B. (2005). Sexuality issues in patients with MS. *Multiple Sclerosis Counseling Points, 1,* 1–9.

Maher, K. (2005). Radiation therapy: Toxicities and management. In C.H.Yarbro, M.H. Frogge & M. Goodman (Eds.). *Cancer Nursing: Principles and Practice* (6th ed.) (pp. 283–314). Sudbury, MA:Jones & Bartlett.

Masters, W.H. & Johnson, V.E. (1966). *Human sexual response.* Philadelphia: Lippincott-Raven.

Masters, W.H., & Johnson, V.E. (1981). Sex and the aging process. *Journal of the American Geriatrics Society, 24*(9), 385–390.

McCabe, M.P. (2002). Relationship functioning and sexuality among people with multiple sclerosis. *The Journal of Sex Research, 39*(4), 302–309.

McCabe, M.P., McKern, S., McDonald, E., & Vowels, L.M. (2003). Changes over time in sexual and relationship functioning of people with multiple sclerosis. *Journal of Sex & Marital Therapy, 29*(4), 305–321.

McInnes, S., & Schilsky, R.L. (1996). Infertility following cancer chemotherapy. In B.A. Chabner & D.L. Longo (Eds.), *Cancer chemotherapy and biotherapy* (2nd ed.) (pp. 31–44). Philadelphia: Lippincott-Raven.

Meston, C.M. (2000). Sympathetic nervous system activity and female sexual arousal. *The American Journal of Cardiology, 86*(2) (Suppl. 1), 30–34.

Meston, C.M. & Gorzalka, B.B. (1996). The differential effects of sympathetic activation on sexual arousal in sexually functional and dysfunctional women. *Journal of Abnormal Psychology, 105,* 582–591.

Mims, F., & Swenson, M. (1978). A model to promote sexual health care. *Nursing Outlook, 26*(2), 121–125.

National Cancer Institute (2007). Sexual and reproductive issues. Retrieved November 22, 2007 from www.cancer.gov/templates/doc.aspx?viewid=829ea02d-5eb8-43e8-b0db-54cb0b0f9bc1&version=0&allpages=1#Section_39

National Institutes of Health (NIH). (1992). Impotence. *NIH Consensus Statement, 10* (4), 1–31.

National Diabetes Information Clearinghouse (NDIC). (2007). Retrieved November 21, 2007 from http://diabetes.niddk.nih.gov/dm/pubs/statistics/#11

Oncology Nursing Society. (2004). *Statement on the scope and standards of oncology nursing practice.* Pittsburgh: Author.

O'Farrell, P., Murray, J., & Hotz, S.B. (2000). Psychologic distress among spouses of patients undergoing cardiac rehabilitation. *Heart and Lung, 29*(2), 97–104.

Roose, S.P., & Seidman, S.N. (2000). Sexual activity and cardiac risk: Is depression a contributing factor?

The American Journal of Cardiology, 86(2A), 38F–40F.

Safarine, M., & Hosseini, S. (2004). Erectile dysfunction, clinical guidelines 1. Retrieved November 22, 2007 from www.unrc.ir/urologyjournal/13_1.pdf

Sands, J.K. (1995). Human sexuality. In W.J. Phipps, V.L. Cassmeyer, J.K. Sands, and M.K. Lehmen (Eds.). *Medical surgical nursing: Concepts & clinical practice* (5th ed.) (pp. 262–284). St. Louis: Mosby.

Sarkadi, A. & Rosenquist, U. (2004). Intimacy and women with Type 2 diabetes: An exploratory study using focus group interviews. *The Diabetes Educator,* 29(4), 641–652.

Shril, R., Koskimaki, J., Hakkien, A., Auvinen, T., Tammela, J., & Hakama, M. (2007). Cardiovascular Drug Use and the Incidence of Erectile Dysfunction. *International Journal of Impotence Research,* 19(2), 208–212.

Steinke, E.E. (2000). Sexual counseling after myocardial infarction. *American Journal of Nursing,* 100(12), 38–44.

Svedlund, M. & Danielson, E. (2004). Myocardial infarction: Narrations by afflicted women and their partners of lived experiences in daily life following an acute myocardial infarction. *Journal of Clinical Nursing,* 13(4), 438–446.

Tilton, M.C. (1997). Diabetes and amputation. In M.L. Sipski & C.J. Alexander (Eds.), *Sexual function in people with disability and chronic illness: A health professional's guide* (pp. 279–302). Rockville, MD: Aspen Publishers.

Wilmoth, M.C. (1994a). Strategies for becoming comfortable with sexual assessment. *Oncology Nursing News* (Spring), 6–7.

Wilmoth, M.C. (1994b). Nurses' and patients' perspectives on sexuality: Bridging the gap. *Innovations in Oncology Nursing,* 10(2), 34–36.

Wilmoth, M.C. (1996). The middle years: Women, sexuality and the self. *Journal of Obstetric, Gynecologic, and Neonatal Nursing,* 25, 615–621.

Wilmoth, M.C. (1998). Sexuality. In C. Burke (Ed.), *Psychosocial dimensions of oncology nursing care* (pp. 102–127). Pittsburgh: Oncology Nursing Press.

Wilmoth, M. C. (2000). Sexuality patterns, altered. In L.J. Carpenito (Ed.), *Nursing diagnosis: Application to clinical practice* (8th ed.), (pp. 837–857). Philadelphia: Lippincott.

Wilmoth, M.C. (2006). Life after cancer: What does sexuality have to do with it? The 2006 Mara Mogenson Flaherty Memorial Lectureship. *Oncology Nursing Forum,* 33(5), 905–910.

Wilmoth, M.C., & Spinelli, A. (2000). Sexual implications of gynecologic cancer treatments. *Journal of Obstetrics, Gynecologic and Neonatal Nursing,* 29, 413–421.

Woods, N.F. (1984). *Human sexuality in health and illness* (3rd ed.). St. Louis: Mosby.

Zaviacic, M., & Whipple, B. (1993). Update on the female prostate and the phenomena of female ejaculation. *The Journal of Sex Research,* 30, 48–151.

Zaviacic, M. & Ablin, R.J. (2000). The female prostate and prostate-specific antigen. Immunohistochemical localization, implications for this prostate marker in women, and reasons for using the term "prostate" in the human female. *Histology Histopathology,* 15, 131–142.

11

Powerlessness

Faye I. Hummel

INTRODUCTION

This was the first time . . . When I woke up the other morning I couldn't get out of bed. I couldn't believe it . . . my body, my legs, they just wouldn't move. I was terrified. I thought I'd had a stroke or something. I called for John but he didn't hear me. I just had to lie there, staring at the ceiling, trying to calm myself. I felt so helpless, so powerless. There was nothing I could do but wait for John to come . . . he helped me into the bathtub where the warmth of the water soothed my aching body. I've always been able to handle my never ending pain . . . the stiffness and rigidity of my body, but that morning . . . that morning was different . . . and now I wonder . . .

Anne, 62-year-old woman with fibromyalgia and
Parkinson's disease

Chronic illness changes one's sense of time and one's sense of self. Living with chronic illness requires one to adapt to a continuous changing of outlooks in which the existence of dualities, such as hope and despair, self-control and loss of power, dependence and independence, can elicit feelings of ambiguity, anxiety, and frustration (Delmar et al., 2006). Chronic illness creates threats to well being and produces multidimensional changes and challenges for the individual and his or her family. Whether these changes occur suddenly or over a long period, chronic illness requires that individuals and families deal with and adapt to an unrelenting altered reality. Managing real and perceived powerlessness is significant. Lack of control and the incapacity to act and change may dominate everyday life for persons with chronic illnesses. Accepting and acknowledging one's limitations as a result of chronic illness may result in a sense of helplessness and loss, as evidenced in the case of Anne:

Last week I watched John working in our garden . . . we have planted a garden for years together. I can't work outside anymore . . . I miss getting my hands in the dirt. I had to quit my job too. I was an accountant for years . . . I really miss my work, my friends, we shared so much. Now . . . now my body is just not able. I have so much pain . . . constant . . . pain is ever with me. My body seems foreign to me . . . I'm losing control of my body. It takes me the better part of the day to get around, to take care of myself . . . I try to cook for us and keep house. I try to plan ahead but I'm just not able to do what needs to be done . . . I don't have a choice. John has to do more around the house now days . . . I'm not much help.

The Phenomenon of Powerlessness in Chronic Illness

At some point in the course of their chronic illness, individuals experience powerlessness. Powerlessness in the absolute sense is the inability to affect an outcome; the inability to have agency in one's own life (Miller, 2000). Powerlessness may be a real loss of power or a perceived loss of power. For some persons, the feelings of powerlessness may be short-lived; whereas for others, it is persistent.

What and who determines powerlessness and what factors facilitate powerlessness? The natural history of chronic illness is highly variable and does not conform to a predictable course of events. The uncertainty of chronic illness, the exacerbation of symptoms, failure of therapy, physical deterioration despite adherence to treatment regimens, side effects of drugs, iatrogenic influences, depletion of social support systems, and the disintegration of the client's psychological stamina can all contribute to powerlessness (Miller, 2000). Chronic illness results in a pronounced loss of functioning over time, disrupts social roles and activities, and limits fulfillment of role expectations (Beal, 2007). Fatigue and inability to participate and engage in social activities contribute to social withdrawal (Asbring, 2001; Beal, 2007) and loss of relationships. Loss of employment, social contacts, and physical and mental function can contribute to disempowerment of individuals with chronic illness. The quintessence of ill health is powerlessness (Strandmark, 2004).

Powerlessness occurs when an individual is controlled by the environment rather than the individual controlling the environment. Therefore, powerlessness is a situational attribute (Miller, 2000). In Anne's story, she experiences powerlessness in part because of the degenerative nature of her disease. Despite her previous life successes, Anne now feels powerless over her own circumstances. Although Anne experienced physical limitations associated with her chronic conditions for a number of years, she was able to successfully adapt and respond to the slow progressive deterioration of her physical condition. Anne maintained power and control over her daily life. When she began to experience the crushing effects of her illness symptoms and physical limitations, Anne felt a loss of control, a sense of powerlessness. No longer was Anne able to maintain her veneer of normalcy, nor was she able to sustain her work and home obligations. Anne resigned from her job and she struggled to keep up with her household demands. When Anne begins to consider herself without worth in terms of social norms and expectations, feelings of powerlessness arise. Her autonomy and existence are threatened. Over time, Anne becomes exhausted from fatigue and grief and feels powerless over her life situation (Strandmark, 2004).

Dorothy Johnson was one of the first to explore the concept of powerlessness in nursing. Johnson (1967) defined powerlessness as a "perceived lack of personal or internal control of certain events or in certain situations" (1967, p. 40) and urged nurses to take into account the concept of powerlessness inasmuch as nursing interventions would not be effective, particularly health education, if the client felt powerless. The work of Miller (1983, 1992, 2000) has also been instrumental in the development of the concept of powerlessness in chronic illness. Miller (1983, 1992, 2000) differentiates powerlessness from similar constructs including helplessness, learned helplessness, and locus of control. Helplessness and locus of control are based on a reinforcement paradigm, whereas powerlessness is an existential construct (Miller, 2000). Miller (2000) categorizes locus of control as a personality trait as opposed to powerlessness, which is situationally determined. The physical and psychosocial outcomes of seeking and gaining control over chronic illness have been the focus of research by social scientists since the late 1960s (Wallston et al., 1999). Locus of control and the beliefs of individuals about whom and what controls their lives (Rotter, 1966) are linked to physical and psychological health (Bandura, 1989).

Powerlessness is associated with loss of personal control. Chronic illness strips away individual control. Progressive physiologic changes resulting from chronic illness may limit mobility and/or diminish cognitive abilities. The continuing nature of chronic illness limits possibilities and opportunities to exert control over daily life events as well as plans for the future. Chronic illness sharply delineates the nature and quality of control, often resulting in a sense of powerlessness in individuals and their families.

Illness is described as the ultimate out-of-control experience (McDaniel, Hepworth, & Doherty, 1997, p. 7). Individuals feel the need to have some control over their lives and are distressed when they lose their ability to control important outcomes (Helgeson & Franzen, 1998). Individuals with greater expectations of control and those who place high importance on the desired outcome, experience greater perceived powerlessness during the times when the individual does not have control of a situation or outcome (Wortman & Brehm, 1975). When individuals have a sense of personal control over their chronic illness, they are more likely to have a positive psychological and physical adaptation to their chronic illness than those individuals who do not (Shapiro, Schwartz, & Astin, 1996). Rånhein & Holand (2006) conducted a hermeneutic-phenomenologic study of women's lived experience with chronic pain and fibromyalgia. The themes of powerlessness, ambivalence, and coping emerged from interviews with 12 women with fibromyalgia. The stories of these women revealed their struggles to manage and control the severe symptoms of their disease and their efforts to reduce their feelings of powerlessness that surfaced with pain, fatigue, and immobility. Individuals with chronic illness who develop effective systems for controlling their most severe symptoms have a more positive outlook and a lessened sense of powerlessness.

Seeman and Lewis (1995) examined the relationship between powerlessness, health status, and mortality. They used data from the National Longitudinal Surveys (NLS) conducted by the U.S. Department of Labor beginning in the mid-1960s. This research found that powerlessness was associated with activity limitations and psychosocial symptoms, and increasing powerlessness was associated with deteriorating health status. Richmond, Metcalf, Daly, and Kish (1992) examined powerlessness and its relationship with health status in a sample of clients with spinal cord injuries. The findings revealed a significant correlation between powerlessness and client acuity. Quadriplegics and persons older than age 60 experienced a higher incidence of powerlessness than their more physically able cohorts. Aujoulat, Luminet, and Deccache (2007) conducted interviews with 40 individuals with various chronic conditions and asked them to discuss their experiences of powerlessness. They found that powerlessness extends beyond medical and treatment issues to feelings of insecurity and threats to their social and personal identities. Desperation and powerlessness were expressed by women with long-term urinary incontinence. Women who lacked control of their urinary incontinence reported their autonomy was threatened, which promoted a sense of powerlessness to control their own bodies (Hägglund & Ahlström, 2007).

The phenomenon of powerlessness in chronic illness is a dynamic and complex issue. Powerlessness in chronic illness can be triggered by individual attributes and perceptions or stimulated by the evolving nature of the chronic disease. Powerlessness is inherent and impending in chronic illness. However, feelings of powerlessness recede and advance throughout the course of the chronic illness as individuals negotiate between control and loss and navigate the changing landscape of their daily realities. Variables such as the degree of physical limitation and ability to manage symptoms of chronic illness can also influence an individual's experience with powerlessness.

The Paradox of Powerlessness in Chronic Illness

The paradox of powerlessness in chronic illness is that power and powerlessness are interrelated. Power takes for granted powerlessness and vice versa (Gibson, 1991; Kuokkanen & Leino-Kilpi, 2000). Power is defined as the "ability to act or produce an effect" and "possession of control, authority, or influence over others" (Merriam-Webster, n.d.). Power can be enabling and enhance one's autonomous ability and capacity. Despite the limiting effects of chronic illness and feelings of powerlessness, individuals continue to exert power and control in areas of their lives through adaptation and accommodation to their evolving abilities and self.

Power is an individual psychological characteristic (McCubbin, 2001), a personal resource inherent in all individuals, and is the ability to influence what happens to one's self (Miller, 2000). Seeking, getting, and preserving power is a dynamic process that reflects a human being's ability to achieve a desired goal in the face of personal, social, cultural, and environmental facilitators and barriers (Efraimsson, Rasmussen, Gilje, & Sandman, 2003).

In our individual-oriented society, power is associated with independence and self-determination. Although we may think of power as an individual quality, in reality, power is a relational attribute. Power has no meaning in the absence of relationships with others and the context of the interaction. Power is developed and maintained in relationships. Power can restrict self-determination with forcefulness or authority by restricting the autonomy of another in personal relationships as well as hierarchical organizations (Moden, 2004). Power is a "social, political, economic and cultural phenomenon, since all these dimensions of human societies determine who has power and what kind" (McCubbin, 2001, p. 76).

Individual power resources include physical strength and physical reserve, psychological stamina and social support, positive self-concept, energy, knowledge, motivation, and hope (Miller, 2000, p. 8). Chronic illness can diminish these power resources. When power resources are significantly altered and affected, an individual with chronic illness may experience feelings of powerlessness. To deal with this powerlessness, persons with chronic illness should direct their energy toward their intact power resources. Power resources facilitate coping with chronic illness. Accordingly when

one power resource becomes depleted, other power components may need to be developed to avert or reduce powerlessness (Miller, 2000).

Theoretical Perspectives of Powerlessness and Power

Persons with chronic illness live in a dual world, that of wellness and sickness, of control and powerlessness, and of hope and despair. The Shifting Perspectives Model of Chronic Illness (Paterson, 2001a, 2003) describes chronic illness as a complex dialectic between the individual and his/her world. This model posits that persons with chronic illness shift between the perspective of wellness in the foreground and illness in the background. Furthermore, this model suggests that the experience of living with a chronic illness is a dynamic process that reflects the elements of both wellness and illness that comprise chronic illness. A perspective shift is a cognitive and affective strategy to negotiate the effects of a chronic illness and to make sense of the experience. The perspectives of wellness and illness are not mutually exclusive, rather it is a fluctuation of the degree to which illness or wellness is in the foreground or background (Paterson, 2001a).

Rather than a static outlook, there is a continual shifting of perspectives (Paterson, 2003). Persons living with chronic illness have a preferred perspective that is assumed most frequently. Therefore, persons with an illness perspective in the foreground focus on their illness, their symptoms, and the negative impact their chronic condition has on them and others. Conversely, from a perspective of wellness in the foreground, the individual views the chronic illness at a distance and focuses on his or her abilities to navigate daily life and to perform roles and responsibilities; the negative aspects of the chronic illness recede to the background. In addition to illness and wellness, this shifting perspectives model acknowledges parallel and simultaneous contradictions in the chronic illness experience such as loss and gain, control, and powerlessness (Paterson, 2003).

Hence, persons with a wellness perspective will likely exert power and control over their daily routines and social interactions.

Both the illness and wellness perspective can be interrupted and changed. Such a shift in perspective can be stimulated by physiologic changes, events, fears, and other people (Paterson, 2003). Social support, competent care providers, hope, and humor are factors that influence a shift from illness in the foreground to wellness in the foreground (Freeman, O'Dell, & Meola, 2003; Haluska, Jessee, & Nagy, 2002; Neville, 1998). Exacerbations of symptoms and other forms of illness intrusiveness such as pain, decreased physical function and mobility, low self-worth, and feelings of loss of life goals and aspirations (Devins, Beanlands, Mandin, & Paul, 1997; Mullins, Chaney, Balderson, & Hommel, 2000), may shift an individual's perspective to his or her disease state and feelings of loss of control and powerlessness may arise. The "relative importance of the illness, physical experiences with the illness and biomedical uncertainties" (Sutton & Treloar, 2007, p. 338) can also trigger a shift in perspective. Clinical indicators of chronic disease progressions may not be congruent with individual perceptions of health and illness inasmuch as health and illness views are constructed within the individual's physical, emotional, and social spheres and may not be compatible with healthcare priorities (Sutton & Treloar, 2007). Although the focus of illness in the foreground can be self-absorbing, this perspective may provide the individual an opportunity to learn more about his or her illness and effective strategies to treat and manage symptoms. Figure 11-1 illustrates the shift of perspectives in chronic illness.

Self-Determination Theory (SDT)

Self-determination theory (SDT) highlights the psychological processes that promote optimal functioning and health. This theory posits three basic, innate psychological needs that are the basis for optimal functioning and personal well-being. These psychological needs—competence, relatedness and

FIGURE 11-1

Shift in Perspectives in Chronic Illness

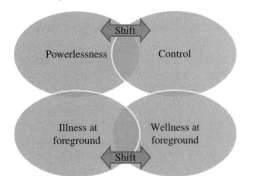

Source: Paterson, B.L. (2001a). The shifting perspectives model of chronic illness. *Journal of Nursing Scholarship, 33,* 21–26A and Paterson, B.L. (2003). The koala has claws: Applications of the shifting perspectives model in research of chronic illness. *Qualitative Health Research, 13*(7), 987–994.

autonomy—are universal and must be satisfied for all people to achieve optimal health. These basic psychological needs provide a framework that specifies the conditions in which people can maximize their human potential. The need for competence results in an individual's ability to adapt to new challenges in a changing context. The need for competency stimulates unique talents of individuals and produces adaptive competences and flexible functioning in the context of changing demands. The need for relatedness is the integration of the individual into the social world in which the individual seeks attachments, security, and a sense of belonging and intimacy with others. The tendencies of relatedness are to cohere to one's group and to feel connection with and care of others. However, the need for relatedness can compete or conflict with autonomy. Autonomy, according to SDT, refers to self-organization and self-regulation, and conveys adaptive advantage. Autonomous individuals function and respond effectively within changing contexts and circumstances. When behavior is regulated by outside pressures and expectations, holistic functioning is precluded. Therefore, autonomous individuals are better able to regulate their actions in accordance with their perceived needs and available capacities as well as coordinate and prioritize courses of action that will maximize self-maintenance (Deci & Ryan, 2000; Ryan & Deci, 2000).

Self-determination theory distinguishes between autonomous and controlled behavior regulation. Behaviors are autonomous when persons experience a sense of choice to act out of personal importance of the behavior. Controlled behaviors, on the other hand, are those performed when persons feel pressured by external forces (Deci & Ryan, 1985, 1991). Autonomous regulation, or the choice to do what is important and relevant to the individual, is associated with subjective experiences of vitality and energized behavior and differentiated controlled and autonomous choice (Moller, Deci, & Ryan, 2006). Clients at a pain clinic who felt more autonomous in seeking treatment reported greater subjective vitality (Ryan & Frederick, 1997), and presumably fewer experiences of powerlessness. Adjustment to chronic illness is influenced by the extent to which individuals believe themselves to be the source of their actions, that is, their feelings of autonomy (Igreja et al., 2000). Healthcare professionals can facilitate self-initiation and increase autonomous self-regulation in individuals with chronic conditions by supporting and acknowledging initiative, providing choice and rationale for treatment regimens, and minimizing controls and pressure to conform (Deci, Eghrari, Patrick, & Leone, 1994).

Cognitive Adaptation Theory

Cognitive Adaptation Theory posits that an individual's attempt to maintain or regain a sense of personal control may be heightened or activated by the psychological challenge that can arise out of an unpredictable illness. The heightened sense of personal control may be used as a way to maintain positive adaptation to chronic illness. An enhanced perception of control may facilitate coping with an illness-related stressor such as exacerbation of symptoms or disease progression (Taylor, 1983), whereas absence of self-control promotes dependency, powerlessness, and erodes client autonomy (McCann & Clark, 2004).

PROBLEMS AND ISSUES ASSOCIATED WITH POWERLESSNESS

Loss

From a medical viewpoint, chronic illness is comprised of physical discomforts and limitations. From a broader perspective, chronic illness brings multiple losses for individuals and their families on the physical as well as psychological level. The diagnosis of a chronic illness may, in and of itself, represent a loss to the individual, and for some, the diagnosis of a chronic illness may be as significant as a death. The diagnosis of the chronic illness may represent the loss of hopes and dreams, income, sexual ability, physical and mental ability, quality of life, or independence (Clarke & James, 2003). The loss of mobility and agility as a result of chronic illness affects one's ability to participate in social activities and to maintain social ties (Beal, 2007; O'Brien, 1993).

Persons with chronic illness have restrictions in their daily lives, experience social isolation, feel they are discounted and are afraid of becoming a burden to others (Charmaz, 1983). Loss of self is felt by many persons with a chronic illness (Charmaz, 1983) in which the serious debilitating effects of chronic illness erode the former self image of the individual. Over time, accumulated loss of self-image can result in diminished self-concept. Loss of self is a result of chronic illness that diminishes control over lives and futures (Charmaz, 1983). Lack of self-confidence and disrupted identity are two major factors of powerlessness. In-depth interviews with clients with various chronic conditions revealed numerous losses including their loss of self control and confidence when their environment and possibilities diminished (Aujoulat, Luminet, & Deccache, 2007).

Uncertainty

Chronic illness generates a wide array of emotions and reactions and engenders anxiety and uncertainty. The uncertainty of chronic illness promotes feelings of loss of control and promotes a sense of powerlessness in individuals and families (Mishel, 1999). Narratives of persons diagnosed with multiple sclerosis revealed concerns about the unpredictable progression of the disease and fear and anxiety relative to the unknown (Barker-Collo, Cartwright, & Read, 2006). Severity of the illness, the erratic nature of symptomatology and the ambiguity of symptoms promotes uncertainty in persons with chronic illness (Mishel, 1999). Anticipating and planning for the future becomes complicated. The unpredictability of physical symptoms and abilities interferes with the individual's ability to schedule activities and events in the future and may result an unwillingness plan in advance. The uncertainty of the chronic illness raises salient concerns for persons about their future, about their ability to control their illness and symptoms, and their ability to garner necessary personal and financial resources to manage their illness.

Chronic Illness Management

Chronic illness management often entails a multifaceted self-management regimen. The complexity of chronic illness has the potential to strip away a client's sense of self-worth and confidence. Clients who lack confidence often are unable to assess their needs accurately, and consequently are at risk of being manipulated or coerced by others and may capitulate to the wishes of family members or healthcare professionals. Self-management of complex chronic disease is often difficult to achieve and is reflected in low rates of adherence to treatment guidelines (Newman, Steed, & Mulligan, 2004). Although some healthcare professionals believe they can inspire persons with chronic illnesses, the motivation to follow a plan of care is internal. Healthcare professionals must acknowledge the personal context of the chronic illness and assess the individual motivators to follow a plan of care (Singleton, 2002). Persons with a chronic illness may not be willing or capable to carry out the complex tasks and activities to manage their chronic illness, and a simple "pep talk"

from one's healthcare professional simply will not suffice. For example, Mrs. Jones, an elderly widow with end-stage renal disease must spend 3 days a week at the local dialysis unit to manage her chronic illness. Even though she has accepted the time involved to adhere to her treatment regimen and has accommodated her lifestyle accordingly, she yearns to visit her extended family that lives some distance from her. At her peril, Mrs. Jones chooses to spend time with her family, to forgo prescribed treatment and to bear the consequences of her decision. In the end, although Mrs. Jones was able to continue her dialysis treatments, her decision was motivated by her personal desire and familial priority, not the prescribed treatment.

Mr. Smith, a young man with AIDS experiences difficulties adhering to a complex pharmacologic regimen because of financial constraints. Mr. Smith finds himself consumed with an ongoing process of seeking resources to maintain his prescribed treatment, which takes away his ability to participate in other areas of his life. The lives of the elderly woman and young man, center around their chronic illness and treatment regimen activities. Each one experiences a loss of control over time management, personal choice, and quality of life. Their chronic illness and treatment regimens consume their daily lives to the detriment of other activities, and feelings of powerlessness arise. What was true for Mrs. Jones and Mr. Smith is also true for other persons dealing with chronic illness. The lack of self-control inherent in their disease and treatment fosters feelings of dependence and powerlessness, and undermines client autonomy (McCann & Clark, 2004).

In contrast, the ability to control one's treatment plan, choose services, and avoid coercion diminishes powerlessness (Nelson, Lord, & Ochocka, 2001). Support is essential to meet the demands and expectations of complex management regimens of chronic illness. Singleton (2002) reported necessary supports as good communication with healthcare professionals, adequate financial resources, time and ability to perform care tasks, and spiritual support.

Another key element to adherence to treatment regimens is meaningful participation in the agencies that provide services (Nelson, Lord, & Ochocka, 2001). Choice of treatment regimen and control of that regimen are central to self-determination in persons with chronic conditions. To provide appropriate information, the nurse must listen to the needs, wants, and desires of the client. When clients feel unheard and have no voice, they feel invalidated and dismissed, and they feel powerless (Courts et al., 2004). As a result of this powerlessness, the opportunity for the nurse to enhance client outcomes diminishes greatly.

Lack of Knowledge

Persons with chronic illness learn about their conditions through daily experiences and by trial and error (Michael, 1996). Although novices during the early stages of their chronic illness, over the course of chronic illness people become highly knowledgeable about their condition and develop effective strategies to manage the daily challenges of their chronic illness.

Knowledge about chronic illness is essential. Lack of knowledge or skills about the disease may impact the dynamics of the disease. Often, information and education about the chronic illness occurs during the acute phase of the illness or during hospitalization, periods when the client and family may not have been able to grasp the concepts at that overwhelming time. Unfamiliar surroundings coupled with the insecurities of a new or recurrent chronic illness diagnosis impact learning. Although the client may have listened intently to the instructions and education, he or she may not have been able to internalize the content. As a result, after discharge from the acute care setting, the client may lack sufficient knowledge to effectively manage issues and problems that arise out of the chronic condition. Lack of information to successfully meet the challenges of daily living further reinforces feelings of powerlessness.

Marginalization/Vulnerability

Knowledge alone is insufficient for management and control of chronic illness. The contextual determinants of health must also be acknowledged. Social determinants of vulnerability include low income, low education, fragile social identity, and limited social networks (Crossley, 2001). Lack of resources contributes to powerlessness. Persons who experience a marginalized sociocultural status and have limited access to economic resources have a greater than average risk of developing health problems and have higher rates of morbidity and mortality associated with chronic illness (Aday, 2001).

The burden of chronic illness disproportionately affects vulnerable populations (Sullivan, Weinert, & Cudney, 2003). Vulnerable clients are the most powerless and the least able to identify and express their needs and desires beyond the completely obvious (Niven & Scott, 2003). Chronic conditions are a significant healthcare challenge, and one's vulnerability is often brought into sharp focus by a chronic disease.

Clients identify that the way healthcare professionals relate to them is the cause for their vulnerability, not their chronic illness (Mitchell & Bournes, 2000). Some clients are viewed as having less social value than others (Glaser & Strauss, 1968). Social value is subjective and influenced by such factors as age, marital status, income, living conditions, hygiene, behavior and so forth. Some clients with chronic illnesses may be perceived as having low moral worth. The nurse may believe the client's illness or condition is the result of behaviors chosen by the client. Clients who do not behave within the prescribed norms and expectations of the institution or agency may be labeled as undesirable and may not have the opportunity to engage in decision-making and control over their healthcare regimen.

Stigma

Persons with chronic illnesses are subject to stigma based on the negative perceptions held by society (see Chapter 3). Stigma is a response to any physical or social attribute or characteristic that devalues a person's social identify and disqualifies him or her from full social acceptance (Goffman, 1963). This stigma and the associated stereotypes and misconceptions about chronic illness lead to a lack of inclusion and powerlessness. Confusion and misinformation about chronic illness can lead to discrimination and stigma and result in unintended, harmful effects for persons with a chronic condition. For example, family and friends of persons with hepatitis C may be fearful and lack knowledge about the virus. For the individual with hepatitis C, the ignorance of others may stimulate feelings of helplessness and infectiousness (Zickmund, Ho, Masuda, Ippolito, & LaBrecque, 2003), or fear of judgment and stigma from those around them (Sutton & Treloar, 2007). In this way, external societal pressures can create and perpetuate feelings of powerlessness in individuals with chronic illness.

Culture

The concepts of powerlessness and power are grounded in the context of cultural values, beliefs, and practices of persons with chronic illness and their families. The traditional power and control culture in the healthcare setting may conflict with cultural customs and beliefs of an individual with a chronic illness. Many cultural groups view the individual as embedded in social relationships, thus the role of the individual in decision-making is not recognized. For group-oriented persons or families, power and control may reside within the family rather than with the individual (Davis, Konishi, & Tashiro, 2003). For example, in some Native American families, healthcare decisions are made by the matriarch of the family rather than the individual with chronic illness. Failure to include the family matriarch in the decision-making process diminishes adherence to prescribed treatment regimens. In some cultures, the oldest male holds the power and control to make decisions. Cultural conflicts may arise when families

are not consulted before an intervention or staff interferes with rituals deemed necessary by the client's family to promote healing.

Conversely, when a client chooses to go against his or her cultural norm or custom, the client must have the power to do so. In situations where families are in disagreement with the client about compliance with cultural customs, the nurse must support the client and give him or her the resources for self-determination in the situation (Zoucha & Husted, 2000). The desires and wishes of the individual client supersede the cultural values, beliefs, and practices of the culture in which the individual and family are in disagreement (Tang & Lee, 2004).

Culture is the context in which individuals, families and groups make healthcare decisions. Power and control in Western society is based on the concept of individualism, a society consisting of autonomous individuals. Western societies promote the actualization of the individual self as the goal, yet other cultures do not. The Western principle of autonomy is self-determination. In other cultures, the principle of autonomy is family-determination, that is, the family is the autonomous social unit in which the entire family, not the individual, has real authority in decision-making. For Chinese cancer patients living in Hong Kong, emphasizing the Chinese cultural beliefs of loyalty to family, letting go, harmony with the universe, and the cycles of life and nature was essential to the development of feelings of empowerment (Mok, Martinson, & Wong, 2004).

Values, beliefs, practices, and responses to chronic illness vary by culture and within culture. Culture impacts and dictates one's responses to normal events of everyday life and is a driving force in the decisions and choices that individuals and families make about health and care (Fletcher, 2002; Salas-Provance, Erickson, & Reed, 2002). Some individuals experiencing chronic illness may remain silent about their experiences and issues with chronic illness. This is not an indicator of indifference or incompetence but a reflection of cultural differences in the use of silence. Eastern cultures value silence, whereas Western cultures value verbal expressions (Poland & Peterson, 1998).

Culturally appropriate care can only occur when culture care values, expressions, or patterns are known and used appropriately (Leininger, 1995). Life experiences and situations of the past influence the present. For many African Americans, religion and spiritual values provide a method for coping with chronic conditions. Their faith and belief in God give them power to endure pain and suffering associated with their chronic conditions (Anthony, 2007). The centrality of cultural values and healthcare decisions is highlighted in the findings of a survey of 1253 African Americans in Alabama churches. This research found that 59% of the respondents reported they believed in fate or destiny in relation to healthcare decisions and health-seeking behaviors. Women who believed in fate or destiny were less likely than those who did not to have breast examinations (Green, Lewis, Wang, Person, & Rivers, 2004). Knowledge of cultural values, beliefs and practices provides an invaluable blueprint for healthcare providers in caring for diverse clients with chronic illness. Furthermore, the promotion of cultural values can help clients with chronic illness mitigate their experiences of powerlessness.

Healthcare System

Clients and their families are vulnerable and powerless in the healthcare power structure (Davis, Konishi, & Tashiro, 2003). Upon entry into the healthcare system, the client relinquishes control over his or her life, loses self-identity and initiative, and becomes distant from supportive networks. The client's voice may be ignored by healthcare professionals or quieted by dwindling energy levels that comes from the disease process itself or the side effects of treatment. The healthcare system is designed for acute, episodic treatment and strives for efficient and cost-effective care. This fast-paced and impersonal care system leaves little time and individual focus for the person with a chronic condition, which requires a more long term, illness management approach.

The procedures and language used by healthcare professionals are foreign and strange to the client and leave many persons with chronic conditions unable and unwilling to be an active participant in their health care (Anthony, 2007). The healthcare system provides fragmented care for persons with chronic illness and leaves individuals feeling isolated and left to care for themselves with inadequate knowledge and resources. Frustration and inability to overcome obstacles in accessing, receiving, and paying for services add to feelings of powerlessness (Dunn, 1998; Walker, Holloway, & Sofaer, 1999).

The healthcare system perpetuates client vulnerability. It has the potential to restrict the autonomy of people and to disable and dominate them by virtue of its bureaucracy, scientific expertise, and technology. Clients surrender their independence to the health care system where the physician is omniscient and the client begins the process of learned helplessness and an inability to speak for themselves (Hewitt, 2002). Today, decisions in the healthcare system are made by power brokers who are neither providers nor consumers of health care, but insurance companies, Wall Street firms, think tanks, consultants, and pharmaceutical companies (Sheridan-Gonzalez, 2000). This type of healthcare system perpetuates client powerlessness.

Powerlessness can be seen in the context of becoming a patient, the expectations of individuals, and the ways in which they play by the rules. It is also a key to understanding the ways in which their horizons change, both as facts—the loss of mobility and contact— and as metaphor—acceptance, control, and changing outlook. It is a response to the limits of the conditions itself, and to the power which is perceived to be vested in the health care system (Gibson & Kenrick, 1998, p. 743).

My life is like a roller coaster . . . some days my life is full of light and joy . . . but those up days are becoming fewer and fewer now that my fibromyalgia and Parkinson's are so much a part of my life. What can I do? The uncertainty of every day makes me so angry, so confused, so sad. I want to escape from all of this but where would I go? You know, I really thought I could beat this. I've done it before but now . . . my pain is relentless! My body is unwilling! What choice do I have?

Anne

INTERVENTIONS

Persons with chronic illness are likely to feel overwhelmed, exhausted, and discouraged at times.

Therefore, one of the most important challenges for nurses working with these clients is to help them overcome feelings of powerlessness. Factors that impact on powerlessness in persons with chronic illness are complex and multidimensional. Nursing interventions to address powerlessness in chronic illness should be equally multifaceted and require attention to the complex nature of the healthcare situation. Appropriate and relevant nursing interventions are based on ongoing assessments and observations of the client with chronic illness in his or her environment, the context in

CASE STUDY

Anne, a Caucasian woman, graduated from the university with a degree in music. She married her high school sweetheart, John, and began her career as a professional pianist and organist. Anne began to notice her fingers on the keyboard of her piano and organ were stiff and slow to respond. She continued to experience increasing symptoms in her hands including numbness and tingling over the course of the next year, and then other symptoms emerged and she was eventually diagnosed with Parkinson's disease. Anne continued her life as usual. She was able to successfully integrate her chronic illness into her daily life. She returned to school and received a degree in accounting, she traveled, and she enjoyed her hobbies and friends. It was when Anne could no longer tolerate extreme muscle pain, fatigue, and difficulty sleeping that she was diagnosed with fibromyalgia. Anne's symptoms continued to increase and her medical regimen became more complex. She began experiencing side effects from her medications. She sought information and knowledge about her illnesses and explored treatment modalities on the Internet. She experimented with alternative treatment and medicines to manage her worsening symptoms. Despite her best efforts,

Anne would spend the entire day managing her symptoms while on other days, she was able to enjoy cooking and engaging in her music and other hobbies. Not knowing what to expect from day to day, Anne began to decline social plans and activities with her family and friends and became increasingly socially isolated. Anne's physical condition worsened. She began spending more time in bed or on the couch. She had neither the energy nor ability to do much more. When Anne did get up, she frequently fell and required assistance from John. Her dwindling abilities to control her own body left Anne with feelings of overwhelming feelings of powerlessness.

Discussion Questions

1. How do the physical and psychosocial challenges experienced by Anne contribute to her sense of powerlessness? How does this affect Anne's family and friends?
2. How would you use theory to guide your nursing plan of care with Anne and her family?
3. What nursing interventions would you recommend to restore and enhance power to Anne? Anne's family?

which the person manages and copes with chronic illness. This includes not only the physical surroundings but the psychosocial dimensions of life as well. Because of the dynamic nature of chronic illness, continuing evaluation of interventions with subsequent modifications to meet the current needs of the client are required. The goals of nursing interventions are to assist the client to manage the realities of one's limitations, to reduce a sense of powerlessness and loss and to create new boundaries for one's changed life.

Nursing interventions to restore client control and increase power resources in clients with chronic illness are discussed. The following are strategies and tools to strengthen the client's power base.

Empowerment

The purpose of the nurse–client relationship is to maintain and restore control to clients. This relationship emphasizes the primacy of the client's own ideas, emotions and beliefs about the chronic illness. The power relationship between the client and the health care professional is a central issue of care. Empowerment is a social process of identification and support of an individual's abilities to attend to one's needs, to problem solve, and to activate necessary resources to control one's own life (Gibson, 1991). Key issues to empowerment are self-awareness and self-determination. Self-determination is the ability to make choices and accept responsibility for one's choices (Aujoulat et al., 2007). Of note, empowerment may not be a desirable outcome or process for all clients, inasmuch as clients may differ in their desire to participate in their healthcare decisions (Loft, McWilliam, & Ward-Griffin, 2001). The nurse must be attentive to the individual beliefs and desires with regard to power and control.

Empowerment strategies and efforts increase power and strengthen individual life circumstances. Two dimensions of empowerment emerge from the literature. One dimension is psychological, which includes self-esteem and self-efficacy.

The other dimension of empowerment is social, action-oriented, and comprised of power, involvement and control over individual life circumstances (Hansson & Bjorkman, 2005).

Empowerment is important for clients with chronic illness because it increases perceived quality of life (Rosenfield, 1992) and promotes self-esteem. It is contingent on social support (Rogers, Chamberlin, Ellison, & Crean, 1997) and results from individual perception of needs for care as met (Roth & Crane-Ross, 2002). Key features of empowering provider–client relationships include continuity of care, patient-centeredness, and mutual acknowledgement and relatedness (Aujoulat et al., 2007).

Health Coaching

Patient-centered strategies can be developed such as incorporating lifestyle changes, engaging in prevention strategies, and making decisions to promote self-management of chronic illness. Although not a new idea in the practice of nursing, the reemergence of the idea of client-centered care is reflected in health coaching. Health coaching is client centered, and clients are actively involved in determining what is important and what they want to accomplish relative to the management of their chronic illness. Health coaching motivates behavior change in clients through collaboration, open-ended inquiry, and questions and reflection (Huffman, 2007).

Discharge Planning

Effective discharge planning is another strategy of empowerment. Discharge planning strengthens the client's position and role in social and healthcare systems. A well-orchestrated discharge plan enhances coping with relocation from one healthcare setting to another. Open and clear communication among all participants including the client, the family, and healthcare professionals is essential for mutual understanding and successful discharge (Armitage & Kavanagh, 1998). Frequently nurses think of discharge planning only from the acute setting to another setting. However, the concept of long-range discharge planning is essential when dealing with clients with chronic illness, where the client transitions from one setting to another.

Collaboration

Successful management of chronic illness and optimal wellness for persons with chronic illness is based on collaboration and partnership with clients to provide necessary information and skills to initiate beneficial behaviors and favorable healthcare decisions. Simplistic approaches to empowering and improving the quality of life in persons with chronic illness are not possible. The lack of a match between a person's readiness and the health-care professional's interventions may result in lack of adherence to the prescribed treatment regimen. Adherence is a dynamic process that is compromised by barriers usually related to different aspects of the chronic illness. Such barriers include social and economic factors, healthcare team and system, characteristics of the disease, therapies, and client-related factors. Solving problems related to each of these is necessary to promote client adherence (WHO, 2003).

The client with a chronic illness must be a full partner with the healthcare professional in decision-making. Imparting knowledge and information to clients is an exchange process and requires active client participation. However, there are times when the clients may not desire information because of fear of the information, information overload, or lack of ability to understand the information. The nurse needs to assess client readiness for information by acknowledging the client's concerns, listening to his/her perspective and respecting the client's desire for new information. Disempowering relationships result from discounting experiential knowledge and provision of adequate resources (Paterson, 2001b).

Self-Management

Persons with chronic illness must be empowered to be managers of their own care within their own realities and settings. The opportunities to manage self-control are dependent on the context in which the clients live their everyday lives (Delmar et al., 2006). In an institutional setting (acute or long-term care), clients with a chronic illness may be highly motivated to manage their own care. However, clients' environment dictates the parameters of activities of daily living and may severely limit the chance to fully operationalize self-management despite ability and desire. In this instance, nurses can be instrumental in altering the institutional structure to accommodate the self-control goals of clients.

Self-management is more than adherence to a treatment regimen but also takes into account the psychological and social management of living with a chronic illness. Chronic illnesses vary in the extent to which they intrude on the psychological and social worlds of individuals. The outcome of empowerment is self-management of chronic illness through the reinforcement of self-determination and control (Aujoulat et al., 2007). Self-management interventions for persons with chronic conditions need to be developed to assist them to better manage their illnesses and to take increasing responsibility for their disease (see Chapter 13).

The difficulty in managing complex treatment schedules of chronic illnesses has led to the development of self-management interventions (SMIs). The key feature of these SMIs is to increase clients' involvement and control in their treatment, and to improve the subsequent impact on their lives (Newman, Steed, & Mulligan, 2004). The skills necessary for clients to develop a self-management intervention are problem solving and goal setting. Even with these skills in place, most persons with chronic illnesses are likely to encounter barriers to care that create major challenges in compliance with SMIs. Those who experience increased barriers are less likely to adhere to plans of care. Frequently reported barriers are time constraints, knowledge deficits, limited social support, inadequate resources, limited coping skills, poor client–provider relationship and low self-efficacy

(Tu & Morrison, 1996). Patient-centered, collaborative nursing strategies reinforce client strengths and ameliorate the impact of these barriers. The nurse becomes a partner with the client to facilitate collaboration in the development of a realistic, self-management program. Failure of the nurse to identify or adequately estimate barriers to self-management will negatively impact adherence to the treatment regimen (Nagelkerk, Reick, & Meengs, 2006).

Control

Perceived control is an antecedent to function, a mediator between social support and psychological wellbeing, and is useful for effective disease self-management (Jacelon, 2007). Perceived control is related to better adjustment to chronic illness. Helgeson and Franzen (1998) discuss two dimensions of perceived control. First, one can believe he or she is personally able to control one's outcomes and secondly, control is achieved by believing that more powerful others can control one's outcomes. The latter, vicarious control can be exerted by physicians, parents, God, or family. To assist the client in achieving optimal functioning, the nurse must assess the client's belief about the source of control: whether within self or from others.

When the professional nurse exerts too much control, the client may relinquish control and put his or her life in the hands of the professional to the detriment of their empowerment (Delmar et al., 2006). Client power is a fundamental element in the client–provider relationship because clients, because of their chronic illness, may become dependent and thus subordinate to healthcare professionals (Efraimsson, Rasmussen, Gilje, & Sandman, 2003). Independence, self-control, and self-responsibility are important elements for increasing patient empowerment. The ability to ask for assistance may be an indicator of self-control and self-management (Delmar et al., 2006).

Self-Determination

Self-determination is a basic human right of individual choice and control. Self-determination ensures that an individual has the autonomy and support to make decisions and to reach personal goals. Self-determination must be balanced with safety and risk of the client and family. Self-determination restores power of choice to the client.

Fostering self-control is integral to promoting wellness in persons with chronic illness, and this control is central to self-determination. To be self-determined, clients must have knowledge and resources to deal with illness-related issues as they arise (McCann & Clark, 2004). Good choices are the result of good possibilities from which to choose. Nurses can give persons with chronic illness adequate and appropriate knowledge as a foundation for making the good choice (Delmar et al., 2006). To manage self-control and live in dignity involves support from health-care professionals and significant others in the decision-making process. Other people can help provide knowledge and expertise as a foundation for making the right choice. Clients with significant physical or mental impairments may be unable to engage in social discourse and may require additional resources to promote self-management. The nurse should provide the client appropriate and relevant resources and work with the client and his or her family to obtain connections and referrals to appropriate community-based services.

Establishing a Sense of Mastery

Powerlessness is reduced and empowerment is facilitated by the development of a sense of mastery. Mastery is helping clients to focus on how they can affect their chronic conditions and can foster a sense of control in an otherwise uncontrollable illness course. Intervention techniques that shift the focus away from uncontrollable aspects of chronic illness, such as use of a wheelchair or dialysis treatments, to the controllable aspects, such as decision-making or self-care activities, can imbue patients with a sense of mastery over their condition (Cvengros, Christensen, & Lawton, 2005). The WHO published guidelines for health-care professionals to facilitate client identification of strategies to reduce barriers to mastery and facilitate integration of self-care into daily activities (WHO, 2003).

Client and Family Education

Persons with chronic illnesses and their families need information, understanding, and competent interventions to help them reformulate their lives, assimilate their losses, and adjust to the changes brought about by their illnesses (Sullivan-Bolyal, Sadler, Knafl, Gillis, & Ahmann, 2003). Information about chronic disease management provides clients with a sense of control and thus increases empowerment (Sommerset, Campbell, Sharp, & Peters, 2001; Wollin, Dale, Spenser, & Walsh, 2000).

Over their lifetimes, persons with chronic illness and their families must shoulder the burden of coordinating medical information and treatment regimens. The need for information must be tailored to meet the needs of the individual client relative to the disease course. The client may not be able to take in information at the time of the diagnosis of a chronic illness; therefore, information should be available to the client and his or her family at a follow-up visit to ensure understanding of information and available services (Barker-Collo, Cartwright, & Read, 2006). The time of diagnosis of a chronic disease is an overwhelming and confusing time for clients and their families. The expectation that clients will be able to assimilate the information given to them about their chronic illness may be unrealistic.

In addition to information and knowledge about the chronic illness, the client needs information about available, accessible, appropriate and affordable resources and services within his or her community. The nurse is the client's link to these resources (Falk-Rafael, 2001). Therefore, it is necessary for the nurse to maintain current information about community resources and services. The nurse assesses the client's needs and preferences, selects appropriate resources for the client, and evaluates the effectiveness and acceptability of the resources to the client. The nurse may also link the client and his or her family to support groups, which can promote empowerment through the expression of shared experiences.

Many clients may also seek information about their chronic illness on the Internet. The ability to obtain this information independent of a healthcare professional can give the client a sense of control and self-determination. As a result, many visit their healthcare providers with requests for specific tests or medications (Corbin & Cherry, 2001). However, this information should be evaluated by the nurse to determine the appropriateness of the suggestion. Online communication and Internet support groups have become not only sources of information for individuals with chronic illness but also sources of social support. Women are more likely to use the Internet for health information and illness-related support than are their male counterparts (Pandey, Hart, & Tiwary, 2003).

Health System Navigation

The concept of patient navigation first appeared in the literature in the 1990s as a means to improve access to health care for medically underserved populations. Patient navigation moves beyond advocacy to identify barriers and challenges to healthcare access and focuses on individual well-being. It is a process in which clients are guided through the bureaucracy of the healthcare system by a nurse advocate in order to complete a specific diagnostic procedure or therapeutic task. By assisting underserved individuals to "navigate" the complex healthcare system, it reduces barriers to healthcare access and treatment. Patient navigators also mobilize appropriate resources for the client. In a study of low income women of color with breast abnormalities, patient navigation was shown to improve the timeliness of diagnosis, compliance with follow-up treatment (Psooy, Schreuer, Borgaonkar, & Caines, 2004), and diagnostic resolution follow-up by healthcare providers (Ell, Vourlekis, Lee, & Xie, 2007). Furthermore, patient navigation has been successful in reducing barriers to care and improving health outcomes in persons with HIV (Bradford, Coleman, & Cunningham, 2007).

Patient navigators promote self-determination in their clients as a means of empowering them. Although patient navigators are charged with helping clients obtain necessary healthcare services, clients must be afforded the respect to choose regarding their individual welfare. The role of patient navigators reveals the essential elements of nursing functions such as liaison and resource mobilization. It also has potential utility for serving at-risk women with high incidences of powerlessness (Ell et al., 2007).

Advocacy

In addition to patient navigation, advocacy is an important tool for increasing empowerment in patients with chronic illness. Advocacy activities seek to redistribute power and resources to people (individuals or groups) who demonstrate a need. Although the ideal of nursing advocacy is to empower clients within the healthcare system, oftentimes institutional, social, political, economic, and cultural constraints prevent clients from accessing health care. When such constraints are present, an advocate is necessary to facilitate procurement. The manner in which the nurse advocate intercedes to increase the client's power depends on the underlying values and beliefs held by the nurse regarding the advocate role. No one wants to be dependent on others, to inconvenience others, or to be a burden to others. Dignity and respect are linked with individual independence. The nurse must take care to ensure the client is still authoritative in his or her own life and is able to maintain responsibility and self-determination. Even when these elements are present, situations may arise in which clients may need help from an advocate to regain dignity and integrity.

Decision Making

When clients make their own decisions and act on them, there may be a difference between the client's choices and those that would have been made by family members or healthcare professionals. Consequently, clients may not only experience disapproval from others regarding their decisions, but also may encounter resistance when attempting to implement them. As previously discussed, Mrs. Jones made a decision to interrupt her dialysis treatments for several days to connect with her family despite protests from her primary care nurse and physician. Upon learning of Mrs. Jones' decision to discontinue treatment for a short time, the primary care nurse contacted the children of Mrs. Jones to persuade them to exert control and interrupt Mrs. Jones' plans. In the end, the sons and daughters of Mrs. Jones agreed to honor the choice and decision made by their mother. This example provides the foundation for further discussions among nurses engaged in client-empowered health care. How much control belongs to the client, the healthcare professional, family members? How do control issues affect the nurse–client, the nurse–family, the client–family relationships? What are the guiding principles in this approach of nursing care of clients with chronic illness?

Nurses must provide clients all information necessary to make a decision. Providing information about the illness and the services that are available will facilitate informed decisions (Aylett & Fawcett, 2003). As clients come to know the nature and meaning of their illnesses, their power tends to be restored and their vulnerability is reduced.

Anticipatory Guidance

Anxiety is triggered by an uncertain future. Uncertainty of the illness trajectory suggests the need for the nurse to offer anticipatory guidance to persons with chronic illnesses. Anticipatory guidance is based on identifying expected future needs and can begin weeks, months, or years before any actual help is required. Future needs can have a profound effect on clients' lives because major life decisions can be influenced by them. Clients need a coach to help them chart an anticipated course throughout their chronic illness (Courts, Buchanan, & Werstlein, 2004). Anticipating future dependency needs allows clients with progressive chronic illnesses to express their own wishes and preferences for care options. Informed anticipation lacks certainty, but it facilitates greater rational future planning for clients and their families, minimizing potentially difficult decisions made during a time of crisis.

Cultural Competence

Cultural competence is a process in which the nurse integrates cultural awareness, cultural knowledge, cultural skills, cultural encounters, and cultural desire to provide care (Campinha-Bacote, 2002). This model assumes variation among persons of different ethnic and cultural groups. For example, in collectivist culture, people may resonate to group norms to experience relatedness and autonomy. In individualist cultures, acting in accordance to the group norm may be viewed as lack of individuality and a threat to autonomy (Ryan & Deci, 2000). It is imperative for nurses to explore potential differences and similarities among clients and their beliefs to ensure culturally competent care (Leininger & McFarland, 2002). Leininger (1995) asserts "clients who experience nursing care that fails to be reasonably congruent with the client's beliefs, values, and care life ways

will show signs of cultural conflicts, noncompliance, stresses, and ethical or moral concerns" (p. 45). When nurses acknowledge and incorporate the client's cultural perspective, an environment of communication and understanding increases feelings of power and control in their client and their families.

OUTCOMES

Outcomes associated with powerlessness in clients with chronic conditions can be measured from three standpoints: self, relationships with others, and client behaviors.

From the first perspective, changes in self are evaluated by measures such as increased self-confidence and self-esteem, which facilitate coping with and management of chronic illness. The best outcomes for persons with chronic illness occur when clients learn to self-manage their chronic illness. The client must monitor and make adjustments in the management of their chronic illness, just as a driver of a car turns the wheel, monitors speed, and applies the brakes while driving a car. Self-management presumes the client is given the opportunity to communicate effectively, seek

EVIDENCE-BASED PRACTICE BOX

Empowerment is the cornerstone of health and well-being, particularly for persons with chronic illness. To establish whether empowerment has attained reliability in meaning and to explore the potential for practice guidelines, Aujoulet, d'Hoore, and Deccache (2007) conducted an extensive literature review of empowerment in relation to the care and education of clients with chronic illness. Using a qualitative method of thematic content analysis they reviewed 55 articles published between 1995 and 2006. Although the results of their study did not result in the development of a well-articulated theory of client empowerment, it did reveal a number of guiding principles and values for healthcare professionals. The application of principle self-determination honors the preferences and priorities of the client within the context of a secure partnership with the healthcare professional. The goals and outcomes of client empowerment must be explored and negotiated with every client in accordance with his or her values and beliefs and within the context of their daily lives.

Source: Aujoulat, I., d'Hoore, W., & Deccache, A. (2007). Patient empowerment in theory and practice: Polysemy or cacophony? *Patient Education and Counseling, 66,* 13–22.

information, collect data, analyze options, and make decisions. Clients need to have information and resources available to them when the need arises, as opposed to when it may be convenient for the healthcare provider to give the information to the client.

The second outcome of measured change of powerlessness is relationships with others. Changes in relationships include improved relationships with family, friends, and healthcare professionals. Relationships are reciprocal in nature. That is, family, friends, and healthcare professionals much play an active role in providing social support and positive interaction with the client with chronic illness. Positive relationships have a powerful impact on the health and well-being of healthcare clients.

The last measurable outcome of reduced powerlessness is behavior. Changes in behavior include health and goal-oriented decisions, which promote personal responsibility for health (Falk-Rafael, 2001). Positive changes in behavior can result in increased treatment regimen adherence, better management of symptoms, and decreases in feelings of powerlessness.

Recommendations for Further Conceptual and Data-Based Work

Chronic illness research with a focus on empowerment interventions is essential not only at the micro-level but at the macro-level. Continued development of knowledge and understanding of the experiences and needs of individuals with serious, chronic, progressive, and largely uncontrollable illnesses is essential to for development of effective strategies for greater self of power and control. The efficacy and appropriateness of social and health policy needs to be evaluated relative to increasing power and control to clients and their families who experience chronic illness. The process of empowerment interventions at the social level would benefit clients with chronic illness, their families, as well as healthcare professionals.

STUDY QUESTIONS

1. Discuss the relationship between chronic illness and powerlessness.
2. Compare and contrast the concepts of power and powerlessness.
3. Discuss the factors that alter power and powerlessness in clients with chronic illness.
4. Explain the association between physiologic and psychosocial factors and powerlessness.
5. How can the theoretical perspectives presented be used to design interventions to reduce powerlessness?
6. Analyze the potential strengths and limitations of nursing interventions to reduce powerlessness.

REFERENCES

Aday, L. (2001). *At risk in America*. San Francisco, CA: Jossey-Bass.

Anthony, J.S. (2007). Self-advocacy in health care decision-making among elderly African Americans. *Journal of Cultural Diversity 14*(2), 88–94.

Armitage, S.K., & Kavanagh, K.M. (1998). Consumer oriented outcomes. *Journal of Clinical Nursing, 7*, 67–74.

Asbring, P. (2001). Chronic illness: A disruption of life – identity-transformation among women with chronic fatigue syndrome and fibromylagia. *Journal of Advanced Nursing, 34*, 312–319.

Aujoulat, I., Luminet, O., & Deccache, A. (2007). The perspective of patients on their experience of powerlessness. *Qualitative Health Research, 17*, 772–785.

Aujoulat, I., d'Hoore, W., & Deccache, A. (2007). Patient empowerment in theory and practice: Polysemy or cacophony? *Patient Education and Counseling, 66,* 13–20.

Aylett, E., & Fawcett, T.N. (2003). Chronic fatigue syndrome: The nurse's role. *Nursing Standard, 17*(35), 33–37.

Bandura, A. (1989). Human agency in social cognitive theory. *American Psychologist, 44,* 1175–1184.

Barker-Collo, S., Cartwright, C., & Read, J. (2006). Into the unknown: The experiences of individuals living with multiple sclerosis. *Journal of Neuroscience Nursing, 38*(6), 435–446.

Beal, C.C. (2007). Loneliness in women with multiple sclerosis. *Rehabilitation Nursing, 32*(4), 165–171.

Bradford, J.B., Coleman, S., & Cunningham, W. (2007). HIV system navigation: An emerging model to improve HIV care access. *AIDS Patient Care and STDs, 21,* S-49-S-58.

Campinha-Bacote, J. (2002). The process of cultural competence in the delivery of health care services: A model of care. *Journal of Transcultural Nursing, 13*(3), 180–184.

Clarke, J.N., & James, S. (2003). The radicalized self: The impact on the self of the contested nature of the diagnosis of chronic fatigue syndrome. *Social Science and Medicine, 57*(8), 1387–1395.

Corbin, J.M., & Cherry, J.C. (2001). Epilogue: A proactive model of health care. In R.B. Hyman and J.M. Corbin (Eds.). *Chronic illness research and theory for nursing practice.* New York: Springer.

Courts, J.F., Buchanan, E.M., & Werstlein, P.O. (2004). Focus groups: The lived experience of participants with multiple sclerosis. *Journal of Neuroscience Nursing, 36*(1), 42–47.

Crossley, M. (2001). The "Armistead' project: An exploration of gay men, sexual practices, community health promotion and issues of empowerment. *Journal of Community and Applied Social Psychology, 11,* 111–123.

Cvengros, J. A., Christensen, A.J., & Lawton, W.J. (2005). Health locus of control and depression in chronic kidney disease: A dynamic perspective. *Journal of Health Psychology, 10*(5), 677–686.

Davis, A.J., Konishi, E., & Tashiro, M. (2003). A pilot study of selected Japanese nurses' ideas on patient advocacy. *Nursing Ethics, 10*(4), 404–413.

Deci, E.L. & Ryan, R.M. (2000). The 'what' and 'why' of goal pursuits: Human needs and the self-determination of behavior. *Psychological Inquiry, 11*(4), 227–268.

Delmar, C., Bøje, T., Dylmer, D., Forup, L., Jakobsen, C., Møller, et al. (2006). Independence/dependence–a contradictory relationship? Life with a chronic illness. *Scandinavian Journal of Caring Sciences, 20*(3), 261–268.

Devins, G., Beanlands, H., Mandin, H., & Paul, L. (1997). Psychosocial impact of illness intrusiveness moderated by self-concept and age in end-stage renal disease. *Health Psychology, 16,* 529–538.

Dunn, J.D. (1998). Powerlessness regarding health-service barriers: Construction of an instrument. *Nursing Diagnosis: The Journal of Nursing Language and Classification, 9*(4), 136–143.

Efraimsson, E., Rasmussen, B.H., Gilje, F., & Sandman, P. (2003). Expressions of power and powerlessness in discharge planning: A case study of an older woman on her way home. *Journal of Clinical Nursing, 12,* 707–716.

Ell, K., Vourlekis, B., Lee, P-J., & Xie, B. (2007). Patient navigation and case management following an abnormal mammogram: A randomized clinical trial. *Preventive Medicine, 44,* 26–33.

Falk-Rafael, A. (2001). Empowerment as a process of evolving consciousness: A model of empowered caring. *Advances in Nursing Science, 24*(1), 1–16.

Freeman, K., O'Dell, C., & Meola, C. (2003). Childhood brain tumors: Children's and siblings' concerns regarding the diagnosis and phase of illness. *Journal of Pediatric Oncology Nursing, 20*(3), 133–140.

Gibson, C.H. (1991). A concept analysis of the concept of empowerment. *Journal of Advanced Nursing, 16,* 354–61.

Glaser, B.G., & Strauss, A.L. (1968). *Time for dying.* Chicago: Aldine.

Goffman, E. (1963). *Notes on management of spoiled identity.* Englewood Cliffs, NJ: Prentice-Hall.

Granger, B.B., Moser, D., Germino, B., Harrell, J., & Ekman, I. (2006). Caring for patients with chronic heart failure: The trajectory model. *European Journal of Cardiovascular Nursing, 5,* 222–227.

Green, B.L., Lewis, R.K., Wang, M.Q., Person, S., & Rivers, B. (2004). Powerlessness, destiny, and control: The influence on health behaviors of African Americans. *Journal of Community Health, 29*(1), 15–27.

Hägglund, D. & Ahlström, G (2007). The meaning of women's experience of living with long-term urinary incontinence is powerlessness. *Journal of Clinical Nursing, 16*(10), 1946–1954.

Haluska, H.B., Jessee, P.O., & Nagy, M.C. (2002). Sources of social support: Adolescents with cancer. *Oncology Nursing Forum, 29*, 1317–1324.

Hansson, L. & Bjorkman, T. (2005). Empowerment in people with a mental illness: Reliability and validity of the Swedish version of an empowerment scale. *Scandinavian Journal of Caring Sciences, 19*, 32–38.

Hewitt, J. (2002). A critical review of the arguments debating the role of the nurse advocate. *Journal of Advanced Nursing, 37*(5), 439–445.

Huffman, M. (2007). Health coaching: A new and exciting technique to enhance patient self-management and improve outcomes. *Home Healthcare Nurse, 25*(4), 271–275.

Igreja, I., Zuroff, D.C., Koestner, R., Saltaris, C., Bropuillette, M.J., & LaLonde, R. (2000). Applying self-determination to the prediction and well-being in gay men with HIV and AIDS. *Journal of Applied Psychology, 30*(4), 686–706.

Jacelon, C. S. (2007). Theoretical perspectives of perceived control in older adults: A selective review of the literature. *Journal of Advanced Nursing, 59*(1), 1–10.

Johnson, D. (1967). Powerlessness: A significant determinant in patient behavior? *Journal of Nursing Education, 6*(2), 39–44.

Kuokkanen, L., & Leino-Kilpi, H. (2000). Power and empowerment in nursing: Three theoretical approaches. *Journal of Advanced Nursing, 31*(1), 235–241.

Leininger, M.L., & McFarland, M.R. (2002). *Transcultural nursing: Concepts, theories, research and practices* (2nd ed.). New York: McGraw-Hill.

Loft, M., McWilliam, C., & Ward-Griffin, C. (2003). Patient empowerment after total hip and knee replacement. *Orthopedic Nursing, 22*(1), 42–47.

McCann, T. & Clark, E. (2004). Advancing self-determination with young adults who have schizophrenia. *Journal of Psychiatric and Mental Health Nursing, 11*, 12–20.

McCubbin, M. (2001). Pathways to health, illness and well-being: From the perspective of power and control. *Journal of Community and Applied Social Psychology, 11*, 75–81.

McDaniel, S.H., Hepworth, J. & Doherty, W.J. (1997). The shared emotional themes of illness. In S.H.

McDaniel, J., Hepworth, & W.J. Doherty (Eds.). *The shared experience of illness: Stories of patients, families, and their therapists.* New York: Basic Books.

Merriam-Webster Online Dictionary (n.d.) retrieved on December 4, 2007 from www.merriam-webster.com/dictionary/power

Michael, S.R. (1996). Integrating chronic illness into one's life: A phenomenological inquiry. *Journal of Holistic Nursing, 14*(3), 251–267.

Miller, J.F. (Ed.). (1983). *Coping with chronic illness: Overcoming powerlessness.* Philadelphia: F.A. Davis.

Miller, J.F. (Ed.). (1992). *Coping with chronic illness: Overcoming powerlessness* (2nd ed.). Philadelphia: F.A. Davis.

Miller, J.F. (Ed). (2000). *Coping with chronic illness: Overcoming powerlessness.* (3rd ed.). Philadelphia: F.A. Davis.

Mishel, M.H. (1999). Uncertainty in illness. *Annual Review of Nursing Research, 19*, 269–294.

Mitchell, G.J., & Bournes, D.A. (2000). Nurse as patient advocate? In search of straight thinking. *Nursing Science Quarterly, 13*(3), 204–209.

Moden, L. (2004). Power in care homes. *Nursing older people, 16*(6), 24–26.

Mok, E., Martinson, I., & Wong, T.K. (2004). Individual empowerment among Chinese cancer patients in Hong Kong. *Western Journal of Nursing Research, 26*(1), 59–75.

Moller, A.C., Deci, E.L., & Ryan, R.M. (2006). Choice and ego-depletion: The moderating role of autonomy. *Personality and Social Psychology Bulletin, 32*(8), 1024–1036.

Mullins, L., Chaney, J., Balderson, B., & Hommel, K., (2000). The relationship of illness uncertainty, illness intrusiveness and asthma severity to depression in young adults with long-standing asthma. *International Journal of Rehabilitation and Health, 5*, 177–186.

Nagelkerk, J., Reick, K., & Meengs, L. (2006). Perceived barriers and effective strategies to diabetes self-management. *Journal of Advanced Nursing, 54*(2), 151–158.

Nelson, G., Lord, J., & Ochocka, J. (2001). Empowerment and mental health in community: Narratives of psychiatric consumer/survivors. *Journal of Community and Applied Social Psychology, 11*, 125–142.

Neville, K.L. (1998). The relationships among uncertainty, social support, and psychological distress in adolescents recently diagnosed with cancer. *Journal of Pediatric Oncology Nursing, 15,* 37–46.

Newman, S., Steed, L., & Mulligan, K. (2004). Self-management interventions for chronic illness. *Lancet, 364,* 1523–1537.

Niven, C.A., & Scott, P.A. (2003). The need for accurate perception and informed judgement in determining the appropriate use of the nursing resource: Hearing the patient's voice. *Nursing Philosophy, 4,* 201–210.

O'Brein, M. (1993). Multiple sclerosis: The role of social support and disability. *Clinical Nursing Research, 13*(4), 434–457.

Pandey, S.K., Hart, J.J., & Tiwary, S. (2003). Women's health and Internet: Understanding emerging trends and implications. *Social Science and Medicine, 56,* 179–191.

Paterson, B.L. (2001a). The shifting perspectives model of chronic illness. *Journal of Nursing Scholarship, 33,* 21–26.

Paterson, B.L. (2001b). Myth of empowerment in chronic illness. *Journal of Advanced Nursing, 34*(5), 574–581.

Paterson, B.L. (2003). The koala has claws: Applications of the shifting perspectives model in research of chronic illness. *Qualitative Health Research, 13*(7), 987–994.

Pedersen, B.D. (2006). Independence/dependence—a contradictory relationship? Life with a chronic illness. *Scandanavian Journal of Caring Science, 20,* 261–268.

Poland, B., & Pederson, A. (1998). Reading between the lines: Interpreting silences in qualitative research. *Qualitative Inquiry, 4,* 293–312.

Psooy, B.J., Schreuer, D., Borgaonkar, J., & Caines, J.S. (2004). Patient navigation: Improving timeliness in the diagnosis of breast abnormalities. *Canadian Association of Radiologists Journal, 55*(3), 145–150.

Rånhein, M. & Holand, W. (2006). Lived experience of chronic pain and fibromyalgia: Women's stories from daily life. *Qualitative Health Research, 16*(6), 741–761.

Richmond, T., Metcalf, J., Daly, M., & Kish, J. (1992). Powerlessness in acute spinal cord injury patients: A descriptive study. *Journal of Neuroscience Nursing, 24*(3), 146–152.

Rogers, E.S., Chamberlin, J., Ellison, M.L., & Crean, T.A. (1997). A consumer constructed scale to measure empowerment among users of mental health services. *Psychiatric Services, 48,* 1042–1047.

Rosenfield, S. (1992). Factors contributing to the subjective quality of life of the chronic mentally ill. *Journal of Health and Social Behavior, 33,* 299–315.

Roth, D. & Crane-Ross, D. (2002). Impact of services, met needs and service empowerment on consumer outcomes. *Mental Health & Mental Health Services Research, 4,* 43–56.

Rotter, J.P. (1966). Generalized expectancies for internal versus external control of reinforcement. *Psychological Monographs, 80,* 1–28.

Ryan, R.M., & Deci, E.L. (2000). Self-determination theory and the facilitation of intrinsic motivation, social development, and well-being. *American Psychologist, 55*(1), 68–78.

Ryan, R.M., & Frederick, C.M. (1997). Nature and autonomy: An organizational view on the social and neurobiological aspects of self-regulation in behavior and development. *Development and Psychopathology, 9,* 701–728.

Seeman, M., & Lewis, S. (1995). Powerlessness, health and mortality: A longitudinal study of older men and mature women. *Social Science in Medicine, 41*(4), 517–525.

Shapiro, D.H., Schwarz, C.E. & Astin, J.A. (1996). Controlling ourselves, controlling our world: Psychology's role in understanding positive and negative consequences of seeking and gaining control. *American Psychologist, 51,* 1213–1230.

Sheridan-Gonzalez, J. (2000). It's not my patient. *American Journal of Nursing, 100*(1), 13.

Singleton, J.K. (2002). Caring for themselves: Facilitators and barriers to women home care workers who are chronically ill following their care plan. *Health Care for Women International, 23,* 692–702.

Sommerset, M., Campbell, R., Sharp, D.J. & Peters, T.J. (2001). What do people with MS want and expect from health care services? *Health Expectations, 4,* 29–37.

Strandmark, M.K. (2004). Ill health is powerlessness: A phenomenological study about worthlessness, limitations and suffering. *Scandinavian Journal of Caring Science, 18,* 135–144.

Sullivan, T., Weinert, C., & Cudney, S. (2003). Management of chronic illness: Voices of rural women. *Journal of Advanced Nursing, 44*(6), 566–574.

Sullivan-Bolyai, S., Sadler, L., Knafl, K.A., & Gillis, C.L. (2003). Great expectations: A position description for parents as caregivers: Part 1. *Pediatric Nursing, 29*(6), 457–461.

Sutton, R., & Treloar, C. (2007). Chronic illness experiences, clinical markers and living with Hepatitis C. *Journal of Health Psychology, 12*(2), 330–340.

Tang, S.T., & Lee, S.C. (2004). Cancer diagnosis and prognosis in Taiwan: Patient preferences versus experiences. *Psycho-Oncology, 13*, 1–13.

Taylor, S.E. (1983). Adjustment to threatening events: A theory of cognitive adaptation. *American Psychologist, 38*, 1161–1173.

Walker, J., Holloway, I., & Sofaer, B. (1999). In the system: The lived experience of chronic back pain from the perspectives of those seeking help from pain clinics. *Pain, 80*, 621–628.

Wallston, K.A., Malcarne, V.L., Flores, L., Hansdottir, I., Smith, C.A., Stein, M.J., et al. (1999). Does God determine your health? The God locus of health control scale. *Cognitive Therapy and Research, 23*(2), 131–142.

Wollin, J., Dale, H., Spenser, N., & Walsh, A. (2000). What people with newly diagnosed MS (and their families and friends) need to know. *International Journal of MS Care, 2*, 4–14.

World Health Organization (WHO). (2003). *Adherence to long-term therapies: Evidence for action.* Geneva, Switzerland: World Health Organization. Retrieved on December 4, 2007 from www.who.int/chp/knowledge/publications/adherence_report/en/.

Wortman, C., & Brehm, J. (1975). Responses to uncontrollable outcomes: An integration of reactance theory and learned helplessness. In L. Berkowitz (Ed.). *Advances in experimental social psychology* (Vol. 8, pp. 277–336). New York: Academic Press.

Zickmund, S., Ho, E., Masuda, M., Ippolito, L., & LaBrecque, D. (2003). "They treated me like a leper": Stigmatization and the quality of life of patients with hepatitis C. *Journal of General Internal Medicine, 18*, 835–844.

Zoucha, R., & Husted, G.L. (2000). The ethical dimensions of delivering culturally congruent nursing and health care. *Issues in Mental Health Nursing, 21*, 325–340.

12

Culture

Pamala D. Larsen and Sonya R. Hardin

INTRODUCTION

Concepts of health and illness are deeply rooted in culture, race, and ethnicity and influence an individual's illness perceptions and health and illness behavior. Adding to this is the fact that cultures are never homogeneous (Helman, 2007), as there are variations and subcultures within each culture, each affecting health and illness perceptions differently. So, although, one may know the "norms" of Chinese culture, Puerto Rican culture, or Indian culture, for instance, there will always be unique differences in each individual from that culture.

According to the Office of Minority Health Web site on cultural competency (www.omhrc.gov/), culture (and language) influence:

- Health, healing, and wellness belief systems
- How illness, disease, and their causes are perceived, both by the patient/consumer and the provider
- The behaviors of patients who are seeking health care and their attitudes toward providers
- Delivery of services by the provider who looks at the world through his/her own "lens" and set of values, thereby potentially

compromising access and care for those of other cultures.

There are factors other than culture that influence health and illness. Factors include, but are not limited to, environment, economics, genetics, age, previous and current health status, personality, social support, and psychosocial factors. Caring for the individual, family, and community, is, therefore, influenced by numerous factors of which culture is only one. In Canada, culture is identified as one of the 12 determinants of health (Racher & Annis, 2007).

Currently in the United States there are continuing disparities in healthcare among those of different cultures, races, ethnicities, and socioeconomic status [Agency for Healthcare Research and Quality (AHRQ), 2008]. Throughout the literature, becoming culturally competent is seen as the first step in decreasing and eventually eliminating those disparities. Although being culturally competent is important on an individual basis, becoming so as an organization is just as important. The National Center for Cultural Competence has identified six reasons that organizations should incorporate cultural competence into policy:

- To respond to the current and projected demographic changes in the United States

- To eliminate long-standing disparities in the health status of people of diverse racial, ethnic, and cultural backgrounds
- To improve the quality of services and health outcomes
- To meet legislative, regulatory, and accreditation mandates
- To gain a competitive edge in the market place; and
- To decrease the likelihood of liability/malpractice claims (National Center for Cultural Competence, n.d.)

Defining Terms

Culture

The literature provides many definitions of culture. Within the nursing literature, each individual with his or her model/theory of transcultural nursing has a different definition. Although there is value in those definitions, perhaps one from medical anthropology offers a broader perspective. Helman (2007) defines culture as "a set of guidelines (both explicit and implicit) that individuals use to view the world and tell them what behaviors are appropriate" (p. 2). Culture is shared, learned, dynamic, and evolutionary (Schim, Doorenbos, Benkert, & Miller, 2007). This evolution is described by Dreher and MacNaughton (2002) as "people live out their lives in communities, where circumstances generate conflict, where people do not always follow the rules, and where cultural norms and institutions are massaged and modified in the exigencies of daily life" (p. 184).

Typically one thinks of culture as being race and ethnicity bound. However, many other cultures exist if a broader definition of culture is used. Examples include the culture of poverty, the culture of cancer survivors, the culture of rurality, and the culture of chronic illness (see Chapter 2) to name a few. Each of these cultures has explicit and implicit guidelines that determine how their members view the world, decide upon appropriate behaviors, and perform those behaviors.

Cultural Competency

Many definitions of culture mandate that there are many definitions of cultural competence. Table 12-1 lists some of the more common definitions found in the literature. The Centers for Disease Control and Prevention National Prevention Information Network (www.cdcnpin.org) lists eight principles of cultural competence. These principles include:

- Define culture broadly
- Value clients' cultural beliefs
- Recognize complexity in language interpretation
- Facilitate learning between providers and communities
- Involve the community in defining and addressing service needs
- Collaborate with other agencies
- Professionalize staff hiring and training
- Institutionalize cultural competence

Cultural competence for systems and organizations may be seen on a continuum (Rasher & Annis, 2007; Srivastava, 2007). The Cultural Competence Continuum was developed by the National Center for Cultural Competence (NCCC) located at Georgetown University, in Washington, DC. There are six levels on the continuum, spanning from cultural destructiveness at level 1 to cultural proficiency at level 6, the highest level. When an organization is culturally proficient, it holds culture in high esteem and uses this perspective to guide its work (Rasher & Annis, 2007, p. 263).

Cultural Awareness and Sensitivity

Oftentimes we hear the terms cultural awareness and cultural sensitivity. What is their relationship with cultural competency? Purnell (2008a, p. 6) explains awareness as an appreciation of the external signs of culture, whereas sensitivity is one's personal attitude toward others of different cultures. Although awareness and sensitivity are part

TABLE 12-1

Cultural Competency Definitions

Author	Definition
Centers for Disease Control and Prevention, 2007	Integration and transformation of knowledge about individuals and groups of people into specific standards, policies, practices, and attitudes used in appropriate cultural settings to increase the quality of services, thereby producing better outcomes
Spector, 2004, p. 8	Within the delivery of care, the provider understands and attends to the total context of the patient's situation, and it is a complex combination of knowledge, attitudes, and skills
Mutha, Allen, & Welch, 2002, p. 25	A set of skills, knowledge, and attitudes that enhance (1) your understanding of and respect for patients' values, beliefs, and expectations; (2) awareness of your own assumptions and value system in addition to those of the US medical system; and (3) your ability to adapt care to fit with the patient's expectations and preference
Purnell, 1998, p. 6	Having the knowledge, abilities, and skills to deliver care congruent with the client's cultural beliefs and practice
Office of Minority Health	A set of congruent behaviors, attitudes, and policies that come together in a system, agency, or among professionals, that enables effective work in cross-cultural situations
Giger & Davidhizar, 2004, p. 8	A dynamic, fluid, continuous process whereby an individual, system, or healthcare agency finds meaningful and useful care-delivery strategies based on knowledge of the cultural heritage, beliefs, attitudes, and behaviors of those to whom they render care

of cultural competence, competency implies that awareness and sensitivity have been operationalized (Schim et al., 2007).

Myths of Culture and Diversity

Myths of culture and diversity must be challenged. Masi (1996) and Srivastava (2007) discuss six myths that can influence caring for culturally diverse clients.

The Myth of Equality

This myth describes that fairness means equal treatment for all (Srivastava, 2007, p. 42). Proponents of this myth cite success stories of individuals of varying ethnic, racial, and gender

backgrounds who have overcome great obstacles and "made it" as individuals. However, this view reflects a lack of awareness to systemic barriers and institutional racism. It is a narrow view that places all responsibility on the individual without acknowledging systemic inequities.

The Myth of Sameness

The assumption of this myth is that someone who shares the client's ethnicity and language will be able to more effectively provide health care and thus eliminate miscommunication (Masi, 1996; Srivastava, 2007). However this "sameness" may be only on the surface, as there may be many other differences that affect the client and healthcare professional relationship. This also presumes a narrow definition of culture (race and ethnicity) as opposed to a broader view.

The Myth That Cultural Differences Are a Problem

Health care has often viewed issues of culture and diversity from a negative perspective, that they were problems or barriers to overcome. Srivastava (2007, p. 46) suggests that culture should not viewed as a problem, but as a leverage point, a point that can affect the health outcome of the client if energy is focused on it.

The Myth That Everything Must Be Acceptable

There is a perception that if something is a cultural value that it must be "accepted." Masi (1996) suggests that respecting an individual's cultural value not be confused with acceptance. He describes that although that society states that child abuse is unacceptable, that defining child abuse may vary with individuals from different cultures. A practice known as "scratching the wind," where bruises are caused by cupping and scratches are created by running a coin on the skin, is used to relieve fevers and illness in some cultures. Respecting this cultural value does not mean acceptance of this practice.

The Myth That Generalizations Are Unacceptable

Masi (1996) and Srivastava (2007) suggest that there is a large difference between generalizations and stereotypes. Generalizations are a necessary starting point to understand groups of individuals as they indicate trends and patterns. These generalizations may help a healthcare professional initiate a conversation with a client. Stereotypes close conversation and knowledge development (Srivastava, 2007, p. 47).

The Myth That Familiarity Equals Competence

Familiarity with cultural differences may make the difference invisible (Srivastava, 2007, p. 48).

This myth dovetails with the one about generalizations, and means that being familiar with a certain culture does not make one competent, as familiarity may not allow for individual differences.

Transcultural Nursing

Transcultural nursing had its beginnings in the 1950s with Madeleine Leininger. With her work over more than 50 years, in addition to other theorists, transcultural nursing has evolved as a specific and unique specialty. Transcultural nursing is defined as "as a formal area of study and practice focused on comparative human-care (caring) differences and similarities of the beliefs, values and patterned lifeways of cultures to provide culturally congruent, meaningful, and beneficial health care to people (Leininger & McFarland, 2002, p. 6).

There are a number of reasons that transcultural nursing is important in health care today. Leininger and McFarland (2002) summarize eight factors that have led to the development and need for transcultural nursing.

- Increase in immigration and migration of people across the world
- Implicit expectation that nurses and other healthcare providers need to know, understand, respect, and respond appropriately to care for others of diverse cultures
- Increase in the use of technologies in caring or curing, with different responses and effects on clients of diverse cultures
- Increased signs of cultural conflicts, cultural clashes, and cultural imposition practices between nurses and those from diverse cultures
- Increase in number of nurses who travel and work in different places in the world
- Anticipated legal defense suits against nurses resulting from cultural negligence, cultural ignorance, and cultural imposition practices in working with diverse cultures
- Rise in gender and the issues and rights of special groups

- Growing trend to care with and for people, whether well or ill, in their familiar or particular living and working environments (Leininger & McFarland, 2002, pp. 13–18)

The Transcultural Nursing Society was founded in 1974 by Leininger as a worldwide organization for nurses and others interested in and prepared to advance transcultural nursing. The society provides a forum to bring nurses together worldwide with common and diverse interests to improve the care for culturally diverse people. The purposes of the society include:

- To learn about the beliefs and healthcare practices of people from diverse and similar cultures.
- To promote and disseminate knowledge related to transcultural nursing care.
- To develop new knowledge that focuses upon diverse lifeways of cultural groups and their nursing care aspects.
- To maintain and improve the nursing care of people whose values, beliefs, and cultures differ.
- To promote and conduct research to advance transcultural nursing worldwide.
- To serve as a forum for discussing issues related to the development of transcultural nursing and its interrelationship with other healthcare providers and disciplines (www.tcns.org).

IMPACT

Changing Demographics

According to the 2000 US Census, approximately 30% of the population is racially and ethnically diverse. The Census Bureau projects that by 2030 this percentage will increase to 40%, with non-Hispanic whites only making up 60% of the US population [Centers for Disease Control and Prevention (CDC), 2007]. Unfortunately our North American healthcare system(s) is based on Western culture, and that includes using a biomedical

TABLE 12-2

Projected Distribution of the Population, Age 65 and Older, by Race and Hispanic Origin, 2000 and 2050

	2000	*2050*
Total	100.0	100.0
Non-Hispanic white	83.5	64.2
Non-Hispanic black	8.1	12.2
Non-Hispanic American Indian and Alaska Native	0.4	0.6
Non-Hispanic Asian and Pacific Islander	2.4	6.5
Hispanic	5.6	16.4

Note: Data are middle-series projections of the population. Hispanics may be of any race. Reference population: These data refer to the resident population. *Source:* US Census Bureau. (2000). Population projections of the United States by age, sex, race, Hispanic origin, and nativity: 1999 to 2100. Retrieved from www.census.gov/population/www/projections/natproj.html

model. With an increasing diverse society, this narrow view will continue to create a mismatch with clients and their healthcare needs and services.

As we age, the potential for having one or more chronic diseases increases significantly, thus the need to look at demographics of aging Americans is paramount. Currently non-Hispanic older adults account for approximately 83.5% of the older adult population. Projections for 2050 indicate that this percentage will decrease by nearly 20–64%. Given these projections, a culturally competent workforce will be needed to meet the needs of individuals from many cultural and ethnic groups (see Table 12-2).

Health Disparities

Although the focus of this chapter is culture and its influence on individuals with chronic illness, health disparities that occur with individuals from different cultures must be noted as well. Race, ethnicity, and culture sharply divide the health and health care of the population in the United States. Although such disparities have been noted for some time, the Institute of Medicine report, *Unequal Treatment* (Smedley, Stith, & Nelson, 2003), was a landmark publication that put these disparities in the forefront. This report demonstrated that racial and ethnic disparities in health care, with a few exceptions, are consistent across a range of illness and healthcare services.

The same year that *Unequal Treatment* was published, the Agency for Healthcare Research and Quality (AHRQ) released the first annual National Healthcare Disparities Report. Their fifth report was released in February of 2008. Overall three themes emerged from their latest report:

▪ Disparities in healthcare quality and access are not getting smaller
▪ Progress is being made, but many of the biggest gaps in quality and access have not been reduced
▪ The problem of persistent uninsurance is a major barrier to reducing disparities (AHRQ, 2008, p. 1)

Some of the biggest disparities noted in this latest report include:

▪ Blacks had a rate of new AIDS cases 10 times higher than whites
▪ Asian adults age 65 and older were 50% more likely than whites to lack immunization against pneumonia
▪ American Indians and Alaska Natives were twice as likely to lack prenatal care in the first trimester than whites (AHRQ, 2008, p. iv)

Another national document that addresses health disparities is *Healthy People 2010*. The two goals of the document are (1) eradicating health disparities, and (2) increasing health-related quality of life. As healthcare professionals, the need is paramount to incorporate appropriate strategies into clinical

practice with an awareness of different cultures to allocate resources fairly within society. Efforts to address racial, ethnic, and other disparities in health care will require nurses to employ creative interventions to assure culturally competent care for these populations.

Beidler (2005) states that health disparities occur in vulnerable patients who are uninsured, racially and ethnically diverse, and frequently speak languages other than English. Maze (2005) refers to health disparities existing among individuals who are disenfranchised, living in poverty, stigmatized, homeless, immigrants, victims of crimes, children, women, prisoners, persons with AIDS, persons with mental illness, and those who have little social support or education. These individuals make up a vulnerable population and may present with a variety of ethical issues for the healthcare professional. For example, illegal immigrants may be hesitant to provide a name, address, and phone number for follow-up care. Should the healthcare provider try to obtain this information from the illegal immigrant? Remember, the client may be fearful that you will "turn them in" to the authorities.

The article *The State of Opportunity in America* (n.d.) confirmed that in 2002, 28% of African Americans, 44% of Hispanic Americans, 24% of Asian Americans and Pacific Islanders, and 33% of American Indians and Alaska Natives were uninsured and more likely to be dependent upon public sources of health insurance. Minorities are more likely to receive inappropriate or insufficient care than are nonminorities (Smedley et al., 2003).

Racial and Ethnicity Classification

In 1997 the Office of Management and Budget (OMB) identified the following categories to be used by federal programs when reporting data: American Indian or Alaska Native; Asian; Black or African American; Hispanic or Latino; Native Hawaiian or other Pacific Islander; and White. American Indian or Alaska Native refers to people of North and South America and those that maintain tribal affiliations (Wallman, 1998). An Asian is a person with origins in the Far East, Southeast Asia, or the Indian subcontinent. Black or African American refers to individuals with origins from any black racial groups of Africa. Hispanic or Latino is an individual of Cuban, Mexican, Puerto Rican, South or Central American, or other Spanish culture or origin. Native Hawaiians or Other Pacific Islanders have origins in Hawaii, Guam, Samoa, or other Pacific Islands. White is a person having origins in any of the original people of Europe, the Middle East, or North Africa. However, with individuals from mixed origins, it may be difficult to assign an individual to one specific ethnic group.

Examples of Different Cultures

The following examples of the Haitian culture, Mexican culture, and Japanese culture are brief overviews and generalizations of what is known about each culture. Disease labels in each of these cultures have different influences and meanings among clients (Turner, 1996).

In addition, the longer that one is a resident in this country (or other countries), subcultures of the original culture evolve, with each one being more unique.

Haitians

Haitians are from Haiti, an island between Cuba and Puerto Rico about the size of the state of Maryland. The Haitian population in the United States is approximately 365,000 (US Census Bureau, 2005); however, Haitian leaders would argue that there are nearly 1.5 million Haitians in the United States (Colin & Paperwalla, 2008).

The influence of France's rule of Haiti from 1697 to 1804 identified two distinct categories of Haitians. Members of the upper class used the marker of *mulatto* (color), the French culture, and the French language to differentiate themselves from the lower class. Those speaking French rose within the social system. The lower class was mostly black and spoke the Haitian Creole language, which is a combination language of multitribe slaves of Africa. Today, Creole is the official language of Haiti (Colin & Paperwalla, 2008).

Traditionally, the man has been considered the head of the household, the primary income provider, the decision maker, and the sexual initiator, whereas women are to be faithful, honest, respectful, and oversee the house (Dash, 2001). However, that may be changing, as a number of families are becoming matriarchal today (Colin & Paperwalla, 2008). The family unit remains an important concept of Haitian culture.

Haitian people are openly demonstrative in their emotions and typically speak loudly. They have a close personal space and may ignore territorial space. Many may pretend to understand, when in reality they are nodding to be nice and not to show a lack of understanding. The use of simple and clear instructions is needed when providing education to enhance the health of the individual. Haitians are private, and if they do not understanding something, will more than likely choose to use a professional interpreter over a family member (Colin & Paperwalla, 2008).

Drinking alcohol and cigarette smoking is culturally approved for men and is the norm. The Haitian diet is high in carbohydrates and fat, with weight loss being a sign of illness. Lifestyle changes needed when faced with a chronic illness will be a challenge for the provider when trying to help clients understand the impact of alcohol, smoking, and diet to a chronic illness (Colin & Paperwalla, 2008).

Even though Haitians are deeply religious, they also have many superstitions. These beliefs include the fear of a loved one not actually dying, but becoming a zombie. If it is believed that an individual is not really dead, they may ask for an autopsy to ensure death. Beliefs of voodooism, with its roots in Africa, are often co-aligned with their religious beliefs. Voodoo occurs when an individual has the power to communicate by trance with ancestors, saints, or animistic deities. This can have an influence on the psychological stance of the client. Hence, illness can be perceived as punishment for being evil or occur from evil spirits (Corrine, Bailey, Valentin, Mortantus, & Shirley, 1992). Given that vodo and folk remedies are used among this group, providers should always ask what prior home interventions have been tried before prescribing (Galembo & Fleurant, 2005).

Mexicans

Hispanic is a term that is commonly used in the United States to designate all those who speak Spanish. This cultural group includes those from Puerto Rico, Cuba, Mexico, Latin America, and other countries as well. Typically many Hispanic people wish to be described by terms that are specific to their culture, thus using the term Mexican American, is more appropriate (Zoucha & Zamarripa, 2008). Because of the poor economy in Mexico, there has been a constant influx of immigrants from that country during most of the 20th century and now into the 21st century. The media consistently reports stories of undocumented aliens who continue to cross the border into the United States to earn money for their families left behind in Mexico.

Religious beliefs are very important to Mexican Americans, who believe that there is a divine power that has ultimate control of their lives, and one must accept what God gives (Berry, 2002, p. 365). The majority of Mexican Americans are Roman Catholics, and although they may not all attend formal church regularly, pictures and statues with a religious theme are evident in many of their homes.

The family and kinship are important social structures to Mexican Americans. In addition, this group is collectively oriented versus the individual orientation so common in North America. Mexican Americans may prefer to live close to their family and extended family, but not necessarily in the same household, as has been seen in the past. Family extends beyond the immediate circle to include fictive kin or compadres, friends who

are chosen for special occasions (Berry, 2002). The elderly are valued and respected, and their knowledge about health information often takes precedence over that of professional healthcare providers (Berry, 2002; Zoucha & Zamarripa, 2008). Younger generations have the obligation to care for the older generations. Typical families are viewed as patriarchal, with males being dominant and females being passive. *Machismo* in the Mexican culture views men as having strength, valor, and self-confidence (Zoucha & Zamarripa, 2008).

Because family is a priority for Mexican Americans, it will take precedence over work issues. Many are sensitive to confrontation and difference of opinion, and will shun those challenges, especially in the workplace. Truth is often tempered with diplomacy and tact (Zoucha & Zamarripa, 2008). As an example, in the workplace when a service is promised for tomorrow even though it cannot be completed by then, that promise is made to please the customer, not to deceive. For some Mexican Americans, truth is a relative concept; whereby for most European Americans, it is an absolute value (p. 314).

Mexican American's concepts of health and illness are a combination of Aztec and Spanish beliefs (Berry, 2002). Within the culture there is a folk belief system, based in part on religion, regarding cause and cure of illnesses. This system stresses the omnipotence of God, the inevitability of suffering, and the lack of personal control (p. 367). Mexican Americans have a fatalistic worldview and an external locus of control. Thus, if someone becomes ill, that's just the way things are. With preventive health care in short supply in Mexico, many Mexican Americans believe that what happens to them is God's will.

A health belief still prevalent today is that illness is caused by a hot and cold imbalance (Gonzalez & Kuipers, 2004). To cure the illness, the opposite quality of the causative agent must be applied (p. 234). Cold diseases or conditions include menstrual cramps, pneumonia, cancer, earaches, arthritis and others. Hot diseases include pregnancy, diabetes, hypertension, infection, and

CASE STUDY

A home health nurse received an angry call from a Mexican American woman after visiting her house the day before. Her infant had been crying and feverish the next morning and the woman recalled the nurse had remarked the child was adorable. The nurse's compliment and the fact that she had not touched the child, led her to conclude that the nurse had given him the evil eye (www.culturediversity.org/hasp/htm).

Discussion Questions

1. How do you, as the nurse, interpret this woman's behavior?
2. What belief of this woman's heritage have you as the healthcare professional offended?
3. How can you avoid offending someone in a similar situation in the future?

kidney and liver conditions. Regarding pain, Mexicans perceive it as a part of life and part of the inevitable suffering (Zoucha & Zamarripa, 2008, p. 321).

Generally, Mexican Americans respect healthcare professionals because of their training and expertise (Zoucha & Zamarripa, 2008). If healthcare professionals demonstrate respect with their clients, can incorporate folk practitioners as necessary and appropriate, and the concept of *personalismo* into their care, the provider will gain the client's confidence and trust.

Japanese

A common stereotype is to categorize those from the Far East and Southeast Asia as Asians, versus Japanese, Chinese, Korean, Malaysian, Vietnamese, Thai, and so forth. In fact, using the US Census as an example, Asians include individuals from 28 Asian countries (Itano, 2005).

Education is highly valued in Japan, and the illiteracy rate is only 1%. Nearly 95% of students in Japan complete the 12th grade, and the standards for this accomplishment are high. As an example, calculus is part of the mandatory junior high school curriculum (Turale & Ito, 2008).

Japanese American immigrants are the only group to refer to themselves by the generation in which they were born. For instance, *issei* refers to first-generation immigrants; *nisei*, to second-generation immigrants; *sansei*, to third-generation immigrants; *yonsei*, the fourth generation; *gosei*, the fifth generation; and *rokusei*, the sixth generation. These generational categories provide a framework for understanding their cultural values (Ishida & Inouye, 2004, p. 335).

Japanese society is both structured and traditional. Politeness, personal responsibility, loyalty, and working together for the greater good are important concepts. Group harmony is stressed above all else. Japan is a collectivist society, where group needs and wants take precedence over individuals. Japanese culture discourages individualism. There is much sensitivity to social status and one's relative position in life (Brightman, 2005; Turale & Ito, 2008).

The culture is also a relatively non–eye-contact culture when communicating. For some it is considered disrespectful to look someone directly in the eye, particularly if that individual is in a superior position (Galanti, 2004). Japanese culture is seen as a nontouch culture (Ishida & Inouye, 2004). Although there is touch and close contact with infants, there is much less touch and physical contact between adults. Lastly, the ideal pattern of communication in Japanese society is silent communication. Japanese do not appreciate aggressive conversation and prefer to remain silent.

The family is important to Japanese Americans. There is a phrase, *kodomo no tame ni* (for the sake of the children), that reflects the sacrifices that parents and adults make for the success of the next generation (Ishida & Inouye, 2004, p. 342).

Pain is a concept that should not be expressed verbally. Bearing pain is seen as a virtue and one of family honor (Turale & Ito, 2008). In fact in Japan, medications to relieve pain are used much less than in the United States. Furthermore, narcotic use, in particular, is restricted.

In Japan today, physicians are clearly in charge of the healthcare team, and are held in high esteem. The majority of hospitals in Japan are managed by physicians as opposed to individuals with a healthcare management background. Because self-care is not highly regarded in Japan, and physicians are held in high regard, being told what to do by the physician is expected (Turale & Ito, 2008).

The Chinese culture has influenced the health care of many Asian groups, including the Japanese. For instance, there must be a balance between hot (*yang*) and cold (*yin*). *Yin* and *yang* are life forces, and it is believed that illness occurs when there is an imbalance between the two forces (Itano, 2005). The approach to care is to restore harmony, order, and control through one's environment. Harmony is highly valued as a healing mode and to control one's emotions (Leininger, 2002, p. 459).

Culture of Poverty

The culture of poverty impacts the health care of a socioeconomic group, which is often faced with numerous barriers such as access, cost of care, health literacy, and a focus on surviving from one day to the next. Individuals living in poverty may place health lower on their list of priorities as they attempt to live day to day without financial resources. The lack of financial resources often results in less diagnostic tests, use of generic drugs, goal setting that is short term, and the challenge of ensuring compliance (Benson, 2000).

Poverty is synonymous with a present-moment orientation, a lack of planning ahead, and a fatalistic future. Generation after generation can perpetuate poverty by basing decisions on previous decisions that have been made by family members, parental employment and earnings, family structure, and parent education. With poverty, chronic health issues such as substance abuse, smoking, obesity, and incarceration (which may result in

diseases such as HIV, hepatitis, or tuberculosis) may emerge (Pearson, 2003).

Poverty impacts migrants such as Mexicans; the North American Indian; and immigrants from the Middle East, India, and China. Providing care to migrants and immigrants poses an added challenge as these individuals are not only impoverished but also from a different cultural orientation. Healthcare professionals need to consider the cultural and social complexities that increase the challenges of managing chronic illnesses. Being uninsured, having a lower income, and lower educational levels have been associated with a decrease in hypertension and cholesterol screening (Stewart & Silverstein, 2002).

INTERVENTIONS

CLAS Standards

In 2000, the US Department of Health and Human Services (DHHS) Office of Minority Health (OMH) released 14 national standards for culturally and linguistically appropriate services (CLAS) as a means to address and correct inequities in the provision of health care to culturally and ethnically diverse groups. These standards are available at the OMH website (www.omhrc.gov/CLAS). These standards are organized by themes: Culturally Competent Care (Standards 1–3), Language Access Services (Standards 4–7), and Organizational Supports for Cultural Competence (Standards 8–14). Some of these standards are mandates, such as 4, 5, 6 and 7, whereas others are guidelines that should be adopted by federal, state, and national accrediting agencies. One standard, Standard 14, is suggested as voluntary.

Standard 4 mandates that healthcare organizations must offer and provide language assistance at no cost to clients during all hours of operation. Standard 5 mandates that healthcare organizations must have a mechanism to provide clients, in their language, information on their rights to receive language assistance. Standard 6 mandates that the language assistance be competent, and

TABLE 12-3

CLAS Standards

Standard 1	Healthcare organizations should ensure that patients/consumers receive from all staff member's effective, understandable, and respectful care that is provided in a manner compatible with their cultural health beliefs and practices and preferred language.
Standard 2	Healthcare organizations should implement strategies to recruit, retain, and promote at all levels of the organization a diverse staff and leadership that are representative of the demographic characteristics of the service area.
Standard 3	Healthcare organizations should ensure that staff at all levels and across all disciplines receive ongoing education and training in culturally and linguistically appropriate service delivery.
Standard 4	Health care organizations must offer and provide language assistance services, including bilingual staff and interpreter services, at no cost to each patient/consumer with limited English proficiency, at all points of contact, in a timely manner during all hours of operation.
Standard 5	Healthcare organizations must provide to patients/consumers in their preferred language both verbal offers and written notices informing them of their right to receive language assistance services.
Standard 6	Healthcare organizations must ensure the competence of language assistance provided to limited English proficient patients/consumers by interpreters and bilingual staff. Family and friends should not be used to provide interpretation services (except on request by the patient/consumer).
Standard 7	Healthcare organizations must make available easily understood patient-related materials and post signage in the languages of the commonly encountered groups and/or groups represented in the service area.
Standard 8	Healthcare organizations should develop, implement, and promote a written strategic plan that outlines clear goals, policies, operational plans, and management accountability/oversight mechanisms to provide culturally and linguistically appropriate services.
Standard 9	Healthcare organizations should conduct initial and ongoing organizational self-assessments of CLAS-related activities and are encouraged to integrate cultural and linguistic competence-related measures into their internal audits, performance improvement programs, patient satisfaction assessments, and outcomes-based evaluations.
Standard 10	Healthcare organizations should ensure that data on the individual patient's/consumer's race, ethnicity, and spoken and written language are collected in health records, integrated into the organization's management information systems, and periodically updated.
Standard 11	Healthcare organizations should maintain a current demographic, cultural, and epidemiologic profile of the community as well as a needs assessment to accurately plan for and implement services that respond to the cultural and linguistic characteristics of the service area.
Standard 12	Healthcare organizations should develop participatory, collaborative partnerships with communities and utilize a variety of formal and informal mechanisms to facilitate community and patient/consumer involvement in designing and implementing CLAS-related activities.
Standard 13	Healthcare organizations should ensure that conflict and grievance resolution processes are culturally and linguistically sensitive and capable of identifying, preventing, and resolving cross-cultural conflicts or complaints by patients/consumers.
Standard 14	Healthcare organizations are encouraged to regularly make available to the public information about their progress and successful innovations in implementing the CLAS standards and to provide public notice in their communities about the availability of this information.

Source: Office of Minority Health. (2008). US Department of Health & Human Services, National Standards on Culturally and Linguistically Appropriate Services (CLAS). Retrieved from www.omhrc.gov/templates/browse.aspx?lvl=2&lvlID=11

that families and friends should not be utilized unless requested by the client. Standard 7 mandates that signs should be posted in a facility that reflect the most commonly encountered language in the service area. These signs and patient materials should be easily understood. The remaining standards are guidelines and recommendations (Table 12-3 includes all of the mandated guidelines and recommendations).

To help implement the standards on an organizational level, the Alliance of Community Health Plans Foundation, with funding from the Merck Company Foundation, developed 13 case studies and a final report about making a "business case" for projects addressing the CLAS Standards. Each of these case studies addresses the business benefits from addressing the cultural and linguistic needs of clients (Alliance of Community Health Plans Foundation, 2007).

Nursing Frameworks for Practice

Currently a variety of models, theories, and frameworks are available to assist nurses in providing appropriate care for diverse populations. The website of the Transcultural Nursing Society (www. tcns.org) provides information about six transcultural nursing theories and models. Models include those by Margaret Andrews and Joyceen Boyle; Josepha Campinha-Bacote; Joyce Giger and Ruth Davidhizar; Madeline Leininger; Larry Purnell; and Rachel Spector. Three of those models are discussed in the following text.

Leininger's Cultural Care Theory of Diversity and Universality

Cultural values, beliefs, and practices impact health and illness and inform and guide the client and his/her family in the choices and patterns of health care. Care is universal; however, patterns of care vary among and between cultural groups with regard to healthcare beliefs and behaviors (Leininger, 2002; Leininger & McFarland, 2002, 2006). Leininger's Culture Care Theory provides a

theoretical framework for healthcare professionals to discover the differences and similarities between and among cultural groups related to their cultural values, beliefs, and practices. The meanings and uses of these diversities and universalities among the cultures of the world need to be uncovered and understood (Leininger & McFarland, 2002, p. 78).

The social structure of the client and his or her family such as economics, religion, and worldview influence cultural care meanings, expressions, and patterns in different cultures (Leininger & McFarland, 2002, p. 78). Embedded within these structures are generic (folk) care practices, which are separate and distinct from professional care practices (Leininger, 1997; Leininger & McFarland, 2002). This theoretical tenet is particularly instructive for healthcare providers. For example, an individual with chronic pain may rely on the home remedies taught by an elder in the family or use a variety of herbs and compounds that have been obtained from a traditional healer to manage pain. The healthcare provider must be vigilant in the belief and use of generic care practices, and incorporate those into the plan of care. The last theoretical tenet of Leininger's theory provides three modes of nursing decisions and actions for culturally congruent care: (1) culture care preservation and maintenance, (2) culture care accommodation and/or negotiation, and (3) culture care restructuring and/or repatterning (Leininger, 2002; Leininger & McFarland, 2002, 2006).

As an example, Mrs. Huerta has degenerative arthritis. Her mother was a traditional healer in the village where she grew up. As a young child, Mr. Huerta learned the healing ways and practices from her mother. As an elderly woman, Mrs. Huerta continues to use these traditional methods to manage her chronic pain. When Mrs. Huerta was admitted to the acute care setting, she brought with her remedies that have brought her comfort and relief in the past. Leininger's three modes of nursing decisions and action are informative and directive for the nurse to provide culturally competent care for Mrs. Huerta. The nurse can incorporate these home remedies into the care within the acute setting, the nurse can talk with Mrs. Huerta, or, in the event the home remedies Mrs. Huerta is taking are known to be unsafe or contraindicated with her present care regime, the nurse can explore alternative comfort and pain relief strategies with Mrs. Huerta. The cultural care values, beliefs, and practices are honored and maintained. Therefore, Leininger advocates cultural holding knowledge by healthcare providers in order to provide culturally competent care and further, to minimize the potential for cultural inappropriate care that has the potential for harm and pain to the healthcare client and his/her family.

Giger-Davidhizar Transcultural Assessment Model

The Giger-Davidhizar Model was developed initially in 1991. The model is built upon concentric concepts with the client, a unique cultural being, in the center. The next circle contains concepts of religion, culture, and ethnicity (2004). The last circle focuses on six cultural concepts: (1) communication, (2) space, (3) social organization, (4) time, (5) environmental control, and (6) biological variation.

Communication refers to all human interaction and behavior, both verbal and nonverbal. Space refers to the distance between individuals when they interact, communicate, or reside together. Time can be past, present, or future oriented. How individuals view this concept is often uncovered through their style of communication. Individuals who focus on the past, attempt to maintain tradition, whereas those focused on the present do not formulate goals. Environmental control refers to the ability of the individual to control nature and to plan and direct factors in the environment that affect them. If persons come from cultural groups where there is external control, there may be a fatalistic view ultimately resulting in the belief that seeking health care is useless. Biological differences, especially genetic variations, exist between individuals. These biologic differences among various racial groups are often less understood (Giger & Davidhizar, 2004).

The Purnell Model for Cultural Competence

Purnell's Model for Cultural Competence is graphically represented in a model that includes both the macro and micro concepts. The model is depicted by four concentric circles, each depicting a macro concept. The outer circle represents global society, and is defined as "world communications and politics; conflicts and warfare; natural disasters and famines; international exchanges in business, commerce, and information technology; advances in the health sciences; space exploration; and the increased ability for people to travel around the world and to interact with diverse societies" (Purnell, 2008b, p. 20).

The second circle is the community, and it is defined as a group of people living that have common interests, but not necessarily living in the same geographic area. It is the physical, social, and symbolic characteristics of the community that enable it to feel connected, not common geography (p. 21). The third circle represents the family that is made up of two or more individuals who are emotionally connected, and who or may not live together. The fourth circle represents the individual who is continually adapting to his or her community (p. 22).

The model's organizing framework comprises 12 microconcepts, or domains, that are interconnected and common to all cultures with implications for health and health care. To assess the ethnocultural attributes of the community, family or person, each of the following domains needs to be addressed:

- Overview, inhabited localities, and topography
- Communication
- Family roles and organization
- Workforce issues
- Biocultural ecology
- High-risk behaviors
- Nutrition
- Pregnancy and childbearing practices
- Death rituals

- Spirituality
- Healthcare practices
- Healthcare practitioners (Purnell, 2008b, p. 22)

Purnell (2008b) also includes barriers to appropriate health care that individuals, families and communities may face. The barriers are termed the 12 A's of which healthcare professionals need to be aware. Barriers include availability, accessibility, affordability, appropriateness, accountability, adaptability, acceptability, awareness, attitudes, approachability, alternative practices, and additional services available.

Communication

Communication is the crux of cultural care. It is important for nurses to be aware of appropriate body stance and proximities, gestures, languages, listening styles, and eye contact when communicating with clients, as different cultural groups, nearly 3000 worldwide, vary widely in their ideas regarding these (Narayanasamy, 2003). Differences in language between the client and healthcare professional impede detection of health needs, treatment, and patient care. For nursing interventions to be effective, it is imperative that nurses give attention to all aspects of the client's care as well as the communication process involving them.

The practice of cultural care requires negotiations and compromise as well as an understanding of how the patient views his health problem. Clients cared for by a nurse who has developed an awareness of cultural care practice have the opportunity to be fully acknowledged. Nurses who have an awareness of appropriate cultural care practice need to encourage their peers and promote the delivery of cultural care nursing by utilizing it in their everyday nursing practice.

Giger and Davidhizar (2004) have developed guidelines for communication (see Table 12-4). Although these are general guidelines, they provide a basis or a starting point. Although all of the guidelines are important, perhaps the initial one that is most important is to assess your own personal beliefs about persons from different cultures.

It is difficult to understand others' beliefs if you do not have an awareness of your own, and how they may influence your attitudes toward others.

The use of symbols to facilitate communication in healthcare facilities can serve as a means to represent a world object, place, or concept. Unfortunately in hospitals, universal symbols on signs are rare; instead text in another language is more often found. The idea of symbols for healthcare signage originated from the subway system in Mexico City, which uses cultural icons to identify destinations. In 2003, Hablamos Juntos utilized a consultant to explore the use of healthcare symbols for wayfinding, including recommendations for future steps (Hablamos Juntos, 2008). The conclusion of the white paper was that symbols were a viable option for wayfinding in health care, that a set of tested symbols, publicly available, would help designers of health facilities increase communication and understanding. A total of 28 symbols were developed, with 17 of them being understood by at least 87% of a subject group of 300 participants from four language groups: English, Spanish, Indo-European, and Asian languages. This information is readily available, but why haven't facilities implemented these symbols?

Communication can be difficult between different cultures because of misunderstandings, inability to speak a language, or the use of technical terminology. Each culture has patterns for word choice, inflection, gestures and facial expressions, eye movement and eye contact, volume and speed of speech, use of silence, directness, and the degree of emotion. Nonverbal cues also impact communication. The amount of personal space, social space, and public space often differ between cultures, and one should always note another person's comfort zone.

Health Assessment

As the initial step in the nursing process, it is critical that healthcare professionals understand certain cultural behaviors related to their physical assessment. Simple things like eye contact and touch can greatly affect an individual's response

TABLE 12-4

Communication Guidelines

1. Assess your personal beliefs surrounding persons from different cultures.
   a. Review your personal beliefs and past experiences
   b. Set aside any values, biases, ideas, and attitudes that are judgmental and may negatively affect care
3. Assess communication variables from a cultural perspective
   a. Determine the ethnic identity of the patient, including generation in America
   b. Use the patient as a source of information when possible
   c. Assess cultural factors that may affect your relationship with the patient and respond appropriately
3. Plan care based on the communicated needs and cultural background
   a. Learn as much as possible about the patient's cultural customs and beliefs
   b. Encourage the patient to reveal cultural interpretation of health, illness, and health care
   c. Be sensitive to the uniqueness of the patient
   d. Identify sources of discrepancy between the patient's and your own concepts of health and illness
   e. Communicate at the patient's personal level of functioning
   f. Evaluate effectiveness of nursing actions and modify nursing care plan when necessary
4. Modify communication approaches to meet cultural needs
   a. Be attentive to signs of fear, anxiety, and confusion in the patient
   b. Respond in a reassuring manner in keeping with the patient's cultural orientation
   c. Be aware that in some cultural groups discussion with others concerning the patient may be offensive and impede the nursing process
5. Understand that respect for the patient and communicated needs are central to the therapeutic relationship
   a. Communicate respect by using a kind and attentive approach
   b. Learn how listening is communicated in the patient's culture
   c. Use appropriate active listening techniques
   d. Adopt an attitude of flexibility, respect, and interest to help bridge barriers imposed by culture
6. Communicate in a nonthreatening manner
   a. Conduct the interview in an unhurried manner
   b. Follow acceptable social and cultural amenities
   c. Ask general questions during the information-gathering stage
   d. Be patient with a respondent who gives information that may seem unrelated to the patient's health problem
   e. Develop a trusting relationship by listening carefully, allowing time, and giving the patient your full attention
7. Use validating techniques in communication
   a. Be alert for feedback that the patient is not understanding
   b. Do not assume meaning is interpreted without distortion
8. Be considerate of reluctance to talk when the subject involves sexual matters
   a. Be aware that in some cultures sexual matters are not discussed freely with members of the opposite sex
9. Adopt special approaches when the patient speaks a different language
   a. Use a caring tone of voice and facial expression to help alleviate the patient's fears
   b. Speak slowly and distinctly, but not loudly
   c. Use gestures, pictures, and play acting to help the patient understand
   d. Repeat the message in different ways if necessary
   e. Be alert to words the patient seems to understand and use them frequently
   f. Keep messages simple and repeat them frequently
   g. Avoid using medical terms and abbreviations that the patient may not understand
   h. Use an appropriate language dictionary
10. Use interpreters to improve communication
    a. Ask the interpreter to translate the message, not just the individual words
    b. Obtain feedback to confirm understanding
    c. Use an interpreter who is culturally sensitive

Source: Giger, J. & Davidhizar, R. (2004). *Transcultural nursing: Assessment and intervention* (4th ed.) (p. 35). St. Louis: Mosby.

TABLE 12-5

Behaviors Related to Health Assessment

Cultural Group	Belief/Practice	Nursing Implication
African Americans	Dialect and slang terms require careful communication to prevent error.	Question the client's meaning.
Mexican Americans	Eye behavior is important. An individual who looks at and admires a child without touching the child has given the child the "evil eye."	Always touch the child you are examining.
American Indians	Eye contact is considered a sign of disrespect.	Recognize that the client may be attentive and interested even though eye contact is avoided.
Appalachians	Eye contact is considered impolite or a sign of hostility. Verbal patter may be confusing.	Avoid excessive eye contact.
American Eskimos	Body language is very important. Individual seldom disagrees publicly with others. May nod yes to be polite, even if not in agreement.	Monitor own body language.
Jewish Americans	Orthodox Jews consider excess touching offensive, particularly from members of the opposite sex.	Establish whether client is an Orthodox Jew and avoid excessive touch.
Chinese Americans	Individual may nod head to indicate yes or shake head to indicate no. Excessive eye contact indicates rudeness. Excessive touch is offensive.	Ask questions carefully and clarify responses. Avoid excessive eye contact and touch.
Filipino Americans	Offending people is to be avoided at all cost; nonverbal behavior is very important.	Monitor nonverbal behaviors.
Haitian Americans	Touch is used in conversation. Direct eye contact is used to gain attention and respect.	Use direct eye contact when communicating.
East Indian Hindu Americans	Women avoid eye contact as a sign of respect.	Be aware that men may view eye contact by women as offensive. Avoid eye contact.
Vietnamese Americans	Avoidance of eye contact is a sign of respect. The head is considered sacred; it is not polite to pat the head. An upturned palm is offensive in communication.	Limit eye contact. Touch the head only when mandated and explain clearly before proceeding to do so. Avoid hand gesturing.

Source: Giger, J. & Davidhizar, R. (2004). *Transcultural nursing: Assessment and intervention* (4th ed.) (p. 15). St. Louis: Mosby.

to the healthcare professional and determine what can and cannot be done regarding the individual's health care. Giger and Davidhizar (2004) have provided a table with some basic cultural variations that may be seen in health assessment (see Table 12-5). Again, as with all cultures, there is uniqueness in each individual, and these behaviors should be seen as general guidelines only.

Professional Education

The need for education about different cultures to progress toward cultural competency is evident. There are an increasing number of resources available online that may provide assistance. For instance, the National Technical Assistance Center at the University of Hawaii provides information about Asian Americans and Pacific Islanders to increase the potential of individuals with disabilities in these groups to gain employment. Their Web site contains overviews of each culture, newsletters, success stories, and training (http://www.ntac.hawaii.edu).

The DHHS OMB has developed Culturally Competent Nursing Modules for nurses to increase awareness, knowledge, and skills in caring for those from diverse populations (Scott, 2008). The content of those modules are focused on the themes of the CLAS Standards. There is no cost for the modules, and continuing education credit is offered.

The National Center for Cultural Competence based at the Georgetown University Center for Child and Human Development (http://www11.georgetown.edu/research/gucchd/nccc) has multiple resources available on their Web site. The center also has a Curricula Enhancement Module Series.

The Commonwealth Fund with their work in cultural competency provides papers, a video, and presentations on their Web site (http://www.commonwealthfund.org). This fund has supported significant research in the area of cultural competency.

Measuring Cultural Competence From the Patient's Perspective

As health care tries to ascertain "best practices" in providing culturally competent care, who better to ask than the patient? The Commonwealth Fund's division of health policy, health reform, and performance improvement has identified five domains of culturally competent care that can best be assessed from the patient perspective. The five components include (1) patient–provider communication, (2) respect for patient preferences and shared decision-making, (3) experiences leading to trust or distrust, (4) experiences of discrimination, and (5) linguistic competency (Ngo-Metzger et al., 2006). The five components have been incorporated into a conceptual framework as well.

Putting the Pieces of the Puzzle Together

Schim, Doorenbos, Benkert, and Miller (2007) view the bigger picture as culturally congruent care versus culturally competent care. Leininger was the first to use the term culturally congruent care, and Schim and colleagues' model builds on Leininger's work and definition. Culturally congruent care is defined as:

> Those cognitively based assistive, supportive, facilitative or enabling acts or decisions that are tailor made to fit with individual, group, or institution cultural values, beliefs and lifeways in order to provide or support meaningful beneficial and satisfying health care or well-being services (Leininger, 1991, p. 49).

Schim and colleagues apply the puzzle metaphor to this care and see the finished puzzle with four constructs (2004, p. 105). These constructs include cultural diversity, cultural awareness, cultural sensitivity, and cultural competence.

- Cultural Diversity

    varies in quality and quantity across place and time; is dynamic, ever-changing

- Cultural Awareness

    cognitive construct; a reality to be contemplated and a corresponding capacity for processing knowledge

- Cultural Sensitivity

    affective or attitudinal construct; attitude about their own person and others

- Cultural Competence

    behavioral construct; is the action that is taken in response to diversity, awareness, and sensitivity

Schim and colleagues suggest that there is one piece missing from their puzzle model and that is the client, whether it be an individual, family, or community. The client "layer" of the puzzle, although essential, is not visualized in the current model (p. 106).

EVIDENCE-BASED PRACTICE BOX

There is consensus that self-care practices play a significant role in the management of chronic illness; however, we don't know how self-care is influenced by culture. This study interviewed 167 African Americans with one or more chronic illnesses from two urban counties in California to determine their self-care practice and influences to those practices. Participants were interviewed three times over the course of a year. The sample included individuals of varying health insurance status and different age groups. The most common illnesses included diabetes, asthma, and heart disease or hypertension. Interview data were divided into low-income and middle-income groups, with a further step of categorizing individuals as uninsured, Medicaid, Medicare, or privately insured. Groups were analyzed separately and then cross-group comparisons were made.

Self-care practices among African Americans were found to be culturally based. The participants described idea systems and behavioral practices that were shared by most in the sample. Three culturally based factors were central to the development of their self-care practices and included: (1) spirituality; (2) social support and advice; and (3) nonbiomedical healing traditions. These factors were present regardless of socioeconomic status (p. 2069).

Spirituality. Almost all participants reported that a belief in God or a higher power helped them to manage their illness. Spirituality was a part of their daily practices. Participants cited the importance of focusing on inner strength derived from their religion and cultural values.

Social Support and Advice. Emotional support was highly valued and came from a variety of sources. Both men and women reported that their mother was a major source of support. In addition, social support came from children to parents as children reminded their parents of medications, treatments, self-care, doctor's appointments, and so on. Friends also reenforced self-care.

Nonbiomedical Healing Traditions. Many times these healing traditions were shared with the participants from their mothers. Although traditional medicine was used, it was augmented with nontraditional remedies.

Nursing Implications. This study underlined the value of being aware of clients' cultural practices and how they influence self-care in chronic illness. Although we have valued self-care as an important component in caring for patients with chronic illness, the cultural component of such care has been underemphasized. With the exception of church-based interventions, public health practice often overlooks the feasibility of building on cultural practices.

Source: Becker, G., Gates, R.J., & Newsom, E. (2004). Self-care among chronically ill African Americans: Culture, health disparities, and health insurance status. *American Journal of Public Health, 94*(12), 2066–2073.

OUTCOMES

The literature is clear that providing culturally competent (or congruent) care is a primary strategy in reducing or eliminating racial and ethnic health disparities in the United States. Thus outcome measures such as the annual National Health Disparities Report produced by the AHRQ and *Healthy People 2010* would provide evidence of decreasing health disparities.

In addition, as suggested by the Commonwealth Fund, giving credence to patients' perceptions of cultural competence makes sense. Healthcare professionals may think they are culturally competent, but do their patients agree? Ngo-Metzger and colleagues (2006) suggest monitoring patient populations through both quantitative and qualitative methods that examine health literacy, English proficiency, language spoken at home, and the use of complementary and alternative medical practices (p. 26).

STUDY QUESTIONS

1. Why does culture matter in the care of an individual, family, or community?
2. How does one become culturally competent?
3. Distinguish between being culturally sensitive, aware, and competent?
4. Standard 12 of CLAS states: Healthcare organizations should develop participatory, collaborative partnerships with communities and utilize a variety of formal and informal mechanisms to facilitate community and patient/consumer involvement in designing and implementing CLAS-related activities. What strategies would facilitate standard 12?
5. Evaluate the barriers to health care in a culturally diverse client you have recently seen using Purnell's identified barriers of availability, accessibility, affordability, appropriateness, accountability, adaptability, acceptability, awareness, attitudes, approachability, alternative practices, and additional services available.
6. How do the different transcultural nursing theories view cultural competence?
7. How are the different cultures (Haitian, Japanese, and Mexican) similar and different in their views of health and illness?
8. Explain how becoming culturally competent might decrease health disparities.

INTERNET RESOURCES

Association of Asian Pacific Community Health Organizations: www.aapcho.org/site/aapcho/section.php?id=10942
Black Health Network: www.blackhealthnet.com
Center for Cross-Cultural Health: www.crosshealth.com
Centers for Disease Control and Prevention National Prevention Information Network: www.cdcnpin.org
Diversity in Medicine: www.amsa.org/div
EthnoMed: www.ethnomed.org
Hablamos Juntos: www.hablamosjuntos.org/signage/symbols/default.symbols.asp
HRSA Health Disparities Collaborative: www.healthdisparities.net/hdc/html/home.aspx
Initiative to Eliminate Racial and Ethnic Disparities in Health: raceandhealth.hhs.gov
Minority Health Program University of North Carolina at Chapel Hill: www.minority.unc.edu
Multicultural Health Communication Service: www.mhcs.health.nsw.gov.au/
Multicultural Audiovisual Resources: ublib.buffalo.edu/libraries/units/hsl/ref/av.html
Multilingual Health Education Net: multilingual-health-education.net
National Center for Cultural Competence: www11.georgetown.edu/research/gucchd/nccc/documents/Materials_ Guide.pdf
National Multicultural Institute: www.nmci.org
National Standards for Culturally and Linguistically Appropriate Services: www.omhrc.gov/CLAS
Office of Minority Health Resource Center Health Resources and Services Administration: www.omhrc.gov
Provider's Guide to Quality and Culture: erc.msh.org/quality&culture
Resources for Cross Cultural Health Care: www.diversityrx.org

REFERENCES

Agency for Healthcare Research and Quality (2008). *National healthcare disparities report 2007.* Rockville, MD: US Department of Health and Human Services. AHRQ Pub. No. 08-0041.

Alliance of Community Health Plans Foundation (2007). *Making the business case for culturally and linguistically appropriate services in health care: Case Studies from the field.* Retrieved on May 31, 2008 from www.achp.org/page.asp?page_id=1059

Becker, G., Gates, R.J., & Newsom, E. (2004). Self-care among chronically ill African Americans: Culture, health disparities and health insurance status. *American Journal of Public Health, 94*(12), 2066–2073.

Beidler, S.M. (2005). Ethical issues experienced by community-based nurse practitioners addressing health disparities among vulnerable populations. *International Journal for Human Caring, 9*(3), 43–50.

Benson, D.S. (2000). Providing health care to human beings trapped in the poverty culture. *Physician Executive, 26*(2), 28–32.

Berry, A. (2002). Culture care of the Mexican American family. In M. Leininger & M.R. McFarland (Eds.). *Transcultural nursing: Concepts, theories, research and practice* (3rd ed.). (pp. 363–373). New York: McGraw Hill.

Brightman, J.D. (2005). *Asian culture brief: Japan.* Retrieved on May 31, 2008 from http://www.ntac.hawaii.edu/

Centers for Disease Control and Prevention. (2007). Cultural competence. Retrieved from www.cdcnpin.org/scripts/population/culture.asp

Centers for Disease Control and Prevention. (2007). Office of Minority Health and Disparity. Retrieved on February 15, 2008 from www.cdc.gov/omhd/

Colin, J.M., & Paperwalla, G. (2008). People of Haitian heritage. In L. Purnell & B. Paulanka (Eds.). *Transcultural health care: A culturally competent approach.* (3rd ed.) (pp. 231–247). Philadelphia: F.A. Davis.

Corrine, L., Bailey, V., Valentin, M., Mortantus, E., & Shirley, L. (1992). The unheard voices of women: Spiritual interventions in maternal-child health. *Maternal Child Nursing, 17*, 141–145.

Dash, J.M. (2001). *Culture and customs of Haiti (Culture and Customs of Latin America and the Caribbean).* Westport, CT: Greenwood Press.

Dreher, M., & MacNaughton, N. (2002). Cultural competence in nursing: Foundation or fallacy? *Nursing Outlook, 50*, 181–186.

Galanti (2004). *Caring for patients from different cultures: Case studies from American hospitals* (3rd ed.). Philadelphia: University of Pennsylvania.

Galembo, P., & Fleurant, G. (2005). *Vodou: Visions and voices of Haiti.* Berkley, CA: Ten Speed Press.

Giger, J., & Davidhizar, R. (2004). (Eds.). *Transcultural nursing: Assessment and intervention* (4th ed.). St. Louis: Mosby.

Gonzalez, T., & Kuipers, J. (2004). Mexican Americans. In J. Giger and R. Davidhizar (Eds.). *Transcultural nursing: Assessment and intervention* (4th ed.), (pp. 221–253). St. Louis: Mosby.

Hablamos Juntos (2008). Language policy and practice in health care. Retrieved on February 15, 2008 from www.hablamosjuntos.org.

Healthy People 2010 – Midcourse Review (2005). Retrieved on March 6, 2008 from www.healthypeople.gov/data/midcourse/default.htm

Helman, C.G. (2007) *Culture, health and illness* (5th ed.). London: Hodder Arnold.

Ishida, D., & Inouye, J. (2004). Japanese Americans. In J. Giger & R. Davidizar (Eds.) *Transcultural nursing: Assessment and intervention* (4th ed.) (pp. 332-361). St. Louis: Mosby

Itano, J.K. (2005). Cultural diversity among individuals with cancer. In C. H. Yarbro, M.H. Frogge & M. Goodman (Eds.). *Cancer nursing: Principles and practice* (6th ed.) (pp.69–94). Sudbury, MA: Jones & Bartlett.

Leininger, M. (Ed.). (1991). *Culture care diversity and universality: A theory of nursing.* New York: National League of Nursing.

Leininger, M. (1995). *Transcultural nursing concepts, theories, research and practices.* New York: McGraw-Hill Inc.

Leininger, M. (1997). Overview of the theory of culture care with the ethnonursing research method. *Journal of Transcultural Nursing, 8*(2), 32–53.

Leininger, M. (2002). Culture Care Theory: A major contribution to advance transcultural nursing knowledge and practices. *Journal of Transcultural Nursing, 13*, 189–192.

Leininger, M.M., & McFarland, M.R. (2002). *Transcultural nursing: Concepts, theories, research & practice* (2nd ed.). New York: McGraw-Hill.

Leininger, M.M., & McFarland, M.R. (2006). *Culture care diversity and universality: A worldwide nursing theory* (3rd ed.). Sudbury, MA: Jones & Bartlett.

Masi, R. (1996). Inclusion: How can a health system respond to diversity. In A.S. Zieberth (Ed.), *Pinched: A management guide to the Canadian health care archipelago* (pp. 147–157). Nepean, ON: Pinched Press.

Maze, C.D. (2005). Registered nurses' personal rights vs. professional responsibility in caring for members of underserved and disenfranchised populations. *Journal of Clinical Nursing, 14*(5), 546–554.

Narayanasamy, A. (2003). Transcultural nursing: How do nurses respond to cultural needs? *British Journal of Nursing, 12*(3), 185–194.

National Center for Cultural Competence. Georgetown University Center for Child and Human Development. Retrieved May 29, 2008 from www11.georgetown.edu/research/gucchd/nccc/resources/cultural5.html

National Prevention Information Network, Centers for Disease Control. Retrieved May 22, 2008 from www.cdcnpin.org/scripts/population/culture.asp.

Ngo-Metzger, Q., Telfair, J., Sorkin, D.H., Weidmer, B., Weech-Maldonado, R., Hurtado, M., et al. (2006). Cultural competency and quality of care: Obtaining the patient's perspective. The Commonwealth Fund. Retrieved May 22, 2008 from www.commonwealthfund.org/publications/publications_show.htm?doc_id=414116   .

Office of Minority Health. (2008). U.S. Department of Health & Human Services, Cultural Competency, Retrieved May 28, 2008 from www.omhrc.gov/templates/browse.aspx?lvl=2&lvlID=11

Office of Minority Health. (2008). U.S. Department of Health & Human Services, National Standards on Culturally and Linguistically Appropriate Services (CLAS). Retrieved from www.omhrc.gov/templates/browse.aspx?lvl=2&lvlID=11

Opportunity Agenda, The. Building the national will to expand opportunity in America (n.d.). *The state of opportunity in America.* Retrieved November 26, 2007 from www.opportunityagenda.org

Pearson, L. (2003). Understanding the culture of poverty. *The Nurse Practitioner, 28*, 4–6.

Purnell, L. (2008a). Transcultural diversity and healthcare. In L. Purnell & Paulanka, B. (Eds.). *Transcultural health care: A culturally competent approach* (3rd ed.). (pp. 1–18). Philadelphia: F.A. Davis.

Purnell, L. (2008b). The Purnell model for cultural competence. In L. Purnell & Paulanka, B. (Eds.). *Transcultural health care: A culturally competent approach* (3rd ed.). (pp. 19–55). Philadelphia: F.A. Davis.

Purnell, L., & Paulanka, B. (1998). *Transcultural health care: A culturally competent approach.* Philadelphia: F.A. Davis.

Rasher, F.E., & Annis, R.C. (2007). Respecting culture and honoring diversity in community practice [Electronic version]. *Research and Theory for Nursing Practice: An International Journal, 21*(4), p. 255–270.

Schim, S., Doorenbos, A., Benkert, R., & Miller, J. (2007). Culturally congruent care: Putting the puzzle together [Electronic version]. *Journal of Transcultural Nursing, 18*(2), 103–110.

Scott, D.E. (2008, January/February). The multicultural health care work environment [Electronic version]. *The American Nurse.* Retrieved May 30, 2008 from www.NursingWorld.org

Smedley, B.D., Stith, A.Y., & Nelson, A.R. (2003). *Unequal treatment: Confronting racial and ethnic disparities in health care.* Washington, D.C.: The National Academies Press.

Spector, R. (2004). *Cultural diversity in health and illness* (6th ed.). Upper Saddle River, NJ: Pearson Prentice Hall.

Srivastava, R.H. (2007). Understanding cultural competence in health care. In R.H. Srivastava (Ed.). *The healthcare professional's guide to clinical cultural competence* (pp. 3–27). Toronto: Mosby Elsevier.

Stewart, S.H., & Silverstein, M.D. (2002). Racial and ethnic disparity in blood pressure and cholesterol measurement. *Journal of General Internal Medicine, 17*, 458–464.

Turale, S., & Ito, M. (2008). People of Japanese heritage. In L. Purnell & B. Paulanka (Eds.). *Transcultural health care: A culturally competent approach* (3rd ed.). (pp. 260–277). Philadelphia: F.A. Davis.

Turner, D.W. (1996). The role of culture in chronic illness [Electronic version]. *American Behavioral Scientist, 39*(6), 717–728.

U.S. Census Bureau (2005). *2005 American Community Survey*. Retrieved April 8, 2008 from www.census. gov/

Wallman, K.K. (1998). Data on Race and Ethnicity: Revising the Federal Standard. *The American Statistician*, 52, 1, 31–33.

Zoucha, R., & Zamarripa, C.A. (2008). People of Mexican heritage. In L. Purnell & B. Paulanka (Eds.). *Transcultural health care: A culturally competent approach* (3rd ed.) (pp. 309–324). Philadelphia: F.A. Davis.

13

Self-Care

Judith E. Hertz

INTRODUCTION

On the surface, self-care is simply taking care of one's self to remain healthy. However, self-care within the context of living with a chronic illness is more complex. Self-care is required for successful management and control of chronic illnesses such as arthritis (McDonald-Miszczak & Wister, 2005; Yip, Sit, & Wong, 2004), heart disease (Burnette, Mui, & Zodikoff, 2004; Chriss, Sheposh, Carlson, & Riegel, 2004; Inglis, Pearsonk, Treen, Gallasch, Horowitz, & Stewart, 2008; Washburn, Hornberger, Klutman, & Skinner, 2005), diabetes (Berg & Wadhwa, 2007), HIV/AIDS (Mendias & Paar, 2007), asthma (Cortes, Lee, Boal, Mion, & Butler, 2004), and fecal incontinence (Bliss, Fischer, & Savik, 2005).

Self-care is also viewed as a pivotal concept in health promotion, disease prevention, and disease-screening programs (Haber, 2002; Resnick, 2001, 2003). Furthermore, self-care has been viewed as essential to "health" in persons with chronic illnesses who receive care in nursing homes (Bickerstaff et al., 2003), home care (Sharkey, Ory, & Browne, 2005), and rehabilitation (Singleton, 2000), and during transitions from one health-care setting to another (Coleman, Smith, Frank, Min, Parry, & Kramer, 2004). Finally, self-care is

applicable globally and transculturally when discussing health status in persons with chronic illnesses (Borg, Hallberg, & Blomqvist, 2006; Cortes et al., 2004; Inglis et al., 2008; Leenerts et al., 2002; McDonald-Miszczak & Wister, 2005; Wang et al., 2001; Yip et al., 2004).

Despite the widespread belief that self-care is integral to persons with chronic illness, there is little agreement about the meaning of self-care. Sometimes self-care is defined as adherence/compliance with treatment regimens (Chriss et al., 2004). whereas other times it is referred to as having the functional ability to carry out activities of daily living (ADLs) and instrumental activities of daily living (IADLs) (Burnette et al., 2004). Other definitions imply that self-care is the belief that one can implement disease-treatment regimens (i.e., self-efficacy) (McDonald-Miszczak & Wister, 2005; Yip et al., 2004) or that one can manage and report symptoms associated with an illness (Chriss et al., 2004; Edwardson & Dean, 1999; Musil et al., 2001). The ability to meet basic holistic human needs and achieve self-actualization provides yet another perspective (Hertz & Rossetti, 2006; Mendias & Paar, 2007). The meaning of self-care becomes even more complex, since often it is equated solely to independent behaviors to care for self (Borg et al., 2006; Burnette, Mui, & Zodikoff,

2004); therefore, if one is dependent on others for assistance, as often happens when living with chronic illnesses, then self-care cannot exist.

Although there is lack of agreement about the definition of self-care, there is implicit and explicit agreement that self-care is vital to individual health maintenance, disease prevention, and health promotion. When persons are living with chronic illnesses, the importance and need to care for self is further underscored.

KEY ISSUES AND FRAMEWORKS FOR VIEWING SELF-CARE WITHIN CHRONIC ILLNESS

The focus of this section is to compare and contrast the many definitions of self-care (or lack of self-care) with evidence to support each view, followed by a working definition of self-care. A self-care framework is presented, and key issues related to self-care in persons living with chronic illnesses are illustrated by reviewing *Healthy People 2010* objectives. The framework and key issues set the stage for application of the nursing process by highlighting important considerations for nurses to address when promoting self-care in clients.

Perspectives on Self-Care

Diverse perspectives of self-care are provided via research on self-care in various populations living with chronic illnesses. These include the idea that self-care means: (1) to comply or adhere to prescribed medical treatments for chronic illnesses; (2) to have a personal belief that one is capable of following disease treatment regimens; (3) to have the functional abilities to carry out daily activities including ADLs and IADLS independently; and (4) to self-determine how to meet one's unique, personal basic human and self-actualization needs. Still others have addressed self-care as being multidimensional. Each perspective will be discussed.

Self-Care as Compliance With Medical Treatments

Haber's (2002) critical analysis of federal initiatives regarding health promotion and aging emphasizes physical aspects and a medical-orientation toward self-care and health promotion. Self-care is implied to be adherence to recommended secondary prevention interventions through disease risk reduction (e.g., smoking cessation) and screening practices (e.g., mammograms).

Edwardson and Dean (1999) explored how selected demographic, social, situational, and symptom experience factors influence the "appropriateness" of self-care responses to symptoms. In other words, the way persons manage symptoms is influenced by many factors. In this study, self-care was equated to medical management of symptoms. Healthcare professionals judged clients' responses to symptoms as either "appropriate" or "inappropriateness," using an evidence-based algorithm. If persons did not seek professional care, used "unsafe" remedies, or did not follow guidelines from professionals, it was "inappropriate."

Sharkey, Ory, and Browne (2005) studied homebound older persons receiving meal delivery in North Carolina to identify the extent that older persons use strategies to reduce out- of-pocket medication expenses when self-managing their medications. From this perspective, lack of self-care was assumed to include noncompliance with medical treatment regimens. Twenty percent admitted to using one or more of the following behaviors to restrict medication use and costs: (1) taking less medicine than the prescribed amount or going without the medication because of cost, or both; (2) getting free drug samples from physicians; (3) obtaining a partial refill of a prescription; (4) taking the drug only when "needed;" or (5) buying only the most important medications. Although these results seem to be "anti-self-management or self-care," they highlight the need to address the concerns and perceptions of patients when trying to promote self-care. Sometimes caring for one's self conflicts with recommended treatment regimens.

Others differentiate self-care from self-management (Barlow et al., 2002). Self-care was identified as tasks performed by healthy people at home, including preventative strategies. Self-management was viewed as daily tasks carried out at home by individuals to control or reduce the impact of disease on physical health. After reviewing the literature on self-management programs for arthritis, asthma, and diabetes, recommendations were made to develop programs to promote self-management of other chronic health conditions.

In summary, self-care has been linked with compliance to recommended medical treatment. However, sometimes self-initiated behaviors may be in conflict with those recommendations. Learning to live with chronic illness most certainly involves following medical recommendations to reduce exacerbations. However, in some situations self-care is not the same as self-management of an illness or compliance with medical recommendations.

Self-Care as Belief in Being Able to Self-Manage

Typical disease self-management programs for arthritis, chronic heart disease, HIV/AIDS, diabetes mellitus, and asthma monitor and report symptoms as well as monitor adherence to medical regimens. Research on self-management programs often attempts to identify how self-efficacy beliefs (i.e., belief that one is capable of self-managing one's treatment regimen) along with other psychological characteristics such as locus of control, perceived threat, or a sense of well-being and situational variables such as demographics, living arrangements, and overall health status influence the ability to self-manage a health condition. Outcomes from these studies often look at symptom relief, functional ability status, changes in self-efficacy beliefs, and laboratory values indicative of "disease control."

An arthritis self-management program with older persons in Hong Kong introduced Tai Chi as a self-management technique. In this study,

self-efficacy was greater, pain decreased, and motor strength increased in the intervention group (Yip et al., 2004) when compared with the control group receiving "usual care." Self-efficacy beliefs were linked to self-care approaches in disease self-management and to positive health outcomes.

A longitudinal study (McDonald-Miszczak & Wister, 2005) with a national Canadian sample also linked self-efficacy with the 11 arthritis self-management "self-care" behaviors of diet, exercise, sleep, self-help group participation, use of alternative remedies, modifications of environment, reading, stress reduction, meditation/prayer, consulting family/friends, and consulting others with the same condition. Self-efficacy beliefs did not predict the use of these 11 behaviors to manage arthritis. However, previous use of these behaviors (i.e., past experience) was a strong predictor of these prescribed self-care behaviors and supplemented self-efficacy beliefs.

Similarly, at the end of 3 months, previous use of self-care behaviors was a significant predictor of self-care in monitoring symptoms, following medical guidelines, reporting symptoms, and seeking help in a self-management program designed for persons with heart failure in a study conducted in the southwestern United States (Chriss et al., 2004). Other characteristics such as social support, education, gender, age, income, comorbidities, and symptom severity were not predictive of this type of self-care.

These studies illustrate that previous lifestyle and experiences are predictive of how persons will manage chronic illnesses in terms of adhering to prescribed behaviors. Although some personal demographic characteristics, emotional state, and personal beliefs about being able to take control and manage a disease on a daily basis had some effect on following the prescribed behaviors, the strongest predictor was previous experience in using the behaviors. This leads one to believe that life experiences and personal values may be very important in determining each individual's self-care behaviors.

Self-Care as Functional Abilities and Independence

Burnette, Mui, and Zodikoff (2004) used functional abilities as an indicator of self-care in their study with a national sample of 597 persons with coronary heart disease (CHD) compared to those without CHD. These researchers proposed that most of the everyday work of managing CHD relied upon self-care as opposed to professional care. Therefore, self-care was defined differently than compliance with prescribed treatment regimens. They defined self-care as the active role persons play in determining outcomes resulting from professional care. The coping strategies of behavioral change, environmental adaptations, and medical equipment use represented self-care strategies in their study. These strategies were also linked to functional abilities related to ADLs, IADLs, and mobility. Impaired functional abilities were indicative of a lack of self-care.

Borg and colleagues (2006) proposed that "older persons who are not able to manage daily life by themselves may have a different view of life satisfaction than those with preserved self-care capacity" (p. 608). Self-care capacity was defined as having functional abilities to carry out activities independently. This study's findings imply that functional limitations are linked to self-care and that functional limitations, more than the presence of a chronic illness, can affect holistic health outcomes such as life satisfaction. Persons with functional limitations might need special assistance and attention to support their self-care practices in order to promote health.

Self-neglect is inability to meet basic needs and is viewed as the opposite of self-care (Dyer, Goodwin, Pickens-Pace, Burnett, & Kelly, 2007). In older clients of the Adult Protective Service in the United States, the prevalence of self-neglect is 50.3% nationally. Dyer and colleagues developed a case definition of self-neglect based on characteristics of 538 cases. The mean age of these clients was 75.6 years, and 70% were women. Executive dysfunction, or the inability to execute specific complex tasks such as ADLs and IADLs independently, was at the root of self-neglect. Executive dysfunction was also associated with several

CASE STUDY

You are the home health nurse assigned to visit Mr. B, an 80-year-old man who lives in a rural area of the United States with his 78-year-old wife. Mr. B has both osteoarthritis and congestive heart failure. He recently was taken to the emergency department of the nearest community hospital by his daughter and son-in-law; his wife noticed that he had sudden loss of speech and was unable to move his left side for a few minutes. Mr. B was admitted to the hospital for diagnostic testing and monitoring. After 2 days, he was discharged and returned to his home. Skilled nursing care was ordered through a home health agency for monitoring of Mr. B's blood pressure and weight; to institute a walking program; and for health teaching on medications, diet, and exercise. He was prescribed

three new medications in addition to the four he was previously taking for arthritis and cardiac disease.

Discussion Questions

1. What is the first area you would assess on your first home visit? Why?
2. Identify at least one self-care goal for this client in each area of health teaching.
3. In doing health teaching on drugs, diet, and exercise, what would be your primary areas of focus and approach as you begin to intervene?
4. List at least three self-care outcomes related to the self-care supportive interventions.

chronic illnesses including dementia, depression, diabetes, psychiatric illness, cardiovascular disease, and nutritional deficiency. This seemingly converse definition of self-care links self-care to the functional ability of acting independently.

Self-Care as Self-Determined Behaviors That Meet the Individual's Unique Needs

Singleton (2000) traced the history of self-care from Nightingale to the present in an eloquent analysis of self-care. The analysis provided a framework for her study on how nurses encourage rehabilitation clients to care for themselves. She emphasized that self-care should be defined by how clients actually care for themselves, and that greater understanding is needed regarding the methods used by nurses to encourage clients to care for themselves in ways that meet their unique needs.

In a nurse-led, home-based multidisciplinary intervention with older persons after hospitalization for heart failure in South Australia (Inglis, Pearsonk, Treen, Gallasch, Horowitz, & Stewart, 2008), the researchers incorporated unique self-determined behaviors in their definition of self-care. Although interventions were aimed at promoting adherence to medical treatments as a means of promoting self-care, the researchers also included special interventions to empower older persons to facilitate their self-determination, that is, self care. Thus, self-determination of self-care was emphasized.

The self-care practices of older persons who had fecal incontinence and who were enrolled in one health maintenance organization were investigated by Bliss and colleagues (2005). On average, these persons reported 2.3 chronic conditions with a range from 0–10, and 1.9 specific self-care practices with a range from 0–7. Self-care activities included diet modifications, use of panty liners, reduction in activities, and use of medications to stop diarrhea. Only 43% reported discussing this problem and their self-care practices with their healthcare provider. Only the self-care practice of diet changes was routinely discussed

with providers. This emphasizes that sometimes the self-care carried out by persons with chronic illnesses truly is unique to meet personal needs, and that often these self-care practices are not discussed with healthcare providers.

In a 27-month longitudinal study with 387 randomly selected older community-dwelling adults (Musil et al., 2001), arthritis and cardiopulmonary symptoms were assessed for consistent recurrence and their effects on well-being and symptom management with self-care. Self-care was defined as the use of home remedies, over-the-counter medications, or changes in lifestyle, but did not include deciding when to seek professional help. There were differences in the use of self-care for persons with each diagnosis. Persons with arthritis and chronic pain complaints across time used self-care, whereas those with cardiopulmonary symptoms did not. It was concluded that patterns differ by the type of symptom and illness and that managing chronic illness is a complex phenomenon.

Essential dimensions of self-care and an integrated model were proposed after reviewing research on self-care conducted in Sweden and Finland (Leenerts et al., 2002). In the model, it was emphasized that self-care activities are related to the individual person's unique view of health and the individual's self-concept. The authors recommended that nurses incorporate the patient's personal beliefs about health into their teaching about self-care activities, and that nurses partner with clients to support meeting their personal needs. They also identified evidence-based outcomes of health promotion in aging individuals as connectedness to others, resource use, transcendence, and well-being. Self-care activities or skills were classified as communication, healthy lifestyle, building meaning in their life, and socializing. They added that self-care takes place within the context of internal and external human environments.

In another study (Bickerstaff et al., 2003), activities that help nursing home residents transcend difficulties and live with contentment and satisfaction in life were identified. In this study, self-care meant activities that promoted holistic health. The 95 respondents, with an average age of 82.2 years, had lived in the nursing home from 3–177 months (M = 35.6 months) and reported a variety of self-care activities. They included (1) generativity activities through helping or reaching out to others and involving family; (2) introjectivity activities such as hobbies, travel, and lifelong learning; (3) temporal integration activities which were past, present, and future based behaviors; (4) body-transcendence activities that incorporated flexibility and making changes in life; and (5) spirituality activities to develop relationships with self, others, and a higher being. These self-care activities encompassed more than a physical orientation to health and well-being and were based on the individual's perception of needs.

Likewise, Wang and colleagues (2001) used focus groups to explore the perceptions of health-promoting self-care in community-dwelling, Taiwanese older adults. All but 4 of the 21 men and women participants were living with some type of chronic illness. The investigators identified five types of self-care activities that these older persons employed in caring for themselves. They included (1) balancing or adjusting one's health, (2) initiating or purposefully using self-care activities, (3) regularizing or maintaining a daily rhythm over time, (4) socializing or involving and connecting with society, and (5) sublimating or seeing the positive side and transcending their situations. They concluded that older adults in Taiwan viewed health and self-care activities as mind–body connections with holistic harmony rather than merely as physical health.

Maddox (1999) conducted a 3-year qualitative study of older women in three different age groups to identify their self-care activities and the meaning they assigned to health. The groups were comprised of (1) 12 nuns ages 72 to 104; (2) eight 55 to 76-year-old women who lived in a single-family dwellings and worked in blue-collar occupations; and (3) five 55 to 86-year-old residents of an urban retirement community who were previously employed as domestic help or worked on farms or in factories. Their reported self-care activities included (1) interactions with a being greater than one's self, (2) acceptance of self, (3) humor, (4) flexibility, and (5) quality of being other-centered. It was pointed out that these self-care activities incorporated more than the traditional physical self-care activities of nutrition, exercise, and relaxation but also included holistic spiritual, social, and emotional behaviors.

Hertz and Rossetti (2007) also found that self-care actions or activities were unique for older persons with chronic illness who lived independently in apartments. In reporting activities, common themes and patterns were identified. These themes, or types of self-care activities, included (1) adapting to life as an older adult by using coping strategies, assistive devices, and avoiding hassles; (2) meeting needs for affiliated-individuation by balancing activities that meet needs for independence and time alone with those that meet needs for dependence and socialization; (3) using self-care knowledge to promote and strive for holistic health by using personal beliefs and values to promote quality of life and self-actualization; (4) self-managing health problems through seeking medical and alternative treatments and by sometimes avoiding medical intervention or treatment; and (5) preventing health problems and issues by following recommendations for screenings and health promotion and by taking safety precautions. The diversity of these individually determined self-care activities also reflect the multidimensionality of self-care.

Self-Care as a Multidimensional Concept

Beattie and colleagues (2003) proposed a model that uses community-based organizations such as Area Agencies on Aging, faith-based organizations, and public health departments to promote health. The dimensions of self-care were implied to include reducing risks to illnesses, managing illnesses, and coping with functional limits.

Lubben and Damron-Rodriguez (2003) analyzed the World Health Organization's Kobe Centre model for organizing health care at the community level for the older adult population. Within this model, self-care was differentiated from professional care (i.e., disease management) and social network care. The authors viewed self-care as multiple activities that prolonged active life and prevented functional declines. Recommendations were made initially to foster the individual's self-care capacity by encouraging productive roles and self-direction, followed by building social network support that accommodates the diverse needs of older adults, and finally engaging community professional services for health care of older adults. Enhancing home and community environments is important because those environments are the contexts in which persons live.

Summary and Working Definition of Self-Care

In summary, there are diverse perspectives about what self-care means and evidence exists to support each perspective. Therefore, the working definition of self-care for this chapter incorporates these diverse perspectives.

Self-care has multiple dimensions, is self-determined, and is unique to each individual based on that person's life experiences, values, beliefs, and personal characteristics and abilities, including biopsychosocial-spiritual and functional abilities. Self-care influences each individual's holistic health. Self-care includes a variety of activities such as following prescribed medical treatments and lifestyle recommendations for chronic illnesses (e.g., take medications, monitor and report symptoms, smoking cessation, diet modifications); carrying out daily activities including ADLs, IADLS, and mobility (e.g., hygiene, dressing, toileting); adhering to recommended guidelines for disease prevention and health promotion (regular screenings, dietary guidelines, exercise); meeting basic needs (e.g., food, shelter, safety, socializing, individuation); and pursuing personal interests that promote spiritual well-being and self-actualization (e.g., meditation, prayer, hobbies, learning).

Self-care includes performing activities both independently and dependently. Furthermore, self-care can be supported and nurtured by nurses and other healthcare professionals. The following framework provides guidelines for promoting self-care in persons living with chronic illnesses.

Self-Care: A Framework for Assessment and Intervention

In nursing, Orem's (2001) theory and perspective on self-care is frequently cited. The original focus of this theory was on patients' self-care deficits or the inability to carry out self-care tasks required for physical health. Conversely, self-care agency is the capability to care for one's self and emphasizes physical abilities. It is implied that healthcare professionals, including nurses, define for clients what self-care is needed and then carry out those activities for the client if the client lacks the capability to do so. Within this definition, there is logical incongruence. If self-care is caring for one's self, then it makes sense that the client, rather than the nurse or other healthcare provider, should be the expert regarding what is needed. Therefore, a theory that is more congruent with the working definition of self-care is presented.

The Self-Care Model (Hertz & Baas, 2006) from Modeling and Role-Modeling (MRM) nursing theory (Erickson, Tomlin, & Swain, 1988; Erickson, 2006) provides a more congruent framework for addressing assessment, interventions, and outcome evaluations of self-care in persons living with chronic illnesses. This perspective takes into account the unique, self-determined, multidimensional nature of self-care based on individual biology, values, and life experiences. It also recognizes that self-care is possible when persons are living with chronic illnesses and when they might be dependent on others for assistance. Finally, the overriding framework of MRM theory provides a focus for interventions that are self-care supportive via the five aims of intervention.

Figure 13-1 illustrates the MRM self-care model. In this model, self-care has three

FIGURE 13-1

Framework for Self-Care in Persons Living with Chronic Illnesses

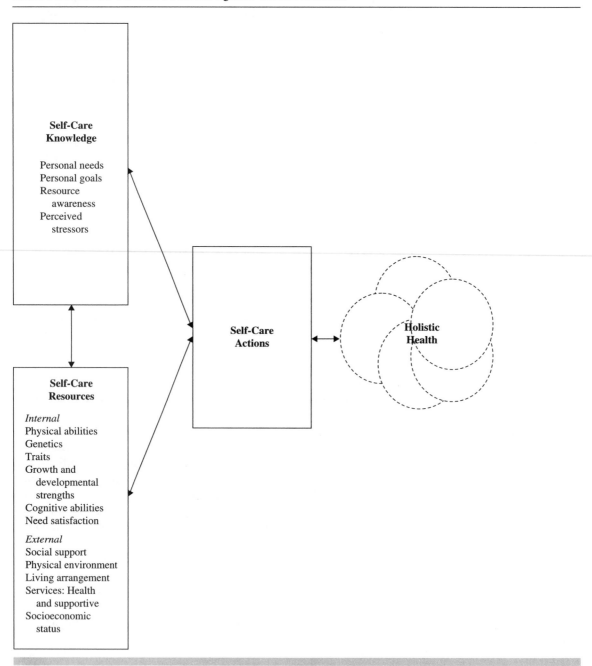

components: self-care knowledge, self-care resources, and self-care actions. Self-care knowledge is the individual's personal knowledge regarding their personal needs and goals. Those personal needs can include basic and higher level human needs as described by Maslow and others (see Erickson et al., 1988; Erickson, 2006) as well as the need for affiliated-individuation, a concept unique to MRM theory and representing the need for persons to sense a separateness and independence from others while at the same time needing to feel connected to and being able to rely on others. Self-care knowledge also incorporates knowledge, either at a conscious or subconscious level, regarding what may have caused a health problem/issue and what will help resolve that issue. This personal knowledge includes perceptions of availability of resources and stressors in the individual's life. Self-care knowledge is the foundation for each individual's "model" or view of that person's world or life situation. Self-care knowledge is interrelated to self-care resources.

Self-care resources are internal and external to the individual. Internal resources include genetic makeup; physical, mental, and cognitive functioning; as well as psychosocial and spiritual characteristics and traits developed over the person's lifetime and as a result of need satisfaction. External resources include persons who provide social supports, the physical environment (e.g., geography, urban vs rural, climate, community design), living arrangements (e.g., type housing, accessibility, safety, neighbors, living alone), service availability (e.g., health care, transportation, social services), and socioeconomic status. These self-care resources are interdependent on self-care knowledge. For example, each person must recognize social support as such; an outsider's view of whether social support is present is less important than the individual's view. Furthermore, the perception of social support as helpful is important because although such support may be available, the client views the behaviors of those persons as not helpful. Both self-care knowledge and resources are interrelated to self-care actions.

Self-care actions are those activities taken by persons to influence health status. Self-care actions require using one's personal self-care knowledge and mobilizing self-care resources to do what is best for one's self. Therefore, self-care actions require that each person perceive a sense of autonomy (Hertz, 1996). To some extent, self-care actions are unique for each individual.

For example, all persons have a need for love and belonging and to affiliate with others. One person might meet this need by purposefully participating in social activities such as a family reunion where one feels they belong and are loved as a member of a family unit; likely, this approach is based on life experiences within the family unit when that person previously felt love and belonging. Another person with different experiences and who has not experienced those feelings within the family unit, might have their personal needs for love and belonging through the caring behaviors of a nurse. For that person, self-neglect of a health problem might lead to reestablishment of a relationship with a home health nurse, which, in turn, could meet the personal need for love and belonging. In both instances, persons are meeting needs for love and belonging and, therefore, are influencing their holistic health status. Obviously, the person who acted in a self-neglectful mode to meet those needs might eventually deplete their resources (physical and other coping resources). Therefore, the nurse can use nursing knowledge of health processes to assist this person to find other means for meeting those needs that will build up rather than deplete resources over the long-term.

According to this model of self-care, health is holistic, meaning that it is more than the absence of physical and mental illness. It incorporates aspects of biopsychosocial-spiritual well-being, quality of life, and self-actualization in addition to addressing and reducing the harmful effects of illnesses. This definition of health is applicable to persons living with chronic illnesses. A high level health and chronic illness can coexist. Nurses can facilitate and nurture self-care through unconditionally accepting the person and that person's unique view or "model" of the world and then by "role-modeling" interventions that fit with that person's model.

There are five aims of interventions that guide the nurse in modeling and role-modeling with each person. They include:

1. Build trust with each client in the nurse–client relationship so that the client trusts others
2. Promote a positive orientation to one's self as a person of worth and to foster hope for the future
3. Facilitate client control so that each person feels and perceives a sense of control over the environment (internal and external) and the person's life situation
4. Build on strengths in terms of building on the person's capabilities and life experiences even in the presence of an illness
5. Set mutual health-directed goals based on the client's model of the world

Structuring interventions around these aims is supportive of self-care.

KEY ISSUES IN PROMOTING SELF-CARE IN PERSONS WITH CHRONIC ILLNESS

According to *Healthy People 2010* [US Department of Health and Human Services (DHHS), 2000], health is determined by biology (genetics, diseases, body functions) and behaviors (those activities people do, e.g., exercise, smoking, sleeping) that result from personal choices or the physical and social environment including health-related policies and interventions and access to quality health care. This definition is also congruent with the MRM self-care framework. The behaviors referred to in the *Healthy People* document are integral to self-care. These self-care behaviors are influenced by the other factors that determine health. Conversely, self-care behaviors can shape the other biological factors to some extent.

In Table 13-1, relevant national objectives and goals from the *Healthy People 2010* (DHHS, 2000) highlight the key issues to be addressed when supporting the self-care of persons with one or more chronic illnesses. Self-care requires taking actions on one's own behalf to influence health states. Self-care goals and objectives found in *Healthy People* are focused on the following key issues: (1) *health education* about key aspects of living with chronic illness (e.g., knowledge about disease processes and management of disease, treatments, monitoring for symptoms), (2) adjustment to or *coping* with the illness (e.g., living with loss of function associated with illness, adaptive equipment, maintaining/improving psychosocial health while living with illness, adjusting to activity limitations), (3) *health promotion* and prevention of other-related physical and psychosocial problems (e.g., health promotion, counseling for healthy behaviors), and (4) development of *support and assistance* from family/friends and others (e.g., support groups, caregiver support and education, ensuring ADLs and IADLs are met).

INTERVENTIONS

There is a lack of evidence-based clinical practice guidelines focused specifically on supporting self-care in persons living with chronic illnesses. However, on the National Guideline Clearinghouse Web site (www.guideline.gov), multiple tangentially related guidelines are identified (see Table 13-2). In particular, there is a guideline to promote self-management in persons living with chronic illnesses. Likewise, several guidelines address the key issues and health problems found in *Healthy People 2010* (DHHS, 2000) and listed in Table 13-1. These guidelines address specific assessment, medical management, intervention strategies, and outcome evaluation.

In addition to these guidelines, programs that support self-care have been studied empirically. What follows are guidelines for assessment and intervention. All are based on the MRM self-care

TABLE 13-1

Relevant *Healthy People 2010* Goals and Objectives That Highlight Key Issues Regarding Self-Care in Persons Living with Chronic Illnesses

Healthy People 2010 *Goals and Objectives*	*Key Self-Care Issues*
1. Access to quality health services *Goal:* To improve access to comprehensive, high-quality healthcare services *Objective:* 1–3 Counseling about health behaviors	Health promotion
2. Arthritis, osteoporosis, and chronic back conditions *Goal:* To prevent illness and disability related to arthritis and other rheumatic conditions, osteoporosis, and chronic back conditions *Objectives:* 2–2 Activity limitations due to arthritis; 2–3 Personal care limitations 2–4 Help in coping; 2–8 Arthritis education	Health promotion; support and assistance; coping; health education
5. Diabetes *Goal:* Through prevention programs, reduce the disease and economic burden of diabetes and improve the quality of life for all persons who have or are at risk for diabetes. *Objectives:* 5–1 Diabetes education; 5–17 Self-blood-glucose monitoring	Health education

Source: US Department of Health and Human Services (DHHS). (2000). *Healthy People 2010: Understanding and improving health* (2nd ed.). Washington, DC: US Government Printing Office.

model, results of empirical studies, and comprehensive literature reviews.

Assessment

Based on the MRM self-care framework (Erickson et al., 1988; Erickson, 2006; Hertz & Baas, 2006) and because the client's model of the world is most important in setting priorities and planning interventions, the client should be the primary source of information when doing an assessment. The initial question should focus on identifying the person's perceived needs and understanding of the health issue for which nursing care is sought or recommended. For example, at the beginning of each encounter, the nurse should ask, "What is your biggest concern right now?" This immediately identifies the client's primary concern(s). In some settings, "Tell me about why you came to the (clinic, hospital, nursing home, rehabilitation setting)," or "Tell me why home health care nurses

were asked to visit you," or "Tell me about what has been happening to you." These questions help the nurse comprehend the client's view of the health problem. Conversely, questions such as "How can I help you?" focus on the nurse by using the word "I" rather than the client. Furthermore, when asking for the client's perspective, the nurse should be prepared for an unexpected response.

Many times the response from clients will be surprising. For instance, the client might believe that hospitalization occurred so that the client can get some sleep, whereas the healthcare professional's reason is to ensure close monitoring of a chronic illness. The nurse must accept the client's response rather than try to explain that the response is "wrong." Indeed, research studies have found that identifying personal needs is a key to promoting and supporting self-care (Leenerts et al., 2002) along with the perception of overall health (Borg et al., 2006; Resnick, 2001, 2003). Those with higher perceived health are more likely

TABLE 13-2

Relevant Clinical Practice Guidelines to Support Self-Care Through Health Education, Coping, Health Promotion, and Support and Assistance

Chronic Care Self-Management

Chronic Care Self-management Guideline Team, Cincinnati Children's Hospital Medical Center, March 2007. *Evidence-based care guideline for chronic care: Self-management* (Guideline no. 30). http://guidelines.gov/ summary/summary.aspx?doc_id=10593&nbr=005535&string=self-management

Arthritis

Institute for Clinical Systems Improvement (ICSI), March 2007. *Diagnosis and treatment of adult degenerative joint disease (DJD)/osteoarthritis (OA) of the knee.* http://guidelines.gov/summary/summary. aspx?doc_id=11081&nbr=005844&string=self-care

Asthma

Kaiser Permanente Care Management Institute, April 2007. *Adult asthma clinical practice guidelines.* http:// guidelines.gov/summary/summary.aspx?doc_id=11247&nbr=005880&string=self-management

Registered Nurses Association of Ontario (RNAO), February 2007. *Adult asthma care guidelines for nurses: Promoting control of asthma: supplement.* http://guidelines.gov/summary/summary.aspx?doc_id=11504&nbr= 005958&string=self-management

Cardiovascular Disease and Hypertension

Health Care for the Homeless Clinicians' Network. 2004. Adapting your practice: treatment and recommendations for homeless patients with cardiovascular diseases. http://guidelines.gov/summary/summary .aspx?doc_id=4851&nbr=003492&string=Self-care

Veterans Administration, Department of Defense, August 2004. *VA/DoD clinical practice guideline for diagnosis and management of hypertension in the primary care setting.* http://guidelines.gov/summary/summary.aspx?doc_id= 6831&nbr=004198&string=Self+AND+care

Chronic Obstructive Pulmonary Disease

Registered Nurses Association of Ontario (RNAO), March 2005. *Nursing care of dyspnea: The 6th vital sign in individuals with chronic obstructive pulmonary disease (COPD).* http://guidelines.gov/summary/summary .aspx?doc_id=7008&nbr=004217&string=self-management

Chronic Pain

Institute for Clinical Systems Improvement (ICSI), March 2007. *Assessment and management of chronic pain.* http://guidelines.gov/summary/summary.aspx?doc_id=10724&nbr=005586&string=self-management

University of Iowa Gerontological Nursing Interventions Research Center, August 2005 http://guidelines.gov/ summary/summary.aspx?doc_id=8627&nbr=004807&string=self-management

Diabetes

Massachusetts Department of Public Health Diabetes Prevention and Control Program, Diabetes Guidelines Work Group, June 2005. *Massachusetts guidelines for adult diabetes care.* http://guidelines.gov/summary/summary. aspx?doc_id=8196&nbr=004571&string=self-management

Diabetes and Chronic Kidney Disease

KDOQI, February 2007. *KDOQI clinical practice guidelines and clinical practice recommendations for diabetes and chronic kidney disease.* http://guidelines.gov/summary/summary.aspx?doc_id=10828&nbr=005653&string= self-management#s23 to also pursue recommended self-care healthy behaviors (e.g., exercise program, eating a healthy diet, regular health screenings).

After the problem or needs are identified, the next focus of assessment should be on gaining an understanding of the client's self-care knowledge regarding what might help relieve this problem. Simply asking, "What do you think will help relieve?" will provide a picture of the client's model of the world. Again, it is important for the nurse to accept the client's response as accurate and realize that it is an important aspect in understanding that client's views. Often the perceptions between providers and clients differ regarding self-care (Cortes et al., 2004). Assessing preferences leads to successful self-care supportive interventions (Mendias & Paar, 2007).

After asking these essential questions, data should be gathered regarding the client's health-related goals, personal values, and internal and external self-care resources. According to research exploring predictors of self-care, information should be asked from family members as well as the client.

Internal resources should be assessed. Age has been found to influence self-care actions. Older community-residing adults participated in more self-care activities that focused on health promotion such as exercise programs, eating a healthy diet, and getting adequate sleep (Resnick, 2001, 2003). The belief that one can carry out self-care actions, in other words, self-efficacy, required for disease management is also important to assess (Callaghan, 2005). Self-efficacy may vary according to ethnicity. Callaghan found that blacks and Hispanics had lower levels of self-efficacy than did white non-Hispanics. Cognitive ability should also be assessed, as those with lower cognitive abilities may not be able to carry out self-care actions or to direct others to assist them (Cortes et al., 2004; Resnick, 2003). Functional abilities to carry out self-care tasks should be assessed as well. Studies have found that individuals who lack functional abilities predicted the number of recommended health-promoting self-care behaviors (e.g., healthy diet, exercise program) more than the presence of chronic illness (Borg et al., 2006; Callaghan, 2005). The presence of medical problems and disabilities can also influence self-care (Callaghan, 2005; Cortes et al., 2004; Resnick, 2001).

External resources found to predict self-care actions include perceived adequacy of income and insurance to pay for health care (Borg et al., 2006; Callaghan, 2005; Cortes et al., 2004). Persons with income levels of between $750 and $1000 per month in the United States at the time of this study were more likely to choose between buying food and medications, were less likely to have supplemental drug coverage, and were more likely to restrict medication use through various means such as taking less than prescribed, taking the drug only in response to symptoms, prioritizing the drugs that were most important, or obtaining a partial refill on prescriptions (Sharkey et al., 2005).

Perceived social support should be assessed (Callaghan, 2005). It is not the number of persons who are available to give support but rather the clients' perceptions of who is supportive in helping them get what is needed that is critical when influencing self-care. This perception of social support should include the assessment of the quality of the relationship with a primary care provider, since a poor relationship might provide a barrier to self-care (Cortes et al., 2004). Finally, transportation is an important resource to assess if recommended self-care includes traveling to support group meetings, formal classes or clinics (Cortes et al., 2004; Mendias & Paar, 2007).

Interventions

Diverse approaches to supporting and promoting self-care have been studied. Interventions discussed here are those that are based on individual reports of nursing interventions but share some commonalities. Self-management programs for discrete chronic illnesses will be addressed, followed by comprehensive programs for individuals with multiple chronic illnesses.

Nursing Interventions

Singleton's (2000) ethnographic study identified methods used by nurses to encourage clients to care for themselves in rehabilitation. Nurses reported that they focused on the individual person and included coordinating care, talking to clients, and teaching. In addition, the investigator observed the nurses taking time with clients, using presence, and building trust to promote the client's control over their own self-care. Oddly, the nurses themselves did not report these activities, but were observed by the investigator. Nonetheless, they are congruent with the MRM self-care framework and aims of interventions.

Washburn, Hornberger, Klutman, and Skinner (2005) examined nurses' knowledge of six key topic areas for educating patients about heart failure management and key self-management principles in a Midwestern US health care system. Topic areas and principles were derived from evidence-based practice guidelines. Nurses (*N* = 51) were mostly registered nurses (RNs) employed in the intensive care unit or general medical unit of the hospital. Only 2 of the 20 questions were answered correctly by 100% of the nurses. Percentages of nurses answering the other questions correctly ranged from 40% for 5 questions to 90% for 6 questions. These findings emphasize the importance of ensuring that the nurse's knowledge base is accurate before teaching clients about self-management of specific chronic illnesses.

Research of self-care globally has pointed out some commonalities regarding self-care supportive interventions globally. Studies have been conducted in Taiwan (Wang et al., 2001), in the United States (Callaghan, 2006; Sharkey et al., 2005; Sullivan, Weinert, & Cudney, 2003), sometimes with minority groups (Cortes et al., 2004); and in Sweden and Finland (Borg et al., 2006; Leenerts et al., 2002). Specific self-care interventions with an emphasis on follow-up after hospitalization have also been assessed globally. These include a nurse-led, multidisciplinary posthospitalization follow-up program for persons with heart failure in South Australia (Inglis et al., 2008), a posthospitalization intervention in the United States for persons with nonspecific illnesses (Coleman et al., 2004; see Evidence-Based Practice Box), and a nurse-led customized program for persons with diabetes also in the United States (Berg & Wadhwa, 2007).

One of the most striking aspects of the studies is that they all recommend basing interventions on the client's model of the world. Assessing the perceived needs of clients is essential and can overcome barriers to "nonadherence." Integrating special self-care activities to manage a chronic illness must fit within the client's day-to-day lifestyle. Another common aspect of these interventions is that they address the holistic health needs of clients, including spiritual and socialization needs, and are not limited to medical diagnoses.

Another commonality is that the programs embrace a multipronged approach to supporting and promoting self-care. For example, teaching is a major component of these interventions but comprehensive skilled assessments, coaching, empowerment, referral, and intermittent follow up contact are also part of the recommended interventions. Finally, the interventions are based on the philosophy that promoting a positive orientation of self-worth fosters hope for the future. This philosophy is operationalized by pointing out the positive, rather than negative or problematic, aspects of the person's situation.

Self-Management Programs

Lorig (2001), a nursing leader in self-management program development and testing, comprehensively summarized findings from more than 20 years of research studies testing self-management programs for arthritis. Characteristics of the programs tested in sequential studies were analyzed to isolate the most important factors when designing these programs to support self-care in terms of disease self-management. First, programs must be focused on the problems and concerns of clients. In other words, modeling the client's world is a key factor. Programs should also be designed for a particular target population. The process of implementing the program is as important as the content to be addressed. Written materials must be included as a reference and for additional reading. Programs should promote self-efficacy by building on the client's strengths; congruent with the self-care model, positive aspects of abilities should be recognized and nurtured. Problem-solving and decision-making by the client should be emphasized rather than relying solely on professional judgment. Skills for communicating with healthcare professionals should be incorporated. Other important aspects include providing a structure for the program that is adhered to during each of its segments, encouraging sharing of ideas and feelings among group members attending the program, employing lay instructors, and recognizing that other education and health teaching are valuable as well.

Chodosh and colleagues (2005) identified similar characteristics through a meta-analysis of 53 randomized trials testing chronic disease self-management programs for older adults with diabetes, osteoarthritis, and hypertension. Although they did not find statistically significant critical elements of these programs, they extrapolated that self-care in the form of self-management requires active participation in decision making and self-monitoring. In addition, programs should be tailored to meet needs, offered in group settings, provide feedback to participants, and emphasize psychological aspects of self-management in addition to medical management.

Rogers, Kennedy, Nelson, and Robinson (2005) identified the importance of the physician–patient relationship style in promoting self-management. Physicians and the health systems in which they practice need to be responsive to patient needs and preferences, and decision making must be shared with the patient. Indeed, the idea of responsiveness to client needs is essential to modeling and role-modeling interventions that promote self-care.

Likewise, the notion of active involvement and participation is also compatible with the self-care model. However, for some clients, active participation might take the form of dependence on others as a self-care action. For example, the person with limited self-care resources might need to depend on others for aspects of self-care to preserve, rather than deplete, their limited resources.

Comprehensive Self-Care Programs

Lynch, Estes, and Hernandez (2005) compared three types of chronic care initiatives for older adults. These comprehensive programs are viewed as alternatives to the traditional medical model of care. The first is the integrated medical, home, and community-based services model, which focuses on providing holistic, integrated health services to persons with complex, chronic care needs in their homes. An example is the Program for All-Inclusive Care for the Elderly (PACE) that has been in place for more than 20 years and has produced many positive health outcomes, despite demanding a high level of ambulatory services.

The second type of chronic care initiation is the disease management programs offered by a variety of providers. An example is the Kaiser Permanente Best Practice Collaborative approach with group clinics and education on disease self-care in primary care settings. The Kaiser programs are interdisciplinary and incorporate motivational interviewing to promote self-care. The benefit is a focus on active participation. But, as previously noted, demanding active, independent participation can be detrimental to some clients' health.

A third and newer model is that of high-risk care management developed by managed care insurers to control costs and to improve the care management of persons living with multiple chronic illnesses. The Guided Care Nurse model represents this approach (Boyd et al., 2007). This model emphasizes coordination and nonduplication of services that are individualized to meet clients' unique needs. A specially educated nurse works in a primary care practice with two to five physicians, and manages care for 50 to 60 older clients. An electronic health record is used to communicate among team members. The focus of guided care nursing interventions is on comprehensive assessment and monitoring of chronic conditions, coaching to aid in self-management of diseases, referral and coordination of services to secure needed resources and to facilitate transitions between healthcare settings, and provision of caregiver education and support. A key component of this model is that the client's highest priority needs for health must be addressed by the nurse. This is a multipronged approach with many client-centered aspects.

There are other types of programs such as case management programs led by social workers, state-funded programs for low-income persons with chronic illnesses, and wellness management programs in senior centers (Lynch et al., 2005). All of these promote self-care in some fashion. However, a limitation is that most of these programs have a very narrow focus. Therefore,

▌EVIDENCE-BASED PRACTICE BOX

Purpose: Tested an intervention to reduce hospitalizations and emergency department utilization by promoting a more active role of older patients and their caregivers in care transitions.

Research design: Quasi-experimental study

Sample: 158 intervention patients and 1235 control patients older than 65 years of age all of whom had recently had a first hospitalization for one of nine conditions (congestive heart failure, chronic obstructive pulmonary disease, coronary artery disease, diabetes, stroke, back condition, hip fracture, peripheral vascular disease, or arrhythmia).

Setting: A large, not-for-profit group-model managed care system with a contracted hospital, skilled nursing facility and home care agency. Providers did not cross settings. All participants resided in the community before and after hospitalization.

Intervention: Comprising four areas: (1) medication self-management, (2) a patient-centered medical record, (3) primary care and specialist follow-up, and (4) teaching red flags warning of worsening condition. A transition coach who was a geriatric nurse practitioner (GNP) with training in chronic disease self-management and a personal health record were used during visits and phone calls. The coach encouraged self-management and communication between the patient or patient's caregiver and primary care provider. The GNP developed rapport in the hospital and then made a follow-up home visit within 24–72 hours post discharge, reconciled the medications, and phoned the patient/caregiver at least three times.

Findings: The intervention group was half as likely as those in the control group to return to the hospital at 30, 90, and 180 days; this was well beyond the 24 days of contact with the transition coach. In addition, the intervention group took a significantly longer period of time until they were rehospitalized and were judged as having a less complicated postdischarge course. No direct costs were measured.

Implications: The intervention demonstrated that a multipronged approach to supporting and promoting self-care via self-management has the potential for reducing healthcare costs after a hospitalization.

Source: Coleman, E.A., Smith, J.D., Frank, J.C., Min, S.J., Parry C., & Kramer, A.M. (2004). Preparing patients and caregivers to participate in care delivered across settings: The care transitions intervention. *Journal of the American Geriatrics Society, 52,* 1817–1825.

the clients' holistic health needs are not always addressed. There is a need for more innovative, comprehensive programs to be developed in the future to help promote self-care in persons living with chronic illnesses. These could be located in housing units or community-based sites where persons with chronic illnesses congregate, for example, churches, shopping centers, and grocery stores. Future models should incorporate the recommended multipronged approaches and address needs related to multiple chronic illnesses. All models need to adopt a client-centered and holistic perspective so that interventions can be tailored to meet clients' unique needs, values, and lifestyles.

OUTCOMES

Grey, Knafl, and McCorkle (2006) developed a framework for describing and organizing outcomes of self-management programs. The categories of outcomes also apply to programs other than ones that promote self-care. The categories are condition outcomes, individual outcomes, family outcomes, and environmental outcomes. Positive outcomes in each category would be optimal.

Condition Outcomes

These outcomes indicate the individual's adherence and responsiveness to treatment regimens. For example, in persons with diabetes, hypertension, and osteoarthritis, outcomes include reduced levels of hemoglobin A1c; decreased systolic blood pressure by 5 mm Hg and decreased diastolic by 4.3 mm Hg; as well as pain reduction, respectively (Chodosh et al., 2005). Following recommended screening procedures (Berg & Wadhwa, 2007) would also be a condition outcome. Other outcomes might include morbidity, mortality, and

improved or stable functional status (Burnette et al., 2004; Grey et al., 2006; Lynch et al., 2005).

Individual Outcomes

Any outcomes that reflect clients' perceptions regarding health status, quality of life, and well-being are included in this category. Connectedness to others, transcendence, a sense of well-being (Leenerts et al., 2002), life satisfaction (Borg et al., 2006), satisfaction with health care, and reports of needs being met (Inglis et al., 2008) are examples. Quality of life and physical, mental and spiritual health ratings (Boyd et al., 2007; Campbell & Aday, 2001), increased health-related knowledge, and a greater sense of being in control of one's situation or sense of autonomy are other individual outcomes (Campbell & Aday, 2001).

Family Outcomes

Outcomes that indicate an effect on the family of the person receiving the promotion intervention are included in this group. Depression in caregivers, improved family functioning, and degree of caregiver burden (Grey et al., 2006) are examples of family outcomes.

Environmental Outcomes

Outcomes that reflect the costs of health care or influence the healthcare system are considered environmental outcomes. For example, cost reductions, unplanned hospital admissions rates, lengths of stay, and frequencies of healthcare utilization (Inglis et al., 2008) fall into this category. In addition, nonduplication of services (Boyd et al., 2007), decreased nursing home admissions, and use of ambulatory services may be included in this category (Berg & Wadhwa, 2007; Lynch et al., 2005).

STUDY QUESTIONS

1. Define self-care as it relates to persons living with one or more chronic illnesses.
2. Identify the relationship between self-care and health outcomes. Why is self-care a key concept to positive health outcomes?
3. How can nurses promote self-care in the clients they care for? Identify the key elements to a self-care supportive intervention.
4. Delineate at least one positive outcome for the individual client, family, and healthcare system as a result of the individual client demonstrating self-care in relation to his or her chronic illness

INTERNET RESOURCES

Center for Self and Family Management of Vulnerable Populations, Yale University School of Nursing: nursing.yale.edu/Centers/ECSMI/
Family Caregiver Alliance, Self-care fact sheet: www.caregiver.org/caregiver/jsp/content_node.jsp?nodeid=847
Guided Care; A new model of care for frail older adults with complex healthcare needs: www.guidedcare.org/index.asp
Modeling and Role-Modeling Nursing Theory: mrmnursingtheory.org/index.html
Self-Care Deficit Nursing Theory: www.scdnt.com/index.html

REFERENCES

Barlow, J.H., Sturt, J., & Hearnshaw, H. (2002). Self-management interventions for people with chronic conditions in primary care: Examples from arthritis, asthma and diabetes. *Health Education Journal, 61*(4), 365–378.

Beattie, B.L., Whitelaw, N., Mettler, M., & Turner, D. (2003). A vision for older adults and health promotion. *American Journal of Health Promotion, 18*(2), 200–204.

Berg, G.D., & Wadhwa, S. (2007). Health services outcomes for a diabetes disease management program for the elderly. *Disease Management, 10*, 226–234.

Bickerstaff, K.A., Grasser, C.M., & McCabe, B. (2003). How elderly nursing home residents transcend losses of later life. *Holistic Nursing Practice, 17*(3), 159–165.

Bliss, D.Z., Fischer, L.R., & Savik, K. (2005). Managing fecal incontinence: Self-care practices of older adults. *Journal of Gerontological Nursing, 31*(7), 35–44.

Borg, C., Hallberg, I., & Blomqvist, K. (2006). Life satisfaction among older people (65+) with reduced self-care capacity: The relationship to social, health and financial aspects [Electronic version]. *Journal of Clinical Nursing, 15*(5), 607–618.

Boyd, C.M., Boult, C., Shadmi, E., Leff, B., Brager, R., Dunbar, L, et al. (2007). Guided care for multimorbid older adults. *The Gerontologist, 47*, 679–704.

Burnette, D., Mui, A.C., & Zodikoff, B.D. (2004). Gender, self-care and functional status among older persons with coronary heart disease: A national perspective. *Women & Health, 39*(1), 65–84.

Callaghan, D. (2005). Healthy behaviors, self-efficacy, self-care, and basic conditioning factors in older adults [Electronic version]. *Journal of Community Health Nursing, 22*(3), 169–178.

Callaghan, D. (2006). The influence of growth on spiritual self-care agency in an older adult population. *Journal of Gerontological Nursing, 32*(9), 43–51.

Campbell, J., & Aday, R.H. (2001). Benefits of a nurse-managed wellness program: A senior center model. Using community-based sites for older adult intervention and self-care activities may promote an ability to maintain an independent lifestyle. *Journal of Gerontological Nursing, 27*(3), 34–43.

Chodosh, J., Morton, S. C., Mojica, W., Maglione, M., Suttorp, M.J., Hilton, L., et al. (2005). Meta-analysis: Chronic disease self-management programs for older adults. *Annals of Internal Medicine, 143,* 427–438.

Chriss, P.M., Sheposh, J., Carlson, B., & Riegel, B. (2004). Predictors of successful heart failure self-care maintenance in the first three months after hospitalization. *Heart & Lung, 33,* 345–353.

Coleman, E. A., Smith, J. D., Frank, J. C., Min, S-J., Parry, C., & Kramer, A. M. (2004). Preparing patients and caregivers to participate in care delivered across settings: The care transitions intervention. *Journal of the American Geriatrics Society, 52,* 1817–1825.

Cortes, T., Lee, A., Boal, J., Mion, L., & Butler, A. (2004). Using focus groups to identify asthma care and education issues for elderly urban-dwelling minority individuals. *Applied Nursing Research, 17*(3), 207–212.

Dyer, C.B., Goodwin, J.S., Pickens-Pace, S., Burnett, J., & Kelly, P.A. (2007). Self-neglect among the elderly: A model based on more than 500 patients seen by a geriatric medicine team. *American Journal of Public Health, 97,* 1671–1676.

Edwardson, S.R., & Dean, K.J. (1999). Appropriateness of self-care responses to symptoms among elders: Identifying pathways of influence. *Research in Nursing & Health, 22,* 329–339.

Erickson, H.C., Tomlin, E., & Swain, M.A. (1988). *Modeling and role-modeling: A theory and paradigm for nursing* (2nd printing). Lexington, SC: Pine Press.

Erickson, H.L. (2006). *Modeling and role-modeling: A view from the client's world.* Cedar Park, TX: Unicorns Unlimited.

Grey, M., Knafl, K., & McCorkle, R. (2006). A framework for the study of self- and family management of chronic conditions. *Nursing Outlook, 54,* 278–286.

Haber, D. (2002). Health promotion and aging: Educational and clinical initiatives by the federal government. *Educational Gerontology, 28,* 253–262.

Hertz, J.E. (1996). Conceptualization of perceived enactment of autonomy in the elderly. *Issues in Mental Health Nursing, 17* (3), 261–273.

Hertz, J.E., & Baas, L. (2006). Self-care: Knowledge, resources, and actions. In H.L. Erickson (Ed.), *Modeling and role-modeling: A view from the client's world* (pp. 97–120). Cedar Park, TX: Unicorns Unlimited.

Hertz, J.E., & Rossetti, J. (2006, March). *Senior apartment residents' reported self-care activities.* Paper presented at the 2006 Midwest Nursing Research Society Conference, Milwaukee, WI.

Inglis, S.C., Pearson, S., Treen, S., Gallasch, T., Horowitz, J.D., & Stewart, S. (2006). Extending the horizon in chronic heart failure: Effects of multidisciplinary, home-based intervention relative to usual care. *Circulation, 114,* 2466–2473.

Kralik, D., & Telford, K. (2005) *Transition in chronic illness: Self-care,* Booklet 10. Australia: RDNS Research Unit. Retrieved March 15, 2008 from www.rdns.org.au/research_unit/documents/Booklet%2010%20%20Self-care.pdf

Leenerts, M. H., Teel, C.S., & Pendleton, M.K. (2002). Building a model of self-care for health promotion in aging. *Journal of Nursing Scholarship, 34*(4), 355–361.

Lorig, K. (2001). Arthritis self-management. In E.A. Swanson, T. Tripp-Reimer, & K. Buckwalter (Eds.), *Health promotion and disease prevention in the older adult: Interventions and recommendations* (pp. 56–80). New York: Springer.

Lubben, J.E., & Damron-Rodriguez, J.A. (2003). An international approach to community health care for older adults. *Family and Community Health, 26*(4), 338–349.

Lynch, M., Estes, C.L., & Hernandez, M. (2005). Chronic care initiatives for the elderly: Can they bridge the gerontology-medicine gap? *Journal of Applied Gerontology, 24,* 108–124.

Maddox, M. (1999). Older women and the meaning of health. *Journal of Gerontological Nursing, 25*(12), 26–33.

McDonald-Miszczak, L., & Wister, A.V. (2005). Predicting self-care behaviors among older adults coping with arthritis: A cross-sectional and 1-year longitudinal comparative analysis. *Journal of Ageing and Health, 17,* 836–857.

Mendias, E.P., & Paar, D.P. (2007). Perceptions of health and self-care learning needs of outpatients with

HIV/AIDS. *Journal of Community Health Nursing, 24*(1), 49–64.

Musil, C.M., Morris, D.L., Haug, M.R., Warner, C.B., & Whelan, A.T. (2001). Recurrent symptoms: Well-being and management. *Social Science & Medicine, 52,* 1729–1740.

Orem, D. (2001). *Nursing: Concepts of practice* (6th ed.). St. Louis, MO: Mosby.

Resnick, B. (2001). Promoting health in older adults: A four-year analysis. *Journal of the American Academy of Nurse Practitioners, 13*(1), 23–33.

Resnick, B. (2003). Health promotion practices of older adults: Model testing. *Public Health Nursing, 20*(1), 2–12.

Rogers, A., Kennedy, A., Nelson, E., & Robinson, A. (2005). Uncovering the limits of patient-centeredness: Implementing a self-management trial for chronic illness. *Qualitative Health Research, 15,* 224–239.

Sharkey, J., Ory, M., & Browne, B. (2005, April). Determinants of self-management strategies to reduce out-of-pocket prescription medication expense in homebound older people [Electronic version]. *Journal of the American Geriatrics Society, 53*(4), 666–674.

Singleton, J.K. (2000). Nurses' perspectives of encouraging clients' care-of-self in a short-term rehabilitation unit within a long-term care facility. *Rehabilitation Nursing, 25*(1), 23–35.

Sullivan, T., Weinert, C., & Cudney, S. (2003). Management of chronic illness: Voices of rural women. *Journal of Advanced Nursing, 44*(6), 566–574.

U.S. Department of Health and Human Services (DHHS). (2000). *Healthy People 2010: Understanding and improving health* (2nd ed.). Washington, DC: U.S. Government Printing Office.

Wang, H-H., Hsu, M-T., & Want, R-H. (2001). Using a focus group study to explore perceptions of health-promoting self-care in community-dwelling older adults. *Journal of Nursing Research, 9*(4), 95–104.

Washburn, S., Hornberger, C., Klutman, A., & Skinner, L. (2005, May). Nurses' knowledge of heart failure education topics as reported in a small midwestern community hospital [Electronic version]. *Journal of Cardiovascular Nursing, 20*(3), 215–220.

Yip, Y.B., Sit, J.W.H., & Wong, D.Y.S. (2004). A quasi-experimental study on improving arthritis self-management for residents of an aged people's home in Hong Kong. *Psychology, Health & Medicine, 9,* 235–246.

14

Client and Family Education

Elaine T. Miller

INTRODUCTION

A chronic illness constitutes a life-changing event that uniquely affects clients and their families as they deal with the associated demands and long-term nature of a particular disease. Chronic illnesses do not always have a similar trajectory of presentation and management (e.g., asthma, depression, cancer, stroke, arthritis, diabetes, and hypertension), and they do not discriminate according to age, race, gender, socioeconomic status, culture or ethnicity, or learning capability. Furthermore, the client and family's response and resources to cope with chronic illnesses may vary tremendously, requiring healthcare professionals (HCPs) to be astute to each client and family's particular needs, expectations, resources, and personal goals.

Essential to the client and family's coping process is enhancing their knowledge, attitudes, and behaviors that contribute to the client, family, and the HCP's approach and subsequent monitoring, management, and evaluation of the progression of the chronic illness.. Given that many clients and their families are likely to experience more than one chronic illness in a lifetime, it is especially important for HCPs to be cognizant of the potential interplay of diverse chronic illnesses that may

influence the client and family's responses to further losses such as incontinence, fatigue, diminishing cognitive function, or mobility.

It is well documented that educating clients and their families is critical to successful coping with chronic illnesses. Although there are frequently some commonalities, each client and family situation has its distinctive characteristics that require HCPs to approach every situation carefully and systematically without making assumptions as to the client and family's capabilities to learn and achieve educational outcomes. Moreover, HCPs must continually assess the factors influencing the client and family's educational needs, the teaching and learning approach, and evaluation of short- and long-term outcomes. Another central element in this educational process is identifying what clients and their families want to learn, their priorities in terms of their educational needs, and having mutual goal setting, so that clients, families, and HCPs are working together to achieve common goals.

Because numerous factors contribute to the success or failure of client and family education pertaining to chronic illness, this chapter will present an overview of the fundamental elements that should be considered and will clarify the state of evidence-based knowledge pertaining to client and family education related to chronic illnesses. Even though much is known regarding client and family education, the literature and research do not suggest simple solutions or approaches that will optimize this educational process in all situations. In addition, the nature of the chronic disease(s) as well as the specific attributes of the learner(s) such as age, gender, race/ethnicity, culture, socio-economic status, motivation, self-efficacy, and learning capability will significantly influence how the HCP approaches and evaluates the success of each client and family educational encounter. The primary focus of this chapter is the adult learner. However, a basic distinction is described regarding key learning differences between adults and children. Finally, since this chapter only purports to present a broad overview of key issues affecting client and family educational processes regarding chronic illnesses, it is highly recommended that additional evidence-based resources be obtained to more specifically target the chronic illness and client population of concern, but also recognize that research and the associated findings continue to expand the science of what is known.

The Teaching–Learning Process

The teaching–learning process is characterized by multifaceted, dynamic, and interactive exchanges that are fundamental to client–family education and nursing practice. Teaching involves a deliberative, intentional act of communicating information to individuals in response to their identified educational needs and with the objective of achieving a desired outcome (Bastable, 2006). Learning, on the other hand, assists the individual to acquire new knowledge, skills, and/or attitudes that can be measured (Bastable, 2006). A review of the literature reveals that there are more than 50 major teaching–learning theories that can shape an educational intervention (The Centre for Teaching and Academic Growth, 2008).

Although many theories and frameworks are applicable to client and family education, behaviorist theory, social–cognitive learning theory,

humanistic learning theory, and constructionist theory have been identified as particularly helpful in shaping educational interventions. Each offers a different orientation of what is most important and the HCP's focus of attention when educating individuals with chronic illness and their families. In addition, each has a particular perspective in terms of how teaching and learning is defined, measured, structured, and the phases of learning.

For example, the behaviorist framework states that learning is the result of connections between the stimuli in the environment and the individual's responses (Skinner, 1974). So if an educator wants a client and/or family to learn new information or alter their attitudes and responses, such as the new need for a client to receive a subcutaneous insulin injection twice daily, the educator would alter the conditions in the environment (e.g., information available on the hospital educational cable system) and reinforce positive new behaviors when they occur (e.g., praise when the injection is given correctly).

On the other hand, social–cognitive theory includes role modeling as a central concept and offers a different approach on teaching clients and their families to perform the same task (Bandura, 1986). In this identical situation, using the social–cognitive theory, the nurse educator would demonstrate how to perform the insulin injection and then have the client, if capable, perform the insulin injection when next scheduled.

Meanwhile, if Maslow's Hierarchy of Needs, one of the best known humanistic frameworks, was applied to this identical scenario, the educator would first need to fulfill lower level needs such as physiologic needs and safety before being concerned about teaching the client how to perform the insulin injection.

Finally, the constructionistic learning theory offers an additional alternative theoretical perspective to guide the HCP's educational encounter, asserting that learners are actively creating meaning as they learn. When viewed from this constructionist orientation, learning is perceived as contextual, requiring not only time, social contact, and motivation, but also creating meanings that foster learning over time and its application (Hein, 1991). In the case of learning how to properly give an insulin injection, the constructionist theory provides a framework to connect the client's understanding/meaning of how the insulin injection should be correctly given, the client's motivation to learn this activity, the time required to correctly perform this task, and the contribution of the HCP who is teaching this skill.

In summary, theoretical frameworks offer alternative ways to approach a teaching–learning situation involving clients and their families. Because there is a myriad of theoretical frameworks, it is important that HCPs determine what is most relevant to their situations, examine available research evidence pertaining to that framework, and then translate that framework to their

particular client–family interactions, and evaluate the efficacy of using that perspective to direct their educational interventions.

In conjunction with the numerous teaching–learning theories that guide the HCP's client–family educational encounters, it is valuable to contemplate several basic assumptions underpinning these interactions. According to Petty (2006), learning involves "an active process of making sense and creating a personal interpretation of what has been learned" (p. 8), rather than simply an exact interpretation of what has been taught. What occurs is more than just a storing of personal interpretations of facts and ideas, it is "also linking them in a way that relates ideas to other ideas, and to prior learning, and so creates meaning and understanding" (p. 8). When viewed from this perspective, learners construct meaning that is more easily applied to solve problems, make

CASE STUDY

Mr. Clark is a 44-year-old African American man, who has a history of diabetes, hypertension, and a stroke 1 year ago. As a result of this stroke, he has right-sided weakness and some expressive aphasia. He lives with his wife of 20 years and 5 children who range in age from 6 to 19 years. In the last 2 months, Mr. Clark and his family moved to a new home that would permit them to be only one hour from his parents and two siblings. Currently, Mrs. Clark works as a dietician in a large metropolitan hospital, but she also juggles this with being the primary caregiver for her children and husband.

Since moving to their new home, Mr. Clark has had several falls. His most recent resulted in a broken left wrist. When Mrs. Clark brings her husband for his scheduled appointment at the doctor's office, she expresses strong concerns that her husband continues to be a fall risk and is very worried that he will fall again and injury himself. Furthermore, although Mr.

Clark is pleasant and tries to be careful, he tends to do more than he should around the home such as trying to start dinner for Mrs. Clark before she returns home from work.

Discussion Questions

1. What appears to be the primary educational objective?
2. What additional assessment data would be helpful in structuring your educational intervention for the husband as well as the wife?
3. What teaching method(s) would be most appropriate and what is your rationale for this decision?
4. What Web sites or national practice standards may be of assistance in helping to develop your teaching plan?
5. Briefly describe what your teaching plan would consist of in terms of objective(s), content, timeline, and teaching strategies?

judgments, and assist clients and their families to perform the numerous tasks associated with living with one or more chronic illnesses. Evidence is steadily expanding to support the constructivism perspective and its positive outcomes (Muijs & Reynolds, 2005). In addition, results from multiple meta-analyses of educational research reinforce the pivotal influence that feedback and reinforcement exert on individual as well as group learning (Petty, 2006).

Significance of Client and Family Teaching to Practice and Healthcare Costs

Practice standards from the American Nurses Association, the American Association of Colleges of Nursing, the National League for Nursing (NLN), specialty nursing practice standards, and other national documents consistently identify health teaching as a fundamental component of nursing practice (ANA, 2004; NLN, 2004). Even in the early writings of Florence Nightingale, teaching was recognized as a prominent nursing activity (Nightingale, 1992). In addition, all state nurse practice acts include teaching within the scope of nursing practice responsibilities and essential to promoting optimal health and disease management of clients and their families.

The underlying premise of *Healthy People 2010* is that "the health of the individual is almost inseparable from the health of the larger community" (p. 3) and is profoundly influenced by the collective beliefs, attitudes, and behaviors of this community. Throughout this comprehensive national health promotion and disease prevention roadmap, there is a recurrent theme emphasizing the improvement of "the availability and dissemination of health related information" (p. 17) pertaining to the leading health indicators of our society. Central to accomplishing these health objectives is education of all stakeholders (i.e., clients, families, HCPs). *Healthy People 2010* data further emphasize how disparities in income and education are associated with higher levels of occurrence of illness and death such as heart disease, diabetes, obesity, and elevated lead levels.

In addition to *Healthy People 2010* emphasizing the importance of client and family education, the Joint Commission on Accreditation of Healthcare Organizations (JCAHO) *2008 Hospital Accreditation Standards* identifies specific critical educational standards that must be achieved by organizations seeking accreditation. The JCAHO standards include:

Standard RI3.10
"Clients are to be given information about their responsibilities while receiving care, treatment and services" (p. RI-177).
Standard PC 6.10
"The patient receives education and training specific to the patient's needs and as appropriate to the care, treatment, and services provided" (p. PC-183).
Standard PC.6.30
"The patient receives education and training specific to the patient's abilities as appropriate to the care, treatment, and services provided by the hospital" (p. PC-184).

The JCAHO patient education standards specify that clients and families assume an active role in this process and have responsibilities just as the educator does. In instances where they do not understand the information, they are to indicate this and must take responsibility for self-management of their needs when capable (e.g., medication, safety, nutrition, pain). Moreover, the educator is expected to consistently and comprehensively assess the client and family's learning needs and barriers affecting the educational outcomes. In addition, JCAHO expects that educational activities be coordinated, tailored according to the clients and families needs/abilities, and evaluated to determine if learning has occurred.

During the 2002 Summit on the Education of Health Care Professionals (Institute of Medicine, 2003), it was emphasized that the education of all HCPs is in serious need of a "major overall" (p. 1) to be better prepared to fulfill the needs of clients and the changing healthcare system. Current nursing graduates must engage in evidence-based practice and integrate research findings pertaining to client and family teaching (IOM, 2003). Building upon this trend of expanding nursing roles, the National League for Nursing Task Group on Nurse Educator Competencies identified core competencies of nurse educators, underscoring their need to engage in scholarly activity pertaining to teaching and learning (2004).

Data from the Centers for Disease Control and Prevention (CDC) highlight the pivotal role that education has in clients' self-management of chronic illness. For instance, the CDC reports that for each dollar invested in diabetic education to assist clients to self-manage their diabetes and prevent hospitalizations, healthcare costs are reduced by $8.76 (CDC, 2005a). With regard to heart disease and stroke, they further emphasize that much of the burden associated with these two diseases can be eliminated by reduction of major risk factors such as high blood pressure, high cholesterol, tobacco use, limited physical activity,

and poor nutrition. By targeting client and family education on those modifiable risk factors, the likelihood of heart disease and stroke can be significantly diminished and personal and financial costs reduced.

Basic Differences Between Child and Adult Learners

The term "pedagogy" is defined as the art and science of teaching children, while "andragogy" refers to adult learning (Bastable, 2006, p. 451, 466). When teaching children versus adults, the key principles operating during the teachable moment are distinctly different, as indicated in Table 14-1.

Quality of Research and Evidence

When developing educational interventions for clients and their families, it is important to first determine the quality of the evidence forming the

---

TABLE 14-1

Comparison of Assumptions Pertaining to Teaching and Learning for Children and Adults

Pedagogy (children)	*Andragogy (adults)*
Rely on others to decide what is important to learn. Teacher is dominant. Learning is teacher led.	Decide for themselves what is important to learn (self-directive).
Expect what they learn will be helpful in the future.	Expect what they are learning to be immediately useful/applicable.
Have little or no experience on which to build knowledge/skill.	Have lots of experience.
Possess little ability to serve as a resource to teacher or classmates.	Possess great ability to serve as a resource to teacher and other learners (active student role).
Expect to be taught and take no responsibility.	Like to take control of the situation.
Not necessarily ready to learn.	Imply their motivation to learn, since they are present in the learning situation.
View learning as a process of acquiring information to be used at a later time.	View learning as a process of increasing competence to achieve a fuller life potential.

Sources: Bastable, S.B. (2006). *Essentials of patient education.* Sudbury, MA: Jones & Bartlett; Conner, M.L. (2005). Andragogy and Pedagogy. *Ageless Learner, 1997–2004.* Retrieved January 12, 2008 from http://agelesslearner.com/intros/andragogy.html; Knowles, M. (1998). *The adult learner: The definitive classic in adult education and human resource development.* Houston, TX: Gulf Publishing; and Mihall, J., & Belletti, J. (1999). Adult learning styles and training methods. *FDIC ADR Presentation Handouts,* Retrieved January 12, 2008 from http://www.usdoj.gov/adr/workplace/pdf/learstyl.pdf

basis for the planned actions. Evidence-based practice (EBP) refers to a problem solving approach used in practice that combines the following three components: the best available evidence, the HCP's clinical expertise, and the client's values and preferences (Melnyk & Fineout-Overhold, 2005). The highest level of evidence is well-conducted meta-analyses and systematic reviews of randomized control trials (RCTs) (Melnyk & Fineout-Overhold, 2005; Craig & Smyth, 2002). However, a review of the literature reveals that a sizable portion of present knowledge directing our educational interventions is of a lower level of evidence quality than preferred such as single randomized trials, nonrandomized studies, consensus opinion of experts, and case studies. Results of a systematic review of 139 educational RCTs involving more than 22,000 clients with diabetes, asthma, or congestive heart failure (CHF) reveal that many of these RCTs draw inappropriate conclusions, with researchers frequently tending to overgeneralize their findings and include their opinions that are not based on research evidence (Boren, Balas, & Mustafa, 2003). Therefore, educators need to carefully scrutinize the level of available evidence that underpins their practice, determine whether stated implications in research studies extend beyond the documented evidence, and recognize the tentative nature of our knowledge.

An excellent illustration of how knowledge evolves is demonstrated by the Internet and the increasing prevalence of online learning that has reshaped, in many instances, the education of clients, families, and HCPs worldwide. In a study investigating clients seeking trends for additional health information regarding their disease/health problem, Rahmqvist and Bara (2007) identified from a sample of 24,800 respondents that young and middle-aged clients primarily use the Internet to expand their knowledge. Despite this Internet access facilitating clients becoming more informed, they stress the inherent quality issues associated with public access to a blend of poor as well as high-quality evidence-based online health information.

Assessment of the Learner

A critical aspect of the client and family educational process is the assessment phase that shapes the other steps in the process, such as planning the educational event/program, its implementation, and evaluating outcomes. However, just as vital signs are obtained to determine the client's physiologic state, so too must certain essential information be obtained in this initial assessment that will affect how the education is structured, delivered, and evaluated. Because it is assumed that the client and family dealing with the chronic illness are equal partners with the HCP, the following are critical questions to ask the client and family:

1. What information do you want provided? Recognize that the client and family may identify different needs. If so, make sure each of their needs is addressed.

2. Are there any new skills that you want to learn or ones you want to review?

3. What are your specific educational goals for the client and family? You may need to give an example (e.g., correctly identify signs/symptoms of hypoglycemic reactions, know what to do when an insulin reaction occurs and how to correctly give an insulin injection). The HCP must recognize that client and family goals can focus on knowledge, attitude (i.e., self-efficacy), and/or skill acquisition.

4. Of the goals identified, what is most important? Once again, the client and family may differ markedly in specific goals and priorities. Listen carefully to both of them.

5. What do you perceive as factors that affect your ability to achieve these educational goals? How will barriers be overcome?

6. Do you feel confident using the information provided to you? If not, how may I assist you in increasing your confidence and ability to use this information?

When clients and family members are providing answers, the HCP must always be an astute listener, nonjudgmental, capable of developing individualized and attainable client and/or family goals, and reflect back to the client and family their understanding of what has been heard (Miller, 2003). While collecting the relevant client and family data, the HCP needs to be organized, perform the assessment in a timely manner, and be aware of readability of assessment materials. In addition, the client who is chronically ill often has associated limitations that affect the assessment (e.g., easily fatigued and diminished hearing and/or vision and/or comprehension).

INFLUENCES ON TEACHING AND LEARNING

Family Structure and Function

Families can vary significantly in structure and function. A chronic illness of a family member can precipitate changes in the family structure and function, as do changes associated with marriage, raising children, or death of a family member. When a family has a member with a chronic illness, the family's response to this change, its capability to adapt and make decisions, can influence their receptiveness to education. When the client and family experience high anxiety, it can markedly interfere with their ability to receive and comprehend information, maintain normal patterns of family functioning, and use appropriate coping skills. Because culture and lifestyle affect the development of family norms and beliefs, differences in these client/family and HCP factors can affect the dynamics of the educational process (Rankin, Stallings, & London, 2005). Once these beliefs and values are identified, they can be addressed through individualized teaching (London, 2002). It is imperative, therefore, that the family structure, function (i.e., roles, resources, strengths, and weaknesses) and norms be considered in the assessment and educational planning process.

According to the 2008 JCAHO standards, the family is to be included in client teaching (e.g., fall reduction strategies, reporting concerns related to care and safety). Because the client's family may be large with varying functions, the HCP must determine the primary family member who should receive the relevant education. Just as in the case of the client, the HCP needs to assess the primary family caregiver's role, expectations, learning needs/goals, learning style, fears, concerns, cognitive and physical abilities, and present knowledge pertaining to the client's healthcare needs (Bastable, 2006). Moreover, the client and the family member may need to receive similar information, reinforcement, and feedback related to their knowledge and/or skill performance. In many instances, the family member is the single most important factor in determining the success or failure of the teaching plan (Haggard, 1989).

Culture

When working with clients and their families, culture can dramatically affect how educational activities are structured, delivered, and evaluated. The client and family's culture comprise "an integral part of each person's life and includes knowledge, beliefs, values, morals, customs, traditions, communication patterns, and habits acquired by members of a society" (Bastable, 2006, p. 455). When educating clients and families, an important initial step is becoming culturally sensitive. This refers to the process of becoming aware of one's own biases and prejudices of another culture or ethnic group. Cultural competence, a higher level, denotes educational interventions reflecting knowledge, understanding, respect, and acceptance of the clients and/or family's culture (Bastable, 2006).

For a successful educational encounter to occur, HCPs and clients and their families must bridge these cultural differences through the use of effective interpersonal communication. This establishment of common understanding between HCPs and clients and their families is facilitated by the HCP performing the following:

■ Explore and respect the clients/family's beliefs, values, meaning of the chronic illness, preferences, and needs.

- Identify what will build rapport and trust. Potential sources of information to assist in this process are other colleagues, family members of the client, community groups, and reputable internet Web sites.
- Determine if there are any common views or interests.
- Identify own biases and assumptions.
- Maintain and convey an unconditional positive regard. Be an excellent listener, open and nonjudgmental, and use consistent perception checks to assess comprehension of what has been communicated.
- Become knowledgeable of the culture and health disparities/discrimination of the particular client/family's culture. Review some of the Web sites identified in this chapter that provide a starting point for resources from reputable sources.
- Use interpreter services when needed.

Cultural differences make each client and family situation unique, but there are also essential considerations in communication, interactions, and the ultimate delivery of any educational activity. Because culture has been linked to cancer-related beliefs and practices, Kreuter and associates (2003) examined the effects of culture on responses to cancer education materials. With a convenience sample of 1227 African American women, it was determined that responses to culturally tailored materials were no different than to other materials, regardless of the women's cultural characteristics. However, for all types of educational materials, women with higher religiosity and racial pride paid more attention to the educational materials. In this study, it appeared that select cultural attributes (e.g., religiosity and racial pride) moderated responses to tailored health education materials.

A number of other contextual factors have been demonstrated to influence health-related attitudes and beliefs of the cancer information–seeking behavior of African American men. One example: living in the South where the Tuskegee

Syphilis Study took place has resulted in distrust of the healthcare delivery system among many African Americans (Freimuth et al., 2001; Green et al., 2000). In a study investigating factors predicting prostate cancer information seeking by 52 African American men, it was discovered that the men increased their awareness by obtaining accurate information regarding the disease, early detection and screening, and treatment. However, negative beliefs such as fear, distrust, and inconvenience of the symptoms and treatment were identified. It was further revealed that peers, siblings, and religious leaders had a significant influence on the study subjects' behaviors.

Viswanathan (2005), in a study with 20 adult African Americans with cardiovascular disease, ranging in age from 45 to 64 years, discovered that the subjects expressed fear. Subjects' fears were related to side effects from their medication, fear of dependence, and worry about forgetting to take their medication correctly. Despite the fears identified, these subjects perceived their medications to be lifesaving, an important part of life, and recognized the necessity to take medication properly to prevent the complications associated with hypertension. As illustrated in this study, compared with the former, the subjects experienced fear, but the stated reasons were distinctly different. This finding emphasizes that not all African Americans experience situations in the same manner, and that individualized assessment and planning needs to occur without making assumptions and applying them to all members of that cultural group.

In an integrative review that focused on Hispanic adults and beliefs about type 2 diabetes, Hatcher and Wittemore (2007) identified several valuable findings that should be considered when developing educational interventions for this population. After reviewing 15 research studies, they identified that generally Hispanic adults' understanding of the etiology of diabetes was an integration of biomedical causes such as heredity and traditional folk beliefs. With knowledge of the importance of heredity and folk beliefs in how Hispanics view diabetes, Hatcher and Wittemore

(2007) recommend this as a starting point to clarify misconceptions and develop individualized plans of teaching and care. Results from this synthesis of the research literature highlight the necessity of obtaining specific knowledge of how race and culture can affect the structure, implementation, and evaluation of educational outcomes.

Determination of the family's sense of burden, ability to cope, and the role of culture is another aspect of the client and family assessment that needs to be taken into consideration when planning individualized educational activities. Cain and Wicke (2000) in a study involving 138 family caregivers of clients with chronic obstructive pulmonary disease (COPD) discovered that African American caregivers experienced less burden than their Caucasian counterparts. Similar levels of burden occurred in men compared with women and

spouse caregivers compared with nonspouse caregivers. In addition, younger caregivers indicated more burden than those 55 and older. Although these findings are not generalizable beyond this study, they acknowledge the importance of educators being cognizant of contextual factors such as caregiver burden and age, and how these factors may affect other activities such as client and family teaching. Table 14-2 provides additional resources to facilitate cultural competence with diverse client and family populations.

Gender and Learning Styles

In addition to cultural background, gender and learning styles have a significant influence on the learner's willingness and ability to respond to and apply educational content. Numerous studies

---

TABLE 14-2

Cultural Competence Resources for Client–Family Education

Center for Human Diversity; provides consulting and training in cultural competence, diversity, and customer service: www.centerforhumandiversity.org/

Joint Commission—Hospitals, Language and Culture; resources on JCAHO standards and Cultural and Linguistically Appropriate Services (CLAS) standards: www.jointcommission.org/PatientSafety/HLC/

Knowledge Path; electronic resource guide to racial and ethnic disparities in health includes information on (and links to) Web sites, electronic and print publications, Web casts, and databases: www.mchlibrary.info/KnowledgePaths/kp_race.html

National Center for Cultural Competence; increase the capacity of health and mental health programs to design, implement, and evaluate culturally and linguistically competent service delivery systems. There is also a Spanish version: www11.georgetown.edu/research/gucchd/nccc/

National Mental Health Information Center; U.S. Dept. of Health and Human Services Substance Abuse and Mental Health Services Administration) SAMHSA: mentalhealth.samhsa.gov/topics/explore/culture/

Network for Multicultural Health; focuses on reducing health disparities in health care through education and training, and by fostering organizational change: futurehealth.ucsf.edu/TheNetwork/Default.aspx?tabid=110

Office of Minority Health: www.omhrc.gov/templates/browse.aspx?lvl=2&lvlID=15

Race, Ethnicity and Health Care: The Basics; the latest data sources and research on racial and ethnic disparities in health care, including information on access and quality, the healthcare workforce, and public opinion: www.kaiseredu.org/topics_reflib.asp?id=329&parentid=67&rID=1

Rural Assistance Center for Minority Health; US Department of Health and Human Services' Rural Initiative Center's resource on issues of minority health in rural communities: www.raconline.org/info_guides/minority_health/

Working Together to End Racial and Ethnic Disparities: One Physician at a Time; AMA toolkit designed to help physicians eliminate health care disparities: www.ama-assn.org/ama1/pub/upload/mm/433/health_disp_kit.pdf

have identified gender differences in the structure of the brain and how it functions (Gur, 1999; Luders et al., 2007; Witelson, Beresh, & Kigar, 2006). Table 14-3 provides an overview of basic gender differences that have been identified, but educators are strongly encouraged to individually determine the applicability of these differences to a particular client and family population (Gurian & Ballew, 2003; Sax, 2005; Connell & Gunzelmann, 2004).

With the increased usage of online courses and Web-based educational materials, research is revealing that there is a variation in learning styles of the online students and students in face-to-face courses (Garland & Martin, 2005). Moreover, these researchers determined that gender is related to learning style and engagement. In their study involving 7 online courses and 168 students (102 female and 66 male), there was a significant relationship with regard to male students who favored abstract conceptualization mode of learning and how many times they accessed the communication area of Blackboard, an online course management

system. Female students, meanwhile, were more highly motivated to perform required class activities than male students. The researchers emphasize that faculty constructing online courses need to be aware of how discussions, chats, and groups are affected by gender, while keeping in mind that postings may be intimidating to some female students. Garland & Martin (2005) further stress the need for additional studies that investigate the relationship between online learning, learning style, and gender, but also the importance of considering gender equity in building and designing online courses and educational programs.

In another study involving an online health-education program, Women-to-Women (WTW), Cudney and colleagues (2005) were interested in determining issues and solutions in a sample of 50 middle-aged women with cancer, diabetes, multiple sclerosis, or rheumatoid arthritis who lived in rural communities. The problems identified included difficulties carrying out self-management programs, negative fears/feelings, poor communication with HCPs, and disturbed relationships

---

TABLE 14-3

Comparison of Brain-Based Learning Differences According to Gender

	Males	*Females*
Deductive and inductive reasoning	Are more inclined to use deductive thinking	Prefer inductive thinking
Abstract and concrete reasoning	Gravitate to abstract arguments	Perform better with concrete analysis
Language usage	Write, read, and speak but usually less than females. In a group of males, one or two tend to dominate	Usually prefer writing, reading, and speaking more words than males
Logic and evidence	Tend to ask for more evidence to support a claim	Tend to be better listeners, more secure in conversation, and require less control of discussion compared with males
Symbolism usage	Respond to pictures with males; more dependent on pictures, diagrams, and graphs in their learning process	Respond to pictures, but not as dependent on pictures, diagrams, and graphs as males to learn

Sources: Gurian, M., & Ballew, A.C. (2003). *The boys and girls learn differently: Action guide for teachers.* San Francisco: Jossey-Bass; Sax, 2005; Connell, D. & Gunzelmann, B. (2004). The new gender gap: Why are so many boys floundering while so many girls are soaring? Retrieved from teacher.scholastic.com/products/Instructor/Mar04_gendergap.htm

with family and friends. Self-identified solutions pertained to problem-solving techniques that were tailored to their rural lifestyle. Although most women indicated that their health-promotion problems were not easily solvable, they continued to identify feasible ways to self-manage their chronic illnesses (i.e., small achievable goals, take one day at a time, taking responsibility for being informed, improving communication with HCP, being proactive in family relationships, being able to say "no"). Results from this study affirm the importance of performing research to expand the best available evidence to guide our practice.

Just as gender differences need to be assessed, many educators indicate that determination of the individual's learning style is equally important. The presumed method by which an individual learns best is defined as one's learning style. The difficulty is that there are more than 80 learning style models and limited scientific evidence to support any of them (Coffield, Moseley, Hall, & Ecclestone, 2004; Stahl, 2002). Despite the controversy over the presence and quality of the evidence, it is still worthwhile to ask clients and families what approach to learning they prefer (e.g., spoken word, reading, writing, doing, or interacting). With this information the HCP can then more effectively plan the teaching interventions. Moreover, age, intelligence, motor skills, degree of impairment, anxiety, and past experiences can significantly affect an individual's ability to learn (Rankin, Stallings, & London, 2005). Along with the aforementioned factors, educational activities must be adapted to clients and families' style of learning and preferences regarding what they need to learn.

Readiness to Learn, Self-Efficacy, and Readiness to Change

Once the learning needs of the client and family are identified, determination of their readiness to learn and self-efficacy are important next steps. Readiness to learn refers to the time when learners are receptive to learning, whereas self-efficacy

indicates that they have confidence in their capability to attain a particular goal (Bastable, 2006). In order for learning to occur, clients and family members must both be ready to learn and possess average to high self-efficacy.

Readiness to learn manifests in a variety of areas such as physical readiness, emotional readiness, experiential readiness, and knowledge readiness (Lichtenthal, 1990). More specifically, physical readiness can be affected by the client's ability to perform the task, the task's complexity, environmental conditions that keep the client's attention and interest, the client's health status, and gender (Lichtenthal, 1990; Bastable, 2006). Research supports that women are more receptive to medical care and less likely to take risks associated with their health compared with men (Bertakis, Rahman, Helms, Callahan, & Robbins, 2000). Emotional readiness to learn, on the other hand, has been demonstrated to be affected by anxiety level, strength of one's support system, motivation, state of mind, and developmental stage (Bastable, 2006). Previous positive as well as negative learning experiences can dramatically affect experiential readiness of clients and family members. Therefore, HCPs planning an educational activity should identify any previous learning successes and failures and prior ways of coping with similar situations, and understand the potential influence of culture and human motivation. Finally, readiness to learn new knowledge can be influenced by what the client or family member already knows, their cognitive ability, any learning disabilities, and general learning style (Bastable, 2006; Rankin, Stallings, & London, 2005; Muijs & Reynolds, 2005).

While assessing clients and family members for readiness to learn, self-efficacy must also be determined. In the research literature, a strong sense of self-efficacy, confidence in one's ability to achieve a behavior, has repeatedly been demonstrated to have significant positive influence on accomplishing a health-promoting behavior change in individuals with chronic illness (Coleman & Newton, 2005; Osborne, Wilson, Lorig, & McColl, 2007; Tung & Lee, 2006).

Readiness to change is another increasingly familiar term applied to chronic illness and reducing unhealthy behaviors. Although readiness to change has varied definitions, the best known emerges from the Transtheoretical Model of Change (TTM), which involves intentional decision making and was developed to promote effective interventions to facilitate positive behavioral change. TTM is a model that reflects an integration of constructs from other theories and describes how individuals modify problem behaviors such as smoking, limited exercise, and overeating to acquire a more positive behavior (Prochaska & DiClemente, 1983; Prochaska, DiClemente, & Norcross, 1992; Prochaska & Velicer, 1997). The central organizing construct is Stages of Change, but the model also includes other variables (e.g., self-efficacy, processes of change, decisional balance, and temptation). TTM focuses on stage-focused interventions pertaining to the individual's readiness to change an unhealthy behavior (e.g., smoking, limited exercise). Within TTM, there are five stages of readiness to change (i.e., precontemplation, contemplation, preparation, action, and maintenance). Measurement instruments with demonstrated reliability and validity can be obtained at the Cancer Prevention Research Center Web site (CPRC, 2008).

Developmental Stage

Chronologic age provides a basic indication of clients and family members' projected physical, cognitive, and psychological state of development. When planning a teaching–learning activity for a client and family member, consideration of the clients' or family members' developmental stage is pivotal, along with past learning experiences, stress level, physical and emotional health, personal motivation, environmental conditions, and available support systems (Bastable, 2006).

Within the literature, there are several prominent developmental theorists who have shaped how HCPs view life stages (Erickson, 1963; Piaget, 1951, 1976). In contrast with childhood where learning is student centered, adult learning tends to be more problem centered, with the primary emphasis on how to apply new knowledge and skills to immediate problems (Bastable, 2006). Adults tend to be more resistant to change, which is why establishing mutual goals and an action plan with HCPs markedly improves the achievement of educational outcomes (Miller, 2003; Rankin, Stallings, & London, 2005).

Table 14-4 provides a brief overview of the developmental stages of adults, the major attributes of the learner, and the most applicable teaching strategies. A common misconception is that older adults cannot learn. When older adults are provided information at a slower rate, material being taught is relevant, and positive feedback is received, they are very capable of learning new knowledge and skills (Bastable, 2006; Mauk, 2006). Because depression, grief, and loneliness are not restricted to older adults, these factors can markedly affect any client or family members' ability to concentrate on content being presented. HCPs, moreover, must be continually aware of other potential cognitive as well as physical limitations (i.e., pain, fatigue, diminished vision, and reduced hearing) that can affect the ability of clients and family members to learn. Table 14-5 provides a listing of recommended resources for HCPs to identify how to optimally structure and evaluate educational activities involving older adults.

Literacy

Health literacy or the ability to understand and apply information to care for one's self is a challenge for approximately 1 in 2 adults in the United States, who cannot read above fifth-grade level (Nielson-Bohlman, Panzer, & Kindig, 2004; Mayer & Vallaire, 2007). Throughout the entire healthcare delivery process, low literacy levels can affect the ability of clients and family members to read and comprehend health information (e.g., discharge instructions, labels on prescription bottles), which serves as an important prerequisite to compliance and overall successful client outcomes (Bastable, 2006; Lasater & Mehler,

TABLE 14-4

Linking Developmental Stage with Learner Characteristics and Teaching Strategies

Developmental Stage	Learner Characteristics	Recommended Teaching Strategies
Young adulthood (18–39.9 years)	Peak body function Self-directive Independent in learning Making decisions about career, education, social roles Competency-based learner If has a chronic illness, tends to want to learn as much as possible to remain independent and lead as normal a life as possible	Immediate application Active participation Learning needs to be convenient, self-paced, and blend of visual and written Tend to like group interaction Organized materials and presentation Use past experiences as a resource for learning Provide practical answers to their problems Give opportunity for immediate application of teaching Seek credible/evidence-based information
Middle age (40–64.9 years)	Well-developed sense of self Usually at career peak Concerned about physical changes Reexamines goals and values Confident in abilities Tends to want to reduce unsatisfying aspects in life May be experiencing mid-life crises	Maintain independence and perhaps reestablish what constitutes normal life patterns Assess prior positive and negative learning experiences Identify potential stressors Provide information that fits to life problems and/or concerns; use past experiences as a resource for learning Provide practical answers to their problems Give opportunity for immediate application of what teaching
Older adult (65 years and older)	Cognitive changes Decreased ability to think abstractly Reduced short-term memory Increased reaction time Focus on past life experiences Motor and sensory losses Auditory and visual changes Hearing loss especially with high pitched tones, consonants, and rapid speech Decreased peripheral vision Decreased risk taking	Use concrete examples Build on past experiences Make information relevant Allow time for processing and responses Use verbal interactions and coaching Encourage active involvement Keep explanations brief (20–40 minutes) Speak distinctly and slowly Minimize distractions while teaching Avoid shouting—if large group, microphone may be needed Use large font in handouts Avoid glares Provide a safe environment Keep teaching sessions short Provide rest periods Rooms where conducted should be neutral temperature (not too hot or cold)

Sources: Bastable, S.B. (2006). *Essentials of patient education.* Sudbury, MA: Jones & Bartlett; Mauk, K.L. (Ed.). (2006). *Gerontological nursing: Competencies for care.* Sudbury, MA: Jones & Bartlett; Rankin, S.H., Stallings, K.D., & London, F. (2005). *Patient education in health and illness* (5th ed.). Philadelphia: Lippincott.

TABLE 14-5

Helpful Resources to Facilitate Teaching and Learning of Older Adults

Organization	Web Site
American Society on Aging	www.saging.org
Association for Gerontology in Higher Education	www.aghe.org
The John A. Hartford Foundation Institute for Geriatric Nursing	www.hartfordign.orh
National Assessments of Adult Literacy	www.nces.ed.gov
National Institute on Aging	www.nia.nih.gov/
National Council on Aging	www.ncoa.org
Osher Lifelong Learning Institute	www.olli.gmu.edu

1998; Nielson-Bohlman, Panzer, & Kindig, 2004). A variety of measurement tools are available to HCPs to assess the readability of written educational materials as well as reading capability of clients and family members. Refer to Table 14-6 for a brief description of several tools that have proved useful.

The following strategies (Mayer & Vallaire, 2007; Bastable, 2006; Petty, 2006; Falvo, 2004) may serve as a starting point when assessing and educating clients and families with low literacy:

- Materials should not be above fifth-grade level and should be culturally appropriate.
- Keep sentences short and limited to 20 words or less if possible.
- Speak and write using short words with only one or two syllables whenever possible. Rely on common words that are easily recognized by more individuals.
- Put the most important information first and limit focus on what the client and family member need to know.
- Clearly and simply define technical words or ones that are unfamiliar (e.g., fasting blood glucose, hypertension), or replace with simpler words (high blood pressure for hypertension).
- Avoid abbreviations (i.e., MI, FBS, I, and O).
- Use consistent words throughout the presentation (e.g., don't switch from diet to menu to dietary prescription).
- Organize information into "chucks" that facilitate recall. Use numbers only when necessary and realize that statistics are usually confusing and meaningless for the low-literate client and family member.
- Keep the number of items in a list to no more than seven.
- Keep teaching sessions short and preferably no longer than 20–30 minutes.
- Use the teach-back method with clients to ensure that they understand their care routine and warning signs if there is a problem (i.e., signs of a wound infection or urinary tract infection, signs of a stroke or heart attack—not myocardial infarction). Never ask "Do you understand? Ask the patient to explain the processes or state the signs of an infection, stroke, or heart attack.
- Have your written materials reviewed by a literacy expert to determine the grade reading level.
- Present information one step at a time to pace instruction and allow clients and family members to understand each step and ask questions before moving on to the next step.

System Factors That Influence the Teaching and Learning Process

To ensure an optimal client, family, and HCP educational situation, certain elements need to be in place. System factors that can significantly contribute to positive educational outcomes include (Edwardson, 2007; Nobel, 2006; Rankin, Stallings, & London, 2005):

- Preparation of the HCP in terms of knowledge of the educational content and teaching capabilities.

TABLE 14-6

Tools to Assess Readability of Educational Materials and Individual's Reading Comprehension

Measurement Tools to Assess Readability of Educational Materials	*Measurement Tools to Assess an Individual's Reading Comprehension*

Flesch Formula

In use more than 50 years to assess news reports, adult educational materials, and government publications. Based on a count of two basic language components: average sentence length in words and average word length measured in syllables per word of selected samples of text (Flesch, 1948; Spadero, 1983). Helpful Web sources to assist with these calculations are: neil.gratton.org/cgi-bin/flesch.cgi and www.csun.edu/~vcecn006/read1.html

Fog Formula

Assesses the reading level of materials from fourth grade to college level. One of the easier tools to use with the calculation based on the average sentence length and percentage of multisyllabic words based on a sample of 100 words (Bastable, 2006; Spadero, 1983). Helpful Web sources: process.umn.edu/groups/ppd/documents/information/writing_tips.cfm and www.thelearningweb.net/fogindex.html

SMOG Formula

This formula has been used primarily to evaluate the grade-level readability of patient educational materials (PEMs) and can measure reading level with as little content as 10 sentences. This formula determines readability from grades four to college level, and is based on number of multi-syllable words (3 or more) within a set number of sentences (McLaughlin, 1969). Helpful Web sources are: www.harrymclaughlin.com/SMOG.htm www.hsph.harvard.edu/healthliteracy/how_to/smog_2.pdf

Wide Range Achievement Test (WRAT)

WRAT is a word-recognition screening test that typically takes about 5 minutes to complete. It assesses the client's ability to recognize and pronounce a list of words out of context to determine reading skills. It has two levels of testing: Level 1 is for children 5 to 12 years; Level 2 is for individuals over 12 years of age (Doak et al., 1996). Helpful Web sources are: findarticles.com/p/articles/mi_g2602/is_0005/ai_2602000563 and www.familylearning.org/tests_wrat.php – 13k

Rapid Estimate of Adult Literacy in Medicine (REALM)

The REALM tests the client's ability to read medical and health-related vocabulary (advantage over the WRAT), takes less time, and has easy scoring (Duffy & Synder, 1998). Although the test has validity, the test offers less precision and reliability than other word tests (Hayes, 2000). Sixty-six medical and health-related words are placed in three columns ranging from short and easy to more difficult. Clients are to begin reading the words from the top and go down. The total number of correctly pronounced words is the raw score that is then converted to a grade range (Doak et al., 1996). Helpful Web source is: www.hsc.wvu.edu/.../Winter%20Spring%202007/

Test of Functional Health Literacy in Adults (TOFHL)

TOFHL is a newer measurement tool to assess clients' literacy skills and actually uses hospital materials (i.e., appointment slips, informed consent documents, and prescription labels). The test consists of two parts: reading comprehension and numeracy (Bastable, 2006). It has demonstrated validity and reliability, takes approximately 20 minutes to administer, and has an English and Spanish version (Quirk, 2000). Helpful Web resource is: www.nifl.gov/nifl-health/2001/0108.html

- Cultural competence and knowledge related to all of the other factors that help to personalize the educational approach (i.e., age, developmental stage, and cognitive and physical status related to the chronic illness).

- Required resources for effective teaching (e.g., equipment/technology, materials—booklets, figures).

- Time limitations that permit updating teaching plans, evaluation tools, and developing/updating educational protocols.

- Coordinating educational activities that are consistent with discharge plans and other important client and family information that needs to be communicated.

- Succinct and timely documentation of what was taught, when, and the outcome, so others can build on and reinforce prior teaching.

- If client and family education is not valued by the system and rewards are not given for educational excellence and positive outcomes.

- If there is inadequate record-keeping and reimbursement policies that reimburse fully for direct hands-on illness interventions, but poorly for client/family education and interventions via telephone and computer.

In conjunction with the system challenges just identified, HCPs must also consider other diverse attributes (i.e., age, gender, culture, developmental stage, literacy, and functional status) that make each client and family educational encounter unique. In addition, what is the best available evidence that will help shape these interventions? Townsend (2006) also asserts that HCPs do not always recognize the tensions and ambiguities permeating clients' experiences, particularly those who have multiple chronic illnesses. Results of his research revealed that clients with chronic illness utilize multiple techniques to manage their symptoms, and frequently felt pressure to manage "well" and have a "normal life" for both their families and HCPs.

Despite the limited strong evidence to support all aspects of HCPs' educational interventions, the research continues to expand as do the meta-analyses and systematic reviews that synthesize the evidence and identify additional areas to be explored. In order to more comprehensively document the specific contribution of nursing to the education and self-care of clients with chronic illness, Edwardson (2007) recommends two focus areas for research. The first is to measure the outcomes of client and family education and have this information included in both the clinical and administrative databases. Whenever possible, the client and family educational process and outcomes should be separated according to type of education, objectives, timing, dose (i.e., strategies, length), and so forth. In addition, systematic reviews and meta-analysis suggest that inpatient education followed by some form of postdischarge intervention may be the most promising approach to reduce hospitalizations (Gonseth, Castillion, Banegas, & Artalejo, 2004). However, for this care system to succeed, databases from ambulatory care, acute care, and after-care services need to be linked to monitor symptoms, monitor adherence to treatment prescription, and to modify treatment plans as needed (Edwardson, 2007).

EDUCATIONAL INTERVENTIONS FOR THE CLIENT AND FAMILY

As indicated in previous sections of this chapter, there are multiple factors to be carefully assessed and considered in the development of an educational plan for the client with chronic illness and their family. Because of the variance in how these elements manifest, the mutually established goals by the client, family, and HCP; associated interventions; and outcomes will need to be uniquely planned, implemented, and evaluated. In most instances, nurses will be the principal HCP who participates in this ongoing educational process and provides the continuity of care for the client with chronic illness and their family.

Development of the Teaching Plan

The teaching plan provides the overall blueprint or outline for instruction that clearly defines the relationship among the behavioral objectives, instructional content, teaching strategies, time frame for teaching, and methods of evaluation (Bastable, 2006). All aspects work together to achieve a predetermined goal that should be mutually agreed upon by the client–family and HCP. The domains of learning that are to be accomplished divide into one of three domains. These are cognitive (knowledge), psychomotor (physical activities), and affective (attitudes or emotions). When constructing teaching plans to address these learning domains for specific chronic illnesses, HCPs should also refer to published practice standards such as those from the Agency for Healthcare Research and Quality (AHRQ), specialty nursing groups, and the American Heart Association, which present evidence-based guidelines. The specific teaching plan includes the following aspects: purpose of the teaching plan; goal(s), broad statement of what is to be achieved; objective(s) that need to be specific and measurable; content covered to achieve each objective; teaching strategies; time required; and evaluation methods to determine if the learning has occurred. A specific example will be provided once key aspects of the teaching plan are described.

Teaching Strategies

Knowing how to use varied teaching strategies to achieve educational objectives can make client and family education more interesting, challenging, and effective for HCPs and learners (Rankin, Stallings, & London, 2005). A general overview of common teaching strategies and their predominant characteristics are presented in Table 14-7. For the client with chronic illness, the research strongly supports that combining multiple teaching methods during several educational sessions consistently produces more positive client outcomes than single teaching methods and events (Bastable, 2006; Beranova & Sykes, 2007; Edwardson, 2007; The Joanna Briggs Institute, 2006). However, the HCP must also remain cognizant of the system factors contributing to the success and/or failure of the teaching and learning process.

A pivotal aspect of any client and family teaching event is preparing measurable objectives that can be achieved in the time frame specified. For example, the client with diabetes may need to learn the signs and symptoms of a hypoglycemic reaction. An appropriate measurable objective could be "Ms. Jones will state four signs/symptoms of a hypoglycemic reaction by the end of this 8-hour shift."

Increasingly, more clients with chronic illness and their family members are receiving education regarding disease management from Web-based sources, with the young to middle aged being the biggest consumers (Beranova & Sykes, 2007; Lee, Yeh, Liu, & Chen, 2007). Approximately 93 million Americans have searched online for health information and services on at least one major health topic (Fox & Falloes, 2003). For clients with chronic illness, the use of the Internet provides a means to encourage behavior change necessitating knowledge sharing, education, and greater understanding of their condition. Results of a meta-analysis comparing Web-based and non–Web-based education of chronically ill adults (mean age 41.2 years) from 1996 to 2003 revealed that there was substantial evidence that Web-based interventions improved behavioral change outcomes (Wantland, Portillo, Holzemer, & Slaughter, 2004). The specific positive outcomes identified were increased knowledge of nutritional status, increased knowledge of asthma treatment, increased exercise time, slower health decline, and 18-month weight-loss maintenance. Web-based interventions that were relevant and individually tailored had more and longer Web-site visits. Wantland and associates further discovered that sites with chat rooms increased social support scores of the users. They caution,

TABLE 14-7

General Overview of Common Teaching Strategies

Teaching Strategy	Learning Domain	Learner Role	Teacher Role	Strength	Weakness
Lecture	Cognitive	Passive	Presents information	Cost-effective; targeted to larger groups	Not individualized
Group discussion	Cognitive; affective	Active, if learner participates	Directs and focuses discussion	Share emotions and ideas	Shy or dominant members affect participation; may lose focus
One-to-one teaching	Cognitive; affective psychomotor	Active	Presents information and encourages individualized learning	Tailored to client or family member's needs and goals	Great diversity; labor intensive; learner isolated
Demonstration	Cognitive	Passive	Modeling of skill or behavior	Preview of skill or behavior, can ask questions	Need individual or small group to visualize
Return demonstration	Psychomotor	Active	Individualized feedback to refine skill performance	Immediate feedback	Labor intensive; anxiety may affect actions
Gaming	Cognitive; affective	Active if client–family participates	Oversees pacing; referee debriefs	Stimulates learners' enthusiasm and participation	May be too competitive; over-stimulating
Simulation	Cognitive; psychomotor	Active	Designs situation; facilitates learning; debriefs	Practice a reality situation in a safe setting	Labor intensive; equipment costs/access; scheduling issues
Online learning	Cognitive; affective	Passive, but can be active if participates in group discussions, problem solving, group projects	Usually designs program/ class presents information provides active learning exercises, discussions, case studies, and group projects	Learners usually at a distance; flexibility when access learning content and activities; learners need to be motivated; feedback provided is usually individualized and immediate	Need equipment to access; lack of personal contact; accessibility; all feedback may not be instantaneous
Computer-assisted instruction	Cognitive; affective	Active	Purchases or designs program; expected to provide feedback to student	Individualized instruction; learner controls pace of the learning; can program to receive feedback; valuable modality if hearing impaired, learning disability, or aphasic	Must have equipment and software

Sources: Bastable, S.B. (2006). *Essentials of patient education.* Sudbury, MA: Jones & Bartlett; Miller, E. (2008). *Theoretical Foundations of Health Promotion, Risk Reduction, and Health Planning (29NURS807): Online Course Manual.* University of Cincinnati; College of Nursing; Wantland, D.J., Portillo, C.J., Holzemer, W.L., & Slaughter, R. (2004). The effectiveness of web-based vs. non-web-based interventions: A meta-analysis of behavioral change outcomes. *Journal of Medical Internet Research, 6*(4), 40–71.

however, that the long-term effects on individual persistence with the chosen therapies and the cost-effectiveness of the Web-based therapies and hardware and software development demand ongoing evaluation.

Learning Curve

Whenever a learner is acquiring knowledge, an attitudinal change, or motor skill, there is a learning curve (Bastable, 2006). Typically individual learning curves are irregular, with fluctuations attributed to changes in the learner such as attention, energy, ability, or situational factors (Gage & Berliner, 1998). In the case of clients with chronic illness, learning to walk again following a stroke may take time and create frustration, as expectations do not match physical capability. Because learning may not always occur in a linear fashion, HCPs must recognize this and assist clients and their families when they experience anger, discouragement, or depression associated with achievement not progressing as anticipated. In addition, research supports that retention of learning is enhanced when there are opportunities to see, hear, observe demonstrations, discuss, and practice as well as teach others (Bastable, 2006; Muijs & Reynolds, 2005; Petty, 2006).

Evaluation

Evaluation of educational outcomes is a critical step in the teaching and learning process. It encompasses a systemic and continuous activity that involves collecting and using information to determine whether the educational objectives have been achieved. This outcome evaluation is labeled summative evaluation, but there can also be formative evaluation. Formative evaluation occurs during the actual teaching process when the implementation is still in process. Formative evaluation permits the HCP to adjust or change aspects of the implementation process that may improve the quality or delivery of the educational program or session. For instance, the HCP may decide to use a Web-based program and face-to-face demonstration of a task to the client and their family. On the basis of immediate negative feedback received regarding the client's unfamiliarity with computers and reluctance to use such a program, the HCP may decide to replace the Web-based education with a small group discussion involving the client and their family.

When performing any type of evaluation, it is also important to identify what outcome is being measured and how and when the data will be collected, and then how it will be interpreted. For example, if the HCP and client have established the outcome objective that the "Client will state three signs/symptoms of hypoglycemia by the end of an 8-hour shift." Determination of achievement for this objective is straight forward. Yet, sometimes barriers occur that hinder the evaluation process. Several barriers that can be particularly problematic are: lack of clarity regarding what is being evaluated, lack of ability to perform the evaluation, and, finally, fear of punishment or low self-esteem (Basable, 2006). With regard to lack of ability, the HCP may not know how to construct a short test to determine if the client and family have a basic understanding of diabetes or feel comfortable orally quizzing them to assess their learning. In other situations, clients may be too ill to learn the information, how to perform a new task, or respond as they anticipate the HCP wants them to.

In many settings, practice guidelines or protocols identify how formative and summative evaluations are to be conducted and what information then needs to be documented. Data from the evaluation process, especially as it applies to the teaching and learning process for the client and family, can be extremely valuable as the chronic illness progresses and additional knowledge, attitudinal, and psychomotor skills need to be developed.

Example of a Teaching Plan

This teaching plan was developed in accordance with the following case situation. You have a newly

TABLE 14-8

Sample Teaching Plan

Objectives	Content (topics)	Time Frame
The client will be able to:		
1. Distinguish the signs and symptoms of hypoglycemia from hyperglycemia. *Cognitive domain of learning	a. Definition of hypoglycemia compared to hyperglycemia b. Signs of hypoglycemia c. Signs of hyperglycemia d. Actions to take when each are present	5 minutes
2. Demonstrate ability to correctly perform a finger stick and reading of glucose level. *Psychomotor domain of learning	a. Purpose of client glucose self-monitoring b. Key aspects in the correct performance of a finger stick and accurate reading of the results	20 minutes
3. Verbalize confidence in performing key elements in glucose monitoring. *Affective domain of learning	Importance of daily monitoring of blood glucose in the continued management of diabetes Accountability and self-monitoring associated with a chronic disease	2 minutes
4. State purpose, dose, time to take, and side effects of single medications prescribed at discharge. *Cognitive domain of learning	Medication prescribed – including purpose, dose, time to take, side effects and other considerations	10 minutes
During the second interaction when this fourth objective is the focus, assess the client's retention of the correct information associated with objectives 1–3.		

diagnosed client with diabetes who is going to be discharged in the next 48 hours. The client is a 43-year-old Hispanic man, who is married and the father of two young children. He has a high school education and has worked as a mechanic for 21 years. As his primary care nurse, you are to make sure that four objectives are accomplished (see Table 14-8).

The specific approach to this client will consider such elements as gender, culture, learning curve, importance of feedback, and reinforcement, as were already described. Given the content and objectives of this specific teaching plan, it is recommended that *not all* of this teaching occur at the same time. The teaching plan pertaining to the first three objectives could be performed, and then teaching of the fourth objective occurs later in the day. During this second educational session, review the key points associated with the first teaching episode. Furthermore, make sure that each teaching session is not interrupted and that there is adequate time to permit questions from the client and family, who should also be present if at all possible.

Teaching Strategy	Evaluation Method
One to one teaching presentation Visual materials: poster listing signs and symptoms of hypoglycemia and hyperglycemia, booklet to keep If client has difficulty getting the content correct, repeat teaching as well as discuss other strategies that may facilitate retention of the information.	Use several vignettes and then ask client to identify signs and symptoms of each from a list. Need 100% correct response. Ask immediate action when each is present. Must get all correct.
One to one teaching-presentation Provide a demonstration of the correct technique Then have client to perform the finger stick and interpretation of results Nurse provides feedback, reinforcement of behaviors, and may have client do this again if needed. May have online or hospital TV channel available so that client and review this again	Client correctly performs the finger stick and glucose interpretation Have a video of incorrect performance of this skill or nurse incorrectly do and client identify incorrect elements performed
One to one teaching and blend brief discussion, reinforcement and feedback	Have rate on a scale of 0 = no confidence to 10 = complete confidence in performing daily glucose monitoring
One to one teaching, poster or other written materials to provide a blend of visual and auditory information is advisable	Orally and/or on paper list the medication's purpose, dose, time to take, prominent side effects and other considerations.
Determine if the client has any questions since had instruction pertaining to objectives 1–3 above	Assess knowledge, actions, and attitudes pertaining to objectives 1–3 with the same evaluation standard as in the first encounter.

SUMMARY AND CONCLUSIONS

Education serves as an essential vehicle to provide the client and family with the knowledge, skills, and confidence to address the many facets associated with living with a chronic illness. Although numerous factors contribute to the success or failure of this educational process, HCPs and nurses in particular play a fundamental role as part of their scope of practice and other national standards such as *Healthy People 2010* and JCAHO benchmarks.

Research evidence continues to expand and guides the assessment of all learners, teaching plan development, and ultimate educational outcomes. Teaching and learning is a complex process and requires consideration of many elements such as family structure and function, culture, gender and learning styles, readiness to learn/change and self-efficacy, developmental stage, literacy, socioeconomic status, resources, and learning capability. In addition, as HCPs partner with the client and their family during this educational process, it is critical that the HCPs assess the client and family's expectations, learning needs/goals, fears, concerns, and present knowledge pertaining to their current healthcare needs. Another central ingredient that is sometimes overlooked is the mutual goal setting that occurs among the client, family, and HCPs. Working together, they are much more inclined to achieve their educational objectives and redirect their actions when needed. Because well over 50% of the US population has at least one chronic illness, the teaching and learning process is paramount to attaining greater quality of life and adapting to the frequently dynamic nature of most chronic diseases.

EVIDENCE-BASED PRACTICE BOX

Purpose: To examine the effects of telephone-delivered empowerment intervention (EI) on outcomes of patients with heart failure (HF), including purposeful participation in goal attainment, self-management of HF, and perception of function and health.

Theoretical Framework: Rogers' Science of Unitary Beings that involves the person and environment interacting in a dynamic manner.

Method: A convenient sample of men and women age 21 and older with a clinical diagnosis of HF were located in a metropolitan hospital in the southwestern United States. The participants were randomly assigned to a control group (n = 45) or EI group (n = 45). All participants received standardized HF patient education. The EI group also received EI delivered via telephone calls from a registered nurse (RN).

Analysis: Repeated measures analysis of variance was used to determine intervention effects.

Results: Telephone-delivered EI group had greater self-management of HF through self-care activities.

Conclusion: Study provided a beginning understanding of strategies to enhance healthcare providers'ability to facilitate self-management of HF among the patients diagnosed with HF.

Source: Shearer, N., Cisar, N., & Greenberg, E.A. (2007). A telephone-delivered empowerment intervention with patients diagnosed with heart failure. *Heart and Lung, 36*(3), 159–169.

STUDY QUESTIONS

1. What level of evidence provides the greatest confidence in the applicability of research findings to practice?

2. What are the pros and cons of three teaching strategies that can be used to educate an individual with a chronic illness?

3. What is the difference between pedagogy and andragogy and what affect does it have on your approach to teaching?

4. What are major factors that should be considered when planning an educational session for a chronically ill client?

5. What is the difference between a formative and summative evaluation?

REFERENCES

Boren, S., Balas, E., & Mustafa, Z. (2003). Evidence-based patient education for chronic care. *Abstract Academy Health* Meeting, 20, abstract no. 788. Retrieved December 11, 2007, from http://gateway.nlm.nih.gov/MeetingAbstracts/102275756.html

Bandura, A. (1986). *Social foundations of thought and action: A social cognitive theory.* Englewood Cliffs, NJ: Prentice Hall.

Bastable, S.B. (2006). *Essentials of patient education.* Sudbury, MA: Jones & Bartlett.

Bereanova, E., & Sykes, C. (2007). A systematic review of computer based software for educating patients with coronary heart disease. *Patient Education and Counseling, 66*(1), 21–28.

Bertakis, K., Rahman, A., Helms, L. J., Callaham, E., & Robbins, J. (2000). Gender differences in the utilization of health care services. *Journal of Family Practice, 49*(2), 147–152.

Boren, S., Balas, E., & Mustafa, Z. (2003). Evidence-based patient education for chronic care. *Abstract Academy Health Meeting, 20,* abstract no. 788. Retrieved December 11, 2007, from http://gateway.nlm.nih.gov/MeetingAbstracts/102275756.html

Bull, S., Gaglio, B., McKay, G., & Glasgow, R. (2005). Harnessing the potential of the internet to promote chronic illness self-management: Diabetes as an example of how well we are doing. *Chronic Illness, 1,* 143–155.

Cain, C.J., & Wicke, M.N. (2000). Caregiving attributes as correlates of burden in family caregivers coping with chronic obstructive pulmonary disease. *Journal of Family Nursing, 6*(1), 46–68.

Cancer Prevention Research Center. (2008). Measures. Retrieved from www.uri.edu/research/cprc/measures.htm

Coffield, F., Moseley, D., Hall, E., & Ecclestone, K. (2004). *Learning styles and pedagogy in post-16 learning: A systematic and critical review.* Retrieved from http://www.Isda.org.uk/files/PDF/1543pdf

Coleman, M., & Newton, K. (2005). Supporting self-management in patients with chronic illness. *American Family Physician, 72*(8), 1503–1510.

Conner, M.L. (2005). Andragogy and Pedagogy. *Ageless Learner, 1997–2004.* Retrieved January 12, 2008 from http://agelesslearner.com/intros/andragogy.html

Craig, J.V., & Smyth, R.L. (2002). *The evidence-based practice manual for nurses.* New York: Churchill Livingstone.

Centers for Disease Control and Prevention. (2005). *Preventing diabetes and its complications.* Retrieved January 3, 2008 from http://www.cdc.gov/nccdhp/publications/factsheets/Prevention/diabetes.htm

Centers for Disease Control and Prevention. (2005). *Preventing heart disease and stroke.* Retrieved January 3, 2008 from http://www.cdc.gov/nccdphp/publications/factsheets/Prevention/cvh.htm

Cudney, S., Sullivan, T., Winters, C., Paul, L., & Orient, P. (2005). Chronically ill rural women: Self-identified management problems and solutions. *Chronic Illness, 1,* 49–60.

Doak, C.C., Doak, L.G., & Root, J.H. (1996). *Teaching patients with low literacy skills* (2nd ed.). Philadelphia: Lippincott.

Evans, P.H., Greaves, R., Winder, R., Smith, J., & Campbell, J. (2007). Development of an educational "toolkit" for health professionals and their patients with prediabetes: The WAKEUP study (Ways of Addressing Knowledge Education and Understanding in Pre-diabetes). *Diabetic Medicine, 24,* 770–777.

Flesch, R. (1948). A new readability yardstick. *Journal of Applied Psychology, 32*(3), 221–233.

Fox, S., & Falloes, D. (2003). *Internet Health Resources.* Washington, DC: Pew Internet & American Life Project.

Freimuth, V.S., Quinn, S.C., Thomas, S.B., Cole, G., Zook, E., & Duncan, T. (2001). African Americans' view on research and the Tuskegee Syphilis Study. *Social Science and Medicine, 52*(2), 797–808.

Gage, N.L., & Berliner, D.C. (1998). *Educational Psychology* (6th ed.). Boston: Houghton Mifflin.

Garland, D., & Martin, B. (2005). Do gender and learning style play a role in how online courses should be designed? *Journal of Interactive Online Learning, 4*(2), 67–81.

Garfield, S., Smith, F., Francis, S., & Chalmers, C. (2007). Can patients' preferences in decision making regarding the use of medicines be predicted? *Patient Health and Counseling, 66,* 361–367.

Gonseth, J., Castillion, G.P., Banegas, J.R., & Artalejo, F.R., (2004). The effectiveness of disease management programmes in reducing hospital re-admission in older adults with heart failure: A systematic review and meta-analysis of published reports. *European Heart Journal, 25*(18), 1570–1590.

Green, B., Partridge, E., Fouad, M., Kohler, C., Crayton, E., & Alexander, L. (2000). African American attitudes regarding cancer clinical trials and research studies: Results from focus group methodology. *Ethics and Disease, 10*(1), 76–86.

Greenlund, K.J., Keenan, N.L., Giles, W.H., Zheng, Z.J., Neff, L.J., Croft, J.B., et al. (2004). Public recognition of major signs and symptoms of heart attack: seventeen states and the U.S. Virgin Islands. *American Heart Journal, 147*, 1010–1016.

Gur, R., Turetsky, B., Matsui, M., Yan, M., Bilker, W., Hughett, P., et al. (1999). Sex differences in brain gray and white matter in healthy young adults: Correlations with cognitive performance. *The Journal of Neuroscience, 19*(10), 4065–4075.

Gurian, M., & Ballew, A.C. (2003). *The boys and girls learn differently: Action guide for teachers.* San Francisco: Jossey-Bass.

Healthy People 2010: Understanding and improving health (2nd ed.). Washington, DC: US Government Printing Office.

Haggard, A. (1989). *Handbook of patient education.* Rockville, MD: Aspen.

Hatcher, E., & Whittemore, R. (2007). Hispanic adults' beliefs about type 2 diabetes: Clinical implications. *Journal of the American Academy of Nurse Practitioners, 19*(10), 536–545.

Hein, G.E. (1991). Constructivist Learning Theory. *Institute of Inquiry.* Retrieved January 14, 2008 from www.exploratorium.edu/ifi/resources/constructivistlearning.html

Knowles, M. (1998). *The adult learner: The definitive classic in adult education and human resource development.* Houston, TX: Gulf Publishing.

Institute of Medicine, Committee on Health Professions Education Summit (2003). *Health professions education: A bridge to quality (Quality Chasm Series).* Washington, DC: National Academies Press.

Keuter, M., & Strecher, V. (1995). Changing inaccurate perceptions of health risk: results from a randomized trial. *Health Psychology, 14*, 56–63.

Kreauter, M., Steger-May, K., Bobra, S., Booker, A., Holt, C., Lukwago, S., et al., (2003). Sociocultural characteristics and responses to cancer education materials among African American women. *Cancer Control: Journal of the Moffitt Cancer Center, 10*(5), 69–80.

Kim, Y. (2006). Application of the transtheoretical model to identify psychological constructs influencing exercise behavior: A questionnaire survey. *International Journal of Nursing Studies, 44*, 936–944.

Lasater, L., & Mehler, P. S. (1998). The literate patient: Screening and management. *Hospital Practice, 33*(4), 163–165, 169–170.

Lee, T., Yeh, Y., Liu, C., & Chen, P., (2007). Development and evaluation of a patient-oriented education system for diabetes management. *International Journal of Medical Informatics, 76*, 655–663.

Lichtenthal, C. (1990). *A self-study model of readiness to learn.* Unpublished manuscript.

Luders, E., Narr, K., Bilder, R., Szeszko, P., Gurbani, M., Hamilton, A., et al. (2008). Mapping the relationship between cortical convolution and intelligence: Effects of gender. *Cerebral Cortex, 18*(9), 2019–2026.

Mauk, K.L. (Ed.). (2006). *Gerontological Nursing: Competencies for Care.* Sudbury, MA: Jones & Bartlett.

Mayer, G.G., & Vallaire, M. (2007). *Health literacy in primary care: A clinician's guide.* New York: Springer.

McLaughlin, G.H. (1969). SMOG-grading: A new readability formula. *Journal of Reading, 12*, 639–646.

Melnyk, B., M., & Finehold-Iverholt, E. (2005). *Evidence-based practice in nursing and healthcare.* Philadelphia: Lippincott.

Mihall, J., & Belletti, J. (1999). Adult learning styles and training methods. *FDIC ADR Presentation Handouts,* Retrieved January 12, 2008 from http://www.usdoj.gov/adr/workplace/pdf/learstyl.pdf

Miller, E. (2008). *Theoretical Foundations of Health Promotion, Risk Reduction, and Health Planning (29NURS807): Online Course Manual.* University of Cincinnati, College of Nursing.

Miller, E. (2003). Readiness to change and brief educational interventions: Successful strategies to reduce stroke risk. *Journal of Neuroscience Nursing, 35*(4), 215–222.

Mulhauser, I. (2005). Evidence-based patient in diabetes and beyond: Application to other chronic diseases. In M. Porta, V. Misell, M. Torento, & V. Jorgens (Eds.), *Embedding education into diabetes practice* (pp. 132–146). Basel, Switzerland: Karger Publishers.

Muijs, D., & Reynolds, D. (2005). *Effective teaching: Evidence and practice* (2nd ed.). Thousand Oaks: Sage Publications.

Nielson-Bohlman, L., Panzer, A.M., & Kindig, D.A. (2004). *Health Literacy: A prescription to end confusion*. Institute of Medicine, Washington D.C.: National Academies Press.

Nightingale, F. (1992). *Notes on nursing: What it is and what it is not*. Philadelphia: Lippincott.

Nobel, J. (2006). Bridging the knowledge-action gap in diabetes: Information technologies, physician incentives and consumer incentives converge. *Chronic Illness, 2,* 59–69.

Osborne, R., Wilson, T., Lorig, K., & McColl, G., (2007). Does self-management lead to sustainable health benefits in people with arthritis? A 2-year transition study with 452 Australians. *The Journal of Rheumatology, 34*(5), 1112–1117.

Petty, G. (2006). *Evidence based teaching: A practical approach*. United Kingdom: Nelson Thornes.

Powell, P. (2001). Randomized control trial of patient education to encourage graded exercise in chronic fatigue syndrome. *British Medical Journal, 322,* 387–390.

Prochaska, J.O., & DiClemente, C.C. (1983). Stages and processes of self-change of smoking: Toward an integrative model of change. *Journal of Consulting and Clinical Psychology, 51,* 390–395.

Prochaska, J.O., & Velicer, W.F. (1997). The Transtheoretical Model of health behavior change. *American Journal of Health Promotion, 12,* 38–48.

Quirk, P.A. (2000). Screening for literacy and readability: Implications for the advanced practice nurse. *Clinical Nurse Specialist, 14*(1), 26–32.

Rankin, S.H., Stallings, K.D., & London, F. (2005). *Patient education in health and illness* (5th ed.). Philadelphia: Lippincott.

Redman, B.L. (2001). *The practice of patient education* (9th ed.). St. Louis: Mosby.

Rahmqvist, M., & Bara, A. (2007). Patients retrieving additional information via the internet: a trend analysis in a Swedish population, 2000–2005. *Scandinavian Journal of PublicHealth, 35*(2), 533–539.

Skinner, B.F. (1974). *About behaviorism*. New York: Merrill.

Spadero, D.C. (1983). Assessing readability of patient information materials. *Pediatric Nursing, 4,* 274–278.

National League for Nursing. (2003). Innovation in nursing education: A call to reform (Position statement). Retrieved January 12, 2008 from http://nln.allenpress.com/nlnonline/?request=get-abstract&issn=1536–5026&volume=25&issue=1&page=47

Skinner, T., Carey, M., Cardock, S., Daly, H., Davies, M., et al. (2006). Diabetes education and self-management for ongoing and newly diagnosed (DESMOND): Process modeling of pilot study. *Patient Education and Counseling, 64,* 369–377.

Stahl, S.A. (2002). Different strokes for different folks? In L. Abbeduto (Ed.). *Taking sides: Clashing on controversial issues in educational psychology* (pp. 98–107). Guilford, CT: McGraw Hill.

The Centre for Teaching and Academic Growth. (2008). Teaching/Learning Theories. Retrieved January 12, 2008 from www.tag.ubc.ca/links/topics/TeachingLearningTheories,php

The Joanna Briggs Institute. (2006). Educational interventions for mental health consumers receiving psychotropic medication. *Best Practice, 10*(4), 1–4.

The Joint Commission on Accreditation of Healthcare Organizations. (2008). *Hospital Accreditation Standards*. Oakbrook Terrace: Illinois.

Wantland, D.J., Portillo, C.J., Holzemer, W.L., & Slaughter, R. (2004). The effectiveness of web-based vs. non-web-based interventions: A meta-analysis of behavioral change outcomes. *Journal of Medical Internet Research, 6*(4), 40–71.

Weingarten, S.R., Henning, J.M., Badamgarav, E., Knight, K., Hasselblad, V., Gano, A., & Ofman, J. (2002). Interventions used in disease management programmes for patients with chronic illness: Which ones work? Meta-analysis of published reports. *British Medical Journal, 325*(26), 1–8.

Williams, F., Beaton, S., Goldstein, P., Mair, F., May, C., & Capewell, S. (2005). Patients' and nurses' views of nurse-led heart failure clinics in general practice: A qualitative study. *Chronic Illness, 1,* 39–47.

Witelson, S., Beresh, H., & Kigar, D.L. (2006). Intelligence and brain size in 100 postmortem brains: Sex lateralization and age factors. *Brain, 129*(2) 386–398.

III

Impact of the Health Professional

15

Health Promotion

Alicia Huckstadt

INTRODUCTION

The single causation theory of morbidity has been largely replaced by multifactorial causation theories and chronicity of conditions. Improved recognition and management of disease processes, better sanitation, immunizations, and other health measures have increased the longevity of Americans. The life expectancy in the early 1900s was the late forties; it has now increased to the late seventies for both genders. Diseases that once brought sudden death have been surpassed by chronic disease. Americans are living longer but not necessarily healthier. Societal influences and individual lifestyle choices have negatively influenced health. In two important research articles describing the actual causes of death (nongenetic), smoking has remained the leading cause of death in the United States for the last two decades (McGinnis & Foege, 1993; Mokdad, Marks, Stroup, & Gerberding, 2004). Poor diet, physical inactivity, alcohol consumption, microbial agents, toxic agents, motor vehicle crashes, incidents involving firearms, sexual behaviors, and illicit use of drugs follow smoking as actual causes of death. It was anticipated that poor diet and physical inactivity would soon become the leading causes of death, replacing smoking (Mokdad et al., 2004); however, the Centers for Disease Control and Prevention

(MSNBC, 2005) later stated the numbers of obesity-related deaths were alarming but not increasing by as many as previously thought (65,000 deaths per year rather than the predicted 100,000 per year), and that the obesity numbers would not overtake smoking as rapidly as first forecasted. As researchers continue to study the condition, long-term obesity has been associated with avoidable hospitalizations and substantial risk for health complications (Schafer & Ferraro, 2007). The CDC has maintained that poor diet, physical inactivity, and smoking are the major underlying causes of death. These factors and the other modifiable behavioral risk factors listed previously are believed to be the genesis of heart disease, malignant neoplasm, cerebrovascular disease, diabetes mellitus, and other chronic diseases. One half of all deaths in the United States could be attributed to a limited number of largely preventable health behaviors and exposures (Mokdad et al., 2004). The escalating healthcare costs, disease, and deaths associated with these factors make health promotion essential for all.

Defining Health Promotion in Chronic Illness

Health promotion is a multidimensional concept and focuses on maintaining or improving the health of individuals, families, and communities.

347

Health promotion for individuals with chronic or disabling conditions is commonly defined as efforts to create healthy lifestyles and a healthy environment to prevent secondary conditions, such as teaching people how to address their healthcare needs and increasing opportunities to participate in usual life activities. These secondary conditions can be the medical, social, emotional, mental, family, or community problems that an individual with a chronic or disabling condition likely experiences. Environmental factors that encompass healthy living include the policies, systems, social contexts, and physical surrounding that facilitate a person's participation in activities, including work, school, leisure, and community events (*Healthy People 2010*).

Health-promoting activities can be implemented at the public level or the personal level, and involve passive or active strategies (Edelman & Mandle, 2006). Passive strategies, such as those used in food industry sanitation, decrease infectious agents in foods and improve public health. National, state, and local public and private agencies are given the responsibility to provide passive strategies to promote health for their constituents. Active strategies, such as engaging in better personal nutrition or activity regimens, are dependent on the individual and/or family becoming involved (Edelman & Mandle, 2006). Although both strategies are essential, this chapter focuses primarily on active strategies for individuals with chronic illness and their families.

Health promotion applies to all individuals regardless of age or disability. The goal of health promotion is to increase the involved person's control over their health and to improve it. Leddy (2006) adds that health promotion is mobilizing strengths to enhance health, wellness, and well-being.

Health promotion in chronic illness involves behavioral change for positive lifestyle activities, accepting one's condition and making the necessary adjustments, decreasing the risk of secondary disabilities and preventing further disease, and striving for optimal health.

Health promotion in chronic illness is important in maintaining and enhancing the function of the individual. It is also critical to prevent recurrence of some conditions. Often families direct their energies toward the illness rather than health. The illness and its cascade of effects alter family dynamics, usual roles, and patterns of life (Heinzer, 1998). Managing medicines, conserving physical and mental energy, keeping appointments with healthcare professionals, adjusting finances, and learning new resources will likely require substantial effort. These new stressors often overtax the individual, and activities to maintain a healthy lifestyle are often ignored. Preventive health screening for other conditions may be forgotten by the client and healthcare professional. Yet, health-promoting behaviors are crucial in the management of chronic conditions and are often the essential aspect in successful management. Chronically ill persons may develop comorbidities that could be avoided or minimized with early detection. Disease-specific preventive care needs and related physical, social, emotional, and spiritual well-being encompass health promotion for those with and without chronic illness. McWilliam, Stewart, Brown, Desai, and Coderre (1996) found in their phenomenological study exploring health and health promotion of 13 select sample participants with chronic illness, "a dynamically changing and evolving endeavor that encompassed four components: fighting and struggling, resigning oneself, creatively balancing resources, and accepting" (p. 5).

Undoubtedly, chronic illness presents numerous challenges to health promotion. The potential for these activities and overall health remains largely untapped in many individuals with chronic illness. Creating new ways of accomplishing health promotion often remains an unfilled goal for nurses and their chronically ill clients. Efforts must go beyond the individual's chronic illness and limitations to include holistic health that focuses on personal goals, evidence-based care tailored to the person, and a willingness to adjust the plan as needed. Determining chronically ill individuals' perceptions of their condition, their aspirations, and their available resources, and supporting their efforts to achieve health promotion is an ongoing process. Leddy (2006) emphasizes that health promotion develops the individual strengths and environmental resources to find solutions rather than focusing solely on illness repair. Chronicity presents challenges to all those involved and can take precedence over other health considerations.

Nurses are ideally suited to promote the health of all individuals and their families. The holistic, caring perspective held by nurses provides opportunities to promote strengths at a time when others may perceive only threats to health. The consequences of failure to promote health are devastating. Additional morbidity; deaths; and financial strain for individuals, families, and society weigh heavy on the healthcare system. The rising healthcare costs and an aging population compound the problem. Sustained increases in out-of-pocket healthcare spending for Medicare recipients could make health care less affordable for all but the highest-income individuals (Neuman, Cubanski, Desmond, & Rice, 2007).

ISSUES AND IMPACT

National Documents

One of the issues surrounding health promotion and disease prevention is compliance with national documents. Initiated almost 30 years ago with the publication of *Healthy People: The Surgeon General's Report on Health Promotion and Disease Prevention (1979)*, and subsequent publications *Healthy People: Objectives for the Nation (1980)*, *Healthy People 2000: National Health Promotion and Disease Prevention Objectives*, and *Healthy People 2010*, Healthy People national documents build on one another and address select areas of health promotion with a vision for achieving improved health for all Americans. Each document was developed through a broad consultative process, made use of the best scientific knowledge available, and was designed to measure progress over time.

Healthy People 2010

Healthy People 2010 identifies a comprehensive set of 10-year health objectives focusing on disease prevention and health promotion to achieve during the first decade of the 21st century. It has two overarching goals—to increase quality and years of healthy life and to eliminate health disparities. The 28 focus areas under the two overarching goals are identified in Table 15-1. Each of the focus areas has specific goals and potential relevance for chronically ill individuals and their families.

One example of relevance for chronically ill individuals and families is Focus Area 6, Disability and Secondary Conditions. The specific goal for this focus area is to promote the health of people with disabilities, prevent secondary conditions, and eliminate disparities between people with and without disabilities in the US population. However, misconceptions are rampant, since disability status has been traditionally equated with health status and the health and well-being of people with disabilities have been addressed primarily within in a medical and long-term–care financing context. Four main misconceptions are identified from this contextual approach: (1) all people with disabilities automatically have poor health, (2) public health should focus only on preventing disabling conditions, (3) a standard definition of "disability" or "people with disabilities" is not needed for public health purposes, and (4) the environment plays no role in the disabling process. These misconceptions have led to an underemphasis of health-promotion and disease-prevention activities targeting people with disabilities and an increase in the occurrence of secondary conditions (medical, social, emotional, family, or community problems that a person with a primary disabling condition likely experiences). Challenging these misconceptions will help to clarify the health status of individuals with disabilities and address the environmental barriers that undermine their health, well-being, and participation in life activities. Health-promotion activities are relevant to all individuals with a disability, whether they are categorized by racial or ethnic group,

TABLE 15-1

Focus Areas for *Healthy People 2010*

1. Access to Quality Health Services	15. Injury and Violence Prevention
2. Arthritis, Osteoporosis, and Chronic Back Conditions	16. Maternal, Infant, and Child Health
3. Cancer	17. Medical Product Safety
4. Chronic Kidney Disease	18. Mental Health and Mental Disorders
5. Diabetes	19. Nutrition and Overweight
6. Disability and Secondary Conditions	20. Occupational Safety and Health
7. Educational and Community-Based Programs	21. Oral Health
8. Environmental Health	22. Physical Activity and Fitness
9. Family Planning	23. Public Health Infrastructure
10. Food Safety	24. Respiratory Diseases
11. Health Communication	25. Sexually Transmitted Diseases
12. Heart Disease and Stroke	26. Substance Abuse
13. HIV	27. Tobacco Use
14. Immunization and Infectious Diseases	28. Vision and Hearing

gender, and primary conditions or diagnoses. *Healthy People 2010* emphasizes that the similarities among people with disabilities are as important as or more important than the differences among clinical diagnostic groups. Developers of the document have also considered caregiver issues as well as environmental barriers. Environmental factors affect the health and well-being of individuals with disabilities in many ways. For example, weather can hamper wheelchair mobility, medical offices and equipment may not be accessible, and shelters or fitness centers may not be staffed or equipped for people with disabilities. Compliance with the Americans with Disabilities Act (ADA) would help overcome some of these barriers.

Throughout *Healthy People 2010*, the US Department of Health and Human Services (DHHS) identifies objectives, such as the previous example of Focus Area 6, to address improvements in health status, risk reduction, public and professional awareness of prevention, delivery of health services, protective measures, surveillance, and evaluation, expressed in terms of measurable targets to be achieved by the year 2010. Full achievement of the goals and objectives of *Healthy People 2010* depends on a healthcare system reaching all Americans and integrating personal health care and population-based public health. The vision of *Healthy People 2010* in healthy communities involves broad-based prevention efforts and moves beyond what happens in physicians' offices, clinics, and hospitals to environments in which a large portion of prevention occurs: to the neighborhoods, schools, workplaces, and families in which people live their daily lives.

Leading health indicators were selected to measure the health of the nation at designated time points. The 10 indicators are: (1) Physical activity, (2) Overweight and obesity, (3) Tobacco use, (4) Substance abuse, (5) Responsible sexual behavior, (6) Mental health, (7) Injury and violence, (8) Environmental quality, (9) Immunization, and (10) Access to health care. These indicators were selected on the basis of their ability to motivate action, availability of data to measure their progress, and their public health importance. *Healthy People 2010* can be accessed at http://www.healthypeople.gov/

Healthy People 2010 *Midcourse Review*

A review assessed the status of the national objectives midway through the decade, and data were made available January 1, 2005. This midcourse review enabled the DHHS, federal agencies, and other experts across the nation to assess the data trends during the first half of the decade, considered new science and available data, and make changes to ensure that *Healthy People 2010* remains current, accurate, and relevant, while concurrently assessing emerging public health priorities. Public comments on the changes at the midcourse to the *Healthy People 2010* objectives and subobjectives were solicited in August and September 2005. The changes to the *Healthy People 2010* objectives and subobjectives included (1) establishing baselines and targets for developmental objectives, (2) changing the wording of objectives and subobjectives, (3) deleting objectives and subobjectives, (4) adding new subobjectives, and (5) revising baselines and targets. The midcourse review also reported progress on objectives with tracking data. From the 467 total objectives in *Healthy People 2010* assessed at midcourse, 281 objectives had tracking data available. From these 281 objectives, 10% met the target, 49% moved toward the target; 14% demonstrated mixed progress; 6% demonstrated no change from the baseline; and 20% moved away from the target.

In all of the 28 focus areas, some objectives were met, exceeded, or moved toward the target. In four focus areas, Cancer (Focus 3), Diabetes (Focus 5), Immunization and Infectious Disease (Focus 14), and Occupational Safety and Health (Focus 20), more than half of the objectives were met or moved toward their targets. In four other focus areas, Environmental Health (Focus 8), Health Communication (Focus 11), Public Health Infrastructure (Focus 23), and Vision and Hearing (Focus 28), the objectives could not be assessed. In Progress for Disability and Secondary Conditions (Focus 6), discussed in the previous example, thirteen objectives were evaluated: four moved toward the target; one demonstrated mixed progress; two moved away from target; and six could not be assessed.

The overarching goal to increase quality and years of healthy life was assessed, and the conclusion was that life expectancy had continued to improve; however, the United States has need for improvement when compared with the rest of the world. Life expectancy for both men and women had increased by about 0.5%. Measuring quality of healthy life was a difficult assessment and resulted in mixed results. It was concluded that clear conclusions for trends in healthy life expectancy could not be reached until data for future years were analyzed. However, some trends were reported. Women can expect to spend 12% of their lives in fair or poor health, 16% with activity limitation, and 39% with one or more chronic diseases. Predictions for men are better, with 10% of their lives in fair to poor health, 15% with activity limitation, and 37% with one or more chronic diseases. It is expected that black Americans will spend a greater proportion of their lives in unhealthy life states compared with whites. It was reported that the black population at birth will spend 15% of their lives in fair or poor health, 18% with activity limitation, and 42% with one or more chronic diseases. Therefore, life expectancy is slightly improving; however, the number of years in unhealthy status is increasing.

Other challenges exist in measuring quality and years of healthy life such as the populations of institutionalized, homeless, and others for whom data are not readily collected. Many of these individuals are likely to have chronic illness and experience overall poor health.

The second overarching goal—to eliminate health disparities that occur by race and ethnicity, gender, education, income, geographic location, disability status, or sexual orientation—was assessed during the midcourse. Disparities between populations were evident for many of the *Healthy People 2010* objectives. There were very few reductions in disparity among populations by education level, income, geographic location, and disability status. Lack of data also existed for population groups such as American Indian or Alaska Native, Asian, and Native Hawaiian or other Pacific Islanders.

Overall, it was emphasized that continued commitment to implementing effective disease prevention and health promotion interventions are essential in increasing quality and years of healthy life. The nation must measure the complex interactions of health, disease, disability, and early death. In addition, it may be more difficult to implement effective health-promotion and disease-prevention programs in some populations. These disparities will need to be further addressed to facilitate progress toward the 2010 goal (*Healthy People 2010 Midcourse Review*).

HealthierUS *and* Steps to a HealthierUS

Another federal initiative, *HealthierUS,* and *Healthy People 2010* share the overarching goal of helping people live longer and healthier lives. *HealthierUS* aims to achieve this goal through four basic components called pillars. The pillars are "physical fitness," "nutrition," "prevention," and "make healthy choices." *HealthierUS* emphasizes that regular physical activity is important for overall health and well-being. People are encouraged to include activities that they enjoy and easily fit into their daily routine such as walking or gardening. Physical activity for 30–60 minutes on most days can help build strength and fitness, relax and reduce stress, gain more energy, and improve sleep. These benefits contribute to decreasing the risk of heart disease and other conditions, such as colon cancer, diabetes, osteoporosis, and high blood pressure. Resources are available through the CDC to accommodate all individuals, such as physical activity for older adults with chronic illnesses http://www.cdc.gov/nccdphp/dnpa/physical/recommendations/older_adults.htm

People who have been inactive for several years or who are currently receiving medical care, need to consult their healthcare professional before starting a new exercise program.

The second pillar, Nutrition, emphasizes the importance of a healthy diet and eating in moderation. Web sites such as http://www.health.gov/dietaryguidelines/dga2005/recommendations.

htm provide helpful nutrition information for the general population. The CDC provides another site http://www.fruitsandveggiesmatter.gov/ to assist people in selecting fruits and vegetables and the US Department of Agriculture, Center of Nutrition Policy and Promotion provides their online MyPyramid Tracker http://www.mypyramidtracker.gov/ as a dietary and physical activity assessment tool that provides information on diet quality, physical activity status, related nutrition messages, and links to nutrient and physical activity information. *HealthierUS* acknowledges that better nutrition can reduce risk for diseases like heart disease, certain cancers, diabetes, stroke, and osteoporosis.

Although *Healthy People 2010* broadly addresses the *HealthierUS* prevention pillar, it is explicitly addressed by a number of objectives within the *Healthy People 2010* focus areas that highlight preventive screenings. *HealthierUS* prevention pillar also encourages all people to learn how to prevent disease and improve their quality of life. The *Healthier US* Web site provides information and recommends that people know their family history and how genes and personal history could put their health at risk.

A variety of screening recommendations are provided from reputable sources such as the American Heart Association, the CDC, National Cancer Institute, National Heart Lung and Blood Institute, and the DHHS Agency for Healthcare Research and Quality (AHRQ). People can review the recommendations and share their history information with their healthcare professionals to determine what tests and screenings are appropriate for them. The make healthy choices pillar is also addressed in several *Healthy People 2010* focus areas, including Tobacco Use, Injury and Violence Prevention, and Substance Abuse. The *HealthierUS* Web site reminds people when faced with choices that may impact their health and the lives of those they love, it is important to remember that there are options and resources to help them make healthy decisions. Related Web sites such as that for the US Food and Drug Administration (FDA) provide information for people to make better informed decisions, for example, in taking medications www.fda.gov/usemedicinesafely, and the Surgeon General in protecting yourself from second hand tobacco smoke www.surgeongeneral.gov/library/secondhandsmoke/factsheets/factsheet3.html

More information about *HealthierUS* is available at www.healthierus.gov.

Steps to a HealthierUS supports evidence-based community programs and interventions focused on reducing the burden of chronic diseases, including diabetes, obesity, and asthma, and related risk behaviors throughout the nation. Like *Healthy People 2010*, this initiative aims to help people live longer and healthier lives. It also links to *Healthy People 2010* directly through DATA2010 (an interactive database system), by explicitly using Healthy People objectives to assess progress. Programs under *Steps to a HealthierUS* work together to guide states and communities throughout the nation toward improving health status. More information is available at www.healthierus.gov/steps

500-Day Plan *and* Priority Activities

The Department of Health and Human Services Secretary Mike Leavitt's *500-Day Plan* and *Priority Activities* are management tools on the agency's primary areas of focus. One of the primary areas is prevention. The prevention priority recognizes that the risk of many diseases and health conditions is reduced through preventive actions, and that a culture of wellness deters or diminishes debilitating and costly health events. The prevention priority does, therefore, build on DHHS prevention policy and programs that are based on the best available evidence on how to prevent or mitigate chronic disease through promotion of healthy lifestyle choices, medical screenings, and avoidance of risky behaviors. *Healthy People 2010* objectives and subobjectives serve as a means of measuring progress in achieving the Secretary's prevention priority. The *500-Day Plan, Priority Activities*, and *250-Day Update* are located at http://www.hhs.gov/secretary/

The following guides are other national documents that serve as recommendations for screening and other preventive health care.

Guide to Clinical Preventive Services

The *Guide to Clinical Preventive Services* includes the US Preventive Services Task Force (USPSTF) recommendations on screening, counseling, and preventive medication topics, as well as clinical considerations for each topic. Sponsored since 1998 by the AHRQ, the USPSTF is an independent panel of experts in primary care and prevention that systematically reviews the evidence of effectiveness and develops recommendations for clinical preventive services. The task force rigorously evaluates clinical research to assess the merits of preventive measures. The clinical categories are cancer; heart and vascular disease; injury and violence; infectious diseases; mental health conditions and substance abuse; metabolic, nutrition, and endocrine conditions; musculoskeletal conditions; obstetrics and gynecologic conditions; pediatric disorders; and vision and hearing disorders. More information is available at www.ahrq.gov/clinic/cps3dix.htm.

Guide to Community Preventive Services

The *Guide to Community Preventive Services* serves as a filter for scientific literature on specific health problems that have a large-scale impact on groups of people who share a common community setting. This guide summarizes what is known about the effectiveness, economic efficiency, and feasibility of interventions to promote community health and prevent disease. The Task Force on Community Preventive Services, an independent decision-making body convened by DHHS, makes recommendations for the use of various interventions based on the evidence gathered in rigorous and systematic scientific reviews of published studies conducted by review teams for the guide. The findings from the reviews are published in peer-reviewed journals and also are made available online. The task force has published more than 100 findings across 16 topic areas, including tobacco use, physical activity, cancer, oral health, diabetes, motor vehicle occupant injury, vaccine-preventable diseases, prevention of injuries due to violence, and social environment. More information is available at www.thecommunityguide.org.

Challenges

These national documents illustrate that health promotion and disease prevention are essential for all Americans. The nation needs to continually work toward the goals; however, to do so will require changes in the healthcare system. Providing chronic health care once the disease has occurred is only a segment of the needed care. Many of the risks to health—obesity, diabetes, hypertension, heart disease, cancer, and other chronic conditions—often result from failure to prevent their occurrence. More closely articulated preventive, public health, and policy programs are needed to promote a healthy life. Other factors, including genetics and environmental risks, contribute to chronic illness.

Health promotion can and should occur before the onset of chronic illness, and as early as possible. Health promotion ideally occurs throughout one's life and in concert with chronic conditions

through the end of life. Health promotion is a lifetime activity and can include end-of-life planning for individuals and their significant others. Preparing for the physical, psychosocial changes that accompany death requires attention before crisis events. Preparation, dissemination, and discussion of advance directives with significant others can help set clear boundaries for honoring the wishes of clients (Rainer & McMurry, 2002).

Barriers

Reported barriers to health screening and other preventive care must be addressed. Unhealthy behaviors continue to increase in the United States, putting people more at risk for initial chronic illness, deters health promotion practices among those with chronic illnesses. The CDC (2007b) reports that more than 50% of US adults do not get enough exercise to receive health benefits, and 25% are not active at all in their leisure time. In 2005, only 23% of US adults and 20% of young people ate five or more fruits and vegetables each day. Cigarette smoking is responsible for about 440,000 deaths in the United States each year. More deaths are caused each year by tobacco use than by all deaths from HIV/AIDS, alcohol use, motor vehicle injuries, suicide, and murder combined. Exercising regularly, eating a healthy diet,

CASE STUDY

L.K. is a 40-year-old woman with type 2 diabetes who lives with her husband of 15 years. Both have been diagnosed as overweight and have elevated blood lipid levels and blood pressure. L.K.'s last hemoglobin AIC was 8.2. She reports that she likes fast, convenient foods, and they both enjoy watching television in the evenings. Neither has a physical exercise regimen. Both speak and write English and dropped out of high school in the 10th grade. L.K. hates to read health information because she thinks it is too complicated. Both L.K. and her husband

work outside the home at sedentary jobs. L.K. does not know why she has diabetes, since no one else in her family has it.

Discussion Questions

1. What are two health literacy implications of the preceding case?
2. How would you tailor a health-promotion program for L.K.?
3. What theoretical framework would be useful for the health-promotion program?

and not using tobacco can help people prevent and manage chronic diseases. However, many people in the United States do not have easy access to healthy foods and safe, convenient places to exercise. These barriers have led to increasingly sedentary lifestyles for the majority of Americans.

Other barriers exist for health screening. Kelly et al. (2007) identified fear and embarrassment as commonly cited client barriers to screening for colorectal cancer. Less than 44% of their study population of Appalachians in the state of Kentucky underwent colorectal cancer screening consistent with guidelines. These researchers identified establishing trust and educating clients, use of resources like educational materials, and finding inexpensive and easy ways to screen as the most productive way to overcome the barriers.

Little is known about how health screening and other preventive care affects outcomes. Norman, Potashnik, Galantino, DeMichele, House, and Localio (2007) emphasized that we do not know what survivors of diseases like breast cancer must do to prevent recurrence. Data are needed on lifestyle change from prediagnosis to postdiagnosis, changes over time after diagnosis, and identification of potential lifestyle risk factors.

Health promotion has not been addressed well in the care of clients with numerous chronic health conditions. Capella-McDonnall (2007) reported that despite the recent focus on health promotion for persons with disabilities, adults who are visually impaired have not received adequate attention. Two conditions, being overweight or obese and not being physically active, are problems for many persons with disabilities including those who are visually impaired.

Problems with health literacy are commonplace in our society. Health literacy is the capacity to obtain, process, and understand basic health information and services needed to make appropriate health decisions (US Department of Health and Human Services, Office of Disease Prevention and Health Promotion, 2007). Nine of 10 adults may lack the skills needed to manage their health and disease prevention. Poor health outcomes and

less frequent use of preventive services are linked with low literacy. Individuals with low literacy are more likely to skip important preventive screening such as colonoscopy, Pap smears, and mammograms, and are less likely to receive protective measures such as flu immunizations. Persons with low literacy are more likely to have chronic illness and are less able to manage effectively. More preventable hospitalizations and use of emergency services are found among clients with chronic illness with limited literacy skills. People with limited literacy skills often lack knowledge about the nature and causes of disease and may not understand the relationship between lifestyle factors such as smoking, lack of exercise and inadequate nutrition, and poor health outcomes.

Other barriers to health screening and preventive care include associated costs; lack of knowledge/understanding; negative beliefs/attitudes; lack of access, especially for those with limited geographical and/or functional ability; and other factors addressed in the models/theories/frameworks discussed in the following.

Models/Theories/Frameworks

An entire body of literature has evolved around the models/theories relating to health behavior change. Considerable research has demonstrated success in changing behavior with smoking cessation, alcohol abuse, and others using these theories. The following examples are theories/models that may be useful in assessing change within chronic illness.

The Transtheoretical Model (TTM) by Prochaska, Redding and Evers (2002) incorporates the processes and principles of change from several major theories in psychotherapy and human behavior. The stages of change within the model include (1) precontemplation (no intention to change in the foreseeable future); (2) contemplation (intention to change in the next 6 months); (3) preparation (intention to take action within the next 30 days and some behavioral steps to change); (4) action (has changed behavior for less than 6 months;

and (5) maintenance (has changed behavior for more than 6 months). These stages represent a temporal dimension to change and are helpful in identifying timing of change interventions. A last stage, (6) termination (individual who possesses total self efficacy is no longer susceptible to temptation of unhealthy behavior), is rarely used, since few individuals reach this level. In the TTM Model, individuals weigh the pros and cons of changing (decisional balance) and determine their confidence (self efficacy) that they can cope with high-risk situations without relapsing to unhealthy or high-risk behavior specific to the situation.

The ten processes of change of the TTM Model are activities that people use to progress through the stages of change. They include (1) consciousness raising (increasing awareness of the behavior); (2) dramatic relief (experiencing increased emotions followed by reduced affect if appropriate action is taken); (3) self-reevaluation (assessing one's image with and without the unhealthy behavior); (4) environmental reevaluation (assessing how one's social environment is affected by the unhealthy behavior); (5) self-liberation (believing and committing to change); (6) helping relationships (building support for healthy behavior change); (7) counterconditioning (learning that healthy behaviors can replace unhealthy behaviors); (8) contingency management (increasing reinforcement and probability that healthy behaviors will be repeated; (9) stimulus control (removing unhealthy behavior cues and adds healthy behavior cues); and (10) social liberation (increasing social opportunities to foster behavior change) (pp. 103–104). The TTM Model has been used in numerous studies including those involving smoking cessation, mammography screening, alcohol avoidance, exercise, and stress management, and others. The TTM Model has been beneficial in tailoring interventions for the most appropriate stage of change.

Theory of Reasoned Action (TRA) and the Theory of Planned Behavior (TPB) offer another framework for examining factors that determine behavioral change. The framework focuses on motivational factors as determinants of the person's likelihood of performing a specific behavior. The TRA provides the rationale that the person's beliefs and values determine if the person intends to change behavior. The TPB adds that perceived behavioral control of facilitating or constraining conditions will affect intention and behavior. Beliefs affecting behavior differ widely among persons, groups, and even specific behaviors of the same individual. Use of the models is helpful in understanding the likelihood of people performing a specific healthier behavior and can provide a framework for interventions. These theories can be applied along with others to design and deliver behavioral change to improve research and practice (Montano & Kasprzyk, 2002).

The Health Belief Model (HBM) has been one of the most widely used conceptual frameworks to explain change in health behavior and to provide a framework for interventions (Janz, Champion, & Strecher, 2002). The components of the HBM have been revised many times since its inception in the 1950s. Once a model to explain readiness to obtain chest X ray screening for tuberculosis, the model has evolved beyond screening behaviors to include preventive actions, illness behaviors, and sick-role behavior. The HBM Model now purports that individuals will take action to prevent, to screen for, or control ill-health conditions if there is Perceived Susceptibility (persons regard themselves as susceptible to the condition), if there is Perceived Severity (persons believe it would have potentially serious consequences), if there is Perceived Benefits (persons believe that a course of action available to them would be beneficial in reducing either their susceptibility to or the severity of the condition), and if the Perceived Barriers can be overcome [persons believe that the anticipated barriers to (or costs of) taking the action are outweighed by its benefits (Janz et al., 2002)]. Determining strategies to activate persons' readiness to change (Cues to action) can include providing information, and awareness campaigns. Like TTM, self efficacy is an integral concept of the HBM. Researchers have tested interventions to increase positive change for each concept.

The Health Promotion Model (HPM) integrates constructs from the Expectancy-Value Theory and Social–Cognitive Theory and provides a nursing perspective to depict the multidimensional nature of persons pursuing health (Pender, Murdaugh, & Parsons, 2002). The HPM purports that behavior change will occur if there is positive personal value and a desired outcome. The HPM has been revised since its initial development in the early 1980s and is considered an approach-oriented or competence model. The authors report that the HPM is different than the HBM discussed earlier, as it eliminates the negative source of motivation, fear or threat, from major motivating sources for health behavior change. The authors emphasize that elimination of the personal threat motivational factor provides applicability of the model across the lifespan. Self efficacy is a major construct of HPM, and assumptions of the model require an active role of the person "in shaping and maintaining health behaviors and in modifying the environmental context for health behaviors" (Pender et al., 2002, p. 63). The HPM has been a framework for studies predicting its general health promoting abilities and for specific health behaviors including hearing protection, exercise, and nutrition (Pender et al., 2002).

INTERVENTIONS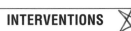

Chronic diseases account for 70% of the 1.7 million deaths that occur in the United States each year. These diseases also cause major limitations in daily living for almost 1 of 10 Americans or about 25 million people. Although chronic diseases are among the most common and costly health problems, they are also among the most preventable. Adopting healthy behaviors such as eating nutritious foods, being physically active, and avoiding tobacco use can prevent or control the devastating effects of these diseases (CDC, National Center for Chronic Disease Prevention and Health Promotion, 2007). "Nurses have been leaders in health promotion since the time of Florence Nightingale, whose pioneering work with the use

of statistics demonstrated the positive effect of improved sanitation on the health of injured soldiers. Nurses have also led the healthcare profession in recognizing that health is a state of physical and mental wellness and that it is impossible to separate the former from the latter" (Calloway, 2006, p. 105). Olshansky (2007), editor of the *Journal of Professional Nursing*, emphasizes that nurses are the most appropriate health professionals to address health promotion. Nursing has role models within our profession such as Nola Pender who developed the HPM described previously. Nursing literature abounds with textbooks, articles, and other publications that include nursing's role in health promotion to individuals, families, communities, and populations. Yet, nurses cannot assume sameness for chronically ill persons, and nurses cannot assume resources are equally available to all. People with chronic illness view health differently and will have different goals defined within their limits of their disability.

Selected Examples

A review of the literature provides examples of health promotion interventions for clients with chronic illness. The following discussion illustrates that much is yet to be examined. In an international study, Huang, Chou, Lin, and Chao (2007) analyzed survey data including the Health-Promoting Lifestyle Profile and quality of life data of 129 outpatients from a medical center who had systemic lupus erythematosus. These researchers found that a health-promoting lifestyle could not enhance the physical component summary of quality of life directly without an improvement in the fatigue disability, but a health-promoting lifestyle had a significant effect on the mental component summary of quality of life. This illustrates that although the physical aspects of the chronic condition may not improve without other physical changes, there can be improvements in psychological health.

Siarkowski (1999) emphasized the importance of including health promotion and illness management when working with insulin-dependent diabetes mellitus in children and their families. Siarkowski's reviewed existing research and revealed factors that put children and their families at risk for poor adaptation. Health promotion is critical to minimize these risks.

Hope has been recommended as a health-promoting force. Hollis, Massey, and Jevne (2007) identified hope-enhancing strategies and sources to improve one's health. Blue (2007) studied 106 adults at risk for diabetes and found the theory of planned behavior to be useful in explaining their healthy eating intentions and physical activity.

Motivational Interviewing

Motivational interviewing incorporates behavior change principles to promote healthy activities. Brodie and Inoue (2005) demonstrated the effectiveness of motivational interviewing over a traditional exercise program in increasing reported physical activity in older adults with chronic heart failure. Jackson, Asimakopoulou, and Scammell (2007) demonstrated in an experimental study of 34 clients with type 2 diabetes that motivational interviewing and behavior change training significantly increased the participants' physical activity and stage of change.

Motivating Factors

In a review of 26 studies (8 randomized controlled trials and 18 observational), use of pedometers have significantly increased physical activity and significantly decreased body mass index and blood pressure (Bravata et al., 2007). The use of pedometers as a motivating factor with chronically ill persons capable of using a pedometer and the long-term effect of pedometers are yet to be investigated. Motivating factors have been identified in theories/models/frameworks, and positive motivators such as those in the HPM are congruent with nursing philosophical bases. Challenges for the future are to continue the testing and use of such frameworks in the health-promoting activities of persons and families with chronic illness.

Health Coaching

Health coaching is emerging as a new approach for preventing exacerbations of chronic illness and supporting lifestyle changes. This method partners with clients to enhance self-management strategies. It is being piloted by Medicare for clients with congestive heart failure and diabetes (Huffman, 2007). Holland, Greenberg, Tidwell, and Newcomer (2003) described the success of the California Public Employees Retirement System (CalPERS) Health Matters program using a community-based health coaching program operating in Sacramento. Criteria for eligibility included one or more qualifying chronic health condition, being 65 or older, and other program criteria. The program uses a menu of disability-prevention strategies, with health coaching, patient education on the self-management of chronic illness, and fitness. The program helps link participants to existing community, health plan, and self-directed programs. It encourages their participation in the programs developed for the project.

Mass Media Campaigns

Beaudoin, Fernandez, Wall, and Farley (2007) used a mass media campaign of high-frequency paid television and radio advertising, as well as bus and streetcar signage to promote walking and fruit/vegetable consumption in a low-income, predominantly African American urban population in New Orleans. These researchers found over 5 months of the campaign, a significant increase in message recall measures, positive attitudes toward walking and toward fruit/vegetable consumption. It is unknown how many persons with chronic illness were included. It is likely many persons were at risk for future chronic illness. These efforts demonstrate population efforts to improve health that may be researched with chronic illness populations.

Snyder (2007) reviewed existing meta-analyses for effectiveness of health communication campaigns, and found that the average health campaign affects the intervention community by about five percentage points. Snyder concluded that successful campaigns that are likely to change nutrition behaviors need to include specific behavioral goals for the intervention, identification of the target population, communication activities and channels that will be used, provision of message content and presentation, and provision of techniques for feedback and evaluation.

Web-Based Programs

Verheijden, Jans, Hildebrandt, and Hopman-Rock (2007) found that Web-based behavioral programs often reach those who need them the least. However, obese people were more likely to participate in follow-up than people of normal body weight. The researchers proposed that the Web-based programs are a nonstigmatizing way of addressing the problem and suggested that weight management is better suited for this delivery method than many other health-related areas. Although this study was based in The Netherlands, it provides a source of potential research for other countries with similar health-promotion problems.

Contracts

Burkhart, Rayens, Oakley, Abshire, and Zhang (2007) found in their randomized, controlled trial of 77 children with persistent asthma that the intervention group who received asthma education plus contingency management, including a contingency contract, tailoring, cueing, and reinforcement, significantly increased adherence to asthma self-management over the control group who received asthma education without the contingency management.

However, in 30 trials involving 4691 participants, Cochrane authors concluded that there is limited evidence that contracts can improve patients' adherence to health-promotion programs.

Large, well-controlled studies are needed to recommend contracts in preventive health programs (Bosch-Capblanch, Abba, Prictor, & Garner, 2007).

Health Literacy

Improving the use of health information is paramount in health-promotion programs. The DHHS, Office of Disease Prevention and Health Promotion (2007) provides a summary of the best practices for healthcare professionals to improve health literacy through providing effective communications and health services that are usable. Table 15-2 outlines these practices.

Nath (2007) reviewed the literature between 1990 and mid-2006 for overcoming inadequate literacy in diabetes self-management and other chronic illnesses. The importance of culturally appropriate health literacy, improvement in self-efficacy, improved communication, and quality computer-assisted instruction were discussed as essential elements in tailoring health education. Nurses were recommended to address barriers related to inadequate literacy by increasing sensitivity to the problem, developing literacy-assessment protocol, creating and evaluating materials for target populations, providing clear communication, including health literacy in nursing curricula, fostering decision making with patients, and conducting research about literacy.

Additional Studies

Using telehealth to improve access, students in a community setting applied self-efficacy theory to help low-income older adults with chronic health problems to increase their practices of health promotion (Coyle, Duffy, & Martin, 2007). Although faculty and students favorably evaluated the activity, measurement of patient outcomes was not conducted. Like Web-based programs, the effects of telehealth require further research.

Program design of health-promotion programs can significantly influence the participation

TABLE 15-2

Improving Health Literacy Interventions

When providing health information, is the information appropriate for the user?	Identify intended users of the information and services. Evaluate the users' knowledge prior to, during, and after the introduction of information and services. Acknowledge cultural differences and practice respect.
When providing health information, is the information easy to use?	Limit the number of messages. Keep it simple and, in general, limit the information to no more than four main messages. Use plain language. Use familiar language and an active voice. Avoid jargon. See www.plainlanguage.gov for more information. Focus on the behavior that you want the person to change Supplement instructions with visuals to help convey your message. Make written communication look easy to read by using large font and use of headings and bullets to break up text; limit line length to between 40 and 50 characters. Improve Internet information by using uniform navigation, organizing information to minimize searching and scrolling, including interactive features. Apply user-centered design principles and conduct usability testing.
When providing health information, are you speaking clearly and listening carefully?	Ask open-ended questions. Use a medically trained interpreter for those who do not speak English or have limited ability to speak or understand English. Use words and examples that make the information relevant to the person's cultural norms and values. Check for understanding using a "teach-back" method to enhance communication.
Improve the use of health services.	Improve usability of health forms and instructions including plain language forms in multiple languages. Improve the accessibility of the physical environment including universal symbols, clear signage, and easy flow through healthcare facilities. Establish a patient navigator program of individuals who can help patients access services and appropriate healthcare information.
Build knowledge to improve health decision-making.	Improve access to accurate and appropriate health information. Increase self-efficacy and facilitate health decision making. Partner with educators to improve health curricula.
Advocate for health literacy in your organization.	Make the case for health literacy improvement. Identify how low health literacy affects programs. Incorporate health literacy into mission and planning. Establish accountability by including health literacy improvement in program evaluation.

of all individuals. Warren-Findlow, Prohaska, and Freedman (2003) demonstrated factors that influenced participation and retention in an exercise intervention study targeted to African American and white older adults with multiple chronic illnesses. These researchers found that eligible participants who did not enroll were more likely to be diabetic and younger than age 60. Seventy percent of the enrolled participants remained in the program after one year. The attrition was related to program site, functional status, and having a high school degree. Attrition was not associated with chronic illness. The researchers concluded that group-specific efforts tailored for the group can be successful in recruiting and retaining participants.

Feldman and Tegart (2003) explored older African American women with arthritis and their motivations and struggles with health promotion. These reflections provide helpful suggestions as nurses develop health promotion programs for clients with chronic illness.

Lindsey (1996) used a phenomenological approach to study health in eight participants living with a variety of different chronic conditions. Lindsey uncovered themes that reflected the adjustment made by participants in a positive way. She suggests transforming nursing care from a problem and deficit focus to a focus on the client's capacity and promotion of health and healing.

Miller and Iris (2002) found that socialization and social support were central to the participation of older adults with chronic illness who participated in a wellness program. In this study, participants recognized that chronic disease did not prohibit living a healthy lifestyle. The White Crane Model of Healthy Lives for Older Adults used in this study contributed to understanding the way older adults view health for themselves. This model is also thought to be helpful in developing program evaluation measures.

A diet and exercise program to reduce cardiovascular disease risk was used with employees regardless of presence of chronic illness. There were significant differences between pre- and post-intervention for lipid profiles and weight. Self-reported levels of participation in the diet were significantly related to improvement in the low-density lipoprotein (LDL) levels (White & Jacques, 2007).

The addition of health promotion to the usual care of frail older home care clients was studied in Canada by Markle-Reid, Weir, Browne, Roberts, Gafni, and Henderson (2006). These researchers found that proactively providing health promotion to older adults with chronic health needs enhanced quality of life but did not increase the overall costs of health care. Better mental health functioning, reduction in depression, and enhanced perceptions of social support were reported in the experimental group. The researchers concluded that their finding underscored the need to provide health promotion for older clients receiving home care.

Many areas remain for further research to measure the effect of health promoting frameworks and interventions with individuals/families with chronic illness. The earlier discussion provides a sampling of the current literature.

Guidelines

There are numerous easily accessible guidelines for health promotion, health screening, and preventive care at the following Web site www.guidelines. gov and other sources. Examples of guidelines are discussed in the following.

Immunizations are one of the most important discoveries in human history. Vaccines have helped save millions of lives worldwide and millions of dollars each year in unnecessary health-care expenditures [Infectious Diseases Society of America (IDSA), 2007]. However, there are unacceptably low rates of coverage among adults and children in the United States. The influenza vaccine alone can save thousands of lives by providing protection for persons with chronic illness. Immunized healthcare providers can decrease transmission of influenza to chronically ill persons. Recommended immunization schedules and information are easily obtained from the CDC.

Several organizations provide guidelines that include health promotion for chronic conditions. Self-management education programs such as the diabetes self-management education (DSME) are outlined in the diabetes national standards (Kulkarni, 2006). Nurses are encouraged to use evidence-based guidelines as they practice.

OUTCOMES

The desired outcome for chronically ill individuals and their families is to maintain and improve their overall health. Health promotion activities should target the major causes of death—tobacco use, poor diet, physical inactivity, alcohol consumption, microbial agents, toxic agents, motor vehicle crashes, incidents involving firearms, sexual behaviors, and illicit use of drugs. These causes are responsible for the majority of deaths in the United States. Measures are needed to research outcomes of health-promoting interventions across populations and disabilities. Further efforts to make activities accessible and studies to evaluate their effectiveness are encouraged. The challenge of the coming years will be to link existing and future research studies to practice.

EVIDENCE-BASED PRACTICE BOX

A shift from preventive home care nursing functions to acute inpatient care functions has resulted in fragmented, expensive care for older adults with chronic illness, rather than comprehensive and proactive care that is more likely to improve health outcomes. Providing the most appropriate services to older adults was the impetus for this study.

A two-armed, single-blind, randomized controlled trial of 288 older frail adults with chronic health needs, aged 75 and older, were evaluated in a Canadian study (Markle-Reid et al., 2006). The model of vulnerability by Rogers (1997) provided the theoretical basis for the study. Participants were randomly assigned to the usual home care or a "proactive" nursing health-promotion intervention that included a health assessment combined with regular home visits or telephone contacts, health education about management of illness, coordination of community services, and use of empowerment strategies to enhance independence. Of the 288 patients randomly assigned at baseline, 242 completed the study (120 with the proactive nursing intervention, 122 in the control group). Results demonstrated that proactively providing the intervention group with nursing health promotion significantly resulted in better mental health functioning ($P = 0.009$), a reduction in depression ($P = 0.009$), and enhanced perceptions of social support ($P = 0.009$), while not increasing the overall costs of health care. Findings supported the need to provide nursing services for health promotion for older patients receiving home care. Implications from this study support that health-promotion efforts are productive in improving health outcomes and can be cost-effective.

Numerous free resources are available through the federal government and other organizations. Many have been described throughout this chapter. Nurses are instrumental in promoting health. Stemming from our earliest work, nurses recognize the importance of health promotion. Like Canada and other countries, health promotion and disease prevention is paramount in our costly, fragmented US healthcare system.

Source: Markle-Reid, M., Weir, R., Browne, G., Roberts, J., Gafni, A., & Henderson, S. (2006). Health promotion for frail older home care clients. *Journal of Advanced Nursing, 54*(3), 381–395.

STUDY QUESTIONS

1. Describe the importance of health promotion in chronic illness.
2. Name the three major actual causes of death in the United States.
3. What is the goal of health promotion?
4. Identify a theory/model framework useful in working with chronically ill individuals who need to change an unhealthy behavior.
5. Discuss national documents that address health promotion and disease prevention.
6. What interventions can nurses use to promote health in persons with chronic illness?

REFERENCES

Beaudoin, C.E., Fernandez, C., Wall, J.L., & Farley, T.A. (2007). Promoting healthy eating and physical activity short-term effects of a mass media campaign. *American Journal of Preventive Medicine, 32*(3), 217–223.

Blue, C.L. (2007). Does the theory of planned behavior identify diabetes-related cognitions for intention to be physically active and eat a healthy diet? *Public Health Nursing, 24*(2), 141–150.

Bosch-Capblanch, X., Abba, K., Prictor, M., & Garner, P. (2007). Contracts between patients and healthcare practitioners for improving patients' adherence to treatment, prevention and health promotion activities. *Cochrane Database of Systematic Reviews 2007, 2,* 1–61.

Brodie, D.A., & Inoue, A. (2005). Motivational interviewing to promote physical activity for people with chronic heart failure. *Journal of Advanced Nursing, 50*(5), 518–527.

Bravata, D.M., Smith-Spangler, C., Sundaram, V., Glenger, A.L., Lin, N., Lewis, R., et al. (2007). Using pedometers to increase physical activity and improve health. *Journal of the American Medical Association, 298,* 2296–2304.

Burkhart, P.V., Rayens, M.K., Oakley, M.G., Abshire, D.A., & Zhang, M. (2007). Testing an intervention to promote children's adherence to asthma self-management. *Journal of Nursing Scholarship, 39,* 133–140.

Calloway, S. (2007). Mental health promotion: Is nursing dropping the ball? *Journal of Professional Nursing, 23*(2), 105–109.

Capella-McDonnall, M. (2007). The need for health promotion for adults who are visually impaired. *Journal of Visual Impairment & Blindness, 101*(3), 133–145.

Centers for Disease Control, National Center for Chronic Disease Prevention and Health Promotion. (2007b). Steps to a HealthierUS program preventing chronic diseases through local community action at a glance 2007. Retrieved December 21, 2007, from http://www.cdc.gov/nccdphp/publications/AAG/steps.htm

Coyle, M.K., Duffy, J.R., & Martin, E.M. (2007). Teaching/learning health promoting behaviors through telehealth. *Nursing Education Perspective, 28*(1), 18–23.

Edelman, C.L., & Mandle, C.L. (2006). *Health promotion throughout the lifespan* (6th ed.). St. Louis: Mosby.

Feldman, S.I., & Tegart, G. (2003). Keep moving: Conceptions of illness and disability of middle-aged African-American women with arthritis. *Women & Therapy,* 127–144.

Heinzer, M.M. (1998). Health promotion during childhood chronic illness: A paradox facing society. *Holistic Nursing Practice, 12*(2), 8–17.

Holland, S.K., Greenberg, J., & Tidwell, L. (2003). Preventing disability through community-based health coaching. *American Journal of the Geriatrics Society, 51,* 265–269.

Hollis, V., Massey, K., & Jevne, R. (2007). An introduction to the intentional use of hope. *Journal of Allied Health, 36*(1), 52–56.

Huang, H.C., Chou, C.T., Lin, K.C., & Chao, Y.F. (2007). The relationships between disability level, health-promoting lifestyle, and quality of life in outpatients with systemic lupus erythematosus. *Journal of Nursing Research, 15*(1), 21–32.

Huffman, M. (2007). Health coaching: A new and exciting technique to enhance patient self-management and improve outcomes. *Home Healthcare Nurse, 25*(4), 271–274.

Infectious Diseases Society of America. (2006). Immunization. Retrieved June 26, 2007, from http://www.idsociety.org/Template.cfm?Section=Immunization.

Jackson, R., Asimakopoulou, K., & Scammell, A. (2007). Assessment of the transtheoretical model as used by dietitians in promoting physical activity in people with type 2 diabetes. *Journal of Human Nutrition and Diet, 20*, 27–36.

Janz, N.K., Champion, V.L., & Strecher, V.J. (2002). The health belief model. In K. Glanz, B.K. Rimer, & F.M. Lewis (Eds.) *Health behavior and health education theory, research, and practice* (3rd ed.). (pp. 45–66). San Francisco: Jossey-Bass.

Kelly, K.M.., Phillips, C.M., Jenkins, C., Norling, G., White, C., Jenkins, T., Armstrong, D., et al., (2007). Physician and staff perceptions of barriers to colorectal cancer screening in Appalachian Kentucky. *Cancer Control: Journal of the Moffitt Cancer Center, 14*(2), 167–175.

Kulkarni, K.D. (2006). Value of diabetes self-management education. *Clinical Diabetes, 24*(2), 54.

Leddy, S.K. (2006). *Health promotion: Mobilizing strengths to enhance health, wellness, and well-being.* Philadelphia: F.A. Davis.

Lindsey, E. (1996). Health within illness: Experiences of chronically ill/disabled people. *Journal of Advanced Nursing, 24*, 465–472.

Markle-Reid, M., Weir, R., Browne, G., Roberts, J., Gafni, A., & Henderson, S. (2006). Health promotion for frail older home care clients. *Journal of Advanced Nursing, 54*(3), 381–395.

McGinnis, J.M., & Foege, W.H. (1993). Actual causes of death in the United States. *Journal of the American Medical Association, 270*, 2207–2212.

McWilliam, C.L., Stewart, M., Brown, J.B., Desai, K., & Coderre, P. (1996). Creating health with chronic illness. *Advances in Nursing Science, 18*(3), 1–15.

Miller, A., & Iris, M. (2002). Health promotion attitudes and strategies in older adults. *Health Education & Behavior, 29*(2), 249–267.

Mokdad, A.H., Marks, J.S., Stroup, D.F., & Gerberding, J.L. (2004). Actual causes of death in the United States, 2000. *Journal of the American Medical Association, 291*, 1238–1245.

Montano, D.E., & Kasprzyk, D. (2002). The Theory of Reasoned Action and the Theory of Planned Behavior. In K. Glanz, B.K. Rimer, & F.M. Lewis (Eds.) *Health behavior and health education theory, research, and practice* (3rd ed.). (pp. 67–98). San Francisco: Jossey-Bass.

MSNBC.com. (2005). CDC corrects error in U.S. obesity risks. Retrieved on January 18, 2005, from MSNBC.com

Nath, C. (2007). Literacy and diabetes self-management. *American Journal of Nursing, 107*(6 Supplement), 43–54.

Neuman, P., Cubanski, J., Desmond, K.A., & Rice, T.H. (2007). How much 'skin in the game' do Medicare beneficiaries have? The increasing financial burden of health care spending, 1997–2003. *Health Affairs, 26*(6), 1692–1701.

Norman, S.A., Potashnik, S.L., Galantino, M.L., DeMichele, A.M., House, L., & Localio, A.R. (2007). Modifiable risk factors for breast cancer recurrence: What can we tell survivors? *Journal of Women's Health, 16*(2), 177–190.

Olshansky, E. (2007). Nurses and health promotion. *Journal of Professional Nursing, 23*(1), 1–2.

Pender, N.J., Murdaugh, C.L., & Parsons, M.A. (2002). *Health promotion in nursing practice* (4th ed.). Upper Saddle River, NJ: Prentice Hall.

Prochaska, J.O., Redding, C.A., & Evers, K.E. (2002). The transtheoretical model and stages of change. In K. Glanz, B.K. Rimer, & F.M. Lewis (Eds.) *Health behavior and health education theory, research, and practice* (3rd ed.). (pp. 99–120). San Francisco: Jossey-Bass.

Rainer, J.P., & McMurry, P.E. (2002). Caregiving at the end of life. *Journal of Clinical Psychology, 58*, 1421–1431.

Rogers, A.C. (1997). Vulnerability, health and health costs. *Journal of Advanced Nursing, 26*, 65–72.

Schafer, M.H., & Ferraro, K.F. (2007). Long-term obesity and avoidable hospitalization among younger, middle-aged, and older adults. *Archives of Internal Medicine, 167*, 2220–2225.

Siarkowski, K. (1999). Children's adaptation to insulin dependent diabetes mellitus: A critical review of the literature. *Pediatric Nursing, 25*(6), 6–27. Retrieved from http://www.gale.cengage.com/Health/

Snyder, L.B. (2007). Health communication campaigns and their impact on behavior. *Journal of Nutrition Education and Behavior, 39*(2) Suppl: S32–40.

U.S. Department of Health and Human Services, Office of Disease Prevention and Health Promotion (2007). Quick guide to health literacy. Retrieved from http://www.health.gov/communication/literacy/quickguide/

Verheijden, M.W., Jans, M.P., Hidebrandt, V.H., & Hopman-Rock, M. (2007). Rates and determinants of repeated participation in a web-based behavior change program for healthy body weight and healthy lifestyle. *Journal of Medical Internet Research, 9*(1), e1. Retrieved from OCLC First Search.

Warren-Findlow, J., Prohaska, T.R., & Freedman, D. (2003). Challenges and opportunities in recruiting and retaining underrepresented populations into health promotion research. *The Gerontologist,* (March 2003), 37–47.

White, K., & Jacques, P.H. (2007). Combined diet and exercise intervention in the workplace: Effect on cardiovascular disease risk factors. *Journal of the American Association of Occupational Health Nurses, 55*(3), 109–114.

16

The Role of the Advanced Practice Nurse in Chronic Illness

Lisa L. Onega

INTRODUCTION

Advanced practice nurses are in a unique position to provide services to individuals with chronic illnesses because of nursing's disciplinary emphasis on holistic, individualized care. They need to consider their role not only from a clinical perspective but also from a conceptual and business perspective. The numbers of people with chronic illnesses are increasing as are their needs, whereas those willing and qualified to provide services to these individuals are decreasing. Advanced practice nurses need to decide whether they will be followers in the healthcare system and continue to let this vulnerable population's need for comprehensive, coordinated, integrated care go largely unmet, or whether they will be leaders in identifying and implementing creative models of care and payment methods that meet the needs of individuals, families, and society.

Philosophical Basis of Care for Individuals with Chronic Illnesses

Advanced practice nurses need to be compassionate and provide hope when caring for individuals

with chronic illnesses. Without these two fundamental qualities, knowledge of the remaining topics of this chapter—entrepreneurial practice, chronic care needs, payment and reimbursement, barriers to meeting the needs of individuals with chronic illnesses, the future of advance practice nursing, interventions, evidence-based research, and outcomes—is meaningless. Compassion provides the lens through which nurses view other human beings, and hope guides nurses' healing interventions.

Compassion

Compassionate advanced practice nurses view individuals and families with chronic illnesses in a thoughtful manner. Compassion enables nurses to understand and respect the suffering, fears, worries, and despair that individuals with chronic illnesses undergo and motivates them to act to relieve distress. Compassion is a pervasive philosophical perspective, not a selected intervention. Consequently, compassionate advanced practice nurses are present with people with chronic illnesses, and that presence is manifest in all aspects of care (Schantz, 2007).

Compassion is different from caring and empathy. Nursing leaders in the early 1900s, such as Lavinia Dock and Lillian Wald, demonstrated compassion and considered it to be an essential component of nursing. Caring, from a nursing perspective, means to be charged with the responsibility of protecting or watching over someone. Although vigilance and concern are aspects of caring, caring does not convey the level of connection, feeling, or understanding that compassion encompasses. Empathy more closely resembles compassion than does caring; however, empathy is detached and situational—it is a targeted strategy used with specific individuals. Compassion is a philosophical perspective that enables a deep connection with people. Advanced practice nurses use compassion to frame their world view (Schantz, 2007).

Advanced practice nurses who choose a compassionate philosophical perspective to guide their practice find themselves in the minority in the healthcare system. Consequently, they may clash with administrators, bureaucrats, and other healthcare providers; however, individuals with chronic illnesses and their families need to be treated with kindness and compassion. Advanced practice nurses who choose compassion have the potential to revolutionize health care for individuals with chronic illnesses (Schantz, 2007).

Hope

Individuals with chronic illnesses need to have a sense of hope. Advanced practice nurses can instill hope that although a condition cannot be cured, individuals and families can find strategies to successfully cope and find meaning and connection in life. Chronic illnesses are discouraging; however, hope-based interventions are inspiring and provide a repertoire of possibilities that enable the person to set and achieve realistic goals. Despite the uncertainties and indignities brought on by chronic illness, hope allows a person to gain a sense of control (Hollis, Massey, & Jevne, 2007; Miller, 2007).

Hope differs from optimism, expectation, and wishful thinking. Optimism may or may not be a realistic perspective; it is the belief that the best outcome will occur. Exacerbations associated with chronic illness often erode an optimistic perspective because the condition is uncertain and fraught with suffering; however, hope offers realistic strategies and ways of coping, even in extremely disheartening situations. Expectation implies an anticipated or certain outcome; and therefore, fails in the face of uncertainty and loss of control. Wishful thinking is passive and unrealistic. Hope is the ability to flexibly and productively cope with any outcome (Hollis et al., 2007).

Advanced practice nurses should utilize hope as a generalized way of viewing problems and also as a strategy for creating possibilities in specific situations. Chronic illness and the healthcare system create obstacles that can be discouraging; the most important armament in providing care for these individuals is to provide them with realistic hope (Miller, 2007).

ISSUES

Advanced practice nurses caring for individuals with chronic illnesses need to be knowledgeable about entrepreneurial practice, chronic care needs, payment and reimbursement, barriers to meeting the needs of individuals with chronic illnesses, and the future of advanced practice nursing.

Entrepreneurial Practice

The healthcare system in the United States is failing to provide adequate care for individuals with chronic illnesses. Advanced practice nurses can either work for change within existing healthcare institutions or create new models of care that better serve individuals with chronic illnesses. Although working within existing healthcare agencies is likely to bring incremental changes, entrepreneurial models of care have the potential to dramatically restructure chronic health care and fill important care gaps.

Self-Examination

Becoming an advanced practice nurse entrepreneur means being a maverick. Entrepreneurship requires self-knowledge, identifying an important niche to be filled, and creating a strategy for filling that niche while being cognizant of business, fiscal, legal, regulatory, and system-wide issues. An advanced practice nurse entrepreneur must deliver compassionate hope-based care that is affordable, cost-effective, and efficient (McCleary, Rivers, & Schneller, 2005, 2006).

Careful examination of oneself is essential to success as an advanced practice nurse entrepreneur. Entrepreneurship requires autonomy, creativity, flexibility, passion about ideas, outstanding problem-solving, excellent planning, and willingness to devote time and take calculated risks (McCleary et al., 2005, 2006). Faced with such a complex and daunting enterprise, entrepreneurs may find it helpful to have mentors, close friends or confidents, and the ability to garner resources (Barry, 2005; McCleary et al.).

Preparation

Taking adequate time, up to 6 months, to explore the market niche to be filled and to gather information about running a business will increase the likelihood of positive results (Barry, 2005; Caffrey, 2005; McCleary et al., 2005, 2006). Gaps in care provide entrepreneurial opportunities. A variety of these will be discussed in the next section, Chronic Care Needs. In separate articles, Caffrey (2005) and McCleary et al. (2005, 2006) identify the following gaps:

- Inadequate services for older adults and diverse populations.
- Lack of continuity of care and fragmented services.
- Insufficient inclusion of individuals and family members in chronic care decisions.
- Failure to respond to the healthcare needs that individuals with chronic illnesses identify.

- The need for technologic advances in documentation and reimbursement systems.
- Health policy factors that inhibit innovations in the care of individuals with chronic illness.

Establishing a business can seem overwhelming. Small Business Association (SBA) development centers, located in each state, provide useful information about cash flow, financial statements, insurance, marketing, recruiting and retaining customers, and regulations (Barry, 2005).

Business Plan

Developing a solid business plan is essential for the entrepreneur. One of the most important aspects of the business plan is determining how individuals with chronic illnesses will be recruited to the practice and retained. Closely related to this issue is deciding what services will be provided. The service aspect of the business plan should address written protocols, documentation procedures, and evaluation of services. It is also essential to ensure regulatory compliance, that services are within the clinician's scope of practice, and that insurance coverage is adequate. For any business to remain viable, it must make money; therefore, close attention to cash flow, revenue generation, budgeting, payment mechanisms, and fiscal sustainability are critical (Dellagiacoma, 2007; DeSilets, 2006; Orton, Umble, Zelt, Porter, & Johnson, 2007).

Chronic Care Needs

In addition to having a philosophical perspective based on compassion and hope and understanding the importance of entrepreneurship, advanced practice nurses, as they consider their roles with individuals with chronic illnesses, need to identify possible market niches, or openings for care. Although it is beyond the scope of this chapter to discuss all of the chronic care needs that exist, several key topics will be addressed: the prevalence and cost of chronic illness, the aging population, chronic mental and physical illnesses, technologic

▌ CASE STUDY

Twyla Bradley, PhD, RN, an advanced practice psychogerontologic nurse, was concerned about the fragmented and impersonalized care that older adults with mental health problems received, so she decided to establish an entrepreneurial business that would provide holistic, individualized care for these individuals and their families. She consulted with a lawyer, an accountant, and the State Board of Nursing to make certain that she understood regulatory and insurance issues. She obtained a business license, a form to name her business, and a tax identification number from the Internal Revenue Service. Twyla set her business up as a sole proprietorship because she planned to start small, would not have any employees, and had malpractice insurance as an advanced practice nurse. As both a clinical nurse specialist in psychiatric nursing and a family nurse practitioner, she needed to understand state law in order to determine which licensure to use in her practice. In her state, clinical nurse specialists were able to have independent businesses but were not able to prescribe medication; nurse practitioners, while permitted to prescribe medications, were required to have clinical protocols on file with the State Board of Nursing and be supervised by a physician. Consequently, she opted to set up her business as a clinical nurse specialist.

Twyla considered the forms, services, and billing that she planned to use in her business. She developed a number of forms or protocols, such as a contract for services, a Health Insurance Portability and Accountability Act (HIPAA) document, consents of different types, a bill for services, and a documentation format for patient baseline and follow-up visits. After she obtained a Medicare number, she realized that Medicare would reimburse her for only 23% of the cost to provide follow-up services, so she rescinded her Medicare provider number and decided to bill patients for the full amount of her services. This was a difficult decision; however, she understood that in order to provide the kind of care that she envisioned, she had to be reimbursed for that service.

Twyla developed a contract with a local retirement community, and the word spread about her service. Some people were unable or unwilling to pay for individualized psychogeriatric services; however, those people who became clients were extremely satisfied with the service. Twyla had a phone dedicated to her business and a home office, but she met with people at their homes. She collaborated with two colleagues about challenging issues that arose and precepted six students. During the second year, the business became profitable. Twyla said that developing an entrepreneurial business was challenging but rewarding.

Discussion Questions

1. What type of an advanced practice entrepreneurial business might you like to establish? Why?
2. What decisions would you need to make to establish your business to ensure legal and fiscal success?
3. How would you market your business?
4. What would you charge for your services? How would you handle reimbursement? How would you handle cash flow? When would you expect your business venture to begin making money?
5. Would you work with employees or other advanced practice nurses?
6. Where would your business be located?

needs, and practice and chronic care issues. As advanced practice nurses identify problems in the healthcare system, the following steps may prove helpful:

- Identify an area of interest or passion.
- Review research and other literature to substantiate problems or needs.
- Plan entrepreneurial services to meet those needs.

Chronic Illness

In 2005, 45% (133 million) of Americans had a chronic illness, and 24% (60 million) had more than one. By 2020, the number of Americans with multiple chronic illnesses is expected to be 81 million (Blue Ribbon Panel of the Society of General Internal Medicine, 2007).

Chronic illness accounts for approximately 80% of direct healthcare costs in the United States, which were $510 billion in 2000 and are anticipated to be more than $1 trillion by 2020. Annual health care cost is $6032 for an individual with a chronic illness, as opposed to $1105 for someone who does not have a chronic illness. Cost for a person with five or more chronic diseases is typically more than $15,000 per year (Blue Ribbon Panel of the Society of General Internal Medicine, 2007). Some of the most expensive illnesses are end-stage renal disease, nephrosis, nephritis, nephritic syndrome, diabetes, and heart failure (Riley, 2007).

Advanced practice nurses who are interested in the prevalence and or cost of chronic illness in general may choose to join agencies within the government or develop their own agency to tackle these issues. For example, a clinical nurse specialist who lives in a rural community that lacks many services for older adults may develop an adult day service for older adults with chronic illnesses.

Aging Population

In 2000, 35 million Americans were older than 65; by 2030 that number is expected to be 71 million (20% of the population). In 2000, 9.3 million Americans were older than 80; by 2030 that number is expected to be 19.5 million (Goldstein, 2006). Advanced practice nurses who enjoy working with older adults with chronic illnesses will find a huge demand for their services and many opportunities for entrepreneurial practice.

Aging and Chronic Illness. An investigation of older adults with chronic illnesses (n = 14,060) was done to compare their satisfaction with health maintenance organizations versus other types of Medicare supplemental coverage, such as fee-for-service. The most common conditions reported were arthritis and hypertension. Clients of health maintenance organizations were less satisfied with overall care and physicians' skills than were other clients. An ongoing client–provider relationship and continuity are important in promoting consumer satisfaction with chronic illness care (Pourat, Kagawa-Singer, & Wallace, 2006). An advanced practice nurse reviewing this research study may find it valuable in determining the type of payment as well as in designing services to be delivered. For example, a fee-for-service payment system may be selected to pay for a case management arthritis service that focuses on the nurse–client relationship and care over time.

Focus groups of older adults (n = 37) uncovered the following strategies to manage chronic illnesses (Loeb, Penrod, Falkenstern, Gueldner, & Poon, 2003): (1) exercising; (2) using religion or spirituality for support; (3) modifying dietary habits; (4) obtaining healthcare information; (5) participating in life, in part by helping others and using diversional strategies; (6) using medications; and (7) working with healthcare providers to maintain control and individuality. Social support was integral to the seven categories. A gerontologic advanced practice nurse considering this study may decide to develop a program in a senior center that provides monthly health education and support for healthy lifestyle maintenance in a group setting. Topics might include diet, exercise, and partnering with healthcare professionals.

Aging and Ethnicity. Loeb (2006) researched African American older adults with chronic illnesses (n = 28) using focus group methodology to identify coping strategies used to deal with their conditions. Findings revealed that they coped by: (1) advocating for themselves; (2) dealing with, or adjusting to, their health problems (often using humor as a strategy); (3) depending on God; (4) exercising; (5) making nutritional modifications; (6) monitoring themselves; (7) obtaining information from a variety of sources; (8) participating and being active in life (frequently using the strategy of helping other people); and (9) using medications (often discontinuing expensive medications or those for which side effects were problematic). All of the coping strategies used were problem-focused except dealing with, or adjusting to, their health problems, which was primarily an emotion-focused strategy. Depending on God was both problem-focused and emotion-focused; the seniors described faith, but they also described actions such as prayer, Bible reading, and church attendance. The gerontologic nurse wishing to promote health education programs should consider ethic cultural centers including parishes, barber shops, and beauty salons. An example of health promotion in beauty salons is Georgia Sadler's successful work in promoting breast cancer and diabetes awareness (Gladwell, 2002).

Access to necessary healthcare services for older adults is a major goal of Medicare that is not being met. Future research should focus on why higher socioeconomic status and being Caucasian leads to better access and a higher quality of care than lower socioeconomic status and nonwhite ethnicity. Services tend to be more prevention-oriented for Caucasian than for African American seniors. For example, African American older adults have 72% fewer coronary artery bypass grafts than Caucasian older adults, and three times the number of lower limb amputations. Advanced practice nurses providing care for older adults with chronic illnesses should seek to ensure that access to basic health services is equal regardless of socioeconomic status and ethnicity (Gornick, 2003). Advanced

practice nurses evaluating this study may work as researchers to better understand disparities or may become administrators of healthcare agencies to ensure that care delivered is equitable.

Aging and Mental Health. By 2030, the number of older adults with mental illnesses is expected to increase almost threefold. Current estimations are that between 65% and 80% of older adults in long-term care institutions have mental illnesses, and only 20% of them are being treated. The psychogeriatric healthcare system is grossly inadequate to meet the mental health needs of older adults; as their numbers grow, the system will be increasingly overwhelmed (Hanrahan & Sullivan-Marx, 2005). A psychogerontologic advanced practice nurse may read these statistics and may establish his or her own entrepreneurial businesses or program to meet the healthcare needs of this population.

In 2000, the U.S. Department of Health and Human Services (DHHS) Administration Center for Mental Health Services identified more than 276,000 mental health providers, including advanced practice nurses, psychiatrists, psychologists, and social workers. Ten percent of these providers submitted mental health claims to Medicare; the submission rate for advanced practice nurses was less than 2% (Hanrahan & Sullivan-Marx, 2005). An advanced practice nurse may become politically active, seeking to educate policy makers about what advanced practice nursing services are, their cost, and the benefits to society of paying for these services.

A study of mental health claims to Medicare (n = 709,221) revealed that 92% had a concomitant physical diagnosis. The majority of the clients of psychiatrists, psychologists, and social worker were age 65 to 74. Primary care physicians provided treatment equally to the 65 to 74-year-olds and the 75 to 84-year-olds, whereas advanced practice nurses cared primarily for the latter group, closely followed by the 85 and older patients. Advanced practice nurses are the clinicians most likely to care for people living in poverty; these individuals comprise almost a third of their caseload

(Hanrahan & Sullivan-Marx, 2005). An advanced practice nurse, aware of this research, may decide to establish a business that provides care to individuals who are 85 and older and live in poverty.

Chronic Mental and Physical Illnesses

Individuals with chronic mental illness often have concurrent physical problems. A study of adults who had a mental health service paid for by Medicaid (n = 787) evaluated their overall health status. Most (83%) rated their health as poor or fair and had a number of physical diagnoses including arthritis, back pain, high blood pressure, migraine headaches, and stomach problems. The majority (78%) said that their quality of life was poor, very poor, or average. Advanced practice nurses should be aware that individuals frequently have both chronic mental and physical illnesses and need to be treated in a holistic manner (Howard, El-Mallakh, Rayens, & Clark, 2007). An advanced practice nurse might establish a practice where the clinician provides integrated care over time for physical and mental health problems.

An investigation of people with chronic mental illness (n = 45), general practitioners (n = 39), and primary care practice nurses (n = 8) using focus group methodology, found that clients preferred to receive mental health care from their primary care provider rather than from a mental health specialist. Conversely, healthcare professionals believed that the healthcare needs of these individuals were too specialized for primary care. Individuals with chronic mental illness wanted a healthcare professional who was an excellent listener, willing to learn, provided hope, had a long-term relationship with them, and enabled quick access to care, especially in times of disease exacerbation (Lester, Tritter, & Sorohan, 2005).

Technologic Needs

Most advanced practice nurses use paper charts, documents, forms, and records, which consume space and are cumbersome for communication transfer, care coordination, and reimbursement. Advanced practice nurses are increasingly using electronic health records for documentation, reimbursement, and evaluation of services, and obtaining information such as practice guidelines. Electronic health records are being developed and modified to facilitate care coordination and thoughtful decision making in caring for individuals with chronic illnesses. Electronic health documentation has the potential to decrease errors, improve communication, and save time (Blue Ribbon Panel of the Society of General Internal Medicine, 2007). An advanced practice nurse who has technologic skills may work for a company that develops and markets electronic health records to healthcare agencies.

Up to 25% of communication with individuals with chronic illnesses could be done by secure e-mail. In addition, secure e-mail might be utilized by healthcare professionals to facilitate care coordination. Expanded use of this medium could increase clinicians' ability to address patients' problems in a timely manner (Blue Ribbon Panel of the Society of General Internal Medicine, 2007). An advanced practice nurse aware of technologic trends may decide to return to school to obtain an undergraduate or graduate degree in information technology.

Practice and Chronic Care

Individuals with chronic illnesses often believe that the healthcare system does not meet their needs. During a physician visit, clients are interrupted by their physicians on average 23 seconds after they begin speaking. More than 90% of clients do not participate in healthcare decision making, and 50% leave their physician's office not understanding diagnostic, treatment, or follow-up discussions. Although clinicians realize that informed, engaged clients and a responsive healthcare team is ideal, they are hindered by time constraints (Bodenheimer, MacGregor, & Stothart, 2005). An advanced practice nurse who is aware of this information may be cognizant of his or practice and ensure that individuals with chronic illnesses are not interrupted, are able to state their concerns, understand their diagnostic and treatment plans, and receive adequate follow-up to their questions and concerns.

In part because of inadequate reimbursement and administrative impediments, care for individuals with chronic illnesses is usually provided by specialists and may be fragmented and inefficient. Thoughtfully considering and understanding complex conditions in the context of the person's life is time-consuming. The clinician should focus on the provider–client relationship, listening, counseling, mutual goal-setting, and problem-solving (Blue Ribbon Panel of the Society of General Internal Medicine, 2007). An advanced practice nurse who understands the overall issues and healthcare problems faced by individuals with chronic illnesses can be valuable to individuals and their families, agencies, and policy makers in identifying and creating solutions that meet the needs of this population.

Advanced practice nurses could be utilized more effectively in the provision of care to individuals with chronic illnesses. For example, advanced practice nurses could complete assessments and review of medical records. The physician could meet with the advanced practice nurse to ensure proper diagnoses, medication management, and disease treatment. The advanced practice nurse could then implement the treatment plan, educate the client and his or her family, and provide follow-up care. The advanced practice nurse could coordinate with other healthcare team members, such as pharmacists, dieticians, and health educators, to provide integrated and comprehensive care (Blue Ribbon Panel, 2007).

An additional role might be directing healthcare management programs. Advanced practice nurses working with individuals with chronic illnesses tend to discuss a broader scope of topics than physicians do, including diet, substance use, and weight management. Individuals with diabetes favor nurse-run diabetes management groups over physician-run groups by 6 to 1 (Bodenheimer et al., 2005).

Payment and Reimbursement

Payment for chronic health care is inadequate from the perspectives of both individuals with chronic illness and healthcare professionals. A person with chronic illness does not want fragmented services that cause him or her to go from one provider to another in a haphazard fashion; he or she wants to be treated as an individual who matters, with seamless and coordinated care. Similarly, healthcare professionals are frustrated with a reimbursement system that inhibits them from providing the care that they know individuals with chronic illness need and deserve. Healthcare costs for individuals with chronic illnesses are extremely expensive; therefore, the majority of Americans are not able to pay for their care out of pocket. This requires that they depend on either governmental or private insurance to pay for the majority of their health care. Insurers are overwhelmed with healthcare claims and are constantly trying to cut costs, resulting in unmet healthcare needs for individuals with chronic health problems. Bureaucratic procedures, intended to decrease spending by identifying system abuses, errors, or fraud, ultimately consume additional time and increase costs to healthcare providers (Blue Ribbon Panel, 2007; Caffrey, 2005; DiPiero & Sanders, 2007; Goldstein, 2006; Hansen-Turton et al., 2006; Kennerly, 2007).

The predominant reimbursement model is a fee-for-service model based on reimbursement for tasks or procedures. This leads to fragmented care because communicating with other care providers, individuals, and families is not reimbursable. Healthcare professionals, who are overworked, donate their time to follow-up on procedures and coordinate care. Consequently, the continuity that is absolutely essential for the care of individuals with chronic illnesses is exceedingly uncommon. Numerous strategies to reform, restructure, and rectify the way that chronic illness care is reimbursed are being considered; however, the fundamental problem is that too many individuals with chronic illness need care that is too expensive for an underfunded system (Blue Ribbon Panel, 2007; Caffrey, 2005).

The Centers for Medicare and Medicaid Services (CMS) proposes to cut the Medicare physician fee schedule 40% between 2007 and 2015. Consequently, changes in reimbursement will occur (Kennerly, 2007). A variety of strategies have been proposed to address the reimbursement dilemma. Some of these strategies include disease management (Goldstein, 2006; Riley, 2007), Composite Measures, pay-for-performance (Kennerly, 2007), and fee-for-condition (DiPiero & Sanders, 2007).

Disease Management

Disease management is a payment strategy used to reimburse healthcare professionals for delivering care to people with a specific disease. Because 5% of Medicare beneficiaries are responsible for more than 25% of Medicare costs, Medicare is evaluating the effectiveness of this newly instituted reimbursement model (Riley, 2007). The CMS has identified the following chronic illnesses as being extremely costly and in need of cost-cutting measures such as disease management programs (Goldstein, 2006):

- Cardiac conditions
- Chronic obstructive pulmonary disease
- Diabetes (insulin dependent and type 2, or adult onset)
- HIV and AIDS
- Uncontrolled hypertension
- End-stage renal disease

Disease management programs include distribution of self-care resources, encouraging medication adherence, and support for behavioral change. Services provided at diabetes management programs typically include blood glucose monitoring; counseling regarding exercise, nutrition, smoking, and lifestyle modifications; early identification and proactive treatment of infections; emphasis on medication adherence; promotion of skin and foot self-monitoring; and routine appointments with specialists (Ahmed & Villagra, 2006).

In 2004, the CMS declared that Medicaid may reimburse disease management programs that are intervention- and outcome-oriented. These programs are typically interdisciplinary and follow individuals for part, or all, of the course of their disease (Goldstein, 2006; Riley, 2007).

Composite Measures

In 2002, the CMS began a sector-by-sector evaluation of quality and reimbursement, first examining nursing homes and then home health. Physician-focused standards are currently being evaluated. The project is developing Composite Measures, which are a grouping of various components of care that are deemed essential in the management of identified chronic illnesses. Using Category II Codes, which are supplemental Current Procedural Terminology (CPT) codes, Composite Measures are being determined. These measures can then be used as national performance standards for disease management. In other words, they would effectively define standards of practice as well as reimbursement (Kennerly, 2007).

Pay-for-Performance

Researchers have developed more than 1500 clinical guidelines for patient care. Many of these guidelines will likely be combined with Composite Measures in a pay-for-performance reimbursement system, where healthcare professionals are held to a national standard for quality, productivity, and reimbursement. Clinicians who exceed the benchmark may receive additional reimbursement, whereas those who fall short of the criterion are likely to be compensated at a lower than average rate (DiPiero & Sanders, 2007; Kennerly, 2007).

Fee-for-Condition

Fee-for-condition is a concept designed to improve quality and reimbursement for individuals with chronic illnesses by providing monthly payments, which are based on condition severity, to chronic care providers. Clinicians would receive a certain amount of money for the client's specific condition and associated health problems and would be able to allocate that money in the most appropriate way to provide comprehensive and coordinated care. Unlike capitation, which provides money for each person in a health plan regardless of disease process and encourages providers to gravitate toward treating healthy people, fee-for-condition provides payment based on each individual's specific health status. Anticipated outpatient services associated with chronic disease, such as clinicians, laboratory work, radiology tests, physical and other rehabilitation therapy, and medications, would presumably be included in the monthly fees (DiPiero & Sanders, 2007).

Advanced Practice Nurses and Reimbursement

The rules of reimbursement, which are critically important, are constantly changing. Third-party payers, private and governmental, ultimately determine compensation and standards of practice. Computer-based programs help clinicians deal with the maze of reimbursement (Goldstein, 2006). Educational programs to help understand reimbursement regulations and avoid legal ramifications of filing or documentation violations abound. For better and for worse, reimbursement dictates practice.

Due in part to declining reimbursement, new physicians are shunning career options that serve people with chronic illnesses. In the last 5 years, the number of physicians specializing in internal medicine has decreased by 50% (Blue Ribbon Panel, 2007). As Medicare reimbursement for physicians continues to diminish, advanced practice nurses (who became eligible to receive Medicare reimbursement in 1997) will likely have more opportunities and more pressures to provide

healthcare services for individuals with chronic illnesses (Chevalier, Steinberg, & Lindeke, 2006). Advanced practice nurses need to understand the complex clinical needs and the complicated and ever-changing reimbursement issues associated with care of the chronically ill (Kennerly, 2007).

Specifically, Kennerly (2007) advises that advanced practice nurses should do the following regarding reimbursement:

■ Use electronic medical records in practice and for reimbursement.
■ Bill insurers under the advanced practice nurse's provider identification number instead of billing under a physician's provider identification number. (The latter method is sometimes referred to as billing "incident to.")
■ Partner with insurers and agencies to institute and evaluate processes and outcomes of new models of care for individuals with chronic illnesses.
■ Monitor developments in reimbursement and outcome-focused research.

Barriers in Meeting the Needs of Individuals with Chronic Illnesses

Barriers to meeting the healthcare needs of individuals with chronic illnesses can be categorized by consumers, other healthcare providers, agencies and institutions, reimbursement, regulations, legal, and nursing (Chevalier et al., 2006).

■ Consumers: Although consumers are becoming more knowledgeable of and comfortable with the various roles of advanced practice nurses, confusion still abounds. The lack of public understanding about the services that advanced practice nurses can provide to individuals with chronic illnesses will continue to require education and marketing (Chevalier et al., 2006; Elsom, Happell, & Manias, 2007; Hanrahan & Sullivan-Marx, 2005).
■ Other Healthcare Providers: Physicians and other healthcare professionals are often

ambivalent about the changes taking place in their professions and how the scope of nursing is expanding to meet healthcare needs. Advanced practice nurses need to respect the knowledge and expertise of other disciplines and retain the core components of nursing (Chevalier et al., 2006; Elsom et al., 2007).

- Agencies and Institutions: Agencies and institutions often underutilize and overwork advanced practice nurses, which leads to role conflict and ethical challenges for the individual nurse. Each advanced practice nurse who wants to care for individuals with chronic illnesses needs to carefully consider the venue in which he or she will be most successful (Chevalier et al., 2006; Elsom et al., 2007; Connelly, Baker, Hazen, & Mueggenborg, 2007; Ulrich & Soeken, 2005).
- Reimbursement: Reimbursement is complex and drives standards of practice. Most insurers reimburse advanced practice nurses at lower rates than physicians (Bodenheimer et al., 2005; Hansen-Turton et al., 2006).
- Regulations: State regulations for advanced practice nurses are restrictive and differ, which makes relocation and business growth challenging. For example, in some states, but not all, advanced practice nurses are legally required to have written protocols with physicians (Chevalier et al., 2006; Elsom et al., 2007; Hanrahan & Sullivan-Marx, 2005; Howard et al., 2007; Miles, Seitio, & McGilvray, 2006).
- Legal: Malpractice and other liability issues are major concerns for almost all clinicians. In an ever-litigious society, the practitioner must be able to withstand any degree of scrutiny and review (Caffrey, 2005; Chevalier et al., 2006; Elsom et al., 2007; Miles et al., 2006).
- Nursing: Within the discipline, advanced practice nurses report lack of autonomy (Elsom et al., 2007; Miles et al., 2006; Ulrich & Soeken, 2005) and collegial support (Caffrey, 2005; Chevalier et al., 2006). Limited numbers of nurses are pursuing advanced practice roles directed toward individuals with chronic illness (Bodenheimer

et al., 2005; DePalma, 2004b; Hanrahan & Sullivan-Marx, 2005), and salaries are often lower than expected (Chevalier et al., 2006). In addition, advanced practice nurses often feel ethical pressure as they attempt to balance the regulatory, reimbursement, institutional, and personal challenges of caring for individuals with chronic illnesses in a society that is allotting too few resources to many people with such extensive needs (Elsom et al., 2007; Miles et al., 2006; Ulrich & Soeken, 2005).

The Future of Advanced Practice Nurses

Two issues facing advanced practice nurses are entry level education and the care role that they will assume.

Entry Level Education

Currently, advanced practice nurses are educated at the post-baccalaureate level and credentialed as clinical nurse specialists, nurse anesthetists, nurse midwives, or nurse practitioners (Chase & Pruitt, 2006; Ervin, 2007; Fawcett & Graham, 2005; Fawcett, Newman, & McAllister, 2004). In 2004, the American Association of Colleges of Nursing proposed that the Doctor of Nursing Practice be the entry level for advanced practice nurses by the year 2015 (Chase & Pruitt, 2006; Lancaster, Chase, & Pruitt, 2006). In keeping with a 150-year history of debate over educational standards, the nursing profession is struggling with entry level education for advanced practice nursing. Although this issue is as important as it is controversial, the more fundamental question that nursing should be addressing is how to best meet the healthcare needs of society.

Advanced Practice Nurse or Physician Extender?

Advanced practice nurses face a choice: whether to remain nurses—with expanded scope—or become mini-physicians. Addressing this issue is fundamental to the discipline's ability to meet the needs of individuals with chronic illnesses (Fawcett & Graham, 2005).

Advanced practice nurses assume medical roles for a variety of reasons. These include increased income for the nurse, cost-savings for medical practices and hospitals, inadequate numbers of physicians in certain regions and specialties, desire for power and prestige, and desire to help individuals with their healthcare problems. Medicine seeks to diagnose and treat disease (Fawcett & Graham, 2005). Nursing is an eclectic discipline, which incorporates medical, nutritional, and psychological knowledge; however, understanding aspects of these other disciplines does not change the focus of nursing. Nursing is a broad discipline that seeks to promote the health and functioning of individuals, families, communities, and society. Concepts that are pivotal to nursing are health promotion, illness prevention, healing, holism, and patient-centered care.

Advanced practice nurses often work as physician extenders to meet institutions' cost-saving goals and because of physician shortages (Fawcett et al., 2004). Some say that exploiting advanced practice nurses in this way is good because it allows nurses to receive some of the societal rewards traditionally reserved for physicians. Unfortunately, when advanced practice nurses stop doing nursing, individuals with chronic illnesses pay the price (Fawcett & Graham, 2005).

People with chronic illnesses are not having their needs met by the existing healthcare system. The discipline of nursing has the knowledge and ability to help these individuals cope with the healthcare challenges that they face (Ervin, 2007; Fawcett et al., 2004; Fawcett & Graham, 2005). Advanced practice nurses should ask themselves whether they will have the courage to advocate for these individuals and provide them with the nursing care that they require, or whether they will succumb to the pressures of institutions and bureaucracies (Fawcett et al., 2004; Fawcett & Graham, 2005). Advanced practice nurses can provide these individuals with compassionate and hope-based care that enables them to find health despite their chronic illnesses.

INTERVENTIONS

Compassion should be the foundation that motivates interventions that advanced practice nurses provide for people with chronic illnesses. Clinicians should always strive to maximize and preserve each individual's functional ability. Interventions are categorized as hope-based, relationship-based, medication use, and fitting into models of care.

Hope-Based Interventions

The language and behavior of advanced practice nurses can help provide a sense of hope to a person with a chronic illness. Individuals and families can be asked what gives them hope, comfort, or peace of mind, and interventions can be tailored that match their responses. Using words such as "yet" and "when" helps the person focus on the temporary nature of disappointments and provides hope for future situations (Hollis et al., 2007).

Hope-related strategies include (Hollis et al., 2007; Miller, 2007):

- Providing comfort and alleviating pain.
- Listening and validating feelings.
- Accepting and respecting the person's individuality and values, and being present for the patient and his or her family.
- Nurturing the person's autonomy, dignity, and quality of life and not providing false hope.
- Helping the individual maintain control over his or her body and environment and facilitating independence, especially with regard to activities of daily living such as feeding and toileting. Comforting routines can help achieve this goal.
- Sharing joy and humor when appropriate and therapeutically using creativity, literature, or music.
- Focusing on meaningful experiences and relationships and minimizing isolation.
- Helping the individual consider alternative options.

- Assisting the person to set attainable goals that are meaningful and promote a sense of worth and mastery.
- Supporting the individual in finding courage, determination, and peace of mind.
- Sharing a sense of confidence in the person's ability to overcome obstacles and inspiring him or her to draw upon inner resources.
- Helping with practical activities that enable goal attainment.
- Focusing on positive experiences and memories as well as helping the person live in the present.
- Identifying resources that assist the individual to problem-solve and cope.
- Supporting spiritual practices such as prayer and meditation.

Relationship-Based Interventions

Relationship-based interventions focus on the nurse–client relationship to reach decisions consistent with the individual's values, resources, and goals. This approach requires listening to how the person makes sense of his or her illness; focusing on the individual's concerns; being genuine; and avoiding interrupting, giving advice, or being judgmental. The therapeutic relationship that advanced practice nurses have with individuals with chronic illnesses can improve quality of life, reduce healthcare costs, and decrease hospitalization (Caffrey, 2005; Perraud et al., 2006).

Communication with individuals with chronic illnesses needs to be patient-centered. This means that advanced practice nurses should be present with individuals and create an unhurried, nurturing environment while attending to complex health problems, promoting adherence, and providing prompt and efficient service. Lack of time is always a concern; however, developing an open and trusting relationship with individuals with chronic illnesses will foster a long-term relationship, may save time in the future, and will lead to improved outcomes (Lein & Wills, 2007).

In addition to focusing on the nurse–client relationship and developing open communication, an advanced practice nurse should also help individuals with chronic illnesses learn to make sense of and cope with their symptoms. When people with chronic illnesses experience a disconcerting symptom, they are often unsure if it is associated with their disease process, related to aging, or fleeting and unimportant. The advanced practice nurse can listen to the individual's perspective about his or her illness, provide information and anticipatory guidance, and help the person develop reasonable criteria for when to contact a clinician. In general, early symptom recognition can minimize suffering, cost, and hospitalization (Fowler, Kirschner, VanKuiken, & Baas, 2007).

Medications and the Role of the Advanced Practice Nurse

Advanced practice nurses need to realize that most individuals with chronic illnesses take one or more medications, which are often extremely expensive. For a small percentage of individuals with chronic illnesses, the cost of medications is not an issue; however, cost is a problem for most patients with chronic illnesses. Medical expenses are even a problem for individuals with insurance.

Advanced practice nurses need to remember that visits to healthcare professionals including physicians, physical therapists, dieticians, mental health counselors, and other clinicians are costly. Diagnostic procedures such as X-rays, computed tomography (CT) scans, magnetic resonance imaging (MRI) scans, and laboratory work are expensive. Transportation and parking may result in additional costs. Furthermore, income may be reduced because of decreased productivity, time away from work, or disability.

The increasing cost of medications can be burdensome for individuals with chronic illnesses. Two research studies demonstrate this point. The first, by Heisler, Wagner, and Piette (2005), is large and provides representative data about the magnitude of this problem. The second, by Loeb and colleagues (2003), is small and provides in-depth and personal insight about how individuals with chronic illnesses cope with the high cost of medications. Advanced practice nurses need to understand both broad and individual implications as they decide what their role will be in designing interventions to address this problem.

Individuals with chronic illnesses are often financially burdened by having to pay out-of-pocket medication costs. A study of randomly selected adults taking prescription medications for one of five chronic illnesses (depression, diabetes, heart problems, high cholesterol, and hypertension) (n = 4055) examined whether their costs led subjects to cut back on necessities such as food or heat, to underuse medications, or to increase debt. Findings revealed that, over the last year, 31% used at least one cost-cutting strategy in order to afford medications, with 22% cutting back on necessities, 18% reducing medications, and 16% increasing debt. Among those who underused medications, 67% also cut out necessities or increased debt. Thirty-six percent of women and 24% of men reported using at least one of the strategies. Even those with high incomes reported making financial adjustments in response to medication costs and using at least one of these strategies. Nonwhite subjects were more than twice as likely as white subjects to cut back on necessities. Strategies were used by individuals from all socioeconomic classifications but were most prominent among those with low-incomes, poor health, and multiple medications. Advanced practice nurses should discuss medication costs with their clients as well as strategies to deal with those expenses (Heisler et al., 2005). In addition, advanced practice nurses who choose to work at the macro-level in agencies or government will find this study useful in educating their constituents and in designing policies that enable people to afford medications.

In the Loeb and colleagues (2003) study of older adults described previously, medications were a primary strategy used to deal with chronic illnesses. Seniors took between 6 and 21 medications. All participants indicated that taking multiple

medications created a financial burden. One subject said that monthly out-of-pocket medication expenses were $2000. Strategies used to cope with the high cost of medications included volunteering at hospitals in order to receive hospital pharmacy discounts, obtaining public assistance, or being part of the Pharmaceutical Assistance Contract for the Elderly. Advanced practice nurses who provide care for individuals with chronic illnesses may ask people regardless of their insurance status, "How much money do you spend out-of-pocket on your medications? What strategies do you use to cope with the cost of your medications?"

Models of Care

Many models for providing care for individuals with chronic illness exist. Three types of models include strategies to frame thinking, service models, and role-related models.

Strategies to Frame Thinking

Many strategies to frame thinking exist; however, it is beyond the scope of this chapter to highlight all of them. Therefore, three strategies that advanced practice nurses can use to organize their thinking will be described. Each advanced practice nurse is likely to be familiar with many useful ways of systematizing information and likely draws aspects from one or more of these in different situations.

An example of a strategy to frame thinking is the Care, Cure, Core Model. Advanced practice nurses use care as the foundation for developing a therapeutic relationship with the patient and attempting to understand the illness from the individual's perspective. Cure involves diagnosing, treating, and educating the individual and his or her family about the illness. Core is reaching the central person and providing emotional and social support that helps the individual find ways to cope with the chronic condition (McCoy, 2006).

Another strategy that an advanced practice nurse may use is the Chronic Illness Trajectory Framework. This perspective postulates that a chronic illness has a path, which can be uncertain. Individuals with chronic illnesses and nurses seek to manage symptoms in order to give a sense of certainty and control to the illness trajectory (Corbin & Strauss, 1992). This framework has been applied to people with cancer (Dorsett, 1992), cardiac illness (Hawthorne, 1992), diabetes (Walker, 1992), human immune deficiency and acquired immunodeficiency syndrome (HIV/AIDS) (Nokes, 1992), mental illness (Rawnsley, 1992), and multiple sclerosis (Smeltzer, 1992).

The Salutogenic Model emphasizes health, not disease. Stressors, such as developing a chronic illness, adversely impact health, whereas generalized resistance resources, such as having health insurance, positively impact health (Antonovsky, 1985). In addition, an individual's sense of coherence, which has three components—(1) comprehensibility, (2) manageability, and (3) meaningfulness—influences his or her health (Antonovsky, 1987). Advanced practice nurses may use this model to assess, intervene, and evaluate care for individuals with chronic illnesses (Onega, 1991).

Service Models

Service models are methods of delivering care to individuals with chronic illnesses. Advanced practice nurses need to select a model of care that is most appropriate for the population, the type of services that they intend to deliver, the setting in which care will be provided, and the personnel who will be part of the team. A variety of models exists and should be carefully examined before one is selected for implementation.

An example of a service model is the Transition into Primary Care Psychiatry Clinical Model, in which a psychiatric nurse and a psychiatrist partner with a primary care provider. Individuals with chronic mental illness who have an exacerbation of symptoms are often hospitalized, stabilized, treated, and then returned to their primary care provider. The goal is a supportive transition between hospital and community-based care, as well as access to treatment, coordination of services, and efficient use of resources. Once

care is resumed by the primary care provider, regular mental health consultations by the psychiatric nurse and psychiatrist occur in the person's home and in an office setting. Psychiatric services include case management, evaluation of relapse potential, focus on adherence, inclusion of the family, home visits, telephone follow-up, vocational services, and wellness promotion. Continuity of care, collaborative planning, and a holistic approach are hallmarks of this model (Haslam, Haggerty, McAuley, Lehto, & Takhar, 2006).

Role-Related Models

Role-related models for advanced practice nurses working with individuals with chronic illnesses are numerous. An example of a role-related model is that of a clinical nurse specialist who is an entrepreneur and owns a dysphagia business. The nurse entrepreneur may start out small by consulting with assisted living centers, nursing homes, and hospitals to assess individuals with dysphagia resulting from illnesses such as multiple sclerosis, Parkinson's disease, and stroke. The advanced practice nurse may do swallow screens to evaluate the four phases of swallowing (the oral preparatory phase, the oral phase, the pharyngeal phase, and the esophageal phase). He or she may prepare inservices and develop practice guidelines for institutions. As the business grows, additional team members may be added, including other advanced practice nurses, speech therapists, or dieticians (Werner, 2005).

Advanced practice nurses should identify colleagues who can serve as mentors and colleagues. They can discuss challenges, opportunities, and ideas with these individuals and establish either a formal or informal support network. They can also influence state and regional politics, participate in research, and help educate advanced practice nursing students.

Evidence-Based Research

Advanced practice nurses providing care for individuals with chronic illnesses need to be knowledgeable about evidence-based research, in particular that which evaluates outcomes. Outcomes research, using assessment instruments and focusing on quality, self-care, the continuum of care, cost, and policy issues, must inform practice (Caffrey, 2005; DePalma, 2004a; DePalma, 2004b; McCleary et al., 2005, 2006). In addition, innovative methods for delivering chronic care services should be tested (Blue Ribbon Panel, 2007). Evidence-based research that evaluates outcomes helps clinicians improve practice and provides consumers and insurers with important data-based information. Evaluation enables advanced practice nurses to compare results with benchmarks and improve services (DePalma, 2004a, 2004b; Goldstein, 2006). Advanced practice nurses may also read integrative reviews and evidence-based practice guidelines and apply these as they deliver care to individuals with chronic illnesses (DePalma, 2004a). Examples of research-related chronic illness management include:

■ An evaluation to determine the effects of treating depression as a chronic disease in primary care settings was done with adults who began treatment for major depression (n = 211). The intervention included nurses managing care over a 24-month period and encouraging patients to be active participants in treatment. Components of the intervention were assessment, education, homework assignments, and follow-up contacts. Findings revealed that symptoms and functioning improved at 24 months, increasing remission by one third (to 74%), improving emotional functioning by 24%, and improving physical functioning by 17% (Rost, Nutting, Smith, Elliott, & Dickinson, 2002).

■ This study sought to understand how time is spent during outpatient appointments for diabetes, as compared with other chronic illnesses and with acute illnesses. Research nurses observed consecutive outpatient visits during two separate days in 138 family physician offices. Time use was categorized into 20 different behaviors using the Davis Observational Code. Time was compared for appointments for diabetes, other chronic conditions, and acute illnesses during visits by patients 40 years old and older (n = 1867). Appointments for chronic illnesses were on average longer than for acute illnesses, and visits for diabetes averaged the most time. During each diabetes appointment, 2.5 problems were addressed, compared with 2.1 problems during other chronic illness appointments and 1.8 problems during acute care appointments. Unlike appointments for other chronic illnesses, visits for diabetes involved more time spent on adherence assessment, discussion about exercise, feedback on test results, health education, health promotion, and nutritional counseling and less time chatting. Compared to acute illness appointments, visits for diabetes were lengthier and involved more encouragement to exercise, evaluation of adherence, health promotion, negotiation, nutritional assessment of adherence, and preventive health care, and less time on procedures (Yawn, Zyzanski, Goodwin, Gotler, & Stange, 2001).

■ The Permanente Medical Group in Northern California examined quality, utilization, and cost for disease management programs for individuals with asthma, coronary artery disease, diabetes, and heart failure. The programs were characterized by multidisciplinary care teams, evidence-based clinical guidelines, self-management education, proactive outreach including telephone follow-up, and care managers trained not only in the specific disease but also in eliciting behavioral change. Decision-making was guided by medication protocols, disease management software, and physician oversight. Quality and utilization improved as a result of disease management programs; however, cost increased (Fireman, Bartlett, & Selby, 2004).

■ Evaluation of a diabetes management program across 10 urban markets in the United

States found that improvements in six quality indicators and lower cost were evident after 6 months of participation. Individuals with diabetes (n = 39,292) were either in the intervention (n = 27,188) or control (n = 12,104) group. Intervention consisted of repeated telephone calls by nurses, dieticians, or health educators; Web-based education; use of scales with remote data transmission capability; reminders; and educational mailings throughout the year. During the baseline nurse telephone call, patients received a structured interview including an assessment of understanding of diabetes, a detailed lifestyle inventory, questions about dietary and activity preferences, and appraisal of the need for adherence to prescription medications. Behavioral and cognitive goals were set for each participant. Follow-up phone calls focused on the American Diabetes Association standards of care and treatment guidelines for comorbidities, adherence to physician treatment plans, healthy lifestyle, and supportive interventions. Cost per month for the treatment and comparison groups were $417 and $554, respectively (a savings of $137), lower medication costs by $9.02, and lower inpatient costs by $17. This investigation demonstrated that a diabetes disease management plan could be delivered remotely with excellent quality and cost results (Ahmed & Villagra, 2006).

▌ EVIDENCE-BASED PRACTICE BOX

More than 250,000 hip fractures occur in the United States each year at a cost on average of $40,000 per person. Total annual expenses are more than $7 billion and are expected to rise to $14 billion by 2040. Hip surgery for fractures is common in older adults.

A gerontologic advanced practice nurse model of care was evaluated in older adults who had a hip fracture (n = 33) by following subjects from hospital discharge for 12 months using a two-group, repeated measures, randomized design. The treatment group received care coordination for 6 months from a gerontologic advanced practice nurse, which included visits and/or phone calls once a week for the first month and twice a week for the remaining 5 months. Care coordination consisted of physical, psychosocial, and functional assessments; medication review; education; referral for appropriate resources; documentation; and communication with patients, families, physicians, and long-term care staff. The control group received standard care.

Ten people did not complete the study: four withdrew and six died. The treatment group (n = 13) scored better than the control group (n = 10) at 12 months on activities of daily living and instrumental activities of daily living, particularly home chores, mobility, and personal care, but had no differences in depression, health, living situation, or pain. Gerontologic advanced practice nurses made an average of 22.5 contacts, lasting 35.6 minutes, with 12 face-to-face visits (60.2 minutes) and 10.5 telephone conversations (7.3 minutes). The treatment cost was $506.50 per patient ($30/hour for the advanced practice nurse's time for a total visit cost of $399, plus transportation at $0.325 for a total transportation cost of $107.50). Although small in scope, this study indicates that gerontologic advanced practice nurses are effective and relatively inexpensive in the care of older adults who have had hip fractures.

Source: Krichbaum, K. (2007). GAPN postacute care coordination improves hip fracture outcomes. *Western Journal of Nursing Research, 29*(5), 523–544.

OUTCOMES

Advanced practice nurses who choose to work with individuals with chronic illnesses will find it challenging to maintain a philosophical perspective based on compassion, which motivates them to deliver hope-based care. They will find establishing entrepreneurial businesses for this population a daunting task. They will often be frustrated with reimbursement issues and barriers to serving people with chronic illnesses. However, advanced practice nurses working with individuals with chronic illnesses know that if they do not find creative ways to meet the needs of and advocate for these people, no one else will. Advanced practice nurses can be inspired by the sacrifices and contributions made by nursing leaders, such as Lavinia Dock and Lillian Wald, that changed lives and changed history, and aspire to improve the lives of patients with chronic illness.

STUDY QUESTIONS

1. Why is it essential for advanced practice nurses working with individuals with chronic illness to have a philosophical perspective based in compassion and hope?
2. Why might advanced practice nurses want to develop entrepreneurial businesses to meet the healthcare needs of people with chronic illnesses?
3. What are some opportunities, gaps, or issues in chronic care?
4. What are some of the challenges regarding reimbursement that the advanced practice nurse providing care to individuals with chronic illness should understand?
5. What are barriers to providing holistic care for people with chronic illnesses?
6. Compare and contrast "advanced practice nurse" and "physician extender."
7. What are some important interventions that advanced practice nurses working with individuals with chronic illness may provide?
8. Why are outcomes essential for advanced practice nurses to consider as they provide care for people with chronic illnesses?

INTERNET RESOURCES

American Academy of Nurse Practitioners: www.aanp.org/Resources+and+Links/Professional+Organizations.htm
Association of Rehabilitation Nurses: www.rehabnurse.org/about/index.html
The Hope Foundation of Alberta: www.ualberta.ca/HOPE/
Institute for Healthcare Improvement; Assessment of Chronic Illness Care Survey: www.ihi.org/IHI/Topics/ChronicConditons/AllConditions/Tools/ACICSurvey.htm\
Improving Chronic Illness Care: www.improving-chroniccare.org/index.php?p=About_ICIC_&_Our_Work&s=6
Medline Plus—Coping with Chronic Illness: www.nlm.nih.gov/medlineplus/copingwithchronicillness.html
National Association of Clinical Nurse Specialists: www.nacns.org/#
National Gerontological Nursing Association: www.ngna.org/
Nurse Entrepreneur Network—Business Solutions for Nurse Entrepreneurs: www.nurse-entrepreneur-network.com/
The Official Business Link to the U.S. Government: www.business.gov
University of Rochester Center for Nursing Entrepreneurship: www.son.rochester.edu/CNE/
U.S. Department of Health & Human Services Centers for Medicare and Medicaid Services: www.cms.hhs.gov/

REFERENCES

Ahmed, T., & Villagra, V.G. (2006). Disease management programs: Program intervention, behavior modification, and dosage effect. *Journal of Consumer Policy, 29*(3), 263–278.

Antonovsky, A. (1985). *Health, stress, and coping.* San Francisco, CA: Jossey-Bass.

Antonovsky, A. (1987). *Unraveling the mystery of health: How people manage stress and stay well.* San Francisco, CA: Jossey-Bass.

Barry, P. (2005). Perspectives on private practice: Questions and answers for the nurse psychotherapist in private practice. *Perspectives in Psychiatric Care, 41*(1), 42–44.

Blue Ribbon Panel of the Society of General Internal Medicine. (2007). *Journal of General Internal Medicine: Official Journal of the Society for Research and Education in Primary Care Internal Medicine, 22*(3), 400–409.

Bodenheimer, T., MacGregor, K., & Stothart, N. (2005). Nurses as leaders in chronic care. *British Medical Journal, 330*(7492), 612–613.

Caffrey, R.A. (2005). The rural community care gerontological nurse entrepreneur: Role development strategies. *Journal of Gerontological Nursing, 31*(10), 11–16.

Chase, S.K., & Pruitt, R.H. (2006). The practice doctorate: Innovation or disruption? *Journal of Nursing Education, 45*(5), 155–161.

Chevalier, C., Steinberg, S., & Lindeke, L. (2006). Perceptions of barriers to psychiatric-mental health CNS practice. *Issues in Mental Health Nursing, 27*(7), 753–763.

Connelly, C.D., Baker, M.J., Hazen, A.L., & Mueggenborg, M.G. (2007). Practice applications of research: Pediatric health care providers' self-reported practices in recognizing and treating maternal depression. *Pediatric Nursing, 33*(2), 165–172.

Corbin, J.M., & Strauss, A. (1992). A nursing model for chronic illness management based upon the trajectory framework. In P. Woog (Ed.). *The Chronic Illness Trajectory Framework: The Corbin and Strauss Nursing Model.* (pp. 9–28). New York: Springer.

Dellagiacoma, T. (2007). Eight essential factors for successful nurse-led services. *Australian Nursing Journal, 14*(10), 28–31.

DePalma, J.A. (2004a). Advanced practice nurses' research competencies: Competency I–Using evidence in practice. *Home Health Care Management & Practice, 16*(2), 124–126.

DePalma, J.A. (2004b). Advanced practice nurses' research competencies: Competency II–Evaluating practice. *Home Health Care Management & Practice, 16*(4), 293–295.

DeSilets, L.D. (2006). What are good business practices, anyway? *Journal of Continuing Education in Nursing, 37*(5), 196–197.

DiPiero, A., & Sanders, D.G. (2007). Condition based payment: Improving care of chronic illness. *British Medical Journal, 330*(7492), 654–657.

Dorsett, D.S. (1992). The trajectory of cancer recovery. In P. Woog (Ed.). *The Chronic Illness Trajectory Framework: The Corbin and Strauss Nursing Model.* (pp. 29–38). New York: Springer.

Elsom, S., Happell, B., & Manias, E. (2007). Exploring the expanded practice roles of community mental health nurses. *Issues in Mental Health Nursing, 28*(4), 413–429.

Ervin, N.E. (2007). Clinical specialist in community health nursing: Advance practice fit or misfit? *Public Health Nursing, 24*(5), 458–464.

Fawcett, J., & Graham, I. (2005). Scholarly dialogue–Advanced practice nursing: Continuation of the dialogue. *Nursing Science Quarterly, 18*(1), 37–41.

Fawcett, J., Newman, D.M., & McAllister, M. (2004). Scholarly dialogue–Advanced practice nursing and conceptual models of nursing. *Nursing Science Quarterly, 17*(2), 135–138.

Fireman, B., Bartlett, J., & Selby, J. (2004). Can disease management reduce health care costs by improving quality? *Health Affairs, 23*(6), 63–74.

Fowler, C., Kirschner, M., VanKuiken, D., & Baas, L. (2007). Promoting self-care through symptom management: A theory-based approach for nurse practitioners. *Journal of the American Academy of Nurse Practitioners, 19*(5), 221–227.

Gladwell, M. (2002). *The tipping point: How little things can make a big difference.* New York, NY: Little, Brown and Company.

Goldstein, P.C. (2006). Impact of disease management programs on hospital and community nursing practice. *Nursing Economics, 24*(6), 308–314.

Gornick, M.E. (2003). Men's health forum—A decade of research on disparities in Medicare utilization: Lessons for the health and health care of vulnerable men. *American Journal of Public Health, 93*(5), 753–759.

Hanrahan, N.P., & Sullivan-Marx, E.M. (2005). Practice patterns and potential solutions to the shortage of providers of older adult mental health services. *Policy, Politics, & Nursing Practice, 6*(3), 236–245.

Hansen-Turton, T., Ritter, A., Begun, H., Berkowitz, S.L., Rothman, N., & Valdez, B. (2006). Insurers' contracting policies on nurse practitioners as primary care providers: The current landscape and what needs to change. *Policy, Politics, & Nursing Practice, 7*(3), 216–226.

Haslam, D., Haggerty, J., McAuley, L., Lehto, J., & Takhar, J. (2006). Collaboration in action—Maintaining and enhancing shared care relationships through the TIPP clinical model. *Family, Systems, & Health, 24*(4), 481–486.

Hawthorne, M.H. (1992). Using the trajectory framework: Reconceptualizing cardiac illness. In P. Woog (Ed.). *The Chronic Illness Trajectory Framework: The Corbin and Strauss Nursing Model.* (pp. 39–49). New York: Springer.

Heisler, M., Wagner, T.H., & Piette, J.D. (2005). Patient strategies to cope with high prescription medication costs: Who is cutting back on necessities, increasing debt, or underusing medications? *Journal of Behavioral Medicine, 28*(1), 43–51.

Hollis, V., Massey, K., & Jevne, R. (2007). An introduction to the intentional use of hope. *Journal of Allied Health, 36*(1), 52–56.

Howard, P.B., El-Mallakh, P., Rayens, M.K., & Clark, J.J. (2007). Comorbid medical illnesses and perceived general health among adult recipients of Medicaid mental health services. *Issues in Mental Health Nursing, 28*(3), 255–274.

Kennerly, S. (2007). The impending reimbursement revolution: How to prepare for future APN reimbursement. *Nursing Economics, 25*(2), 81–84.

Krichbaum, K. (2007). GAPN postacute care coordination improves hip fracture outcomes. *Western Journal of Nursing Research, 29*(5), 523–544.

Lancaster, J., Chase, S.K., & Pruitt, R.H. (2006). DNP discussion continues..."The practice doctorate: Innovation or disruption?" *Journal of Nursing Education, 45*(8), 295–296.

Lein, C., & Wills, C.E. (2007). Using patient-centered interviewing skills to manage complex patient encounters in primary care. *Journal of the American Academy of Nurse Practitioners, 19*(5), 215–220.

Lester, H.E., Tritter, J.Q., & Sorohan, H. (2005). Patients' and health professionals' view on primary care for people with serious mental illness: Focus group study. *British Medical Journal, 330*(7500), 1122–1127.

Loeb, S.J. (2006). African American older adults coping with chronic health conditions. *Journal of Transcultural Nursing, 17*(2), 139–147.

Loeb, S.J., Penrod, J., Falkenstern, S., Gueldner, S.H., & Poon, L.W. (2003). Supporting older adults living with multiple chronic conditions. *Western Journal of Nursing Research, 25*(1), 8–29.

McCleary, K.J., Rivers, P.A., & Schneller, E.S. (2005/2006). A diagnostic approach to understanding entrepreneurship in health care. *Journal of Health and Human Services Administration, 28*(3/4), 550–577, 582.

McCoy, M.L. (2006). Care of the congestive heart failure patient: The care, cure, and core model. *Journal of Practical Nursing, 56*(1), 5,6,30.

Miles, K., Seitio, O., & McGilvray, M. (2006). Nurse prescribing in low-resource settings: Professional considerations. *International Nursing Review, 53*(4), 290–296.

Miller, J.F. (2007). Hope: A construct central to nursing. *Nursing Forum, 42*(1), 12–18.

Nokes, K.M. (1992). Applying the Chronic Illness Trajectory Model to HIV/AIDS. In P. Woog (Ed.). *The Chronic Illness Trajectory Framework: The Corbin and Strauss Nursing Model.* New York, NY: Springer Publishing.

Onega, L.L. (1991). Theoretical framework for psychiatric nursing. *Journal of Advanced Nursing, 16*(1), 68–73.

Orton, S., Umble, K., Zelt, S., Porter, J., & Johnson, J. (2007). Management academy for public health: Creating entrepreneurial managers. *American Journal of Public Health, 97*(4), 601–605.

Perraud, S., Delaney, K.R., Carlson-Sabelli, L., Johnson, M.E., Shephard, R., & Paun, O. (2006). Advanced practice psychiatric mental health nursing, finding our core: The therapeutic relationship in the 21st century. *Psychiatric Care, 42*(4), 215–226.

Pourat, N., Kagawa-Singer, M., & Wallace, S.P. (2006). Are managed care Medicare beneficiaries with chronic conditions satisfied with their care? *Journal of Aging and Health, 18*(1), 70–90.

Rawnsley, M.M. (1992). Chronic mental illness: The timeless trajectory. In P. Woog (Ed.), *The Chronic Illness*

Trajectory Framework: The Corbin and Strauss Nursing Model, (pp. 59–72). New York: Springer.

Riley, G.F. (2007). Long-term trends in the concentration of Medicare spending. *Health Affairs, 26*(3), 808–816.

Rost, K., Nutting, P., Smith, J.L., Elliott, C.E., & Dickinson, M. (2002). Managing depression as a chronic disease: A randomized trial of ongoing treatment in primary care. *British Medical Journal, 325*(7370), 934–939.

Schantz, M.L. (2007). Compassion: A concept analysis. *Nursing Forum, 42*(2), 48–55.

Smeltzer, S.C. (1992). Use of the Trajectory Model of Nursing in multiple sclerosis. In P. Woog (Ed.), *The Chronic Illness Trajectory Framework: The Corbin and Strauss Nursing Model* (pp. 73–88). New York: Springer.

Ulrich, C.M., & Soeken, K.L. (2005). A path analytic model of ethical conflict in practice and autonomy in a sample of nurse practitioners. *Nursing Ethics, 12*(3), 305–316.

Walker, E.A. (1992). Shaping the course of a marathon: Using the trajectory framework for diabetes mellitus. In P. Woog (Ed.), *The Chronic Illness Trajectory Framework: The Corbin and Strauss Nursing Model* (pp. 89–96). New York: Springer.

Werner, H. (2005). The benefits of the dysphasia clinical nurse specialist role. *Journal of Neuroscience Nursing, 37*(4), 212–215.

Yawn, B., Zyzanski, S.J., Goodwin, M.A., Gotler, R.S., & Stange, K.C. (2001). Is diabetes treated as an acute or chronic illness in community family practice? *Diabetes Care, 24*(8), 1390–1396.

17

Symptom Management

Linda L. Steele and James R. Steele

INTRODUCTION

Symptom management is the hallmark of an effective treatment plan to control symptoms related to chronic disease and to improve the quality of life (QOL) and day-to-day living. MacDonald (2002) points out that although symptoms such as nausea, shortness of breath, and pain can play a warning and protective role for the body in acute illness, symptoms lose their purpose over time when present in chronic illness. In the context of a nursing perspective, symptom management requires an understanding of the individual patient experience as well as the meaning associated with each symptom.

A holistic approach to symptom management is well suited to the increasing number of people with chronic illness (Haworth & Dluhy, 2001). The management of symptoms related to chronic illness requires a holistic and individual approach, with the focus being the individual, not the symptom. Nurses play a key role in the assessment and management of symptoms and in promoting quality of life in patients with chronic illness.

According to Taylor (2000), symptoms are the most common reason that individuals seek care. However, those already living with a chronic illness seek relief. The symptoms related to chronic illness are vast and complex. Dodd and colleagues (2001a) state that the experience of symptoms, minor to severe, results in millions of patient visits to healthcare professionals each year. Symptoms create distress as well as changes in social functioning. Patients and their families have the burden of dealing with the distress caused by symptoms related to chronic illness. Developing symptom management strategies that can be applied across acute and home care settings is difficult because few models of symptom management have been tested empirically.

It is rare that patients with a chronic illness experience one symptom, but more often, experience symptom clusters related to their particular disease process. To date, the majority of research on symptoms has been directed toward studying a single symptom, such as pain or fatigue, or toward evaluating associated symptoms, such as depression and sleep disturbance. Although this approach has advanced our understanding of some symptoms, a more generic symptom management model is needed to provide direction for determining appropriate interventions, directing future research, and synthesizing a number of symptoms associated with chronic diseases and conditions, such as rheumatoid arthritis, diabetes, chronic obstructive pulmonary disease (COPD), and HIV (Dodd et al., 2001a).

Interest is growing in a common biological mechanism underlying a group of symptoms (Cleeland et al., 2003). The term "underlying mechanism" in the context of symptom management conjures the idea of physiologic mechanisms. Sickness behavior has been described by a symptom profile that can include anorexia, cachexia, fever, nausea, fatigue, anhedonia (loss of pleasure), pain, and impaired learning (Lee et al., 2004). Bower et al. (2000) studied fatigue in almost 2000 breast cancer survivors and found it was associated with pain, depression, and insomnia. Glover, Dibble, Dodd, and Miaskowski (1995) studied pain in 200 patients with cancer with a variety of diagnoses and treatments and demonstrated that pain was associated with depression, fatigue, and anxiety.

In an integrative review of 35 journal articles reporting on 32 studies, O'Neill and Morrow (2001) examined how women interpret, cope with, and manage chronic illness symptoms. The analysis identified important gender differences in the experience of symptoms. They discovered that women with chronic illness report more symptoms and poorer physical health than men. Women also enter the healthcare system later and more ill than their male counterparts. The authors concluded that although individual symptoms are well documented in the literature, symptom management strategies and the cultural meaning of symptoms are understudied.

Although there is little research addressing interventions for symptom clusters, Homsi et al. (2006) examined the systematic assessment of multiple symptoms with an open-ended assessment question "What symptoms are you having now?" The median number of symptoms obtained was 10, with a range of 0–25. Several other studies have tested the efficacy of systematic symptom assessment, and a few studies demonstrated that providing clinicians with systematic assessment information has a beneficial effect on QOL (McLachlan et al., 2001). Sarna (1998) concluded that systematic assessment

of symptoms delayed an increase in symptom distress.

In a study that examined symptom distress in older women with and without breast cancer, Heidrich and colleagues (2006) concluded that women in both groups most often attributed the cause of their symptoms to aging, chronic illness, or the unknown, but rarely to breast cancer. Attributing symptoms to chronic illness or breast cancer was significantly related to more pain, depression, role impairment, and poorer mental health. The individual's perception of purpose in life, poorer social functioning, less energy, and higher levels of depression and anxiety were related to not knowing the cause of symptoms. They suggest that a broader assessment of symptoms is needed to assist older breast cancer survivors with symptom management and that symptom interventions in older women should address patients' beliefs about symptoms so that QOL can be enhanced.

Barsevick (2007) conducted a systematic review of the literature from 1995 to 2007 to include the definition and importance of the symptom cluster; theoretical frameworks that may explain clusters; analytical strategies to identify clusters; interventions to alleviate symptoms clusters; and suggestions for future research. Four symptoms were examined as a candidate symptom cluster for this analysis: fatigue, insomnia, pain, and depression. Although the findings suggested that fatigue, insomnia, pain, and depression constitute a viable cluster for further study, more research is needed to define the cluster and describe underlying mechanisms.

Addressing multiple symptoms is beneficial in reducing negative patient outcomes. When conducting symptom assessment, healthcare professionals should address the four symptoms (fatigue, insomnia, pain, and depression) targeted in this review because evidence of clustering exists. Guidelines provided by the National Comprehensive Cancer Network (http://www.nccn.org/) for fatigue and distress provide algorithms and decision trees for assessment and management of these symptoms.

Symptom Management Models

Dluhy (1995) wrote that fatigue, pain, symptom management, day-to-day living with illness, and social support are promising areas to begin building a mid-range theory of chronic illness, and believes that developing a cumulative knowledge base narrows the gap between theory and practice. Although several models of symptom management are described in the literature, there has been

little empirical testing completed. The following four models are described.

Symptom Management Model

The Symptom Management Model (Figure 17-1) is based on the interrelationship of three components: the symptom experience, symptom management strategies, and patient outcomes (Dodd et al., 2001a). The symptom experience is a patient's perception of the frequency, intensity, distress, and meaning of a single symptom or multiple symptoms. This model describes symptom management

FIGURE 17-1

Symptom Management Model

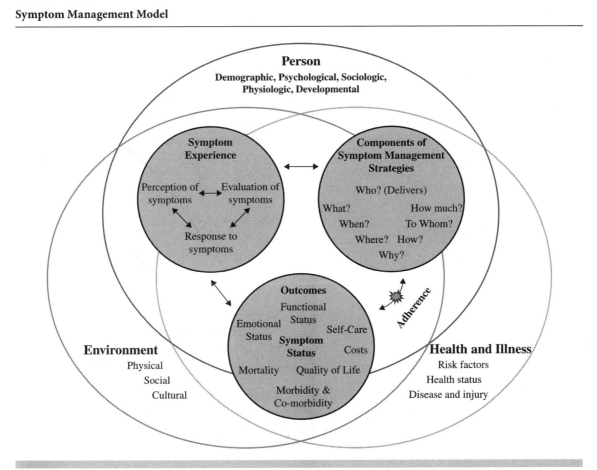

Source: Dodd, M., Janson, S., Facione, N., Faucett, J., Froelicher, E.S., Humphreys, J., et al. (2001). Advancing the science of symptom management. *Journal of Advanced Nursing, 33,* 668–676.

as a dynamic process in which management strategies evolve and change over time. The primary outcome of symptom management is symptom status, which is improved, remains stable, or worsens. Other outcomes include functional status, emotional state, self-care, QOL, cost, mortality, and morbidity.

Because there are few empirically tested models of symptom management, healthcare professionals have difficulty developing symptom management strategies that can be applied across settings. Therefore, to advance the knowledge of symptom management and improve the practice of healthcare professionals and outcomes for individuals, a nursing research team at the University of California, San Francisco, initiated the Research Center for Symptom Management. From this Center, the Symptom Management Model, as described previously, was developed and published in 1994, having been derived from faculty research and practice in a variety of settings. According to Dodd and colleagues (2001a) their model focuses on patient symptom experiences, interventions, and outcomes. The model is based on assumptions that include:

■ The gold standard for the study of symptoms is based on the perception of the individual experiencing the symptom and his or her self-report; and

■ Symptom management is a dynamic process that is modified by individual outcomes and the influences of the nursing domains of person, health/illness, or environment.

This model is based on the premise that in order to achieve effective management of patient symptoms, the three dimensions of symptom experience, symptom management strategies, and outcomes must be considered (Dodd et al., 2001a). Although previous research has focused on the management of single symptoms such as pain, or dyads such as nausea/vomiting, the Symptom Management Model can be used to direct care and research with a variety of symptoms or clusters that result from a variety of diseases and conditions. The dynamic nature of symptom expression means that the primary symptom within a cluster may be subject to rapid change and thus pose a challenge in managing interventions.

The goal of symptom management is to prevent or delay a negative outcome by implementing interventions based on management therapies, and/or self care strategies. Symptom management should begin with assessment of the symptom experience from the individual's perspective, followed by identifying the focus for intervention. Interventional strategies may focus on one or more components of the individual's symptom experience to achieve one or more desired outcomes. Symptom management is a dynamic process, and may require changes in strategies over time or in response to the effectiveness of the strategies. The nature of the intervention depends on the state of the science and supporting evidence for the treatment of particular symptom and/or symptom clusters (Dodd et al., 2001a).

Outcomes emerge from symptom management strategies as well as from the symptom experience. The duration of symptom evaluation depends upon the symptom's persistence, need for continued intervention, and response to treatment. A key question in the evaluation of symptom management is who evaluates symptom outcomes? Is it the patient, family, or healthcare professional, and/or others? (Dodd et al., 2001a, 2001b).

The Theory of Unpleasant Symptoms

The Theory of Unpleasant Symptoms is based on symptoms that begin with antecedents that shape the symptom experience (Lenz, Pugh. Milligan, Gift, & Suppe, 1997). Symptoms can occur as separate entities or concurrently as a symptom cluster. Characteristics of symptoms include intensity, distress, quality, and duration. The effects of the symptom experience include effects on functional status, cognitive functioning, and physical activity, with each component of the model having a feedback loop with other components.

The Symptoms Experience Model

The Symptoms Experience Model (Armstrong, 2003) builds on the Theory of Unpleasant Symptoms and the Symptom Management Model. This model is based on understanding the meaning of the symptom experience through encompassing the perception of the impact of a symptom(s) on daily life and the capacity of the patient's ability to cope with it.

Symptom Interaction Model

Parker and colleagues (2005) proposed a Symptom Interaction Framework based on the possibility of relationships or interactions between symptoms, and defined a symptom as the subjective perception of an alteration in a bodily process or function.

Outcomes for Interventions for Symptom Clusters

Gaston-Johansson and colleagues (2000) targeted pain, fatigue, psychological distress, and nausea as outcome measures in patients with breast cancer who underwent autologous bone marrow transplantation (BMT). The intervention for the study was a comprehensive coping strategy program that was compared with "usual care." The program was effective in reducing nausea, as well as nausea combined with fatigue, 7 days after BMT, when side effects of treatment are most severe.

Given and colleagues (2004) used a cognitive–behavioral intervention to reduce symptom severity during chemotherapy for solid tumors. A significant interaction was found between the study group and baseline symptom severity. Patients in the experimental group who had higher symptom severity at study entry had significantly lower severity at weeks 10 and 20. Participants with worse baseline symptoms had the most benefit from the intervention. Both of these studies demonstrated a decrease in symptoms from interventions targeted at multiple symptoms, rather than treating each single symptom.

Pearson and colleagues (2006) studied the effects on morbidity and mortality at 6 months in a cohort of patients with chronic illness randomly assigned to an intensive, multidisciplinary home-based intervention (HBI) designed to improve management of chronic disease beyond the initial 6-month intervention. A home visit by the study nurse and pharmacist occurred at week 1 to: (1) assess the patient's physical, clinical, and psychosocial status; (2) optimize home medication management; (3) increase patient and/or caregiver vigilance for clinical deterioration; and (4) improve liaison with community-based services thereafter. Strategies including education, counseling, and the introduction of reminder cards and medication compliance devices. Patients with more complex problems were referred to a community pharmacist for a regular review of potential long-term problems. Patients and family members were also counseled regarding the importance of recognizing early signs of clinical deterioration or adverse effects of medications and alerting their healthcare team. Plans for more intensive follow-up were also arranged when required. Active study follow-up lasted 6 months. At this stage, the study suggested that this form of intervention provided long-term cost benefits, owing to reduced recurrent hospital stays associated with a range of chronic illnesses, except COPD. Other studies (Hallerbach, Francoeur, & Pomerantz, 2008; Inglis, Pearson, & Treen, 2006) have also demonstrated that patients exposed to HBI experienced significantly fewer hospital admissions and fatal events during 6 months of follow-up with heart failure patients.

Common symptom profiles relevant to chronic illness that will be discussed in this chapter include: (1) chronic pain; (2) depression; (3) fatigue; and (4) anorexia, cachexia, and wasting. The purpose of this chapter is to describe common symptoms experienced by patients with chronic illness, discuss assessment and management of those symptoms based on evidence-based guidelines, and develop and evaluate holistic plans of care.

CASE STUDY

Dawn Summers is a 26-year-old woman who was diagnosed with HIV 4 years ago. Her children are 12, 10, and 7 years. She began using intravenous drugs while away at college at the age of 18. Her weight was 136 pounds at the time of diagnosis and today it is 97. Currently she is hospitalized for significant weight loss and anorexia. She is also experiencing joint pain, fatigue, and depression. During the interview she also expresses regret and fear of what will happen to her children, "after I die."

Identified Problems

Assessment of her symptoms using the Symptom Management Model: Dawn has a symptom cluster related to her chronic illness. The short-term needs revolve around her anorexia and resultant weight loss. This may be, in part, due to the medication regimen she is taking to control her underlying disease process. The treatment of patients with chronic disease will require that the several symptoms related to her disease process (symptom cluster) be addressed simultaneously. Algorithms to assess and manage her symptoms with evidence-based research should be implemented. Ms. Summers' symptoms, including lack of appetite, joint pain, and fatigue, are related to her disease process, and the emotional distress she is experiencing surrounding the care and well-being of her children now and when and if she approaches the end of life.

Interventions

Her medication regimen should be assessed and evaluated for effective symptom management without undesirable side effects that contribute to the burden of coping with chronic illness. Often a simple reduction or increase in the dosing will reduce the adverse symptoms or deliver more effective relief. Medication levels should be determined and doses adjusted. In addition she has lost weight, which would in all likelihood lead to her body requiring less medication to achieve therapeutic levels. Higher doses of the medications could build to toxic levels, thereby further complicating her care.

Pain interventions should be concentrated on nonpharmacologic measures in addition to pharmacologic methods, particularly with regard to the joint and muscle pain. The use of any and all measures to alleviate the discomfort that is preventing her from an adequate caloric intake would have to be implemented. Selecting from the medications available for anorexia will help maintain current weight and/or help in increasing her appetite.

Emotional support should be provided for her personally and for her children. The involvement of social service agencies and other support will help to provide Ms. Summers with real information about the options available to her for her own care and that of her family. Involving her in that discussion and decision process will tend to provide her with the maximum possible psychological support and reenergize her self-management strategies to empower her to make collaborative decisions related to her care.

Discussion Questions

1. What specific nonpharmacologic interventions would you use to control Dawn's pain? What is the evidence to support your choices?
2. What can be done to control her anorexia and weight loss?
3. Would you consider depression as part of the symptom cluster for Dawn? If so, why, and what treatment options would you design for her?
4. Apply the Symptom Management Model to summarize a holistic approach to the assessment and management of Dawn Summers and her family.

CHRONIC PAIN

Chronic pain is not uncommon. Approximately 35% of Americans have some element of chronic pain, and approximately 50 million Americans are disabled partially or totally due to chronic pain (Singh & Jashvant, 2005). The International Association for the Study of Pain defines pain as "an unpleasant sensory and emotional experience associated with actual or potential tissue damage, or described in terms of such damage" (Merksey, 1986, p. S217). Melzack (1973) describes pain as "a highly personal experience depending on cultural learning, the meaning of the situation, and other factors that are unique to each individual" (p. 22). McCaffery and Pasero (1999) state that pain is a subjective experience and relies heavily on the patient's self-report whenever possible. Pain should be defined in the context of whatever the person experiencing the pain says it is, existing whenever the person says it does. It is essential that healthcare professionals understand this concept in order to effectively gain insight into the complex nature of pain and thereby develop methods to assess and manage pain in chronic illness.

Chronic pain is defined as persistent pain, which can be either continuous or recurrent and of sufficient duration and intensity to adversely affect a patient's well-being, level of function, and QOL. Pain is not time dependent; however, at 6 weeks (or longer than the anticipated healing time), patients should be evaluated thoroughly for the presence of chronic pain [National Guideline Clearinghouse (NGC), 2007]. Pain is chronic when it occurs at intervals for months or years, and/or is associated with chronic pathology (McCaffery & Pasero, 1999; Wall & Melzack, 1999; Warfield & Bajwa, 2004). When an individual has chronic pain, the body's adaptive physiologic and autonomic responses are usually absent. Chronic pain can be continuous, intractable, intermittent, or recurrent. Even when mild, it can be sufficiently pervasive that it becomes a condition unto itself that requires daily management. Although persons who have chronic health problems can experience either acute and/ or chronic pain, it is the ever-present nature of chronic pain that controls much of their lives.

Pain is regularly undertreated by healthcare professionals. Many healthcare professionals have a poor understanding of pain assessment and pain management. They are often frustrated with patients who do not manifest symptoms of their pain or who do not respond well to treatment (Green et al., 2002; Lazarus & Neumann, 2001; McCaffery, Ferrell, & Pasero, 2000; Shvartzman et al., 2003; Weinstein et al., 2000). Contributing to undertreatment are the negative stereotypes that healthcare professionals often have of those with chronic pain. Professionals do not always give credence to pain complaints, unless there is identifiable pathology or clients demonstrate autonomic or behavioral responses (Turk, 1999; Weinstein et al., 2000). Healthcare professionals often assume that all patients have the same pain perception threshold and, therefore, perceive the same intensity of pain from the same stimuli (Voerman, van Egmond, & Crul, 2000). Many have become desensitized to their patients' pain experience and rate pain as less important than patients do (Shvartzman et al., 2003).

Knowledge is limited about the specific mechanism(s) for transmission and perception of pain. However, several theories have been proposed, some of which are briefly noted herein. The specificity theory, one of the oldest theories that serves to explain pain transmission, is based on the concept that there is always a cause and effect relationship. It proposes that specific pain receptors (nociceptors) project impulses over specific neural pain pathways (A-delta and C fibers) via the spinal cord to the brain.

However, chronic pain is often quite different, although no less severe than acute pain, and thus a more subtle scientific understanding of pain is required to treat it. Unfortunately, many healthcare professionals try to extend the specificity theory to patients with chronic pain. The theory assumes that if surgery or medication can eliminate the alleged "cause" of the pain, then the chronic pain will disappear. This is often not true for those patients who experience chronic pain.

For example, if the specificity theory is applied to a patient's chronic pain problem, the patient may be at risk for receiving unnecessary and ineffective diagnostic procedures, drugs, and surgical treatment as the search for the source of the pain is the main objective (Deardorff, 2004).

The theory most widely used in clinical practice today is the gate control theory proposed by Melzack and Wall (1965), even though it is not fully supported by incontrovertible experimental evidence. According to this theory, a gating mechanism in the dorsal horn of the spinal cord permits or inhibits the transmission of pain impulses. Peripheral nerve fibers that synapse in the gray matter of the dorsal horn serve as a gate. When the gate is closed, pain impulses are prevented from reaching the brain. Therefore, pain must reach a conscious awareness before it is perceived; if awareness can be prevented, then the perception is decreased or eliminated.

Assessment of Pain

All patients have a right to adequate assessment of their pain [Institute for Clinical Systems Improvement (ICSI), 2007]. Pain assessment is now the fifth vital sign as designated by the Joint Commission on Accreditation of Healthcare Organizations (JCAHO) by standards that were implemented January 1, 2001 (Douglas, 1999; Krozek & Scoggins, 2001a, 2001b; JCAHO, 2001). All patients should be asked if they are having pain and, if so, to rate its intensity. Initial assessment includes history taking, observation, and physical examination.

Subjective factors from the history, such as patient perceptions and responses to the pain, should be assessed. This includes documentation of pain location, intensity, quality, onset/duration/variations/rhythms, manner of expressing pain, pain relief, what makes it worse, and the effects of pain on the patient's QOL and ability to perform activities of daily living, employment, and social interests. Also included should be number of prior treatments for pain and responses, as well as inquiring about sleep and diet. It is also critical to take a complete history to elicit any history of depression or other psychopathology that may affect the perceptions of pain. Inquire specifically about any current physical, sexual, or emotional abuse.

A history of chemical dependency is of particular interest in patients with chronic pain. The CAGE questionnaire by Ewing (1984) is a useful tool for brief alcohol screening (NGC, 2007). The CAGE questionnaire includes the following four questions:

> Have you ever felt that you should **C**ut down on your drinking?
> Have people **A**nnoyed you by criticizing your drinking?
> Have you ever felt bad or **G**uilty about your drinking?
> Have you ever had a drink first thing in the morning to steady your nerves or to get rid of a hangover (**E**ye opener)?

The pain assessment tool in Figure 17-2 is useful in any setting and type of pain and can be easily adapted to patient needs. Because of the strong influence a family can have on patients, the family system should be part of the assessment as well. Objective findings from the physical examination should be part of the assessment, since chronic pain frequently involves the musculoskeletal and nervous systems. Table 17-1 summarizes aspects of the physical examination related to pain assessment.

Although there are no specific diagnostic tests for chronic pain, it is important to remember that even if pathology is found on diagnostic tests, that information does not necessarily support that the identified pathology is causing the patient's pain. However, diagnostic testing is useful in chronic pain patients to direct treatment and referral. X-ray is helpful in musculoskeletal pain to rule out pathology that might require more immediate attention. Magnetic resonance imaging (MRI) and computed tomography (CT) are frequently used in spine-related pain. Electromyography (EMG) and nerve conduction studies should be used in patients suspected of having lower motor neuron

FIGURE 17-2

Initial Pain Assessment Tool

INITIAL PAIN ASSESSMENT TOOL Date ____________

Patient's Name ______________________________ Age ______ Room ______

Diagnosis ______________________ Physician ______________________

Nurse ______________________

I. LOCATION: Patient or nurse mark drawing.

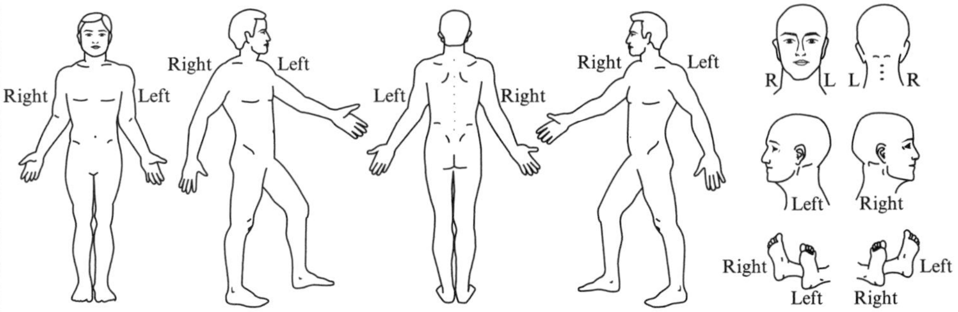

II. INTENSITY: Patient rates the pain. Scale Used ______________________

Present: ______________________

Worst pain gets: ______________________

Best pain gets: ______________________

Acceptable level of pain: ______________________

III. QUALITY: (Use patient's own words, e.g., prick, ache, burn, throb, pull, sharp) ______________________

IV. ONSET, DURATION, VARIATIONS, RHYTHMS: ______________________

V. MANNER OF EXPRESSING PAIN: ______________________

VI. WHAT RELIEVES THE PAIN: ______________________

VII. WHAT CAUSES OR INCREASES THE PAIN? ______________________

VIII. EFFECTS OF PAIN: (Note decreased function, decreased quality of life)

Accompanying symptoms (e.g., nausea) ______________________

Sleep ______________________

Appetite ______________________

Physical activity ______________________

Relationship with others (e.g., irritability) ______________________

Emotions (e.g., anger, suicidal, crying) ______________________

Concentration ______________________

Other ______________________

IX. OTHER COMMENTS: ______________________

X. PLAN: ______________________

Source: McCaffery, M., & Pasero C. (1999). *Pain: Clinical manual for nursing practice* (2nd ed.). St. Louis: Mosby, p. 60.

TABLE 17-1

Objective Assessment of Pain—Information Obtained From the Physical Examination

Vital signs	Note presence of increased blood pressure, rapid pulse rate, or increased respiratory rate
Inspection	How does the patient look? Facial expression, color, diaphoretic?
	Cyanosis or pallor of an extremity
	Is there obvious deformity or atrophy? If present it should be measured
Palpation	Asymmetry of bones, extremities, joints
	Observe posture, gait, and station
	Examine joints for redness and swelling and signs of effusion, instability, and ligament or cartilage pathology
	Is there hemiplegia or paresis present?
	Check muscle strength and sensation
	Evaluate deep tendon reflexes
	Is there pain, guarding, or muscle spasm or tenseness when the affected area is palpated?
	What is the temperature and texture of the skin?
	Check range of motion

---

dysfunction, nerve or nerve root pathology, or myopathy (NGC, 2007).

Functional assessment and pain assessment tools are necessary components of a complete pain assessment. Baseline functional ability assessment can provide information about a patient's QOL and ability to participate in desired activities. Personalized goal setting, such as regaining ability to perform a specific job task, hobby, or family activity, may also be used. Tools to assess chronic pain have limitations, owing to lack of scoring consistency and failure to provide useful information for healthcare professionals. According to the National Institutes of Health, patient self report is the most reliable indicator of the existence and intensity of pain and is a key component of chronic pain assessment (NGC, 2007). The Assessment Algorithm from the Institute for Clinical Systems Improvement is shown in Figure 17-3.

Management of Chronic Pain

Management of patients with chronic pain is the responsibility of the entire healthcare team,

including the individual and family. Nurses plan and provide interventions that are individually appropriate through an understanding of chronic pain. In a concept analysis of pain, Davis (1992, p. 81) defines pain management as "success in taking care of or handling the pain by using certain actions and by directing and controlling one's own use of these actions." In addition, three distinct attributes that comprise pain management are identified:

- Pain relief is easing or alleviating the pain.
- Pain modulation is adjusting to or softening the effects of the pain under a variety of circumstances.
- Self-efficacy is the individual's capacity to take care of or handle the pain.

In a study by Davis and White (2001), when those with chronic pain spoke of managing their pain, they generally described the use of specific strategies such as medicine, heat application, and distraction. Some persons believed that they would probably never be able to control their pain, but

FIGURE 17-3

Assessment of Pain Algorithm

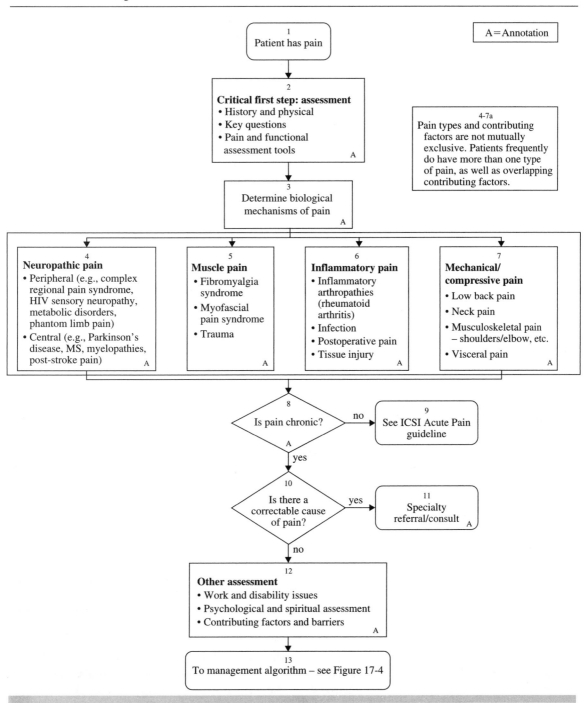

A = Annotation

1
Patient has pain

2
Critical first step: assessment
• History and physical
• Key questions
• Pain and functional
  assessment tools
                              A

4-7a
Pain types and contributing
factors are not mutually
exclusive. Patients frequently
do have more than one type
of pain, as well as overlapping
contributing factors.

3
Determine biological
mechanisms of pain
                    A

4
Neuropathic pain
• Peripheral (e.g., complex
  regional pain syndrome,
  HIV sensory neuropathy,
  metabolic disorders,
  phantom limb pain)
• Central (e.g., Parkinson's
  disease, MS, myelopathies,
  post-stroke pain)   A

5
Muscle pain
• Fibromyalgia
  syndrome
• Myofascial
  pain syndrome
• Trauma
                  A

6
Inflammatory pain
• Inflammatory
  arthropathies
  (rheumatoid
  arthritis)
• Infection
• Postoperative pain
• Tissue injury   A

7
**Mechanical/
compressive pain**
• Low back pain
• Neck pain
• Musculoskeletal pain
  – shoulders/elbow, etc.
• Visceral pain   A

8
Is pain chronic?   no → 9
                          See ICSI Acute Pain
                          guideline
       A
      yes

10
Is there a
correctable cause   yes → 11
of pain?   Specialty
                          referral/consult A
      no

12
Other assessment
• Work and disability issues
• Psychological and spiritual assessment
• Contributing factors and barriers
                                      A

13
To management algorithm – see Figure 17-4

Source: Institute for Clinical Systems Improvement. (2007). Assessment and management of chronic pain. Bloomington, MN: Institute for Clinical Systems Improvement.

that they could realistically expect to manage it. This distinction is an important factor to consider when implementing a pain management strategy. A written plan of care is an essential tool for ensuring a comprehensive approach to treatment of a patient with chronic pain and should include the following personal goal statements:

- Improvement of sleep
- Increased physical activity
- Management of stress
- Decreasing pain

Treatment approaches suggested by the National Guideline Clearinghouse (NGC) (2007) incorporate two levels in managing chronic pain. Level I treatment includes standard methods of pain management such as pharmacologic and nonpharmacologic methods, and complementary medicine management. These approaches should be implemented as the first steps toward rehabilitation.

Level II treatment includes referral for multidisciplinary pain rehabilitation or surgery for placement of a spinal cord stimulator or intrathecal pump. These treatments may be effective for patients with chronic pain who have not responded to previous treatment options. However, Level II treatments are designed for the most complex and challenging chronic pain patients, and these options are expensive and require a significant investment on the part of the patient to be effective.

Cognitive Behavioral Strategies

Cognitive–behavioral approaches in the management of patients with persistent and unremitting chronic pain are considered to be among the most helpful available (NGC, 2007). The goal of cognitive–behavioral strategies is for patients to question and reappraise thoughts, feelings, and behaviors that they have related to their pain. The role of the healthcare professional is as educator, trainer, and coach. This process is well described by Turk and Okifuji (2003, 2004) and Winterowd, Beck, and Gruener (2003).

Patients may be referred to a therapist, counselor, social worker, or psychologist for this treatment, but there are many cognitive–behavioral steps that can be implemented by primary care providers. Patients can make gains toward significant rehabilitation goals by changing the contingencies of reinforcement, with the help of their healthcare professionals. The goals of cognitive–behavioral strategies in the management of those with chronic pain are to improve physical functioning, assist patients in returning to work, reduce disability, reduce pain-related fear/avoidance, and reduce psychological distress and depression (NGC, 2007).

The effectiveness of cognitive–behavioral programs is not universal, and like other interventions for individuals with chronic pain, some interventions work better for some than for others. Cognitive–behavioral strategies work best in combination with other interventions and, as with other noninvasive methods, for persons who are motivated to control their pain. In addition, many clinicians do not recommend cognitive–behavioral strategies for those persons with psychiatric problems, clinical depression or significant problems with mood or affect.

Pharmacologic Management

Opioids. Opioids are an important class of drugs for pain management. Opioids work not only by modifying central nervous system perception, but also by interrupting the mechanisms responsible for causing the pain, increasing the pain threshold, blocking peripheral nervous system input, or relieving anxiety or depression. Pain control can often be achieved by nonopioids, adjuvant analgesics (antidepressants, anticonvulsants, muscle relaxants, corticosteroids, antibiotics, and vasodilators, and so on. However, only general information about opioids, nonopioids, and antidepressants is discussed in this section.

Prior to consideration of opioid use for the patient with chronic pain, a thorough evaluation of the patient's appropriateness for opioid therapy is recommended (NGC, 2007). It is appropriate to consider opioid therapy for patients with persistent moderate-to-severe pain; however, healthcare professionals should not feel compelled to prescribe opioids or any drug if it is against their best judgment or if they feel uncomfortable prescribing the drug.

Clinical evidence suggests opioids are likely to be effective in neuropathic pain that is not responsive to first-line therapies such as tricyclic antidepressants (TCAs) or gabapentin. Opioids are rarely beneficial in the treatment of inflammatory or mechanical/compressive pain and are not indicated for chronic use in treatment of headache. They have an equal or better therapeutic index than alternative therapies.

Opioid therapy is considered part of the overall management for management of a pain syndrome. The goal of opioid therapy is to provide partial analgesia, and maintain or improve function with acceptable side effects. According to the NGC guidelines (2007), the Four A's, analgesia, adverse drug effects, activity, and adherence, should be evaluated when using opioid therapy. Is there significant relief of pain with this medication? Are there any side effects? If so, do they impact functional status, activity, and QOL? Finally, is the patient able to be compliant with the medication regimen? If not, examine the factors impacting adherence to the medication regimen.

Several factors contribute to the effectiveness of opioids: (1) client-related factors (e.g., age, gender, psychological distress, prior opioid use); (2) pain-related factors (e.g., usual intensity, breakthrough pain, tempo of pain escalation); and (3) effects of the specific medication (Shalmi, 2004). The use of an equianalgesic chart can guide the amount and route of drugs that are used for pain control (e.g., Lipman & Jackson, 2004, p. 585) as can information about what to consider when prescribing narcotics (e.g., Berde & Masek, 2003, pp. 545–558; Sweeney & Bruera, 2003, pp. 382–385).

Healthcare professionals have no difficulty decreasing medication when necessary, but they typically are not comfortable with increasing doses, especially if greater than usual amounts are needed or if their patients are not getting adequate relief. Professionals may need re-education to relieve their fear of "addicting" clients; clients do not become addicts as long as medication is being used to control pain. Table 17-2 lists a number of behaviors that are often mistaken as indicators of addiction.

Another strategy recommended by Fishman and associates (1999), and based on a review of 90 pain centers, is an opioid contract or written agreement (Canadian Pain Society, 1998; McCaffery & Pasero, 1999; Sweeney & Bruera, 2003). This contract provides healthcare professionals with confidence that the planned opioid administration does not put patients at risk and provides patients with a clear picture of their pain management, one that they have had a part in negotiating. Although the format of contracts is diverse, the goal is the same—to increase the quality of pain management.

Morphine, the standard opioid for severe acute pain and chronic cancer pain (American Pain Society, 1987; Gourlay, 1998), is one of four commonly used opioids (morphine, hydromorphone, levorphanol, and methadone) that are equally capable of relieving pain. Various reasons for selecting one or the other include: prior pain experience, the number and severity of side effects experienced, the concentration or volume of doses available, and the characteristics of the medication (e.g., rate of onset, duration, accumulation).

Nonsteroidal Anti-inflammatory Drugs. Nonsteroidal anti-inflammatory drugs (NSAIDs), are best known for their anti-inflammatory effect, but they can also be used to manage chronic pain (Simon, 2004). Their pain-relieving effects are often underestimated. These drugs can provide additional pain relief when given with an opioid. Giving them together poses no more danger than alternating them. The peak effect of NSAIDs is about 2 hours after oral administration, about the time that the effectiveness of an intramuscularly administered narcotic tends to decrease. When

(*Text continues on page 404*)

TABLE 17-2

Misconceptions: Behaviors Indicating Addiction

Behaviors That Are Often Mistaken as Indicators of Addiction	*Correction/Comments—What Else Could It Be?*
1. The patient requests analgesics by name, dose, interval between doses, and/or route of administration; e.g., "I'll need two Vicodin every 4 hours." "Morphine, 10 mg IV, works best for my headache."	This is likely to be a well-educated patient who probably has had pain previously or has chronic pain. Patients need to be educated about all their medications, including analgesics. If this patient were a diabetic talking about insulin requirements, it would be welcomed information. This patient is providing helpful information for the pain treatment plan.
2. The patient is "a frequent flyer," frequently visiting several emergency departments (EDs) to obtain opioid analgesics.	This is not desirable behavior, but it may be caused by inadequate pain treatment. If treatment at the ED results in poor pain relief or if staff convey that the patient comes too often, the patient may go to another ED for additional pain relief or to decrease the frequency of visits to a single ED. The patient may have a chronic pain problem that is not well managed by the private physician, so the patient is forced to seek help in the ED. If patients return often to the ED, a plan should be developed and on file to document previous assessments, the effectiveness of treatments, and recommendations for initiating pain relief on subsequent ED visits.
3. The patient obtains opioids from more than one physician.	This is not desirable behavior but, like the aforementioned, may reflect poor pain management. For example, a patient's physician may prescribe an opioid/nonopioid oral analgesic (e.g., Percocet or Tylenol No. 3). The patient may find that one dose in the morning effectively relieves his pain and helps him get moving so that he can work through the day. If the physician refuses to prescribe more than 30 tablets every 3 months and suggests no other methods of pain relief, the patient may seek drugs from another physician. Improved assessment and pain treatment, including use of nonopioids and other modalities, may remedy this situation.
4. The patient requires higher doses of opioids than other patients. "He's hitting his PCA button too much."	There is no set dose of opioid that is safe and effective for all patients. Even a patient who has not received opioids regularly (opioid naive) may require 6 times more opioid than another patient. A patient who is tolerant to opioid analgesia may require 100 times more opioid than the opioid-naive patient. Some conditions, such as sickle cell crisis, are more painful than others. A patient may require much more opioid for a sickle cell crisis than for major abdominal surgery. Frequent use of the PCA button indicates that the pump parameters need to be adjusted.
5. The patient has been taking opioids frequently for a long time.	Length of time on opioids does not appear to increase the likelihood of developing addiction. Many patients with cancer or noncancer pain have taken opioids for months or longer and ceased taking them when the pain subsided. Physical dependence and tolerance may develop with prolonged use, but they are not the same as addiction.

(Continued)

TABLE 17-2

Misconceptions: Behaviors Indicating Addiction (*Continued*)

Behaviors That Are Often Mistaken as Indicators of Addiction	*Correction/Comments—What Else Could It Be?*
6. The patient is a "clock watcher" and may ask for the analgesic in advance of a specified time. The patient may say, "I'll need my next dose in about 30 minutes."	Sometimes analgesics are prescribed at intervals longer than their duration. When the patient asks for a dose before the interval elapses, the clinician often tells the patient how much time he must wait. For example, "You can't have your next pill for 2 hours." Because the patient must wait in pain for 2 hours, he is likely to note the time and ask for the medication as soon as the 2 hours pass. The patient may then find that it takes the nurse another 30 minutes to deliver the dose. The patient may work with these realities by calculating when the next dose can be given and asking for it 30 minutes in advance. This situation strongly suggests that the patient's opioid prescription should be changed to a longer acting opioid or the intervals between doses should be shortened.
7. The patient "prefers the needle to the pill."	When the same dose given parenterally is given orally, the pain relief is likely to be much less. Using an equianalgesic chart often explains the problem. For example, if a patient has been receiving morphine, 10 mg IM or IV q4h, switching the patient to an opioid/nonopioid combination, such as one Tylenol No. 3, provides only one-sixth to one-fifth as much pain relief. The solution may be to use a single entity oral opioid such as morphine. A dose of 30 mg will provide approximately the same pain relief. If pain has decreased by 50%, morphine, 15 mg PO, is indicated.
8. The patient "enjoys his Demerol."	Once pain is relieved, it is natural for the patient to feel happier and engage in more activities, such as talking and ambulating. By contrast, it may look like the patient is "high" or euphoric, but it is simply a return to normal mood, perhaps with some elation at being in less pain.
9. The patient says he is allergic to everything except one particular opioid.	Allergy to opioids is rare, but patients often mistake side effects such as nausea, vomiting, and itching for an allergy. These may have been poorly managed side effects, or the patient may have more severe side effects with some opioids than others. If the patient has more side effects with certain opioids, they should be avoided. If the patient is more convinced of the effectiveness of one opioid over others, it is possible that the patient will try to avoid the others by saying he is allergic to them. Even when an analgesic is not terribly effective, the patient may be afraid to try another analgesic for fear the results will be even worse. If it is not necessary for the patient to change to another opioid, the patient should receive what he prefers. If a change is necessary, perhaps because the opioid preferred by the patient has an active metabolite that is accumulating (a common problem with meperidine), then selection of another opioid will depend on careful assessment to determine whether the patient is allergic or whether he has experienced unmanaged or unmanageable side effects.

combined, a lower dose of opioid may be effective, with the added benefit of a decrease in side effects (Portenoy, 2000).

NSAIDs are indicated for the treatment of mild-to-moderate inflammatory or nonneuropathic pain. All NSAIDs inhibit the enzyme cyclooxygenase-1 (COX-1), which in turn impedes the production of prostaglandins that cause pain and inflammation. However, the newer COX-2 inhibitor drugs do not block the COX-1 enzyme, but selectively block the COX-2 enzyme. These drugs appear to have fewer gastrointestinal side effects than the COX-1 inhibitors. However, high dose, long-term use of COX-2 inhibitor agents have a higher rate of cardiovascular adverse effects.

The NGC (2007) offers the following guidelines:

- All NSAIDs have gastrointestinal (GI) risks of gastritis and possible bleeding. Risk benefits should be weighed especially when treating older adults or those at higher risk for GI adverse effects. Consider using in combination with the gastroprotective agent misoprostol or a proton pump inhibitor.
- Use with caution in patients with coagulopathies or thrombocytopenia and those at risk for bleeding.
- Chronic NSAID use increases the risk of renal insufficiency, especially in patients with diabetes, and patients should be monitored for signs of reduced renal function.
- Ketorolac should not be used for longer than 5 days and, therefore, is not an appropriate choice of NSAID in the treatment of chronic pain.
- NSAIDs have significant opioid dose-sparing properties and in turn may reduce opioid-related side effects.

Monitor all NSAID use including patient use of nonprescription drugs to prevent duplication of therapy and adverse effects (NGC, 2007, p. 25).

Topical Agents. Topical lidocaine 5% patches (Lidoderm) have recently been approved for pos-

therpetic neuralgia, but have also shown efficacy in other neuropathic pain syndromes. Systemic absorption of lidocaine is minimal, and the patch has a good safety profile with a dosage schedule of 12 hours on and 12 hours off. Topical creams and solutions can be used in treating both neuropathic pain and arthritic pain. Capsaicin used topically depletes the pain mediator substance-P from afferent nociceptive neurons and should be applied for at least 6 weeks to determine the full benefits (NGC, 2007).

Antidepressants. Tricyclic antidepressants (TCAs) are being used more frequently in conjunction with opioid and nonopioid analgesics in the management of chronic pain (Jackson & St. Onge, 2003; Macres, Richeimer, & Duran, 2004; Monks & Merskey, 2003). Although the mechanism of action of antidepressants is controversial, they have been found to reduce pain in both depressed and nondepressed clients (Ansari, 2000; Richeimer et al., 1997). Both tricyclic and serotonin reuptake inhibitors can be effective, but results are specific to individuals and the medication used, as is true with most groups of medications (Ansari, 2000). It is also interesting to note that when patients with chronic pain report difficulty sleeping, one of the side effects of many antidepressants, even at low doses, is falling asleep more easily and staying asleep at night. These medications are most effective if they are used in a regimen with analgesics and other strategies to manage pain (Jeffrey, 1996).

Noninvasive Methods of Pain Control

There are many noninvasive, nonpharmacologic modalities or methods that can be used to control chronic pain (Laliberte, 2003). In general, physical methods include: counterirritation, vibration, percussion, local application of heat and cold, nerve fatigue from repetitive stimulation, triggerpoint stimulation, acupuncture, therapeutic touch, physiotherapy, occupational therapy, and neuromodulation. Most of the physical methods involve application of the therapy or modality locally,

TABLE 17-3

Selection and Use of Nondrug Pain Treatments

1. Clarify the relationship between the use of nondrug pain treatments and the use of analgesics.

   - In most clinical situations (e.g., postoperative pain or cancer pain) nondrug pain treatments should be used in addition to analgesics.
   - Emphasize to the patient that nondrug therapies do not replace analgesics.

2. Assess the patient's attitude toward and experience with nondrug pain treatments.

   - If the patient has used nondrug methods, find out whether they were successful and what, if any, problems were encountered.
   - Find out whether the patient feels that personal attempts at nondrug therapies have been exhausted and that more conventional pain therapies are now appropriate.
   - Find out whether the patient is using nondrug methods to avoid using analgesics. If analgesics are appropriate, discuss the patient's concerns.

3. Ask the patient what, besides taking pain medicine, usually helps with the pain.

   - Try to identify nondrug treatments that are similar to the patient's coping style.
   - Some patients simply want more information about pain or its management, whereas others want to divert their attention away from pain.
   - Many patients naturally use distraction to cope with pain. For these patients, providing a selection of music or videotapes may be helpful.

4. Assess the patient's level of fatigue, cognitive status, and ability to concentrate and follow instructions.

   - Optimal functioning in these areas is desirable to learn and to use a technique such as relaxation imagery but is unnecessary if a cold pack is used.
   - Some patients barely have enough time to perform required activities of daily living. Adding a lengthy relaxation technique may simply increase stress and decrease the patient's sense of control.

5. Ask the patient's family/friends if they wish to be involved in nondrug pain treatments.

   - In home care, the primary caregiver may already be overburdened and have no time or energy to help the patient with a technique such as massage.
   - Some family/friends may welcome a technique like massage that allows them to touch the patient and "do something." However, not all patients or family members are comfortable with techniques that involve touch.

6. Provide the patient and family with adequate support materials.

   - Whenever possible, supply written or audiotaped instructions for even the simplest techniques.
   - Determine whether the appropriate equipment is available. If not, can the patient afford to purchase it? If not, identify less expensive nondrug materials or therapies.

although a systemic effect may occur (e.g., acupuncture). Central methods, which help individuals accept and live with their pain include the doctrines of yoga and transcendental meditation, distraction, and relaxation (progressive muscle relaxation or guided imagery), psychotherapy, operant conditioning, and behavior modification. These methods can be effective, although research is limited.

Determining the effectiveness of noninvasive methods for each client requires a trial-and-error approach to determine what works in each unique situation (Table 17-3). Open communication is essential between patients and professionals to identify modalities and to evaluate their effectiveness. Believing the client is essential. Use of multiple modalities or techniques may be more effective than a single method. Only a few of the myriad methods are reviewed here. For further details, please see McCaffery and Pasero (1999) or any of the other references cited on this topic.

Cutaneous Stimulation. Cutaneous stimulation refers to stimulating the skin for the purpose of relieving pain, especially localized pain. Although the exact mechanism is unknown, the gate control theory suggests that stimulation of the skin may activate the large-diameter fibers that close the gate to pain messages carried by small fibers. Cutaneous stimulation may also work by increasing endorphins and/or decreasing sensitivity to pain.

Cutaneous stimulation is not curative. Although the effects are variable and unpredictable, the intensity of pain is usually reduced during or after stimulation. Some kinds of stimulation work best with acute localized pain; whereas other methods are effective with chronic pain. Many methods of cutaneous stimulation require little participation or action on the part of patients, which makes them appropriate for people who have limited physical or mental energy (see Table 17-4 for a description of cutaneous stimulation methods). Potential benefits include decreased pain intensity; relief of muscle spasm that is secondary to underlying skeletal or joint pathology, or nerve root irritation; and, increased physical activity (Kubsch, Neveau, & Vandertie, 2000).

Distraction. Distraction from pain is achieved by focusing attention on a stimulus other than the pain sensation. Just as children can be distracted by involving them in other activities, family can provide distraction for either adults or children who have chronic pain (Rapoff & Lindsley, 2000). Reading, singing, listening to music, and humor are some of the methods used for distraction (Mobily, Herr, & Kelley, 1993). Distraction works by relegating the pain to the periphery of awareness, but does not eliminate it.

Distraction is easy to learn and is effective as long as the distracting stimulus is present. Even if pain is severe, the pain is less intense if the focus is on another sensory input or on the less bothersome qualities of the pain sensation, such as pressure or warmth. Not only does distraction help to ease pain, but focusing on pleasant things also improves mood, which helps to counteract depression and leads to a sense of control over the painful experience. Any form of distraction requires clients to understand instructions, have the physical ability and energy to perform the activities, and have the ability to concentrate on the stimulus or stimuli being presented.

Relaxation. Relaxation should be used as an adjunct to other pain relief methods. It is not a substitute for medications or other methods, because it does not relieve pain directly. The goals of relaxation are to facilitate the reduction of physiologic tension (in muscles and other structures) and to provide psychologic calming or unwinding. Relaxation breaks the cycle of stress, pain, muscle tension, and anxiety. Ideally, clients achieve the relaxation response: normal blood pressure; decrease in respiratory rate, heart rate, and oxygen consumption; reduction in muscle tension; increase in the brain's alpha waves; and improvement of mood (Laliberte, 2003; McCaffery & Pasero, 1999; Schaffer & Yucha, 2004).

All relaxation methods have been found to be effective for some persons some of the time (Carroll & Seers, 1998). However, to be effective, these methods must be practiced daily. Just as muscles become weak without daily exercise or use, the effectiveness of these methods are lost without regular practice.

Progressive muscle relaxation is an example of one relaxation technique that has proven helpful. It has been practiced for centuries as part of meditation but currently is also used to reduce pain intensity. It can be self-taught, but is usually easier to learn if another person provides verbal direction. Books and videotapes that can be used when there is no one to read instructions, can be found in the health sections of most large bookstores. Tables 17-5 and 17-6 include characteristics of various techniques and guidelines for their use.

TABLE 17-4

Pointers on Selecting a Method of Cutaneous Stimulation

▪ Massage	Minimal side effects and contraindications. Backrubs or body massage can be time consuming and may relieve only mild pain, but pain need not be localized and most patients enjoy it. Modest patients may object to touch or disrobing. Massage of feet and hands may be more accessible, acceptable, and even more effective.
▪ Pressure, sometimes with massage	Massage/pressure to trigger points or acupuncture points may be very effective but is briefly uncomfortable. Initially it requires time to locate the points. But then patients can learn to work on some trigger points on their own.
▪ Vibration	A more vigorous form of massage that may be more effective. Low risk of tissue damage. Check on availability or cost of a vibrator. May be used for trigger points. May be unacceptable due to noise or intensity of stimulation if vibrator is not adjustable. Sometimes this is a less expensive substitute for TENS.
▪ Heat and cold	Probably works best for well-localized pain. Both may be done with a minimum of equipment and both should be applied at a comfortable level of intensity. Cold has more advantages than heat. Unwanted side effects (e.g., burns, and contraindications—bleeding and swelling) are more frequent with heating than with cooling. When cold relieves pain, it tends to be more effective than heat. However, patients usually prefer heat to cold, and use of cold often requires some persuasion.
▪ Ice application/massage	A frozen substance applied to the skin is uncomfortable, but only for a few minutes before numbness occurs. Continuous use for ten minutes or less. Pain must be well localized. May relieve severe pain. Simple, low-risk technique for brief, painful procedures. Especially effective in obliterating needle-stick pain. May be used on trigger points. Sometimes this is a very inexpensive substitute for TENS.
▪ Menthol	Refers to menthol-containing substances for application to skin. Intensity increases with amount of menthol; may be uncomfortable at higher concentrations. Odor offensive to some people. Use influenced by culture; more restricted use by Americans than other cultures (e.g., Asians). Inexpensive. Once it is applied, it provides continuous stimulation without additional effort. Well suited for nighttime use.
▪ TENS	Compared with above methods, much more expensive, less available, and more time needed to teach nurse and patient, but supported by more research and regarded by many as more "scientific."

Source: Reproduced by permission from McCaffery, M., & Beebe, A. (1989). *Pain: Clinical manual for nursing practice.* St. Louis: The C.V. Mosby Company.

Participants are asked to focus on specific muscle groups, to tense or tighten them for 5 seconds, to relax them, and then to focus on the relaxed muscles. This process is repeated in a systematic pattern for the entire body (Laliberte, 2003; Schaffer & Yucha, 2004).

Imagery. Imagery is the interpretation of what humans intentionally visualize and what is experienced in a symbolic manner. Through the use of imagery, patients can learn to modify their outlook, which can be helpful in reducing pain (Burte, 2002; Lewandowski, 2004). Imagery is not a strategy that all patients can use or that all healthcare professionals can teach. When used as a form of distraction from pain, it increases tolerance; when used to produce relaxation, it decreases distress. Imagery can also produce an image of pain relief that decreases the perceived intensity of the pain. Hypnosis, which requires additional training on

TABLE 17-5

Practical Guidelines for Matching Relaxation Techniques to Patients and Situations

1. Consider the *amount of time* the patient will experience pain vs. the time involved in teaching and using the technique. Usually:

   ■ Use the less time-consuming techniques for brief episodes of pain (e.g., jaw relaxation or slow rhythmic breathing for procedural or postoperative pain).
   ■ Be willing to invest more time for patients with chronic pain (e.g., peaceful past experiences or meditative relaxation for cancer pain or recurrent headaches).
   ■ Beware of introducing time-consuming techniques to patients who are already under considerable stress, even if they have chronic pain, since this may add another stressor.

2. Consider how pain, fatigue, anxiety, and other factors influence the *patient's general ability to learn or engage in an activity.* Usually:

   ■ Use brief, simple techniques or massage during severe pain, lack of concentration, or along with other pain relief measures (e.g., deep breath/tense, exhale/relax, yawn), when narcotic is given, such as for renal colic.

■ Teach more time-consuming techniques when the patient is alert and comfortable (e.g., meditative relaxation when severe back pain is in remission).
■ Even if the patient says relaxation is not helpful during pain or the anticipated pain will be too severe for him to use relaxation, suggest he use it before and after pain.

3. Note if the patient has *energy that needs to be dissipated* (e.g., restless, "up-tight," or the "fight or flight" response—meaning that he has generated energy to fight or flee but has nowhere to go). Use a technique that releases energy (e.g., progressive relaxation).

4. For the *patient who misunderstands the purpose of relaxation*, use other terminology and suggest humor, peaceful past experiences, or passive recipient techniques such as a back rub.

5. *Consider whether the focus is inward on the body or outward on peaceful scenes.* An inward focus can increase distress about changes in body image or feelings of failure about physical limitations. Be cautious about using an exclusively inward body focus for patients who are distressed about changes in body appearance or function, severely depressed, or have difficulty maintaining contact with reality.

Source: Reproduced by permission from McCaffery, M., & Beebe, A. (1989). *Pain: Clinical manual for nursing practice.* St. Louis: The C.V. Mosby Company.

the part of the professional, often uses imagery as a technique (Holroyd, 1996). No form of imagery should be used with resistant patients, regardless of the good intentions of qualified healthcare professionals.

Complementary or Alternative Therapies. Although complementary or alternative therapies remain controversial, they are often used by persons with chronic pain, typically in conjunction with traditional treatment (Haetzman et al., 2003). There is growing scientific evidence that alternative therapies can reduce chronic pain (Berman & Swyers, 1999; Lee, 2000; NIH, 1995). Two of the

therapies that have been evaluated are acupuncture and therapeutic touch. Acupuncture, used for centuries in "Eastern medicine," can reduce pain intensity for adults (Ezzo et al., 2000; Leibing et al., 2002; Nabeta & Kawakita, 2002) and for children (Kemper et al., 2000). Therapeutic touch has been shown to decrease both pain and anxiety for older adults with degenerative arthritis (Lin & Taylor, 1998; Smith, Arnstein, Rosa, & Wells-Federman, 2002). Clinical research with randomized, placebo-controlled trials supports the use of acupuncture for certain chronic pain conditions such as fibromyalgia, headache, back pain, neck pain, and osteoarthritis of the knee (NGC, 2007).

TABLE 17-6

Characteristics of Specific Relaxation Techniques and Indications for Use

Deep breath/tense, exhale/relax, yawn	This takes only a few seconds; is easily learned by patient; is appropriate to introduce when patient is already tense and in pain (e.g., during a procedure) or may be taught prior to brief painful procedures or preoperatively.
Humor	This takes very little of the nurse's time to suggest to patients; patients may spend as much time as they wish using it. It may be appropriate for patients who are elderly; who resist or misunderstand the idea of relaxation; who are depressed or easily lose contact with reality; who have little time or energy for learning the skill of relaxation; or who are from a different culture (assuming a tape from that culture can be obtained). It may be used to relieve boredom of prolonged pain under confining circumstances; also appropriate for brief procedural pain.
Heartbeat breathing	The nurse may have to teach the patient how to find and count the radial pulse, and some patients may have difficulty with this. If not, it takes very little of the nurse's or patient's time. Heartbeat breathing has an internal focus but is used only briefly. It may relieve a sudden, sharp increase in fear or anxiety and may be used without others noticing. It may be very helpful to patients who are aware of a sudden increase in heart rate during stress.
Jaw relaxation	This takes very little time for the nurse to teach or for the patient to use. It is considered an abbreviated form of progressive relaxation. Its effectiveness may be due to relaxation of one area of the body, leading to relaxation of the rest of the body. Useful for brief moderate to severe pain (e.g., postoperative pain), especially if taught in the absence of severe pain and tension. Effective with elderly patients.
Slow rhythmic breathing	This takes very little of the nurse's time to teach. It is very adaptable; patient can use for 30 to 60 seconds (a few breaths without others noticing) or for up to 20 minutes. It is also a useful technique for initial relaxation prior to engaging in more complex relaxation techniques.
Peaceful past experiences	This may prove to be the best of all approaches to relaxation since it relies on what the patient has already found relaxing. It is usually an outward focus (i.e., not focused on the present body state). Recalling a peaceful experience is often a therapeutic process, and this approach may be the most appropriate for patients with chronic pain, particularly those with terminal illness. Remembering certain past experiences may serve many purposes (e.g., releasing or letting go of treasured events or reinforcing the conviction that a valued event will occur again). However, the sharing of a valued past experience may require a trusting relationship between the nurse and patient. This may take a considerable amount of the nurse's time, but not always. Give *priority* to this for terminally ill patients, and tape record it.
Meditative relaxation script	This usually takes a minimum of three contacts with the patient. The first two take about 15 minutes each. The second usually involves tape recording the script. The third is a follow-up and may take only a minute unless problems occur. The script is highly effective in producing relaxation in English-speaking, middle-class Americans. It is permissive enough that patients can individualize it on their own, and it combines an inward focus (breathing techniques and modified progressive relaxation) with an outward focus (peaceful place). Even when patients say that certain options in the script are not helpful to them, it is seldom necessary to rerecord the tape, since patients usually say they simply ignore what does not help them.

(Continued)

TABLE 17-6

Characteristics of Specific Relaxation Techniques and Indications for Use (*Continued*)

Progressive relaxation script	Give *priority* to this (or peaceful past experiences or progressive relaxation) for patients with prolonged pain. It takes more time than you may have and it is not a miracle, but it often makes a significant difference.
	This also usually takes a minimum of three contacts with the patient for a total of 35 minutes or more. The first two contacts take about 15 minutes. The second usually involves tape-recording the technique. The third is a follow-up and may take only a few minutes, unless problems have occurred.
	Its potential advantages are that it involves physical activity that gives a sense of "doing something" (e. g. , muscle contraction, dissipates energy), is focused inward without the necessity of keeping the eyes closed, does not rely exclusively on mental activity, and easily gets the patients' attention by asking them to perform specific tasks.
	Give this *priority* for patients with prolonged pain who exhibit signs of moderate to severe anxiety or "fight or flight," especially if they cannot engage in their customary physical exercise. They need to get rid of that muscular energy. Later they may benefit from a more meditative approach.
Simple touch, massage, or warmth	This may be done by the nurse or the patient's family or friends. It need not take much time and is indicated for patients who do not have time or energy to do for themselves whatever would produce relaxation. Loved ones who want to feel useful may benefit themselves and the patient by committing to body rubs of only 3 minutes (e.g., back, feet, hands). Help family and friends identify definite times for performing body rubs. This gives structure for the patient and the loved ones

Source: Reproduced by permission from McCaffery, M., & Beebe, A. (1989). *Pain: Clinical manual for nursing practice.* St. Louis: The C.V. Mosby Company.

Healthcare professionals need information about the most common alternative therapies to understand and support the decisions made by their patients. Maintaining open communication is important so patients feel comfortable talking about all interventions/strategies they are using to manage their pain. These therapies are numerous and beyond the scope of this chapter to describe (see Chapter 18).

Pain Management Programs

Pain management programs are not new. Aronoff (2004) describes the inception of such programs 35 years ago when there was a shift in focus from traditional medical treatment (e.g., medications, nerve blocks) to treating chronic pain different from acute pain. Growth in the numbers and types of pain management programs is an indicator of the need for more effective pain management strategies for those with chronic pain. Pain management programs help patients better manage their pain and regain some control of their lives. Such programs seek to: decrease pain intensity and pain-related disability; improve mood and decrease depression; decrease use of the healthcare system and medications; and increase independence in activities of daily living, involvement with family, and social activities.

A multidisciplinary/interdisciplinary (M/I) approach for the treatment of noncancer chronic pain has become very popular. The implementation of interdisciplinary pain management is a relatively new concept in Japan. A recent study by Kitaha, Kojima, and Ohmura (2006) evaluated the effectiveness of multidisciplinary/interdisciplinary pain treatment in Japanese patients with chronic noncancer pain. Results demonstrated: (1) 68.9% of patients reported a significant decrease in pain; (2) 92% stopped using inappropriate medication including NSAIDs, benzodiazepines, and muscle relaxants; (3) 51.4% were able to perform their usual daily activities without being disturbed by pain; and (4) 75% who had been unemployed because of pain returned to work. Overall, the treatment succeeded in 56.8% of the patients. The results suggest that interdisciplinary treatment based upon the biopsychosocial model of pain is associated with significant improvement in multiple outcomes in this sample of Japanese patients with chronic pain.

FIGURE 17-4

Pain Management Algorithm

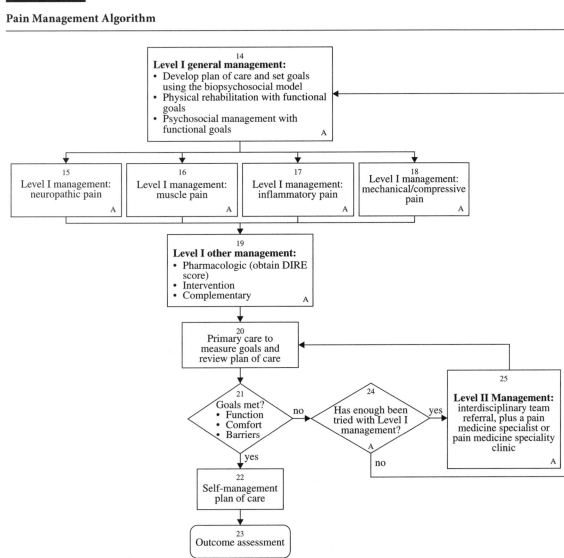

Source: Institute for Clinical Systems Improvement (ICSI). (2007). *Assessment and management of chronic pain.* Bloomington, MN: Institute for Clinical Systems Improvement.

Outcomes for Pain Management

According to Davis and White (2001), the nurse or healthcare professional should assist patients in setting realistic expectations regarding the outcomes of various pain management methods. For example, individuals generally expect some relief of pain within a given period of time when taking medication. An important role for nurses and other healthcare professionals is making patients aware of other methods discussed in this chapter that may be appropriate for their use and then assisting them to use the methods correctly. Being aware of and learning to use a variety of different management methods is important so that the best combination for each patient can be selected at any given time. Given this conceptualization of pain management, determining what management strategies are being used, how well they are perceived to be working, and the individual's confidence about using them is an essential component of outcome evaluation.

Pain control and/or management must be evaluated by the patient. Being pain free may be an achievable outcome in acute pain, but in chronic pain, the level of pain that is determined to be achievable and acceptable may not be a 0 on a 10-point scale. Patients are encouraged to set goals with their healthcare professionals. For some, this will be low pain intensity, and for others, it may be the ability to be involved in activities of daily living, even with pain present. The key to a successful outcome of the individual's pain management program is an ongoing evaluation and dialog between the patient and provider. It is not a static or linear process, but rather an ongoing strategy that is flexible and revised as needed according to patient responses, needs, and desires. If a treatment plan fails to achieve the desired outcomes when the patient is following the plan, then the plan needs to be modified. If the patient is not able to adhere to the plan, then the nurse should address barriers, and further evaluate stressors, life events, or motivation. Attainable goals can lead to "restructuring a life that has often been significantly altered by chronic pain" (NGC, 2007).

Figure 17-4 is the pain management algorithm that has been developed by the Institute for Clinical Systems Improvement.

DEPRESSION

Definition

Depression is defined by the Dana Farber Cancer Institute (2007) as a mental condition marked by ongoing feelings of sadness, despair, loss of energy, and difficulty dealing with normal daily life. Other symptoms of depression include feelings of worthlessness and hopelessness, loss of pleasure in activities, changes in eating or sleeping habits, and thoughts of death or suicide.

Diagnosis of Depression

The *Diagnostic and Statistical Manual of Mental Disorders*, 4th Edition (*DSM IV*) states that five of the following criteria must be present at the same time for a diagnosis of depression:

One of the following two must be present:

■ Depressed mood most of the day or every day
■ Markedly diminished interest or pleasure in most activities

Plus four of the following (three, if both criteria above are present):

■ Significant weight gain or loss
■ Insomnia or hypersomnia
■ Fatigue
■ Feelings of worthlessness
■ Diminished capacity to concentrate
■ Recurrent thoughts of death or suicide

The PHQ-9 form (Figure 17-5) is a form from Pfizer that is free to download and may be used to assess patients for depression.

Treatment

According to the National Institute for Clinical Evidence (2004), the most appropriate method

FIGURE 17-5

Patient Health Questionnaire (PHQ-9)

NAME:_____ DATE:_____

Over the last 2 weeks, how often have you been
bothered by any of the following problems?
(use "✓" to indicate your answer)

	Not at all	Several days	More than half the days	Nearly every day
1. Little interest or pleasure in doing things	0	1	2	3
2. Feeling down, depressed, or hopeless	0	1	2	3
3. Trouble falling or staying asleep, or sleeping too much	0	1	2	3
4. Feeling tired or having little energy	0	1	2	3
5. Poor appetite or overeating	0	1	2	3
6. Feeling bad about yourself—or that you are a failure or have let yourself or your family down	0	1	2	3
7. Trouble concentrating on things, such as reading the newspaper or watching television	0	1	2	3
8. Moving or speaking so slowly that other people could have noticed. Or the opposite—being so fidgety or restless that you have been moving around a lot more than usual	0	1	2	3
9. Thoughts that you would be better off dead, or of hurting yourself in some way	0	1	2	3

add columns: _____ + _____ + _____

TOTAL: _____

10. If you checked off any problems, how difficult have these problems made it for you to do your work, take care of things at home, or get along with other people?

Not difficult at all _____
Somewhat difficult _____
Very difficult _____
Extremely difficult _____

Source: Adapted from PRIME MD TODAY, developed by Drs Robert L. Spitzer, Janet B. W. Williams, Kurt Kroenke, and colleagues, with an educational grant from Pfizer Inc. For research information, contact Dr Spitzer at rls8@columbia.edu. Use of the PHQ-9 may only be made in accordance with the Terms of Use available at http://www.pfizer.com. Copyright 1999 Pfizer Inc. All rights reserved. PRIME MD TODAY is a trademark of Pfizer Inc.

for treating depression in chronic disease is to use the Step Method. This progressive model establishes five steps in the progression of depression and uses a matrix format to identify and address all the stressors and available resources for each individual. The five steps begin with the basics and add complexity and intensity as they increase in number. It should be noted that the progression assumes that each of the tasks in the previous step have been addressed adequately.

The Step Method includes the following steps (National Institute for Clinical Evidence (2004):

1. Recognition of depression in primary care and hospital settings
2. Managing recognized depression in primary care—mild depression
3. Managing recognized depression in primary care—moderate to severe depression
4. Involvement of specialist mental health services including crisis teams treatment-resistant, recurrent, atypical, and psychotic depression, and those at significant risk
5. Depression needing inpatient care

Step 1: Recognition of Depression in Primary Care and Hospital Settings

Patients do not usually present with complaints of depression. Most present with some form of somatic complaint without an apparent cause. Patients with chronic illness should be routinely screened for depression, as they require medications and treatments that in and of themselves may be the etiology of some of the depression (National Institute for Clinical Evidence, 2004).

Step 2: Recognized Depression in Primary Care Settings–Mild Depression

The majority of people with mild to moderate depression are treated by their primary care provider. Many will respond to distraction or self-help guidance. Others will require more structured

therapies, such as personal problem-solving, periods of cognitive–behavioral therapy (CBT), or counseling.

General Measures to Help Patients Cope. Rest is nature's way of restoring a person's sense of balance. Patients with chronic diseases face disruption in the normal sleep cycle due to complications of their disease process and bouts of depression. Care should be afforded to offer advice to ensure proper rest. Adding a medication or therapeutic intervention to established regimens may further burden the patient and family and only exacerbate the situation. Sometimes it is best to give the "episode" time and see if it will pass.

Exercise is another natural method to reestablish a patient's personal balance. Aside from the established health benefits surrounding exercise, persons with depression may experience a sense of self-actualization by becoming a more active participant in their therapeutic regimen. It also serves in the distraction of negative thoughts to more positive ideas. Exercise should take the form of structured sessions spread out over the course the week.

A program of guided self-help should consist of take-home materials that providers distribute to patients. These should be discussed when they are given to the patient and should be reviewed periodically to ensure that the patient is performing them and receiving and/or attaining the desired outcomes.

Psychological Interventions. For mild depression, a number of brief psychological interventions are effective. The choice of treatment should reflect the patient's preference based on informed discussion, past experience of treatment, and the fact that the patient may not have benefited from other brief interventions. For all treatments the strength of the therapeutic alliance is important in ensuring a good outcome. Problem-solving is a brief treatment that can readily be learned by practicing nurses.

Antidepressant Drugs. The use of medications in patients with chronic illnesses is not considered a first-line therapy, owing to the existing debilitated states and complex medication regimens already used to treat the underlying conditions. The potential of drug interactions and risks associated with the individual medications must be considered first. However, with depression, in randomized controlled trial evidence, in patients with mild to moderate depression, there is little clinically important difference between the therapeutic effects of antidepressants and placebo. Medications should be considered after failure of alternative therapies or in those who are displaying medical or psychological problems associated with their depression (National Institute for Clinical Evidence, 2004).

Step 3: Recognized Depression in Primary Care Settings—Moderate or Severe

Moderate or severe depression can be treated in the primary care setting but is more likely to require the addition of care provided by practitioners with advanced and specialized training. The greatest fear and/or risk with deepening depression can be the risk of suicide. Along with this consideration is the risk that depressed patients with chronic diseases pose to others.

Antidepressant Drugs. There is an extensive body of research about the effectiveness and use of medications to treat more severe depression. Classic risk–benefit calculations offer greater latitude in the justification of drug use when the condition is more severe. Some medications are known to increase the severity of the depression for a time before they get to therapeutic levels. Therefore, monitoring for the presence of side effects is crucial in the early stages of drug therapy. These patients will often have had previous therapies and these should form the base of the decision as to type, dose, and length of drug therapy. Antidepressants may take a long period to attain therapeutic levels and also require equally lengthy periods to discontinue. They also pose problems is not taken as directed (National Institute for Clinical Evidence, 2004).

Step 4: Specialist Mental Health Services— Treatment-Resistant, Recurrent, Atypical, and Psychotic Depression, and Those at Significant Risk

Some of the depression associated with chronic disease will not respond to therapy. The underlying conditions or the depression itself may be so severe or advanced that even specialized interventions will be limited in their scope and effectiveness.

Treatment-Resistant Depression. This is defined as depression that fails to respond to two or more antidepressant medications given at an adequate dose for an adequate time. Such patients could benefit from psychological interventions such as counseling and/or the more radical treatments like electroconvulsive therapies (National Institute for Clinical Evidence, 2004).

Step 5: Depression Needing Inpatient Care

When patients have not responded to efforts performed outside of the specialized in-patient settings, they are, by definition, candidates for inpatient care. There are some interventions that can be performed only as an inpatient, such as the electroconvulsive therapy. Patients that pose threats to themselves or others are required by law to be placed in these specialized settings, either voluntarily or on an involuntary basis.

Treatment often takes the form of a combination of medication and therapeutic communication, in either an individual or a group setting. Healthcare professionals may be able to help mildly depressed persons through their depression by helping them understand it. Persons with chronic disease are already using the majority if not all their coping mechanisms and often will require medications to control the symptoms particular to their depression.

Drugs that treat the symptoms of depression are selected according to the patient's current issues. Many new drugs have entered the markets that address specific components of behavior. One major issue with these medications are their costs, interaction with the medications that patients are already taking to treat their underlying conditions, and the side effects (National Institute for Clinical Evidence, 2004).

An alternative to classic medication intervention for depression is the use of cognitive therapy. Sadovsky (2002, p. 1902) defined cognitive therapy as "a focused, structured, collaborative, and usually short-term psychological therapy that aims to facilitate problem solving and to modify dysfunctional thinking and behavior." This type of therapy has documented success in dealing with mood disorders and fatigue. Self-management and collaboration are important principles of therapy and emphasize building skills with which the patient can manage psychological problems. A key principle of cognitive therapy in the treatment of depression is recognizing the interrelationship of behavior, mood, thoughts, beliefs, and physical feelings. Cognitive therapy usually includes homework that involves cognitive and behavioral strategies designed to diminish factors that cause symptoms and help the patient control both physical and psychological feelings.

Summary

Depression associated with chronic illness is estimated to occur in roughly one third of these individuals. Depression can often appear at the time of diagnosis, as the patient must address the reality of a chronic illness, while attempting to form a plan for addressing the illness and the life-changing processes that will inevitably follow. The diagnosis may trigger depression as the emotional and coping mechanisms the individual possesses are overwhelmed by the realities of the disease and the doubts posed for the future.

In the population as a whole, the rate of diagnosed depression is estimated at 10–25% for women and 5–12% for men. According to Cleveland Clinic findings (2002), the rate of depression occurring with physical illnesses is quite high:

- Heart attack: 40–65%
- Coronary artery disease (without heart attack): 18–20%

- Parkinson's disease: 40%
- Multiple sclerosis: 40%
- Stroke: 10–27%
- Cancer: 25%
- Diabetes: 25%

These chronic illnesses themselves are often aggravated by depression. Symptoms such as pain and fatigue are magnified and cause greater disruption in the patient's life, making treatment more difficult. Depression also tends to make people withdraw from normal activities causing social isolation.

FATIGUE

Fatigue is a common term used to describe that time of the day or period during one's life where they lack the vigor and/or energy they perceive as normal. However, according the Glaus, Crow, and Hammond (1996), persons with known chronic disease perceive this sensation of fatigue as more intense, and it forms a greater threat to the individual's sense of well-being. Dittner, Janson, Facione, Wessley, and Brown (2004) postulate that fatigue should not be described in terms of a linear measurement from absence to one of debilitation, but a more complex analysis of fatigue on the physical plane, how the patient perceives the threat, and how it affects the patient's emotional well-being and their ability to perform activities of daily living.

Fatigue is a nonspecific symptom that is common in individuals with chronic diseases or conditions (McPhee & Schroeder, 1999). For many chronic diseases, fatigue is present every day to some degree and often worsens with increased disease activity. Fatigue affects every aspect of a client's life and may interfere with his or her ability to carry out activities of daily living related to self-care as well as the ability to perform family and societal roles.

The goal in caring for the individual with fatigue is to find ways to reduce fatigue or assist the client in managing its effects. Care of the individual with fatigue involves the active participation of the client, who is in charge of living with and managing the illness and symptoms on a daily basis.

Significance of Fatigue

Fatigue commonly occurs with illnesses that induce pain, fever, infection, diarrhea, bed rest, extreme stress, disturbed sleep, anxiety, or depression. Fatigue is recognized as a side effect of cancer treatment (Meek et al., 2000; Stone, Hardy, Huddart, A'Hern, & Richardson, 2000; Stone, Richardson, A'Hern, & Hardy, 2000). Reduced physical activity can lead to fatigue, but, conversely, fatigue can lead to reduced physical activity. When manifested in a clinical situation fatigue in its mildest form may represent a sense of resistance to initiating or performing tasks that are possible to overcome. Although on the opposite end of this continuum, fatigue represents a sense of total exhaustion with an overwhelming lack of desire or capacity to perform tasks, which leads to inactivity.

Defining Fatigue

Multiple factors contribute to the experience of fatigue, and the pattern of onset, duration, and the progression of fatigue may vary with specific disorders (Piper et al., 1989). With multiple factors involved, defining fatigue has been a challenge. Fatigue has been described from different perspectives (Aaronson et al., 1999). At the cellular level, studies have been conducted with muscle fatigue—a condition in which recovery can occur after rest (MacLaren, Gibson, Parry-Billings, & Edwards, 1989). From a neurologic perspective, fatigue has been described as central (malfunction of the central nervous system) and peripheral (impaired neuromuscular transmission). From a psychological perspective, fatigue has been described as a product of boredom or reduced motivation (Lee, Hicks & Nino-Murcia, 1991). Clients often experience difficulty describing their fatigue, relying on metaphors to describe their experience (Potter, 2004). Further complicating definitions of fatigue is the fact that the exact mechanism that causes fatigue in many chronic diseases is unknown. Fatigue can be documented subjectively and objectively, but little is known about the pathophysiology involved.

Problems and Issues with Fatigue

Fatigue affects physical functioning and can interfere with performance of self-care activities of daily living such as dressing, bathing, and eating. If fatigue interferes with the preparation or eating of food, malnutrition and weight loss can occur, which can increase the level of fatigue. Decreasing one's level of physical activity contributes to development problems associated with immobility, such as constipation, decreased muscle strength and loss of muscle mass, and lower overall physical and social isolation.

Fatigue can cause social isolation. The fatigued client may avoid contact with others, feeling that it takes too much energy to communicate effectively or participate in group activities. This normal reaction may remove the client from those who could be most supportive. Invitations to social events may diminish or cease completely if the ill person consistently declines such invitations. This leaves the person isolated, with a sense of loss, and may initiate the grief process. Grief can manifest itself in many forms, such as denial, pain, depression, loss of appetite, disturbed sleep, and/or guilt.

Fatigue may have an impact on spirituality, especially if the fatigue occurs in the context of terminal illness. Results of a study examining the fatigue experience in patients with advanced cancer revealed that patients used fatigue as an indicator of where they were in the process of their illness (Potter, 2004). Potter suggests that the meaning of fatigue may be integrated into the process of coping with a terminal illness and impending death, and may determine reactions to fatigue.

Fatigue may have an impact on QOL. Fatigue has been negatively associated with global QOL in clients with prostate cancer receiving hormone therapy (Stone et al., 2000) and with different aspects of QOL in patients with ankylosing spondylitis, with different domains of QOL explained by different dimensions of fatigue (Claudepierre, 2005).

Measurement of Fatigue

Measurement of fatigue is important because measurement determines whether interventions have been effective in decreasing fatigue levels. There are a number of instruments that have been developed to measure fatigue. Instruments include: (1) Fatigue Severity Scale (Krupp, LaRocca, Muir-Nash, & Steinberg, 1989); (2) Visual Analog Scale for Fatigue (Lee, Hicks, & Nino-Murcia, 1991); (3) Multidimensional Assessment of Fatigue (Tack, 1990); (4) Profile of Mood States short form fatigue subscale (McNair, Lorr, & Droppleman, 1992); (5) Short Form-36 Vitality Subscale of the Short Form Health Survey; and (6) Fatigue Questionnaire (Chalder et al., 1993). A discussion of these instruments is beyond the scope of this chapter, but Neuberger (2003) provides a thorough description and critique of many of them.

Fatigue and Other Symptoms

Fatigue does not occur in isolation from other symptoms of chronic illness, and other symptoms may affect the experience of fatigue (Dodd, Miaskowski, & Paul, 2001; Gift, Stommel, Jablonski, & Given, 2003). Symptoms such as anorexia and/or cachexia, leading to weight loss, can affect the energy available for daily activities. Other symptoms such as breathlessness or dyspnea (Oh, Kim, Lee, & Kim, 2004; Potter, 2004), negative mood states such as anxiety or depression (Oh et al., 2004; Phillips et al., 2004), and poor sleep quality (Phillips et al., 2004) can increase the severity of fatigue. A holistic approach is necessary to assess all of the factors that may be contributing to the fatigue of each patient.

Coping with pain takes both physical and mental energy. Research supports a positive relationship between pain and fatigue in clients with rheumatoid arthritis (RA) (Belza et al., 1993; Huyser et al., 1998; Neuberger et al., 1997), and in clients with ankylosing spondylitis (Claudepierre, 2005).

Cultural Influences

Each culture has a different activity orientation, referring to a group's perception of themselves as "doing" or "being." People from "doing"-oriented cultures value achievement, whereas, persons from "being"-oriented cultures value inherent existence (Giger & Davidhizer, 2004). Compared with persons from a being-oriented culture, a person from a doing-oriented culture may have a more difficult time coping with fatigue and may find it more difficult to set personal limits on activities.

Patients may use a variety of approaches to help reduce or limit the effects of fatigue. A variety of alternative and complementary therapies are available and attractive to such persons. Examples of such therapies include acupuncture, biofeedback, meditation, diet-based therapies, homeopathic treatments, folk medicine, massage, hypnosis, therapeutic touch, aromatic therapy, and guided imagery. According to the National Center for Complementary and Alternative Medicine (2004), approximately 36% of adults are using some form of complementary and alternative medicine in the United States, and the percentage increases to 62% when megavitamin therapy and prayer specific for health reasons are added. In addition, many people consult the Old Farmer's Almanac or the Zodiac to determine the best time to perform activities or receive health-related procedures; others may depend on dreams as a reliable source of guidance (Giger & Davidhizer, 2004). By the time some patients with fatigue seek conventional medicine, the nurse might correctly assume that every home remedy known to the client, as well as a variety of alternative and complementary therapies, has been tried.

Nurses and other healthcare professionals should assess the remedies that patients have used to reduce the level of fatigue, and try to determine if the practices are harmful, neutral, or beneficial. To determine whether a current practice is harmful, Giger and Davidhizer (2004) suggest that the nurse ask the patient if the practice has worked. If the patient answers "no," the nurse may suggest that a different approach be tried. If the client believes that the harmful practice is beneficial, the nurse must provide education on the potential consequences of the harmful practice (Giger & Davidhizer, 2004).

Assessment of Fatigue

Potential interview questions about fatigue include the following (Dzurec, 2000):

- In your own words, how would you describe your experience with fatigue?
- How long have you been bothered with fatigue?
- Has fatigue had any effect on your relationships with other people, especially with family or significant others?
- What time of day does your fatigue occur?
- What activities increase your fatigue?
- Has anything helped your fatigue?

Encourage the client to keep a diary of their daily activities for one week and write down the times when fatigue occurs. These data can assist the healthcare professional and the patient in planning appropriate interventions. At follow-up in a busy clinical setting, nurses may simply ask clients to rate their level of fatigue on a scale of 0 to 10. Recording these verbal assessments at each patient visit or contact will aid the nurse in assessing whether interventions are helpful in reducing fatigue.

Wearden (2006) discusses the use of pragmatic rehabilitation, supportive listening, and general treatment measures to control fatigue. Pragmatic rehabilitation involves providing patients with a detailed explanation of their symptoms in terms of such physiologic explanations as the effects on their circadian rhythm alteration through disrupted sleep patterns. Patients are encouraged to address these issues that are within their control and increase knowledge of those outside their scope. The aim of the supportive listening treatment arm is to provide emotional support and validation for the patient through the development of a collaborative relationship in which the patient is held in unconditional positive regard and encouraged to talk about his or her experiences.

General Measures for Managing Fatigue

Nursing interventions for the patient with fatigue focus on educating the patient on interrelated energy-conservation and exercise strategies; setting priorities; delegating; planning; acting during times of peak energy; and pacing (Whitmer, Tinari, & Barsevick, 2004). Setting priorities involves making a list of daily activities each day and identifying which are essential, desirable, transferable, and optional. At first, patients may overestimate the number of tasks that can be achieved in a day, but eventually they will learn to be more realistic.

Delegating activities may be difficult, and patients may need counseling to determine which activities should be delegated and how to request help from others (Whitmer et al., 2004). Sometimes roles within the family can be modified or shared. When a particular task is bothersome for the patient, it needs to be reassigned to another family member. For example, vacuuming is a strenuous task for a person with arthritis that affects the wrists and small joints of the fingers. If the patient lives alone, a cleaning service may be the answer, or trading vacuuming for another more manageable task with a neighbor or friend.

Planning refers to the process of anticipating needed resources and determining the easiest way to carry out the most important activities (Whitmer et al., 2004). It involves rearranging home and work environments to minimize obstacles in performing tasks and to consolidate similar tasks. One example is arranging items in home or office work areas to have items used frequently closer to the workspace. Occupational therapists have special expertise in these areas and should be consulted when indicated (Mahowald & Dykstra, 1997). Acting during times of peak energy involves planning to complete high-priority tasks when energy is at its peak.

Pacing involves planning for periods of rest and exercise, breaking up big tasks into smaller more manageable ones, and spreading out the smaller activities over the week. An example of pacing is to teach the patient to lie down for 20–30 minutes after arriving home from work in the late afternoon before starting to prepare dinner for the family. Rest periods can involve reading or listening to music; naps should be limited to avoid a dysfunctional diurnal rhythm (Whitmer et al., 2004). Regular exercise at low or moderate intensity can increase endurance and decrease fatigue (Burnham & Wilcox, 2002). Increasing physical activity has been recommended by the CDC National Arthritis Action Plan (CDC, 1999) as one strategy to preserve function and independence among people with arthritis.

Maintaining one's role as a spouse or significant other, including sexual intimacy, is important for both the patient and partner. Open discussion, negotiation, and compromise between sexual partners as to time, place, and alternate positions for intimacy are necessary to preserve this important aspect of a couple's life together.

Knowledge of the results of studies about fatigue in specific patient populations can help the nurse assess factors that may be modified to help reduce or manage fatigue. For example, in patients with multiple sclerosis, heat has been found to exacerbate fatigue. Cooling therapies may be beneficial for those clients (Ward & Winters, 2003). Young-McCaughan et al. (2003) state that more than 40 studies have demonstrated that both overall functional capacity and QOL were improved in patients with chronic illnesses after participation in an organized program of exercise. Most often utilized and tested was a 12-week phased cardiac rehabilitation program.

The nurse or healthcare professional can educate patients with newly diagnosed cancer to anticipate that fatigue may occur and what measures they can take to alleviate its effects. The nurse can teach the patient that pain can increase fatigue; therefore, it is important that pain is adequately controlled. Remind patients to be assertive in asking for help if their pain is not under control. It may also be helpful to suggest that patients allow extra rest periods on treatment days but continue to do some light exercise such as walking on nontreatment days to help maintain muscle strength and endurance. Explore with patients activities that elevate their mood, such as music, reading, or visiting an art museum, and encourage them to schedule these activities to help elevate their mood

and help them remain positive. Remind patients to report problems with nausea and to eat healthy, nutritious meals to avoid weight loss, which can increase fatigue. Eating small snacks more frequently may be better tolerated by patients than eating three large meals.

It is important that patients understand the mechanisms that medications and/or other treatments provide in decreasing fatigue. Patients may tend to reduce the number of medications taken as their fatigue and other symptoms improve. Some may do this to save money or because they are reluctant to take medications on a regular basis. Therefore, it is important to teach patients how other treatments may help lessen fatigue.

Insomnia or disrupted sleep secondary to pain or other discomfort may contribute to fatigue. Validate with the patient that he or she is taking pain medication properly. If pain is unrelieved, obtain an order for new or additional medications. Teach the patient sleep hygiene methods such as avoiding caffeine, use of their bed only for sleeping or napping and not for reading or doing work, and establishing a regular time for sleep and awakening. If these measures are not effective, the patient may need an antidepressant or nonaddictive sedative to promote sleep.

When fatigue is present, patients tend to reduce physical activity and increase rest periods to eliminate the feeling of fatigue. Such inactivity contributes to increased fatigue levels. Teach the patient to increase performance of appropriate aerobic exercises that will increase muscle strength and endurance (Mahowald & Dykstra, 1997). Consultation with a physical therapist may be indicated when specific therapeutic exercises are indicated (e.g., for patients who have had a stroke or have multiple sclerosis).

Regardless of the type of chronic illness causing fatigue, a healthy nutritious diet is vital. Being underweight or overweight can contribute to fatigue. Therefore, it is important to teach the patient the effect of nutrition on fatigue. Consultation with a dietician may be indicated.

Fatigue management programs may be beneficial for some patients. Ward and Winters (2003), for example, found evidence that a fatigue management program designed for patients with multiple sclerosis was effective in reducing the impact of fatigue on patients' lives, and increased performance and satisfaction in everyday living. The program focused on energy-conservation techniques and provided opportunities for patients with multiple sclerosis to interact with one another, socialize, and share personal experiences with respect to fatigue.

Outcomes for Fatigue Management

- The patient's fatigue lessens or occurs later in the day.
- The patient's family is able to describe how to prioritize daily activities to avoid or decrease fatigue.
- The patient has more restful sleep.
- The patient maintains normal body weight.
- The patient increased muscle strength and cardiopulmonary endurance.
- The patient displays positive affect and denies feelings of depression.

ANOREXIA, CACHEXIA, AND WASTING

Unintentional weight loss, loss of appetite, cachexia, and/or wasting continue to be nutritional problems in the treatment of HIV/AIDS, cancer and many other chronic diseases. Although wasting is a general sign of energy imbalance, the relative contribution of increased energy demands and decreased energy intake remains incompletely understood. Physical symptoms other than pain often contribute to suffering in those with chronic illness and those near the end of life. In addition to pain, the most common symptom in the terminal stages of an illness such as cancer or acquired immunodeficiency syndrome (AIDS) are fatigue, anorexia, cachexia, nausea, vomiting, constipation, delirium, and dyspnea (Ross & Alexander, 2001).

Cachexia is an involuntary weight loss of 10% of premorbid weight and is associated with muscle wasting and hypoproteinemia. Lipid stores are depleted, and serum albumin and pre-albumin diminish as serum acute-phase reactants increase. Gastric dysmotility leads to anorexia and associated early satiety, which results in reduced caloric intake. Anorexia and cachexia may also have psychological and social consequences. The physiologic consequences and the psychologic anguish of weight loss and weakness can be as great as those of uncontrolled pain. Anorexia and cachexia have not received the attention in the literature that pain and nausea have (Davis & Dickerson, 2000).

External factors, such as aging, physical activity (disuse), and decreased essential foodstuffs intake, create a praxis or cycle of poor nutrition. Prolonged anorexia leading to cachexia (independent of food intake) has been associated with the release of the cytokine tumor necrosis factor (TNF), formerly known as cytokine tumor necrosis factor-alpha (TNFα). Tumor necrosis factor, along with other cytokines, is released from monocytes and macrophages in response to cancer, sepsis, and severe traumatic events that progress to systemic inflammatory response syndrome (SIRS) and multiple-organ dysfunction syndrome (MODS) (Childs, 2003).

The treatment for anorexia and cachexia has been reactive rather than proactive, initiated after the patient has had significant weight loss and nutritional depletion. Anorexia may be related to increased plasma tryptophan, which is a precursor to serotonin, as a result of catabolism of somatic muscle. The direct result of weight loss and anorexia is nausea. There is also a correlation of weight loss and anorexia with reduced hemoglobin and hematocrit levels; glycemia; and reduced pre-albumin, sodium, and serum creatinine. In some cases the loss of appetite is caused by depression or psychological stress. Opioid analgesics cause nausea in one third of patients by central MU2 receptor agonist activity and by gastroparesis. Constipation complicates opioid therapy and accompanies dysmotility resulting from weight loss, leading to nausea and the opioid bowel syndrome. Depression-induced anorexia will, in fact, respond to tricyclic antidepressants with weight gain. Depression has long been associated with weight loss, a decreased appetite, and a history of anhedonia, guilt, and a sense of worthlessness (Davis & Dickerson, 2000).

It is essential to identify the underlying causes before choosing the best treatment for the patient. Finding medications to reverse the cachectic spiral will decrease or minimize weight loss and muscle weakness, improve performance status and immune function, and improve tolerance to therapy.

Assessment

A complete history with physical examination is necessary to determine the underlying cause of anorexia and cachexia.

History

- What is the primary cause of the symptom?
- Are there any secondary or tertiary causes of the symptoms?
- What are the patient's food preferences and is altered taste or smell present?
- Are there mouth sores or is the mouth dry?
- Are there problems with chewing or swallowing?
- Is nausea and/or vomiting present?
- How often does the patient have a bowel movement?
- What are the patient's current medications?
- Is there alcohol or drug use?

Physical Examination

- Observe the patient for nutritional deficiencies.
- Is oral candidiasis present?
- Are bowel sounds increased or decreased?
- Is succession splash present?
- Is hepatosplenomegaly present?

- Is ascites present?
- Is fecal impaction present?

Laboratory Studies

- Blood glucose
- Serum electrolytes
- Calcium
- Total protein, serum albumin, and pre-albumin
- Acute-phase reactants (Davis & Dickerson, 2000).

Interventions

Aggressive nutritional support in the form of either enteral or parenteral nutrition has been studied in cancer patients undergoing antitumor therapy. Meta-analysis of published trials in patients undergoing chemotherapy showed no improvement in survival, and perhaps reduced survival and poor tumor response including significant infectious complications (Ovesen et al., 1993).

Both megestrol acetate and medroxyprogesterone acetate have been used to treat cancer cachexia to stimulate appetite. Megestrol acetate at 160 mg. three times a day, improves appetite, activity, and well-being in patients with advanced cancer. Short-term benefits include improved appetite and decreased fatigue, and in the long term it increases weight. Side effects include dependent edema, dyspnea, and, upon rapid, withdrawal, an addisonian reaction and venous thromboembolism, which is more frequent than with corticosteroids (Jatoi et al., 2004).

A Cochrane review of research confirms that megestrol acetate is a good choice to increase appetite and weight gain in cancer patients compared with placebo. Although some authors have suggested that there may be a tendency toward greater efficacy with higher doses, this update demonstrated that clinical effects of megestrol acetate appear not to be dose related. The adverse event profiles of megestrol acetate have shown edema to be the only one significant difference between placebo and megestrol acetate, suggesting that megestrol acetate is a safe treatment option in these patients. Megestrol acetate may be prescribed in patients with cancer to increase appetite and weight gain (Berenstein & Ortiz, 2005).

In a large randomized trial of cyproheptadine, a serotonin antagonist, there appears to be mildly enhanced appetite, but the trial failed to reduce progressive weight loss (Kardianl et al., 1990). Metoclopramide has been shown to be effective in the treatment of nonspecific nausea, early satiety, and constipation that leads to reduced caloric intake. Patients with gastrostasis of a nonmechanical nature respond to metoclopramide with minimal side effects. Corticosteroids have been used frequently as appetite stimulants in cancer patients. However, there is no prolonged benefit, with any benefit lost within a month of treatment. The ability of dexamethasone to stimulate appetite is equivalent to that of megestrol acetate, but it does not produce weight gain. Dexamethasone is relatively inexpensive compared with megestrol acetate, but has more pronounced long-term side effects, including peptic ulcer, glucose intolerance, myopathy, cataracts, and osteoporosis, in addition to opportunistic infections and psychosis. It can be useful for patients with a short-term prognosis, or for those who may benefit from the use of corticosteroids such as those with dyspnea, bronchospasm, bone pain, or cerebral metastases (Hardy, 1998).

Cannabinoids are C21 compounds extracted from cannabis. Dronabinol, the commercially available form, is 90% absorbed but has a high first-pass clearance. Appetite-stimulating effects last for 24 hours, whereas the antiemetic qualities last for 4–6 hours. Dronabinol reduces anorexia and nausea and increases weight in patients with advanced cancer. Doses such as 2.5 mg, two to three times a day are typical (Hardy, 1998).

Jatoi and Winschitl (2002) conducted the first study to compare megestrol acetate with dronabinol in the treatment of cancer-associated anorexia and/or weight loss. Their findings demonstrate that megestrol acetate is superior to dronabinol in the treatment of cancer-associated anorexia and

that the addition of dronabinol to megestrol acetate does not provide any additional benefit. These results are important because they may influence oncologists' viewpoints on the medical uses of cannabinoid derivatives, since the study shows that dronabinol does little to promote appetite or weight gain among advanced cancer patients compared with megestrol acetate. Another noteworthy aspect of this trial was the improvement in QOL with the use of megestrol acetate as compared with dronabinol alone.

Davis and Dickerson (2000) synthesized the evidence-based literature into a four-step approach in the treatment of anorexia and cachexia:

- Treatment of potentially reversible causes of anorexia, such as anxiety, constipation, depression, dysphagia, nausea, vomiting, oral candidiasis, and pain.
- If a patient has reduced appetite associated with early satiety or evidence of gastroparesis, a trial of metoclopramide at 10–20 mg before meals and at bedtime, up to 120 mg per day.
- Failing this, a trial of megestrol acetate, starting at 160 mg/day and increasing doses up to 800 mg/day for patients with a relatively good prognosis, or the use of dexamethasone 8–10 mg twice a day in patients with a poor prognosis or other symptoms. Megestrol acetate should not be combined with chemotherapeutic agents.
- Based on promising, although small, trials of dronabinol, thalidomide, eicosapentaenoic acid, and melatonin: dronabinol 2.5 mg two to three times a day, thalidomide 100 mg at night, eicosapentaenoic acid at 2–3 g/day, and melatonin 20–40 mg/day (Davis & Dickerson, 2000).

Nutritional counseling should be based on eating high calorie meals of small portions that are pleasant for the patient. It is important to include the patient's family in such discussions. It is useful to clarify that an excess of calories is unlikely to benefit the patient, by explaining that

EVIDENCE-BASED PRACTICE BOX

Symptom Management in Patients with Heart Failure

Godfrey et al. (2007) conducted a study to determine whether pain was reported by a cohort of individuals with heart failure at the time of discharge from hospital, and at 2 and 6 weeks post discharge. This study was part of a larger randomized controlled trial with 3-month follow-up data obtained from 169 individuals diagnosed with heart failure. At the time of discharge, 68% (n = 115) of the cohort reported pain. For these subjects, the occurrence of pain fluctuated throughout the 6 weeks, decreasing to 68% (n = 78 of 115) at week 2, and increasing again to 72% (n = 83 of 115) at week 6. The severity of pain also varied throughout the 6-week period with 69% (n = 79 of 115) of these individuals rating their pain as moderate or severe at discharge, and by week 6, just over half, 59%, (n = 47 of 79) continued to experience pain at this intensity. Throughout the 6 weeks, 63 individuals (37%) consistently reported pain and 23 (14%) never reported pain. These results support findings of other studies.

Differences in health-related quality of life (QOL) were found between those who reported pain and those who did not at discharge and week 2. In addition, depression, worry, feeling a loss of control over one's life, and feeling as if one was a burden to family were significantly more prevalent in individuals who reported pain. Differences were also found in self-rated health status and number of prescription medications taken daily.

The results of this study have several implications for evidence-based nursing practice. A comprehensive approach to successful symptom management in patients with heart failure is critical for desired outcomes. The role of the nurse in the hospital setting is to direct careful discharge planning for the patient and family. Information is needed to address the issues of the individual's ability to both monitor and manage their symptoms, including pain, daily weights, changes in energy levels, and fluctuations in the severity of dyspnea. Any breakdown in this process of self-management may contribute to an exacerbation. It seems likely that the symptom of pain would compromise an individual's capacity to maintain the delicate balance required for symptom management. The impact of symptoms and the ongoing cycle of exacerbations with hospital readmission clearly places additional burden upon individuals and their families.

The study found that individuals diagnosed with heart failure do experience pain. Pain is an important symptom and although it may not be consistent, when pain is experienced, it does affect QOL and activities of daily living. The experience of pain needs to be monitored in patients with heart failure, as it may also be indicative of their overall health status. Addressing the issue of pain is necessary for advanced practice nurses who may follow heart failure patients in primary care practices, as well as for home health nurses. The assessment and monitoring of pain is beneficial not only for the individuals experiencing it, but also as a way to reduce the rate of hospital readmissions, thereby decreasing the strain on economic resources. Pain may also affect the capacity of individuals to care for themselves at home. Particular attention should be given to female patients with heart failure, as they appear more vulnerable, especially if they are older and living alone.

Source: Godfrey, C.M., Harrison, M.B., Friedberg, E., Medves, J.M. & Tranmer, J.E. (2007). The symptom of pain in individuals recently hospitalized for heart failure. *Journal of Cardiovascular Nursing, 22*(5), 368–374.

his/her metabolic system does not have the ability to use these calories in the same way as that of a healthy person. Although cachectic, the patient is not "starving." Patients who are unable to swallow because of severe dysphagia (e.g., head and neck cancers and neurologic disorders) and who complain of hunger or express concerns related to malnutrition may benefit from nutrition via a gastrostomy tube (Davis & Dickerson, 2000).

SUMMARY AND OUTCOMES

Optimal patient outcomes emerge from symptom management strategies as well as from the symptom experience. In the symptom management model, there are no arrows indicated directionality between the multidimensional indicators and symptom status. The duration of symptom evaluation depends upon its persistence, need for continued intervention, and response to treatment. If a symptom is successfully treated and completely resolved, the model is no longer relevant. However, if continued intervention is necessary to control recurring symptoms, then the model continues to be applicable, and direct symptom management and measurement of outcomes continues (Dodd, Miaskowski, & Paul, 2001).

Although research is sufficient to build a case that the symptom cluster has validity as a scientific construct and a clinically relevant problem, many unanswered questions remain (Barsevik, 2007). More research needs to be done to understand the efficacy of interventions for symptom clusters. Developing new tools for studying symptom clusters and testing the mechanisms by which pharmacologic and nonpharmacologic therapies influence symptoms is needed. Working collaboratively to provide full and clear descriptions of the symptom cluster and developing symptom cluster interventions to achieve the most favorable patient outcomes are essential.

STUDY QUESTIONS

1. Discuss the symptom management concepts, models, and theories presented in this chapter. Which are the most relevant for providing a meaningful framework to assess and manage the patient with chronic illness? Why?
2. Analyze the components of pain assessment algorithms in development of a comprehensive pain management plan.
3. Differentiate pain management principles to consider in the use of narcotics and non-narcotic analgesics for the management of patients with chronic pain.
4. Compare the following methods of managing chronic pain in terms of evidence-based research, effectiveness, benefit, cost, and ease of delivery:
   a. Cutaneous Stimulation
   b. Distraction
   c. Relaxation
   d. Imagery

5. What are the advantages and disadvantages of a pain management program? What criteria should healthcare providers advise that their clients consider in the selection of such a program?
6. What are the three benefits of nonsteroidal anti-inflammatory drugs?
7. What common disease or illness states and alterations in health induce fatigue?
8. What psychosocial factors are associated with fatigue?
9. How is fatigue assessed?
10. What interventions can be used to relieve fatigue?
11. What factors put clients with chronic illness at greater risk for development of depression?
12. At what point on the depression diagnostic continuum does the National Institute for Clinical Evidence recommend the use of medications?

13. What four techniques can be used by primary care physicians to care for patients with chronic diseases?

14. Why is it important to consider fatigue, depression, and anxiety for clients who have chronic pain?

15. What factors are to be considered when using analgesics to manage chronic pain?

16. How do these factors influence selection and administration of narcotic and nonnarcotic analgesics to children, adults, and the elderly?

17. What aspects of pain assessment are essential for management of chronic pain? Why?

18. How can healthcare professionals assist clients in selecting an appropriate pain management program?

19. Analyze the symptom experience of a patient with depression related to living with diabetes.

20. Give examples of the eight components of symptom management strategies in a patient with chronic pain caused by rheumatoid arthritis.

21. Using the Symptom Management Model, what would be the outcomes of effective management strategies for a patient with chronic anorexia and fatigue resulting from terminal cancer?

REFERENCES

Aaronson, L.S., Teel, C.S., Cassmeyer, V., Neuberger, G.B., Pallikkathayil, L., Pierce, J., et al. (1999). Defining and measuring fatigue. *Image, 31*(1), 45–50.

American Pain Society. (1987). *Principles of analgesic use in the treatment of acute pain and chronic cancer pain: A concise guide to medical practice.* Washington DC: Author.

American Psychiatric Association (2000). *Diagnostic and statistical manual of mental disorders* (4th ed.). Washington DC: American Psychiatric Association.

Ansari, A. (2000). The efficacy of newer antidepressants in the treatment of chronic pain: A review of current literature. *Harvard Review of Psychiatry, 7,* 257–277.

Armstrong, T.S. (2003). Symptoms experience: A concept analysis. *Oncology Nursing Forum, 30*(4), 601–606.

Aronoff, G.M. (2004). The role of pain clinics. In C.A. Warfield & Z.H. Bajwa (Eds.), *Principles & practice of pain medicine* (2nd ed.) (pp. 813–824). New York: McGraw-Hill.

Barsevick, A. (2007). The elusive concept of the symptom cluster. *Oncology Nursing Forum, 34*(5), 971–980.

Belza, B.L., Henke, C.J., Yelin, E.H., Epstein, W.V., & Gilliss, C.L. (1993). Correlates of fatigue in older adults with rheumatoid arthritis. *Nursing Research, 42*(2), 93–99.

Berde, C.G., & Masek, B., (2003). Pain in children. In R. Melzack & P.D. Wall (Eds.), *Handbook of pain management: A clinical companion to Wall and Melzack's textbook of pain* (pp. 545–558). Philadelphia: Churchill Livingstone.

Berenstein, E. & Ortiz, Z. (2005). Megestrol acetate for treatment of anorexia-cachexia syndrome. *Cochrane Database of Systematic Reviews 2005, 2.* Art. No: CD004310. DOI:10.1002/14651858. CD004310.pub2.

Berman, B. M., & Swyers, J.P. (1999). Complementary medicine treatments for fibromyalgia syndrome. *Best Practice Research in Clinical Rheumatology, 3,* 487–492.

Bower, J. E., Ganz, P.A., Desmond, K.A., Rowland, J.H., Meyerowita, B.E., & Belin, T. R. (2000). Fatigue in breast cancer survivors: Occurrence, correlated, and impact on quality of life. *Journal of Clinical Oncology, 18*(4), 743.

Burnham, T. R., & Wilcox, A. (2002). Effects of exercise on physiological and psychological variables in cancer survivors. *Medicine and Science in Sports and Exercise, 34*(12), 1863–1867.

Burte, J. M. (2002). Psychoneuroimmunology. In R.S. Weiner (Ed.), *Pain management: A practical guide for clinicians* (6th ed.) (pp. 807–816). Boca Raton, FL: C.R.C. Press.

Canadian Pain Society (1998). Use of opioid analgesics for the treatment of chronic pain: A consensus statement and guidelines from the Canadian Pain Society, *Pain Research Management, 3,* 197–208.

Carroll, D.C. & Seers, K. (1998) Relaxation for the relief of chronic pain: A systematic review. *Journal of Advanced Nursing. 27*(3), 476–487.

Centers for Disease Control and Prevention. (1999) National arthritis action plan: A public health strategy. Retrieved November 1, 2004 from www.cdc.gov/nccdphp/naap_executive_summary.pdf

Chalder, T., Berelowitz, G., Pawlikowska, T., Watts, L., Wessely, S., Wright, D. et al. (1993). Development of a fatigue scale. *Journal of Psychosomatic Research, 37,* 147–153.

Childs, S. (2003). Cachexia in chronic kidney disease: Role of inflammation and neuropeptide signaling. *Orthopedic Nursing, 22*(4), 251–257.

Claudepierre, P (2005). Spa therapy for ankylosing spondylitis: Still useful? *Joint, Bone, and Spine, 72*(4), 283–285.

Cleeland, C.S., Bennett, G.J., Dantzer, R., Dougherty, P.M., Dunn, A.J., Meyers, C.A., et al. (2003). Are the symptoms of cancer and cancer treatment due to a shared biologic mechanism? A cytokine-immunologic model of cancer symptoms. *Cancer, 97,* 2919–2925.

Cleveland Clinic (2002). Chronic illness and depression. Retrieved November 15, 2007 from www.cchs.net/health/health-info/docs/2200/2282.asp?

Dana Farber Cancer Institute (2007). Dictionary of medical terms. Retrieved on November 8, 2007 from www.dana-farber.org/can/dictionary/?index=d

Davis, G.C. (1992). The meaning of pain management: A concept analysis. *Advanced Nursing Science, 1,* 77–86.

Davis, M., & Dickerson, D. (2000). Cachexia and anorexia: Cancer's covert killer. *Support Care Cancer, 8,* 180–187.

Davis, G.C., & White, T.L. (2001) Nursing's role in chronic pain management with older adults. *Topics in Geriatric Rehabilitation, 16*(3), 45–55.

Deardorff, W.W. (2004). Depression and chronic back pain. Retrieved on November 10, 2007 from www.spine-health.com/topics/cd/depression/depression01.html

Dittner, A.J., Janson, S, Facione, N., Wessely S.C., & Brown R.G. (2004). The assessment of fatigue; A practical guide for clinicians and researchers. *Journal of Psychosomatic Research, 56,* 157–170.

Dluhy, N. (1995). Mapping knowledge in chronic illness. *Journal of Advanced Nursing, 21*(6), 1051–8.

Dodd, M., Janson, S., Facione, N., Faucett, J., Froelicher, E.S., Humphreys, J., et al. (2001a). Advancing the science of symptom management. *Journal of Advanced Nursing, 33,* 668–676.

Dodd, M. J., Miaskowski, C., & Paul, S.M. (2001b). Symptom clusters and their effect on the functional status of patients with cancer. *Oncology Nursing Forum, 28*(3), 465–470.

Douglas, M. (1999). Pain as the fifth vital sign: Will cultural variations be considered? *Journal of Transcultural Nursing, 10,* 285.

Dzurec, L.C. (2000). Fatigue and relatedness experience of inordinately tired women. *Image, 32,* 339–345.

Ewing, J.A. (1984). Detecting alcoholism: The CAGE Questionnaire. *Journal of the American Medical Association, 252,* 1905–1907.

Ezzo, J., Berman, B., Hadhazy, V. A., Jadad, A. R., Lixing, L., & Singh, B.B. (2000). Is acupuncture effective for the treatment of chronic pain? A systematic review. *Pain, 86,* 217–225.

Fishman, S.M., Bandman, T.B., Edwards, A., & Borsook, D. (1999). The opioid contract in the management of chronic pain. *Journal of Pain and Symptom Management, 8,* 27–37.

Gaston-Johansson, F., Fall-Dickson, J.M., Nanda, J., Ohly, K.V., Stillman, S., Krumm, S., et al. (2000). The effectiveness of the comprehensive coping strategy program on clinical outcomes in breast cancer autologous bone marrow transplantation. *Cancer Nursing, 23*(4), 277–285.

Gift, A. G., Stommel, M., Jablonski, A., & Given, W. (2003). A cluster of symptoms over time in patients with lung cancer. *Nursing Research, 52*(6), 393–400.

Giger, J.N., & Davidhizar, R.E. (2004). *Transcultural nursing: Assessment and intervention* (4th ed.). St. Louis, MO: Mosby.

Given, C., Given, B., Hohammad, R., Sangchoon, J. McCorkle, R, Cimprich, A., et al. (2004). Effect of a cognitive behavioral intervention on reducing symptom severity during chemotherapy. *Journal of Clinical Oncology, 22*(3) 507–516.

Glaus A., Crow R., & Hammond S. (1996). A qualitative study to explore the concept of fatigue/tiredness in cancer patients and in healthy individuals. *European Journal of Cancer Care, 5,* 8–23.

Glover, J., Dibble, S.L., Dodd, M.J., & Miaskowski, C. (1995). Mood states of oncology outpatients: Does pain make a difference? *Journal of Pain and Symptom Management, 10,* 120–128.

Godfrey, C.M., Harrison, M.B., Friedberg, E., Medves, J.M. & Tranmer, J.E. (2007). The symptom of pain in individuals recently hospitalized for heart failure. *Journal of Cardiovascular Nursing, 22*(5), 368–374.

Gourlay, G. K. (1998). Sustained relief of chronic pain. Pharmacokinetics of sustained release morphine. *Clinical Pharmacokinetics, 35*(3), 173–190.

Green, C.R., Wheeler, J.R.C., LaPorte, F., Marchant, B., & Guerrero, E. (2002). How well is chronic pain managed? Who does it well? *Pain Medicine, 3*, 56–65.

Haetzman, M., Elliott, A.M., Smith, B.H., Hannaford, P., & Chambers, W. (2003). Chronic pain and the use of conventional and alternative theory. *Family Practice, 20*, 147–154.

Hallerbach, M., Francoeur, A., & Pomerantz, S. (2008). Patterns and predictors of early hospital readmission in patients with congestive heart failure. *American Journal of Medical Quality, 23*, 18–23.

Hardy, J. (1998) Corticosteroids in palliative care. *European Journal of Palliative Care, 5*, 46–50.

Haworth, S. & Dluhy, N. (2001). Holistic symptom management: Modeling the interaction phase. *Journal of Advanced Nursing, 36*(2), 302–310.

Heidrich, S.M., Egan, J., Hengudomsub, P., & Randolph, S.M. (2006). Symptoms, symptom beliefs, and quality of life of older breast cancer survivors: A comparative study. *Oncology Nursing Forum, 33*(2), 315–322.

Holroyd, J. (1996). Hypnosis treatment of clinical pain: Understanding why hypnosis is useful. *The International Journal of Clinical and Experimental Hypnosis, 44*(1), 33–51.

Homsi, J., Walsh, D., Rivera, N., Rybicki, L.A., Nelson, K.A., Legrand, S.B., et al. (2006). Symptom evaluation in palliative medicine: Patient report versus systematic assessment. *Supportive Care in Cancer, 14*, 444–453.

Huyser, B.A., Parker, J.C., Thoreson, R., Smarr, K.L., Johnson, J.C., Hoffman, R. (1998). Predictors of subjective fatigue among individuals with rheumatoid arthritis. *Arthritis & Rheumatism, 41*, 2230–2237.

Inglis, H., Pearson, S., & Treen, S. (2006). Extending the horizon in chronic heart failure: Effects of multidisciplinary, home-based intervention relative to usual care. *Circulation, 114*, 2466–2473.

Institute for Clinical Systems Improvement (ICSI). (2007). Assessment and management of chronic pain. Bloomington, MN: Institute for Clinical Systems Improvement.

Jackson, K.C., & St. Onge, E.L. (2003). Antidepressant pharmacotherapy: Considerations for the pain clinician. *Pain Practice, 3*, 135–143.

Jatoi, A., & Windschitl, H. (2002). Dronabinol versus megestrol acetate versus combination therapy for cancer-associated anorexia. *Journal of Clinical Oncology, 20*(2), 567–573.

Jatoi, A., Rowland, K. Loprinzi, C., Sloan, J.A., Dakhil, S.R., MacDonald, N., et al. (2004). An eicosapentaenoic acid supplement versus megestrol acetate versus both for patients with cancer-associated wasting: A North Central Cancer Treatment Group and National Cancer Institute of Canada collaborative effort. *Journal of Clinical Oncology, 22*, 2469–2476.

Jeffrey, J. (1996). Role of nursing in the management of soft tissue rheumatic disease. In R.P. Sheon, R.W. Moskowitz, & V.W. Goldberg (Eds.). *Soft tissue rheumatic pain: Recognition, management, prevention* (3rd ed.) (pp. 329–350). Sudbury, MA: Jones & Bartlett.

Joint Commission on Accreditation of Healthcare Organizations Pain Standards for 2001. (2001). Retrieved from www.jcaho.org/standards_frm.html.

Kardinal, C., Loprinzi, C. & Schaid, D. (1990) A controlled trial of cyproheptadine in cancer patients with anorexia and/or cachexia. *Cancer, 65*, 2657–2662.

Kemper, K.J., LicAc, R.S., Silver-Highfield, E., Xiarhos, E., Barnes, L., & Berde, C. (2000). On pins and needles? Pediatric pain patients' experience with acupuncture. *Pediatrics, 105* (Suppl), 941–947.

Kitahara, M, Kojima, K.K., & Ohmura, A. (2006). Efficacy of interdisciplinary treatment of chronic nonmalignant pain patients in Japan. *Clinical Journal of Pain, 22*(7), 647–655.

Krozek, C., & Scoggins, A. (2001a). Patient rights . . . amended to comply with 2000 JCAHO standards. Glendale, CA: CINAHL Information Systems.

Krozek, C., & Scoggins, A. (2001b). Patient and family education amended to comply with 2000 JCAHO standards. Glendale, CA: CINAHL Information Systems.

Krupp, L.B., LaRocca, N.G., Muir-Nash, J., & Steinberg, A.D. (1989). The fatigue severity scale: Application to patients with chronic fatigue syndrome. *Archives of Neurology, 46*, 1121–1123.

Kubsch, S.M., Neveau, T., & Vandertie, K. (2000). Effect of cutaneous stimulation on pain reduction in emergency department patients. *Complementary Therapies in Nursing and Midwifery, 6*(1), 25–32.

Laliberte, R. (2003). *Doctor's guide to chronic pain: The newest, quickest, and most effective ways to find relief.* Pleasantville, NY: The Reader's Digest Association.

Lazarus, H., & Neumann, C.J. (2001). Assessing under treatment of pain: the patients' perspectives. *Journal of Pharmaceutical Care in Pain and Symptom Control, 9*(4), 5–34.

Lee, B.N., Dantzer, R., Langley, K.E., Bennett, G.J., Dougherty, P.M., & Dunn, A.J. (2004). A cytokine-based neuroimmunologic mechanism of cancer-related symptoms. *Neuroimmunomodulation, 11*, 279–292.

Lee, K.A., Hicks, G., & Nino-Murcia, G. (1991). Validity and reliability of a scale to assess fatigue. *Psychiatry Research, 36*, 291–298.

Lee, T.L. (2000). Acupuncture and chronic pain management. *Annals of Academic Medicine of Singapore, 29*(1), 17–21.

Leibing, E., Leonhardt, U., Köster, G., Goerlitz, A., Rosenfeldt, J.A., & Ramadori, G. (2002). Acupuncture treatment of chronic low-back pain—a randomized, blinded, placebo-controlled trial with 9-month follow-up. *Pain, 96*, 189–196.

Lenz, E.R., Pugh, L.C., Milligan, R.A., Gift, A., & Suppe, F. (1997). The middle-range theory of unpleasant symptoms: An update. *Advances in Nursing Science, 19*(3), 14–27.

Lewandowski, W.A. (2004). Patterning of pain and power with guided imagery. *Nursing Science Quarterly, 17*, 233–241.

Lin, Y., & Taylor, A.G. (1998). Effects of therapeutic touch in reducing pain and anxiety in an elderly population. *Integrative Medicine, 1*(4), 155–162.

Lipman, A.G., & Jackson, K.C. (2004). Opioid pharmacotherapy. In C.A. Warfield , & Z.H. Bajwa. (Eds.), *Principles & practice of pain medicine* (2nd ed.) (pp. 583–600). New York: McGraw-Hill.

MacDonald, N. (2002). Relationship of cancer symptom clusters to depressive affect in the initial phase of palliative radiation. *Journal of Palliative Medicine, 5*, 301-304.

MacLaren, D.P.M., Gibson, H., Parry-Billings, M., & Edwards, R.H.T. (1989). A review of metabolic and physiological factors in fatigue. *Exercise and Sport Science Review, 17*, 29–66.

Macres, S., Richeimer, S., & Duran, P. (2004). Adjuvant analgesics. In C.A. Warfield & Z.H. Bajwa (Eds.), *Principles & practice of pain medicine* (2nd ed.) (pp. 627–638). New York: McGraw-Hill.

Mahowald, M.D., & Dykstra, D. (1997). Rehabilitation of patients with rheumatic diseases. In J.H. Klippel, C.M. Weyland, & R.L. Wortmann (Eds.), *Primer on the rheumatic diseases* (pp. 407–412). Atlanta: Arthritis Foundation.

McCaffery, M., & Beebe, A. (1989). *Pain: Clinical manual for nursing practice.* St. Louis: Mosby.

McCaffery, M., & Ferrell, B. R. (1999). Opioids and pain management: What do nurses know? *Nursing 1999, 29*(3), 48–52.

McCaffery, M., Ferrell, B.R., & Pasero, C. (2000). Nurses' personal opinions about patients' pain and their effect on recorded assessments and titration of opioid doses. *Pain Management in Nursing, 1*, 79–87.

McCaffery, M., & Pasero C. (1999). *Pain: Clinical manual for nursing practice* (2nd ed.). St. Louis: Mosby.

McLachlan, S.A., Allenby, A., Matthews, J., Wirth, A., Kissane, D., Bishop, M., et al. (2001). Randomized trial of coordinated psychosocial interventions based on patient self-assessments versus standard care to improve the psychosocial functioning of patients with cancer. *Journal of Clinical Oncology, 19*, 4117–4125.

McNair, D. M., Lorr, M., & Droppleman, L. F. (1992). *Profile of mood states manual* (2nd ed.). San Diego, CA: Educational & Industrial Testing Service.

McPhee, S.J., & Schroeder, S.A. (1999). General approach to the patient: Health maintenance, disease prevention and common symptoms. In Tierney, L.M., McPhee, S.J., & Papadakis, M.A. (Eds.). *Current medical diagnosis and treatment.* Stanford, CT: Appleton & Lange.

Meek, P.M., Nail, L.M., Barsevick, A., Schwartz, A.L., Stephan, S. & Whitmer, K., et al. (2000). Psychometric testing of fatigue instruments for use in cancer patients. *Nursing Research, 49*(4), 181–190.

Melzack, R. (1973). *The puzzle of pain.* New York: Basic Books.

Melzack, R., & Wall, P. D. (1965). Pain mechanisms: A new theory. *Science, 150*, 971–979.

Melzack, R., & Wall, P.D. (2003). *Handbook of pain management: A clinical companion to Wall and Melzack's textbook of pain.* Philadelphia: Churchill Livingstone.

Merskey, J. (1986). Classification of chronic pain: Descriptions of chronic pain syndromes and definitions of pain terms. *Pain,* Suppl. 3, S1–S225.

Mobily, P.R., Herr, K.A., & Kelley, L. S. (1993). Cognitive-behavioral techniques to reduce pain: A validation study. *International Journal of Nursing Studies, 30,* 537–548.

Monks, R., & Merskey, H. (2003). Psychotropic drugs. In R. Melzack, & P.D. Wall (Eds.). *Handbook of pain management: A clinical companion to Wall and Melzack's textbook of pain.* (pp. 353–376). Philadelphia: Churchill Livingstone.

Nabeta, T., & Kawakita, K. (2002). Relief of chronic neck and shoulder pain by manual acupuncture to tender points—A sham-controlled randomized trial. *Complementary Therapies in Medicine, 10,* 217–222.

National Center for Complementary and Alternative Medicine (2004). Retrieved October 7, 2004 from nccam.nih.gov/news/camsurvey_fs1.htm

National Institute for Clinical Excellence (2004). *Depression: management of depression in primary and secondary care.* London (UK): National Collaborating Centre for Mental Health.

National Guideline Clearinghouse (2007). Assessment and management of chronic pain. Retrieved November 30, 2007 from www.guideline.gov/summary/summary.aspx?doc_id=11507&nbr=005960&string=chronic+AND+pain

National Institutes of Health. (1995). *Integration of behavioral and relaxation approaches into the treatment of chronic pain and insomnia.* Technology Assessment Conference Statement. Bethesda, MD.

Neuberger, G.B., Press, A.N., Lindsley, H.B., Hinton, R., Cagle, P.E., Carlson, K., et al. (1997). Effects of exercise on fatigue, aerobic fitness, and disease activity measures in persons with rheumatoid arthritis. *Research in Nursing and Health, 20,* 195–204.

Neuberger, G.B. (2003). Measures of fatigue. *Arthritis Care and Research, 49*(5S), S175–S183.

Oh, E., Kim, C., Lee, W., & Kim, S. (2004). Correlates of fatigue in Koreans with chronic lung disease. *Heart & Lung, 33*(1), 13–20.

O'Neill, E.S. & Morrow, L.L. (2001). The symptom experience of women with chronic illness. *Journal of Advanced Nursing, 33*(2), 257–268.

Ovesen, L., Allingstrup, L., Hannibal, J., Mortensen, E.L., & Hansen, O.P. (1993). Effect of dietary counseling on food intake, bodyweight, response rate, survival and quality of life in cancer patients undergoing chemotherapy: A prospective, randomized study. *Journal of Clinical Oncology, 11,* 2043–2049.

Parker, K.P., Kimble, L.P., Dunbar, S.B., & Clark, P.C. (2005). Symptom interactions as mechanisms underlying symptom pairs and clusters. *Journal of Nursing Scholarship, 37*(3), 209–215.

Pearson, S., Inglis, S., McLennan, S., Brennan, L., Russell, M., Wilkerson, D., et al. (2006). Prolonged effects of a home-based intervention in patients with chronic illness. *Archives in Internal Medicine, 166*(6), 645–650.

Phillips, K.D., Sowell, R.L., Rojas, M., Tavakoli, A., Fulk, L.J., & Hand, G.A. (2004). Physiological and psychological correlates of fatigue in HIV Disease. *Biological Research for Nursing, 6*(1), 59–74.

Piper, B.F., Lindsey, A.M., Dodd, M.J., Ferketich, S., Paul, S., & Weller, S. (1989). The development of an instrument to measure the subjective dimension of fatigue. In S.G. Funk, E.M. Tornquist, M.T. Champagne, L.A. Copp, & R. Wiese (Eds.), *Key aspects of comfort* (pp. 199–208). New York: Springer.

Portenoy, R.K. (2000). Current pharmacotherapy of chronic pain. *Journal of Pain and Symptom Management, 10* (Suppl), S16–S20.

Potter, J. (2004). Fatigue experience in advanced cancer: A phenomenological approach. *International Journal of Palliative Nursing, 10*(1), 15–23.

Rapoff, A.J., & Lindsley, C.B. (2000). The pain puzzle: A visual and conceptual metaphor for understanding and treating pain in pediatric rheumatic disease. *Journal of Rheumatology Suppl, 58,* 29–33.

Richeimer, S.H., Bajwa, Z.H., Karhamann, S.S., Ransil, B.J., & Warfield, C.A. (1997). Utilization patterns of tricyclic antidepressants in a multidisciplinary pain clinic: A survey. *Clinical Journal of Pain, 13,* 324–329.

Ross, D., & Alexander, C. (2001). Common symptoms in terminally ill patients: Fatigue, anorexia, cachexia, nausea and vomiting. *American Family Physician, 64*(5), 807–814.

Rothman, A., Anderson, M., & Wagner, E. (2003). Chronic illness management: What is the role of primary care? *Annals of Internal Medicine, 138*(3), 256–261.

Sadovsky, R. (2002). Cognitive behavior treatment of chronic disease. *American Family Physician, 65*(9), 1902.

Sarna, L. (1998). Effectiveness of structured nursing assessment of symptom distress in advanced lung cancer. *Oncology Nursing Forum, 25,* 1041–1048.

Schaffer, S.D., & Yucha, C.A. (2004). Relaxation and pain management: The relaxation response can play a role in managing chronic and acute pain. *American Journal of Nursing, 104*(8), 75–82.

Shalmi, C. L. (2004). Opioids for nonmalignant pain: Issues and controversy. In C.A. Warfield & Z.H. Bajwa. (Eds.), *Principles & practice of pain medicine* (2nd ed). (pp. 601–611). New York: McGraw-Hill.

Shvartzman, P., Friger, M., Shani, A., Barak, F., & Yoram, C., Singer, Y. (2003). Pain control in ambulatory cancer patients—can we do better? *The Journal of Pain and Symptom Management, 26,* 716–722.

Simon, L.S. (2004). Nonsteroidal anti-inflammatory drugs. In C.A. Warfield & Z.H. Bajwa (Eds.), *Principles & practice of pain medicine* (2nd ed). (pp. 616–626). New York: McGraw-Hill.

Singh, M., & Jashvant, P. (2005). Chronic pain syndrome. Retrieved from www.emedicine.com/pmr/topic32.htm on November 10, 2007.

Smith, D.W., Arnstein, P., Rosa, K.C., & Wells-Federman, C. (2002). Effects of integrating therapeutic touch into a cognitive behavioral pain treatment program: Report of a pilot clinical trial. *Journal of Holistic Nursing, 20,* 367–387.

Stone, P., Hardy, J., Huddart, R., A'Hern, R., & Richardson, M. (2000). Fatigue in patients with prostate cancer receiving hormone therapy. *European Journal of Cancer, 36*(9), 1134–1141.

Stone, P., Richardson, M., A'Hern, R., & Hardy, J. (2000). A study to investigate the prevalence, severity and correlates of fatigue among patients with cancer in comparison with a control group without cancer. *Annals of Oncology, 11*(5), 561–567.

Sweeney, C., & Bruera, E. (2003). Opioids. In R. Melzack & P.D. Wall (Eds.), *Handbook of pain management: A clinical companion to Wall and Melzack's textbook of pain.* (pp. 377–396). Philadelphia: Churchill Livingstone.

Tack, B. (1990). Self-reported fatigue in rheumatoid arthritis: A pilot study. *Arthritis Care and Research, 3*(3), 154–157.

Taylor, D. (2000). More than personal change: Effective elements of symptom management. *Nurse Practitioner Forum, 11*(2), 79–86.

Turk, D.C. (1999). The role of psychological factors in chronic pain. *Acta Anaesthesiologica Scandinavica, 43,* 885–888.

Turk, D.C., & Okifuji, A. (2003). A cognitive-behavioral approach to pain management. In R. Melzack & P.D. Wall (Eds.), *Handbook of pain management: A clinical companion to Wall and Melzack's textbook of pain.* (pp. 533–542). Philadelphia: Churchill Livingstone.

Turk, D.C., & Okifuji, A. (2004). Psychological aspects of pain. In C.A. Warfield and Z.H. Bajwa (Eds.), *Principles and practice of pain medicine.* (pp. 134–147). New York: McGraw Hill.

Voerman, V.F., van Egmond, J., & Crul, B.J.P. (2000) Elevated detection thresholds for mechanical stimuli in chronic pain patients: Support for a central mechanism. *Archives of Physical Medicine and Rehabilitation, 81,* 430–435.

Wall, P.D., & Melzack, R. (Eds.). (1999) *Textbook of pain* (4th ed). Edinburgh: Churchill Livingstone.

Ward, N., & Winters, S. (2003). Results of a fatigue management programme in multiple sclerosis. *British Journal of Nursing, 12,* 1075–1080.

Warfield, C.A., & Bajwa, Z.H. (Eds.) (2004). *Principles & practice of pain medicine* (2nd ed). New York: McGraw-Hill.

Wearden, A.J. (2006). Fatigue intervention by nurses evaluation – The FINE Trial. A randomized controlled trial of nurse led self-help treatment for patients in primary care with chronic fatigue syndrome. *BMC Medicine , 4,* 9.

Weinstein, S.M., Laux, L.F., Thornby, J.I., Lorimor, R.J., Hill, C.S., Thorpe, D.M., et al. (2000). Physicians' attitudes toward pain and the use of opioid analgesics: Results from a survey from the Texas Cancer Pain Initiative. *Southern Medical Journal, 93,* 479–487.

Whitmer, K., Tinari, M.A., & Barsevick, A. (2004). How do we manage fatigue in cancer patients? *Rehabilitation Nursing, 29,* 112–113.

Winterowd, C., Beck, A.T., & Gruener, D. (2003). *Cognitive therapy with chronic pain patients.* New York: Springer.

Young-McCaughan, S., Mays, M.Z., Arzola, S.M., Yoder, L.H., Dramiga, S.A., Leclerc, K.M., et al. (2003). Research and commentary: Change in exercise tolerance, activity and sleep patterns, and quality of life in patients with cancer participating in a structured exercise program. *Oncology Nursing Forum, 30*(3), 441–454.

18

Alternative, Complementary, and Integrative Therapies

Lisa L. Onega

INTRODUCTION

When clinicians caring for individuals with chronic illnesses consider alternative, complementary, and integrative treatments, a scientific and humanistic perspective is invaluable (Chez & Jonas, 2005). What motivates a person with a chronic illness to try non-traditional therapies? If the traditional allopathic approach is not able to provide a treatment that relieves human suffering and improves quality of life, should healthcare practitioners help individuals with chronic illnesses find nonallopathic treatments that may help? In a free society, what is the role of government in balancing the safety of healthcare treatments with an individual's right to access alternative, complementary, or integrative treatments? Perhaps the most important question that clinicians who provide care for individuals and families coping with a chronic illness need to ask themselves is: how important is it for individuals with chronic illnesses to have hope? Addressing these questions in a scholarly and compassionate manner will assist advanced practice nurses to provide improved health care for their clients with chronic illnesses.

Definitions

The terms allopathic, conventional, and traditional are used interchangeably to describe standard healthcare practices. Alternative, complementary, and integrative are labels used to describe nonstandard healthcare practices (Cuellar, Cahill, Ford, & Aycock, 2003; Cuellar, Rogers, & Hisghman, 2007; National Center for Complementary and Alternative Medicine [NCCAM], 2004; Oguamanam, 2006) (see Table 18-1). In general, alternative, complementary, and integrative treatments are thought to work by curing or decreasing the effects of a chronic illness, reducing anxiety and pain, and providing a feeling of wellness and involvement in care (Helms, 2006).

Users

Americans (n = 31,044) were interviewed about health and illness in the National Health Interview Survey, completed in 2002. This survey found use of alternative, complementary, and integrative treatments increased 20% in 4 years to 36% of the subjects. These results excluded prayer and multivitamins; including these as therapies, the percentage was 62% (Burke, Ginzburg, Collie, Trachtenberg, & Muhammad, 2005; Helms, 2006; NCCAM, 2004; Saydah & Eberhardt, 2006; Sommers & Porter, 2006). Most individuals who use nonstandard therapies have at least one chronic illness (Saydah & Eberhardt, 2006). The most frequently cited therapies were prayer for

TABLE 18-1

Definitions

Alternative Treatments	*Complementary Treatments*	*Integrative Treatments*
"practices are used in place of mainstream healthcare practices" (College of Registered Nurses of British Columbia, 2006, p. 20)	"practices are used alongside the mainstream healthcare system" (College of Registered Nurses of British Columbia, 2006, p. 20)	"a healthcare system in which physicians and nonconventional providers work in tandem to offer patients both biomedical and [complementary and alternative medicine] options" (Boozang, 2003, p. 251)
"used alone in place of conventional medical practices. A term for nonconventional therapies usually given by individuals who do not have a medical qualification and are not accepted by mainstream or Western medical establishments" (Cuellar et al., 2003, p. 129, 130)	"used in conjunction with conventional medical practices. They do not replace conventional biomedical treatments and may be used alone or as a non mainstream modality in addition to standard medical practice" (Cuellar et al., 2003, p. 129)	"includes conventional, complementary, and alternative approaches, as practiced by qualified providers working in respectful collaboration to offer effective patient-centered care" (Integrated Healthcare Policy Consortium, 2007)
"refers to treatments that replace traditional therapies" (Helms, 2006, p. 118)	"refers to therapies used in conjunction with conventional medicine" (Helms, 2006, p. 118)	"conventional, and complementary and alternative healthcare . . . options for addressing the body, mind and spirit, as well as the environment and relationships with others. It focuses on wellness, health promotion, and the healing process" (Integrative Health Institute at Mount Royal, 2007)

self (43%), prayer for others (24%), natural products (19%), and breathing exercises (12%). The most commonly reported health problems treated nonallopathically were anxiety, back or neck pain, colds, depression, or joint pain or stiffness (NCCAM, 2004). Annual costs, most of which are out-of-pocket expenses to the consumer, are thought to range from $21 to $47 billion (Burman, 2003; Sommers & Porter, 2006).

A study of rural-dwelling older adults diagnosed with diabetes [n = 698, with Native-Americans (n = 181), African Americans (n = 220), and Caucasians (n = 297)] examined the amount of and reasons for home remedy use. Findings revealed that 53% consumed food-related home remedies

and 57% employed non–food-related home remedies. Food-related home remedies were consumed by 60% of the Native American older adults, 59% of the African American older adults, and 43% of the Caucasian older adults. Non–food-related home remedies were employed by 68% of the Native American older adults, 65% of the African American older adults, and 45% of the Caucasian older adults. Reasons for home remedy use were unclear and require further study; however, the researchers suspect that culture and ethnicity may influence the meaning and value of self-care to older adults with chronic illnesses and influence home remedy selection and use (Grzywacz et al., 2006).

Reasons for Use

Individuals with chronic illnesses often feel frustrated with disease-focused, fragmented, time-limited traditional allopathic care. As a result, they may turn to alternative, complementary, and integrative practitioners, who take time to listen and evaluate not only their health problems but their entire life. Specifically, these nontraditional healthcare services are noted for extensive clinical evaluations that focus on understanding individuals and their experiences in dealing with a chronic illness; continuity with care providers over time; active participation in care by clinicians, patients, and their family members; choice of individualized services; provision of hope; open communication and information sharing; and an emphasis on the meaning and spiritual components of dealing with chronic illnesses (Bezold, 2005; Burman, 2003; Helms, 2006; Oguamanam, 2006; Saydah & Eberhardt, 2006).

More than 70% of users of alternative, complementary, and integrative treatments do not tell their allopathic healthcare providers about their use of other types of therapies (NCCAM, 2004; Saydah & Eberhardt, 2006). Perhaps this is because when clients do tell their clinicians about their choices, these providers often scold them, become angry and defensive, and dismiss their reasons for seeking additional care instead of exhibiting caring, compassionate, and understanding behaviors. This lack of empathy may result in future reluctance to tell conventional practitioners about nonstandard treatments as well as loss of trust in allopathic providers (Oguamanam, 2006; Sleath, Callahan, DeVellis, & Sloane, 2005).

Common Treatment Modalities

A national initiative established in 1991 to evaluate alternative treatments led to the establishment of the Office of Alternative Medicine (OAM) at the National Institutes of Health (NIH). In 1998 the OAM became the National Center for Complementary and Alternative Medicine (NCCAM) (Helms, 2006; NCCAM, 2004). The NCCAM identifies five major categories of alternative and complementary treatments including: (1) biologically-based treatment; (2) energy-based therapies; (3) manipulative and body-based approaches; (4) mind–body interventions; and (5) whole medical systems. Each of these categories of alternative and complementary treatments encompasses a wide variety of subcategories (Burman, 2003; Cuellar et al., 2007; Helms, 2006; NCCAM, 2004).

Biologically Based Treatment

Herbal medicine includes the use of various herbs such as echinacea, ginger rhizome, ginkgo biloba extract, ginseng root, wild chrysanthemum flower, and witch hazel. Practitioners use individualized combinations of herbs to treat people's chronic conditions. Herbal combinations are designed to interact with each other and with the body to provide a holistic sense of wellness.

Diet, nutrition, and lifestyle changes include the Gerson diet (raw foods and juices), macrobiotics (diets based on brown rice and vegetables), megavitamins, and nutritional supplements. Goals of nutritional therapies are to provide healthy energy sources and eliminate toxins. Pharmacologic and biological treatments include antioxidizing agents, chelation therapy, metabolic therapy, and oxidizing agents such as ozone. These therapies provide alternative ways to rid the body of toxins, strengthen the immune system, and treat chronic illnesses.

Energy-Based Therapies

This category includes bioelectromagnetic applications, such as blue light treatment, electroacupuncture, electromagnetic fields, and neuromagnetics, and healing life-force therapies, exemplified by Johrei, Qi gong, Reiki, and therapeutic touch (see Table 18-2). Bioelectromagnetic treatments are based on the interactions between living beings and electromagnetic fields, and are characterized as either ionizing or nonionizing electromagnetic radiation therapy. These applications may be used

TABLE 18-2

Energy-Based Therapies

Approach	Therapeutic Method	Rationale
Johrei	Noninvasive healing energy is transmitted from one person to another by tapping into a universal spiritual and healing energy or vibration.	Spiritual and healing energy cleanse the body and mind, promote healing, and enable a person to enjoy beauty and happiness.
Qi gong	A series of breathing exercises, meditation, and rhythmical movements is incorporated into one's life.	A smooth flow of energy promotes health and healing.
Reiki	Selected hand positions and placement are applied on various body parts.	Life energy is transmitted from the practitioner to the individual with a chronic illness to promote healing.
Therapeutic touch	The palms are held two to three inches away from a person's body to sense energy imbalances, correct imbalances, and facilitate energy flow throughout the body.	Energy does not stop where the physical body does and can be used to promote healing, increase functioning, and decrease pain.

Sources: The Johrei Institute. (2003). Frequently asked questions.Retrieved November 18, 2007, from http://www.johrei-institute.org/faq.asp#1, and National Center for Complementary and Alternative Medicine. (2003). *Research report: questions and answers about homeopathy*. (Publication No. NCCAM D183). NCCAM, National Institutes of Health. Retrieved March 14, 2008, from nccam.nih.gov/health/homeopathy/

for bone repair, immune system stimulation, nerve stimulation, neuroendocrine modulation, osteo-arthritis, and wound healing. Healing life-force therapies remain poorly understood from a scientific perspective but may be useful in clinical practice.

Manipulative and Body-Based Approaches

Manual healing methods include acupressure, Alexander technique, chiropractic medicine, cranial–sacral therapy, kinesiology, osteopathy, and reflexology (see Table 18-3). These methods incorporate physical manipulation to provide the individual with improved strength and flexibility, pain relief, and a feeling of overall wellness.

Mind–Body Interventions

Mind–body interventions are based on the interconnection between the mind and the body and include aerobic exercise; art, dance, and music therapy; biofeedback; counseling; hypnosis; imagery; meditation; prayer; relaxation; tai chi; and yoga. These therapies enable individuals to improve their physical health and reduce pain through participation in interventions that combine mental, physical, and spiritual activities.

Whole Medical Systems

Alternative medical systems of healing include acupuncture, Ayurvedic medicine, Chinese medicine, community-based healthcare practices such as shamanism and Native American Indian practices, environmental medicine, homeopathic medicine, and naturopathic medicine (see Table 18-4). Each system is based on its own philosophical and therapeutic perspective and provides holistic interventions designed to maintain wellness and treat chronic illnesses.

TABLE 18-3

Manipulative and Body-Based Approaches

Approach	Therapeutic Method	Rationale
Acupressure	The fingers are used to apply pressure to the same points in which needles are used in acupuncture.	Manipulation is used to change the energy flow in the body and lead to symptom relief.
Alexander technique	Verbal and tactile guidance is used to enable individuals to rebalance postural sets such as physical alignment by mentally focusing on the correct alignments.	Proper body mechanics reduce pain, improve functioning, and facilitate health.
Chiropractic medicine	Adjustments, high-velocity, low-amplitude thrusts, are made on the spinal column.	Replacing displaced structures promotes healing, improves functioning, and decreases pain.

Digging Deeper: Gaining Knowledge about a Specific Area

The purpose of this chapter is to provide an overview of alternative, complementary, and integrative treatments and to foster introspection that enables advanced practice nurses to consider their relationship with these therapies in the care of individuals with chronic illnesses. Some advanced practice nurses may want to learn more about a nonallopathic treatment than can be provided in this chapter. To whet the appetite, this section provides information about homeopathy. However, it is recognized that to become proficient in any area of interest that an advanced practice nurse may have, he or she should consider taking courses or clinical training with an expert.

An advanced practice nurse working with individuals with a chronic illness such as fibromyalgia may be concerned about fragmentation or inadequacy of allopathic care. He or she may become interested in nonallopathic treatments such as homeopathy and may choose to learn more about these therapies in order to offer these options.

What Is Homeopathy?

Homeopathy is a whole medical system or a different philosophical way of viewing individuals and illnesses that was developed in Germany in the 18th century by Samuel Hahnemann. He was concerned about the inadequacy of accepted medical treatments, which included blood-letting, blistering, and the use of mercury, and sought to find gentler, more conceptually appealing therapies (NCCAM, 2003).

Hahnemann was a chemist, a linguist, and a medical doctor. In his work as a linguist, when translating a book, he read about cinchona bark, an herbal remedy used to treat malaria. He obtained some cinchona bark and noted that when ingested, it caused symptoms of malaria. Based on this, Hahnemann hypothesized that substances that produced symptoms similar to a disease might be useful in treating that disease. He tested, observed, and recorded this hypothesis on many herbal and chemical substances, and these findings formed the foundation of the discipline of homeopathy. He reported that diluting these substances, using small quantities of substances, and shaking the mixture during dilution yielded the best results. Hahnemann also believed in treating the entire individual—paying attention to nutrition, sleep, exercise, emotional states, and cognition. Because of this individualized approach, two people matched on gender and age with the same disease

| TABLE 18-4 | | |

Whole Medical Systems

Approach	Therapeutic Method	Rationale
Acupuncture	Thin needles are inserted superficially on the skin in various patterns and left in place for 8 to 20 minutes.	Points along channels of energy are manipulated to restore balance.
Ayurvedic medicine	Herbs, lifestyle modification, meditation, nutrition, oil massages, and yoga are used to balance three core principles or elements (vata dosha, movement in body; pitta dosha, digestion of food and liquids; and kapha dosha, protection and stability).	Balancing the three core principles will form an inner state of harmony, spiritual realization, and self-healing.
Chinese medicine	All aspects of the person are interconnected and interacting with the environment. Acupuncture, herbs, and nutrition are used to promote health and internal and external balance.	Health and healing result from determining and resolving imbalances of energy flow in the body.
Community-based health practices	Shamanism and American Indian healthcare practices are examples.	Culturally relevant approaches are necessary to treat health problems.
Environmental medicine	Testing of environmental factors such as the quality of air, food, and water is done.	Illness frequently derives from environmental causes.
Homeopathic medicine	Remedies made from naturally occurring substances are given in small doses to produce a cure. High doses of the remedy would produce the illness.	This system was developed in the late 18th century and is based on the Law of Similars. The symptom is part of the cure.
Naturopathic medicine	Natural treatments such as acupuncture, exercise, herbal preparations, and nutrition are provided.	A healthy state is maintained to prevent illnesses and to facilitate healing.

Sources: The Ayurvedic Center. Discovering your ayurvedic constitution. Retrieved November 18, 2007, from www. holheal.com/ayurved3.html; National Center for Complementary and Alternative Medicine. (2004). *Expanding horizons of health care: strategic plan 2005–2009.* (Publication No. NIH 04–5568). US Department of Health and Human Services National Institutes of Health. Retrieved November 18, 2007 from nccam.nih.gov/about/plans/2005/ index.htm, and National Center for Complementary and Alternative Medicine. (2007). *What is ayurvedic medicine?* (Publication No. NCCAM D287). US Department of Health and Human Services National Institutes of Health. Retrieved November 18, 2007, from nccam.nih.gov/health/ayurveda/

could have very different homeopathic treatments (NCCAM, 2003).

Educational Preparation for Homeopathic Practitioners

Educational preparation for becoming a homeopath consists of three elements: formal theory instruction, individualized learning, and clinical supervision. Curricula and format vary; however, a consensus document developed by the Council for Homeopathic Education recommending that educational standards should guide homeopathic programs (Council for Homeopathic Education, 2008; Standards and Competencies for the Professional Practice of Homeopathy in North America, 2006).

Homeopathic educational options include certificate and diploma programs. Typically, licensed health-care professionals such as physicians, advanced practice nurses, or chiropractors augment their professional expertise by obtaining additional education as homeopaths (NCCAM, 2003).

Homeopathic Practice

Homeopathic practitioners spend between 1 and 4 hours comprehensively assessing an individual with chronic illnesses. Several days to a week later they have a follow-up appointment and discuss the treatment plan with the individual and his or her family. Routine follow-up appointments occur as therapeutic adjustments are needed (NCCAM, 2003).

Substances, or remedies, are prescribed to treat individuals. Remedies must be labeled and list their name, the ingredients, the dilutions required, and the instructions for use. The Homeopathic Pharmacopoeia of the United States, which is published by homeopathic experts, serves as the primary clinical and prescribing source for information about remedies. Research indicates that homeopathic remedies are safe; however, some people report initial exacerbation of disease symptoms, which soon subsides. Studies evaluating the effectiveness of homeopathic treatments are inconclusive (NCCAM, 2003).

INFORMATIONAL ISSUES

Informational issues concerning alternative, complementary, and integrative therapies include research, dissemination of information, legislative matters, and quackery.

Research

In 2004 the budget of the NCCAM was $117.8 million; however, through collaborative partnerships with other Institutes at NIH, overall funding for alternative, complementary, and integrative research was estimated to be $305 million. Despite what may seem like a large budget, NCCAM funded only 17% of the proposals that it received. The goals of the NCCAM are to fund research that establishes a scientific knowledge base about alternative, complementary, and integrative treatments; educate researchers; and disseminate information to professionals and the public. By the end of 2004, NCCAM had funded more than 1000 research studies at more than 200 institutions on a wide variety of clinically applicable topics. Research areas included cancer, endocrinology, mental health, and pain. Most funded projects examined biologically-based treatment or whole medical systems; however, NCCAM is seeking increased research in mind–body interventions as well as the other categories (NCCAM, 2004).

There are challenges to designing accurate and rigorous research studies to evaluate alternative, complementary, and integrative therapies. Determining the correct therapy, amount to be administered, and population to receive the treatment is essential in order to test effectiveness, but is particularly challenging when these parameters are not standardized in the practice arena. Another concern related to variability arose when analyzing biologically-based products such as herbs and nutritional supplements; NCCAM now requires that these products be research-grade. Most studies have evaluated the effectiveness of single aspects of whole medical systems; however, new methodologies that enable researchers to examine the entire system need to be developed (Kligler, 2004; National Center for Complementary and Alternative Medicine, 2004).

Criticisms of research on alternative, complementary, and integrative treatments include the following: studies often do not use hypothesis testing, large numbers of subjects, or randomly assign subjects to treatment and control groups; and they often rely on subjective responses from clients rather than objective measures. Strategies to address these concerns include use of individuals as their own controls over time and a focus on patient satisfaction. To provide more population-

CASE STUDY

Mrs. Martin, a 70-year-old woman, developed rheumatoid arthritis when she was 18 years old. Her first symptoms were swelling in her left knee and ankle. She had just relocated from a rural community to a college town, where she worked as a secretary full-time and attended college part-time. She was in a great deal of pain when she went to see a physician. The physician drained her knee, performed various diagnostic tests, and informed her that she had rheumatoid arthritis. She was told to take 12 aspirin throughout the course of each day. No education regarding her illness, prognosis, or the potential side effects of her medication were provided. She was shy, deferred to authority figures, and was unprepared to advocate for herself.

She took a leave of absence from her job for a month, returned to the rural community in which she was raised, and rested. Her father had died when she was 4 years old. Her mother had an eighth-grade education. Her two older brothers and sisters lived nearby but were not actively involved in her life. After she had rested and began to feel a little better, she returned to her secretarial job and continued taking classes. Her left knee and both of her ankles remained swollen and painful, and the same symptoms developed in her fingers, wrists, and elbows. She had her knee drained and injected with steroid medication every other month; however, in a short time it would swell again. She felt fatigued and in pain.

Several years after her diagnosis, she married and had two children. During the course of her pregnancies, her arthritis symptoms totally resolved. After each of her children was born, her symptoms immediately came back. As the years went by, she was followed closely by her primary care physician and saw a number of internists and rheumatologists. She took many different nonsteroidal anti-inflammatory agents.

Her joints were periodically drained and injected with a steroid. She tried gold shots without any relief. She went to physical therapists and was careful to eat a healthy and well-balanced diet. Over time, her wrists, elbows, fingers, and feet developed joint deformities and contractures. Despite the deformities and pain, she maintained an active lifestyle and balanced her household and maternal duties.

When she was 35, Mrs. Martin's symptoms became so severe that she was unable to do any household work and was bedridden for 6 months. Because of her severe pain, she cried most of the time that she was awake. Her primary care doctor was empathetic but unable to help her. He referred her to a rheumatologist who failed to help relieve her suffering, but told her, "You're doing fine for having a case of rheumatoid arthritis that is so aggressive."

Mr. Martin began to actively read about arthritis and search for ways to help relieve some of his wife's suffering. The couple tried a number of dietary programs without success. One day a friend mentioned to Mr. Martin that he knew of a woman with rheumatoid arthritis who had been in a wheelchair and was now walking. Mr. Martin tracked the woman down, and she told him about an alternative treatment for arthritis that seemed miraculous and had changed her life.

Because this was an alternative treatment, governmental regulations prohibited it from being provided in the United States. Against the advice of her rheumatologist, Mr. and Mrs. Martin went to Canada for therapy. Within 3 days, Mrs. Martin's pain and swelling were reduced. She was walking, had resumed her household duties, and felt more energetic and in less pain than she had felt in her adult life. The contractures that had developed did not go away. However, with the use of her alternative treatment

(Continued)

■ CASE STUDY (*Continued*)

and an array of vitamins, healthy nutrition, exercise, and rest, she was functioning again. Mrs. Martin has been on this alternative regimen for 35 years. She adjusts her dosage daily in response to the presence of symptoms and continues to walk a half a mile each day, drive a car, do much of her own housework, and participate in social activities such as going to the opera.

Over the years, primary care physicians have not been willing to prescribe Mrs. Martin's alternative treatment, requiring her to travel yearly to get her medication. However, they have been amazed at the change in her health status. Currently, although several newer allopathic treatments for rheumatoid arthritis are available, she does not see a rheumatologist. In order to determine if any of these allopathic treatments were appropriate for her, Mrs. Martin consulted with seven different rheumatologists. Each chastised her for her long-term use of an alternative, unproven therapy and was unwilling to discuss transitioning her to one of the newer allopathic treatments unless she completely stopped her existing medication (in order for them to do several months of work-up). Consequently, since she is functioning well, considering the severity and length of time that she has had her disease, Mrs. Martin has opted to continue alternative treatment and also has

weekly massages to help with mobility, muscle relaxation, and pain minimization.

Discussion Questions

1. What motivated Mrs. Martin to begin using alternative treatment for her rheumatoid arthritis?
2. What worked well for Mrs. Martin in the allopathic healthcare system, and what did not work well?
3. Advanced practice nurses were absent from Mrs. Martin's care; what are some of the ways that they could have—or should have—been involved in her care?
4. How will you help individuals who have chronic illnesses and choose to use alternative treatments to meet their healthcare needs?
5. What would you do if you or one of your family members developed a chronic illness that was continuing to cause worsening disability and suffering and allopathic healthcare providers were unable to offer effective treatment options?
6. What is the advanced practice nurse's role in advocating for expanded practice, changes in the healthcare system, and an open-minded, hope-based approach with regard to alternative treatments for individuals with chronic illnesses?

---

specific knowledge, research that examines the effects of nonstandard treatments on children, older adults, and vulnerable populations needs to increase. In addition, qualitative research investigating patients' experiences is necessary (Boozang, 2003; Kligler, 2004; NCCAM, 2004; Oguamanam, 2006).

Barriers to research of nontraditional treatments include limited funding; lack of needed

research skills among practitioners; lack of access to computers, academic libraries, and statistical support; problems obtaining suitable numbers of subjects; difficulty in comparing and interpreting research; and methodological issues such as individualized treatment and lack of control subjects for comparison. Ultimately, allopathic medicine demands scientific validation of the efficacy of a treatment on composite groups of patients using experimental and control groups, whereas, nonallopathic therapies emphasize holistic, individualized treatment that is qualitative in nature. Therefore, the two therapeutic paradigms may lend themselves to different types of evaluative research (Boozang, 2003; Oguamanam, 2006).

Individuals with chronic illnesses who have had positive outcomes using nontraditional therapies believe their experiences to be valid and significant. They reject the dismissal of their results as anecdotal and inconsequential and support increased case study methodology to validate and explain their experiences (Boozang, 2003; Isaacs, 2007).

Dissemination of Information

Journals developed for healthcare practitioners to address alternative, complementary, and integrative treatments include: *Alternative Therapies in Health and Medicine, Complementary Therapies in Medicine, Evidence Based Complementary and Alternative Medicine, Journal of Alternative and Complementary Medicine, Journal of Holistic Nursing,* and *Research in Complementary Medicine* (American Holistic Nurses Association, 2007a; Coelho, Pittler, & Ernst, 2007; Helms, 2006). The Internet is another useful source of information (see Internet Resources at the end of this chapter).

Coelho et al. (2007), in an effort to categorize knowledge dissemination and compare it with previously published categorizations from 1995 and 2000, examined the 2005 contents of six major journals that publish research on alternative, complementary, and integrative treatments. Fewer articles than in previous years were clinical trials (1995 had 28%, 2000 had 23%, and 2005 had 22%). Several additional journals were also reviewed, which had not previously been included in the 2000 and 1995 investigations. With these articles included (n = 363), only 19% of the manuscripts were classified as clinical trials. None of the journals published meta-analyses, and only 4% of the articles were a systematic review of the state of the science. The most common

articles were about general alternative, complementary, and integrative topics (20%), phytomedicine (standardized herbal treatments) (14%), and homeopathy (11%). This survey of the literature indicates that although the number of individuals with chronic illnesses is increasing, the evidence-based literature testing nonallopathic therapies to treat these individuals is decreasing. Clinicians who want to provide safe and effective options for their clients and families are in a quandary because they know that hope and options are essential both for treatment of disease and for healing the human spirit; however, they also know that scientific evaluation of treatment modalities is necessary.

Legislative Matters

Legal matters related to alternative, complementary, and integrative therapies are discussed in two sections: overall paradigm issues and those specific to advanced practice nurses.

Paradigm Issues

Some critics of allopathic health care have argued that physicians, out of self-interest, have convinced legislators to restrict the scope of practice of alternative, complementary, and integrative healthcare providers and limit choices for individuals with chronic illnesses. They believe that because physicians work closely with hospitals, pharmaceutical companies, and reimbursers, they have persuaded these organizations to avoid partnering with nontraditional healthcare providers. Therefore, according to these critics, physicians, hospitals, pharmaceutical companies, and reimbursers have influenced policy and legislation to limit these practices and, when possible, to prosecute nonphysician practitioners who offer competitive healthcare services (Boozang, 1998; Cuellar et al., 2003).

Ultimately, a clash exists between proponents of the allopathic healthcare paradigm and proponents of the alternative, complementary, and integrative healthcare paradigm. Advocates of the allopathic healthcare paradigm believe that governmental regulation is based on scientific evidence, promotes safety, and ensures that the treatment provided to persons with a chronic illness is effective. Advocates of the nonallopathic healthcare paradigm believe that individuals should have access to information and treatment, the freedom to evaluate benefits and risks, and ultimately decide for themselves their form of health care (Cuellar et al., 2003; Oguamanam, 2006).

Advanced Practice Nursing Issues

Advanced practice nurses providing care for individuals with chronic illnesses are often concerned about whether activities related to alternative, complementary, and integrative treatment fall within acceptable legal parameters. In addition, they are worried about liability protection as it relates to nontraditional therapies (College of Registered Nurses of British Columbia, 2006; Cuellar et al., 2003; NCCAM, 2004). For example, individuals with a chronic illness who feel that they have exhausted allopathic options may ask advanced practice nurses to prescribe or administer nonallopathic treatments. Clinicians may feel persuaded by anecdotal evidence, compassion for clients and their families, and the belief that the treatment is in their scope of practice; however, they may be concerned about how the Board of Nursing or their malpractice insurer would view their prescribing or administering the requested treatment. Contacting the Board of Nursing and their malpractice insurer to obtain other perspectives may provide useful feedback about the desired treatment and assist advanced practice nurses in making wise decisions (Cuellar et al., 2003).

Advanced practice nurses should know that states differ regarding licensure of nonallopathic practitioners. For example, acupuncturists must be licensed in 34 states, massage therapists in 27 states, naturopaths in 14 states, and

homeopaths in 4 states. Nonallopathic treatment comprises only 5% of malpractice insurance policies and is offered by less than 50 underwriters. Therefore, advanced practice nurses should be aware that such coverage may not be included or available under their existing malpractice policy (Cuellar et al., 2003).

Quackery

Although research verifying the effectiveness of most alternative, complementary, and integrative treatments is inadequate, practitioners have the responsibility to provide information regarding the known benefits and risks of the treatment (Chez & Jonas, 2005; Cuellar et al., 2003). When healthcare providers misrepresent treatments to consumers, they are committing fraud (Cuellar et al., 2003).

Boozang (1998) defines quackery as treatment that is implausible, unscientific, unproven, or disproved. She notes, however, that some nonallopathic treatments, although not yet adequately evaluated (unproven), may be helpful to clients. She emphasizes the importance of heightened informed consent for any treatments outside of the accepted standard of care. Cuellar and colleagues (2003) state that clinicians have a duty to present both traditional and nontraditional perspectives and assert that informed consent means providing information about allopathic and nonallopathic treatment options along with benefits, risks, and uncertainties associated with each choice.

CONCEPTUAL ISSUES

The way that advanced practice nurses view individuals with chronic illnesses will help them empathize with the difficult treatment choices that these people make.

Cultural Factors

Individuals with chronic illnesses can be characterized as a unique cultural group whose daily life is influenced by unpredictable exacerbations and remissions of their disease. To provide culturally sensitive care, clinicians need to understand the experience of living with a chronic illness from the point of view of clients and family members. This requires empathy that is not stressed in many allopathic educational programs. Rather, the focus of most allopathic training programs is on understanding symptoms, diseases, and treatments—not on understanding the human experience of living with a chronic illness (Baker, 2007; Burman, 2003; Chez & Jonas, 2005; Oguamanam, 2006; Wagner, Bennett, Austin, Greene, Schaefer, & Vonkorff, 2005).

Advanced practice nurses who are educated to think about the implications of dealing with a chronic illness on a 24-hour basis are in a unique position to consider individuals with a chronic illness as being members of a distinct cultural group. Although advanced practice nurses frequently either lead support groups or refer their patients to support groups designed to enable individuals with similar health problems to listen to each other, share coping strategies, and nurture each other; they may not carry this cultural perspective into the allopathic care that they provide. Using a cultural perspective may enhance empathy and understanding and enable advanced practice nurses to strengthen their therapeutic relationship with patients who have chronic illnesses (Burman, 2003; Chez & Jonas, 2005; Wagner et al., 2005).

Recognition that the advanced practice nurse who is providing care is an outsider is an essential component of this perspective. Rather than expecting individuals with chronic illnesses to fit into the pervasive acute illness, disease-focused model that characterizes much of health care, practitioners should acknowledge to their patients the complexity of living with a chronic illness. Advanced practice nurses who understand the culture of an individual with a chronic illness can better comprehend and assist with treatment choices (Baker, 2007; Burman, 2003; Chez & Jonas, 2005; Wagner et al., 2005).

Professional Education

Medical schools are realizing the importance of including alternative, complementary, and integrative therapies in curricula. In 1998, 63% of medical schools offered at least one course dedicated to this content and 37% offered two or more (Helms, 2006).

Nursing schools have been slower to include classes in alternative, complementary, and integrative treatments. This material is often integrated throughout graduate and undergraduate curricula; however, few schools provide dedicated courses. Several schools have made a noteworthy commitment to nonallopathic theories. The University of Minnesota has incorporated alternative, complementary, and integrative content and research into its undergraduate, masters, and doctoral programs in nursing. The University of California at San Francisco was the first nurse practitioner program in the country to include this material in its curriculum. In order to prepare advanced practice nurses to properly care for individuals with chronic illnesses, nursing education needs to instruct students about these therapies (Helms, 2006).

Ethical Decision Making

Advanced practice nurses working with individuals who have chronic illnesses may experience ethical decision-making challenges related to the use of nonallopathic treatment. Two examples are provided in subsequent text; however, advanced practice nurses who care for people with chronic illnesses will face a number of ethical issues that are almost impossible to predict. Thinking about one's values, beliefs, and rationale for decision-making will help prepare the advanced practice nurse for those unexpected and difficult challenges.

Dr. Litton—A 58-Year-Old with Amyotrophic Lateral Sclerosis

Dr. Ezra Litton is a 58-year-old man who has postdoctoral education and is a mathematician. He is a professor and owns a successful mathematical consulting business. Ezra has been happily married for 32 years to his wife, Ursula, who is a geologist. They have three children, Samuel, who is 30, married, has two children, and lives across the country; Jenna, who is 27, married, and lives in another state; and Ben, who is 25 and in graduate school in another state. Although their children are grown and do not live nearby, Ezra and Ursula maintain a close relationship with them.

Throughout his adult life, Ezra has tried to maintain a healthy balance between work and family. He visits relatives once a year, has several good friends, and has many acquaintances. He eats healthy foods and exercises at a gym twice a week. He has never smoked cigarettes, used illegal drugs, or used alcohol excessively. He describes himself as a "high energy person" and functions well on about 6 hours of sleep a night.

Ezra has been seeing Ms. Zareau, a family nurse practitioner, for physical examinations and episodic visits for 28 years. He has excellent preventive health care and health habits. Ezra is known to Ms. Zareau to always be on time for appointments, prepared, cooperative, and highly motivated. Ms. Zareau considers him to be, "the model patient, just an all around great guy." She provides care for the entire family and says that, "the whole family is special." She feels that long-term relationships like these are what make being an advanced practice nurse meaningful and rewarding.

About 2 years ago, Ezra set up an appointment with Ms. Zareau because he was feeling weak, had tripped over carpet several times, and was dropping things (Amyotrophic Lateral Sclerosis Association [ALSA], 2008a). Ms. Zareau did a neurologic and muscle evaluation, laboratory work (including blood and urine studies with high resolution serum protein electrophoresis, thyroid and parathyroid hormone levels, and 24-hour urine collection for heavy metals), and X-rays. She also referred him to a neurologist for further evaluation (ALSA, 2008b). The neurologist diagnosed him with amyotrophic lateral sclerosis (ALS), also known as Lou Gehrig's disease.

Ezra has been a model patient in coping with his ALS; however, his illness has progressed. About a year and a half ago he took disability from his job at the university, and several months later closed his consulting business. Ursula took family medical leave for 6 months to modify their house for a person with a disability, made sure that business and legal matters such as power of attorney and advance directives were updated, and hired around the clock live-in care. She has gone back to work out of financial necessity. Ezra's treatment team includes physical, occupational, and speech therapists; rehabilitation specialists; and two neurologists. He now uses a motorized wheelchair and is unable to feed himself or do any activities of daily living on his own.

Ezra's mind remains active, and he and his wife have used the Internet to look for treatment options. They recognize that gold treatment is a long-shot but have spoken to three individuals with ALS in different states who have experienced remission using gold treatment. These individuals have sent information regarding their dosage and where they obtained their medication. In addition, Ezra and Ursula have read information from homeopathic, alternative, and anecdotal sources that explain the rationale, procedures, dosing, and prescribing for gold in ALS treatment. They have provided this information to their two neurologists, who have dismissed their requests to have this information reviewed (Smith, 2008; Earth Clinic, 2008).

Ezra and Ursula have a long-standing relationship with Ms. Zareau; they trust her and know that she cares about them as individuals, so they share the information that they have gathered with her and ask her if she would be willing to order gold treatment for Ezra. They say that they understand that she may feel uncomfortable with this request, but they ask her to put herself in their position, think about the evidence that they have provided, and make a fair-minded, and hope-based decision. They also state that they will be happy to sign any type of form stating that they understand that this is not the usual treatment but that under the circumstances, they want to take the risk because they feel that the risk of not trying this treatment outweighs the benefit of trying the treatment (Atkinson, 2008).

Nurse practitioners in the state in which Ms. Zareau works are independent. They are governed exclusively by the Board of Nursing. They do not practice under the supervision of physicians or as physician extenders. They are expected to abide by the regulations of the Board of Nursing and provide care within their scope of practice. Ms. Zareau contacts the Board of Nursing to obtain further clarification. The Board representative says that if she is knowledgeable about a treatment and deems it to be appropriate, she should document her rationale and provide the treatment. Ms. Zareau contacts her malpractice insurance company, but is unable to speak with a lawyer. The service representative tells her that careful documentation of care is necessary. She consults a trusted colleague and asks him about the case. He says that there is "no way" that he would ever prescribe a medication that was not approved by the Food and Drug Administration (FDA).

Ms. Zareau cares about Ezra. She has worked with him for 28 years and knows that he is a thorough, reliable, and careful person. She understands that he is suffering from an incurable disease and that allopathic treatments offer no hope. She believes that trust and offering hope are the most valuable interventions that an advanced practice nurse can provide to a person with a chronic illness. She has talked to both Ezra and Ursula and know that they are not looking for a cure or a miracle; they are looking for some relief of suffering, improved quality of life, and a little extra time together. She worries that other practitioners may question her judgment and even file a complaint against her to the Board of Nursing. Since she has not spoken to Ursula and Ezra's children about this treatment, she is concerned that one of them may be angry about their father's illness and may file a law suit against her at some point in the future. What should she do? What would you do? Why?

Ms. Bispiki—A 76-Year-Old with Dementia, Depression, and Osteoporosis

Ms. Marie Bispiki, a 76-year-old woman, has just moved to an assisted living facility. She was admitted because of wandering at night, constant weeping, periodic agitation, and occasional falls. She had been living at home with her 78-year-old husband, Jimmie. Her three children are supportive, live in neighboring counties, and have chronic health problems.

Marie has seen her primary care physician for about 35 years and has a good relationship with him. She was diagnosed with osteoporosis after menopause and was treated by her primary care physician. She was also diagnosed with depression after menopause and has seen two endocrinologists, one neurologist, five psychiatrists, three psychologists, and a massage therapist. None of these professionals substantially improved her symptoms: crying; sadness; lethargy; lack of interest; irritability; agitation; anxiety; somatic concerns; insomnia; loss of appetite; and feeling hopeless, lonely, and worthless. Two years ago Marie had difficulty doing crossword puzzles, which had previously been one of the few activities that she continued to enjoy. She was also unable to concentrate when reading. Her primary care physician did a number of tests and referred her to a neurologist, who confirmed a diagnosis of dementia, probably of the Alzheimer's type. She was followed by this neurologist and was also seen by a geropsychiatrist.

Faced with Marie's deteriorating condition and an absence of tangible benefit from the many allopathic specialists seen, her family decided to have her evaluated by a homeopath/naturopath. Because they had such a long-standing and good relationship with her primary care physician, they planned to continue seeing him and asked him if he would be comfortable working with an alternative healthcare provider. He said that he thought that this arrangement would be good and welcomed the ideas of the homeopath/naturopath. Jimmie, Marie, the three children, and their spouses went in two cars on a 2-hour one way trip to see the homeopath/naturopath, Dr. Miller, who was also a medical physician. The first assessment visit lasted 4 hours and was quite thorough. That appointment was followed by another 2-hour visit in which a treatment plan was proposed. A follow-up appointment was scheduled one month later and then every 3 months thereafter.

The day after the second visit to Dr. Miller, Marie moved into the assisted living facility. Jimmie had told the administrator that Marie was seeing a homeopath/naturopath and that treatment recommendations were pending. He was assured that this was not a problem. Upon admission, Jimmie brought a sheet with orders stating the name of the medication, dose, route, time, frequency, and purpose of each supplement or tincture. He also delivered information about each of the supplements or tinctures that included purpose, composition, desired effect, side effects, contraindications, acceptable dosages, and other pertinent facts. In addition, he brought medications, supplements, and tinctures that the homeopath/naturopath had provided.

Six days later, Mr. Peters, the clinical nurse specialist at the assisted living center, was doing an assessment on Marie and identified that her Mini-Mental State Examination had gone from a 10 of 30 to a 13 of 30 (Dellasega & Morris, 1993; Tombaugh & McIntyre, 1992) and that her Hamilton Rating Scale for Depression had gone from a 28 of 52 to a 23 of 52 (Miller, Bishop, Norman, & Maddever, 1985). He asked the registered nurse (RN) on day shift how she thought that Marie was doing. The nurse expressed concern about administering medications that were not FDA approved. The nurse said that she was worried about her license because she did not know what all of these medications were and that she was not sure that they were safe to administer. She also pointed out that over the course of the day, Marie was taking 84 different pills and said, "It is no wonder she is not eating much. She does not have room in her stomach for anything but all of those pills."

Mr. Peters asked other medication nurses [licensed practical nurses (LPNs) and RNs] on all three shifts what their perspective was about Marie's homeopathic/naturopathic medication regimen. Responses varied. Some nurses thought that she was doing better as a result of the medications, whereas others disagreed. Some felt comfortable giving the medications and believed that they had enough information about the medications to safely administer them, whereas others did not.

Mr. Peters contacted the Board of Nursing, which told him that homeopaths and naturopaths were licensed professionals in his state. However, in this situation the homeopath/naturopath was also a medical physician. The Board of Nursing representative said that nurses are legally obligated to administer medication that a physician orders. Mr. Peters raised concerns that the supplements and tinctures were not FDA approved, information about the medication had only been provided by the homeopath/naturopath, and that 84 pills were taken each day. He also pointed out that the patient's cognitive and affective status seemed to be improving. The Board of Nursing representative said that nurses need to follow the regulations that govern their practice and that this was a complicated situation.

Mr. Peters talked with the assisted living administrators and family, who felt that the nurses should provide the supplements and tinctures. As a clinical nurse specialist, Mr. Peters is responsible for assessing individuals and families as well as facilitating staff and agency functioning. Staffing is limited, and only one LPN or RN is often available to administer medications; therefore, maintaining staffing rotations that ensure that a nurse who believes that it is acceptable to administer these supplements and tinctures is not feasible. Coming in each shift to administer the supplements himself for the rest of her stay at the assisted living facility is not a good use of Mr. Peters' time and is also not feasible. What should he do? What would you do? Why?

INTERVENTIONS

Advanced practice nurses considering the role of alternative, complementary, and integrative treatment in the care of individuals with chronic illnesses need to be aware of their life experiences and feelings, promote wise decision-making, deliver safe and effective care, and be informed about legal issues.

Self-Awareness

Advanced practice nurses need to be aware of their feelings about alternative, complementary, and integrative treatments as they relate to chronic illness. Typically, most advanced practice nurses are comfortable with complementary and integrative treatment; however, personal experience influences how they view alternative therapies that replace allopathic methods. Understanding one's own experiences and beliefs is essential in order to be present with individuals with chronic illnesses and understand their fears, concerns, motivations, and needs, without burdening them with personal biases that may inhibit them from making the wisest choices for their circumstances (American Holistic Nurses Association, 2007b; Burman, 2003; College of Registered Nurses of British Columbia, 2006).

Decision Making

Advanced practice nurses espouse individualized, holistic, and healing care; this requires considering the unique aspects, goals, and needs of each individual with a chronic illness. It is essential to partner with patients and view them as human beings, not cases with diseases (Burman, 2003; Chez & Jonas, 2005; Helms, 2006; Sleath et al., 2005; Wagner et al., 2005). Care should be accessible, affordable, compassionate, effective, efficient, evidence-based, patient-focused, safe, and timely (Bezold, 2005; Chez & Jonas, 2005). To facilitate wise decision-making, advanced practice nurses can ask individuals with chronic illnesses

considering alternative, complementary, and integrative treatments to address the following (Burman, 2003; College of Registered Nurses of British Columbia, 2006; Cuellar et al., 2003, 2007):

■   What is your goal in searching for an appropriate alternative, complementary, or integrative treatment (control over symptoms, cure, lengthening of life, or improved quality of life)?

■   Are you willing to accept responsibility for obtaining information and making choices about alternative, complementary, and integrative treatments?

■   Are you confident that you have been accurately diagnosed? Do you understand the benefits and risks of conventional treatments for your chronic illness?

■   What are the qualifications of those who are for and against nonallopathic treatments that you are considering? Do you have confidence in the providers of the therapies that you have selected?

■   Are you comfortable with the underlying principles of the nontraditional treatments that you are considering?

■   What side effects and interactions may occur with the therapies that you are examining?

■   Are the alternative, complementary, and integrative treatments that you are considering thought to be safe and effective for your specific illness?

■   Are you willing to invest needed time and money?

■   How long will it take to determine whether the treatments are working?

■   Are the benefits greater than the potential risks?

Safe and Effective Practice

Advanced practice nurses who provide alternative, complementary, and integrative therapies for individuals with chronic illnesses need to monitor their protocols and quality of care. Participation in relevant continuing education programs is essential. Merge practice, education, and research to promote discourse and evaluation of services. Develop educational programs for clinics, communities, and hospitals to foster knowledge and decision-making among patients and staff. Nursing education should use an integrated, holistic curriculum to enhance students' understanding and appreciation of alternative, complementary, and integrative treatments (Burke et al., 2005; Burman, 2003; Cuellar et al., 2003; Cuellar et al., 2007; Flannery, Love, Pearce, Jingyu, & Elder, 2006). Advanced practice certification examinations should include questions regarding these types of therapies (Burman, 2003).

Advanced practice nurses who provide alternative, complementary, and integrative treatment for individuals with chronic illnesses need to consider:

- Implementing quality improvement programs to promote safe protocols as well as evaluation of outcomes (Burman, 2003; Cuellar et al., 2003, 2007; NCCAM, 2004).
- Ethical and legal matters, such as informed consent, promotion of healthcare choices, maintenance of malpractice insurance, and professional accountability (Burman, 2003; Cuellar et al., 2003, 2007; Oguamanam, 2006; Sleath et al., 2005).
- Practice issues, including scope of practice and maintenance of standards of care (Burman, 2003; Cuellar et al., 2007; NCCAM, 2004).
- Education and information to ensure provider skills and competencies and to provide knowledge to individuals and families dealing with chronic illnesses (Burman, 2003; Chez & Jonas, 2005; Cuellar et al., 2003, 2007; Flannery et al., 2006; Sleath et al., 2005).
- Administrative matters, such as documentation of the treatment and its outcomes (Burman, 2003; Cuellar et al., 2003).

Advanced practice nurses providing alternative, complementary, and integrative treatments need to identify their intended outcomes. Clinical goals often include controlling pain, relaxation to foster health and healing, maintaining a healthy state to protect against illness, promoting optimal body function, and facilitating a feeling of internal and holistic connectedness (Burke et al., 2005; Burman, 2003; Cuellar et al., 2003).

Legal Implications

Advanced practice nurses wishing to incorporate alternative, complementary, and integrative treatments in their activities should be certain that therapies comply with federal, state, and local licensure and regulatory requirements. Close adherence to governmental requirements is challenging but necessary, as many of the individuals monitoring adherence to these requirements may have little understanding of nontraditional therapies (Burman, 2003; College of Registered Nurses of British Columbia, 2006; Cuellar et al., 2003; Helms, 2006; NCCAM, 2004).

Although individuals with chronic illnesses often use alternative, complementary, and integrative treatments, advanced practice nurses are challenged to maintain a balance between providing these therapies and protecting the public from potentially harmful interventions. Education about nonallopathic treatments can enable advanced practice nurses to intelligently differentiate between clinical innovations that do not harm individuals and offer them hope and fraudulent or harmful treatments that rob individuals of dignity and economic resources (Burman, 2003; College of Registered Nurses of British Columbia, 2006; Cuellar et al., 2003; Cuellar et al., 2007; NCCAM, 2004; Sleath et al., 2005).

Advanced practice nurses should share conceptual and data-based information about alternative, complementary, and integrative treatments with colleagues, legislators, and reimbursers. Regulatory reform to facilitate a flexible scope of practice with rigorous competency requirements will not only ensure public safety but will also enable clinicians to practice to the full extent of their preparation, improve access to nontraditional therapies, and promote cost-effective treatment options. Although existing state practice acts vary, they do not prohibit advanced practice nurses from providing nonallopathic treatments. As knowledge increases, state practice acts need to be revised to incorporate advanced practice nurses' rights to provide these services (Burman, 2003; Cuellar et al., 2003; NCCAM, 2004).

Evidence-Based Research

In evaluating the risks and benefits of alternative, complementary, and integrative therapies, advanced practice nurses should be guided by evidence-based information such as national guidelines, quality improvement data, research, and relevant opinions and perspectives (expert and otherwise) (College of Registered Nurses of British Columbia, 2006). Advanced practice nurses should be knowledgeable about nontraditional interventions related to their specialty. Examples of evidence-based research evaluating a variety of nonallopathic treatments follow.

- To explore alternative and complementary treatment use, Magin, Adams, Heading, Pond, and Smith (2006) performed semi-structured interviews with individuals with acne (n = 26), eczema (n = 7), and psoriasis (n = 29) (total n = 62). Findings revealed that the majority of participants used nonallopathic treatments. Subjects with acne employed these therapies to promote natural and generalized skin health and to feel a sense of control over treatment. Conversely, people with eczema and psoriasis tried a variety of disease-specific, nontraditional treatments, often switching because of lack of efficacy.
- To examine alternative and complementary therapy use, Matthews, Sellergren, Huo, List, and Fleming (2007) surveyed breast cancer survivors who had completed allopathic treatment at least one year previously (n = 115). Findings revealed that 69% used

nontraditional treatments, with 73% identifying their diagnosis of breast cancer as their rationale.

- To determine the effect of wet cupping on lipid levels, Niasari, Kosari, and Ahmadi (2007) studied 18- to 25-year-old men (n = 47). Wet cupping is a puncture-drainage technique aimed at removing toxins. Results showed that low density lipoprotein levels decreased significantly; however, triglyceride, total cholesterol, and high density lipoprotein levels did not change significantly.
- Robinson, Chesters, Cooper, and McGrail (2007) developed a new instrument, Perspectives on the Use in Communities of Complementary and Alternative Medicine Questionnaire. The purpose of the tool was to measure individuals' attitudes, concerns, and demographic data related to 23 nontraditional therapies. Rural and urban individuals in Victoria, Australia (n = 459) were surveyed, and solid preliminary reliability and validity results were obtained.
- Sarnat, Winterstein, and Cambron (2007) compared clinical and cost outcomes of integrative medicine providers with traditional medicine providers from 1999 to 2005 using health maintenance organization (HMO) member months (n = 70,274). Results showed the following reductions: 85% in medication costs, 62% in outpatient surgeries and procedures, 60% in hospital admissions, and 59% in hospital days.
- Spence, Thompson, and Barron (2005) evaluated self-reported health status in individuals with chronic illness who received outpatient homeopathic care in the United Kingdom (n = 6544). Findings revealed health improvement was better or much better for 51%, some better for 20%, unchanged for 23%, worse for 3%, and not reported for 3%.
- Wu, Lin, Wu, and Lin (2007) studied the effects of acupressure in individuals with chronic obstructive pulmonary disease in Taipei, Taiwan (n = 44). Acupressure decreased depression and dyspnea and increased oxygen saturation.

EVIDENCE-BASED PRACTICE BOX

Sampling clients using public health services over a 6-month period (n = 222), Sommers and Porter (2006) examined price elasticities associated with a 17% price increase for acupuncture, Chinese herbal consultations, and shiatsu. Their hypothesis was that the demand for acupuncture was inelastic, meaning that the demand for acupuncture would decrease to a lesser extent than the percentage of price change (price elastic coefficient [PEC] <–1). Findings revealed that although the demand for each service decreased, the demand for acupuncture was inelastic (PEC = –0.35). Conversely, there was an elastic demand for Chinese herbal consultation (PEC = –1.31) and more so for shiatsu (PEC = –2.34). The researchers were, therefore, correct in their prediction that most clients would continue to pay for acupuncture despite a significant price increase. They suggested that this might be explained by the perception of immediate and effective results from acupuncture.

Price elasticity research, although uncommon, is useful in evaluating clients' degree of commitment to specific nonallopathic therapy. Price elasticity helps to distinguish whether a product or service is viewed as a necessity or a luxury. In general, a nurse entrepreneur working with individuals with chronic illnesses would do well to specialize in areas of greater price elasticity. It is worth noting, however, that nontraditional health care is a dynamic and evolving market, so today's luxury may be tomorrow's necessity.

Source: Sommers, E., & Porter, K. (2006). Price elasticities for three types of CAM services: Experiences of a Boston public health clinic. *The Journal of Alternative and Complementary Medicine, 12*(1), 85–90.

OUTCOMES

Advanced practice nurses caring for individuals with chronic illnesses need to balance an open-minded, hope-based view of alternative, complementary, and integrative treatments with a scientific, evidence-based perspective. Advanced practice nurses are in a unique position to bridge the gap between allopathic and nonallopathic health care by melding compassion, flexibility, and commitment to scientific and clinical excellence with common sense.

People with chronic diseases are not having their needs met by the existing healthcare system, which is hampered by the dichotomous relationship between traditional and nontraditional schools of thought. The disciplinary perspective of advanced practice nurses enables them to offer these individuals alternative, complementary, and integrative options that address their specific circumstances.

STUDY QUESTIONS

1. What are alternative, complementary, and integrative treatments?
2. How many Americans use nonallopathic therapy?
3. Why do individuals with chronic illnesses use nontraditional treatments?
4. What are the five categories of alternative and complementary treatments outlined by the NCCAM?

5. Why is researching alternative, complementary, and integrative treatments challenging?
6. What journals and Web sites provide useful information for obtaining further knowledge about nonallopathic therapy?
7. What are some of the legislative issues associated with nontraditional treatments?
8. Why does Boozang recommend a "heightened" level of informed consent for alternative, complementary, and integrative therapy?
9. Why are advanced practice nurses in a unique position among allopathically trained clinicians to consider individuals with chronic illnesses from a cultural perspective?
10. How do nursing and medical school curricula differ regarding alternative, complementary, and integrative treatments?

11. How does self-awareness regarding nonallopathic therapies relate to providing unbiased care for individuals with chronic illnesses?
12. How can advanced practice nurses help individuals with chronic illnesses make decisions regarding alternative, complementary, and integrative treatments?
13. What factors need to be considered when providing safe and effective nonallopathic interventions to individuals with chronic illnesses?
14. What legal issues do advanced practice nurses need to consider when providing nontraditional treatments?
15. What does it mean to examine evidenced-based and outcome-based information about alternative, complementary, and integrative therapies?

INTERNET RESOURCES

American Holistic Nurses Association: www.ahna.org/home/home.html
Arthritis Consulting Services, Inc.: www.stoparthritis.com/
Complementary and Alternative Medicine (general information: en.wikipedia.org/wiki/Complementary_and_alternative_medicine
Complementary Healthcare Plans: www.chpplans.us/index.asp
How to Start an Alternative and Complementary Healthcare Business in Ontario: www.canadabusiness.ca/servlet/ContentServer?cid=1089652224388&lang=en&pagename=CBSC_FE%2Fdisplay&c=GuideHowto
Mayo Clinic, Complementary and Alternative Medicine Center: www.mayoclinic.com/health/alternative-medicine/CM99999
National Center for Complementary and Alternative Medicine: nccam.nih.gov/
National Center for Homeopathy: nationalcenterforhomeopathy.org/
New York Online Access to Health, Complementary and Alternative Medicine: www.noah-health.org/en/alternative/
The Skeptic's Dictionary: www.skepdic.com/althelth.html
Alternative Medicine Therapies, Ayurveda Medicine: library.thinkquest.org/24206/ayurveda-medicine.html
The Well Being Journal: www.wellbeingjournal.com

REFERENCES

American Holistic Nurses Association. (2007a). About AHNA. Retrieved November 18, 2007, from linkhttp://www.ahna.org./Aboutus/tabid/1158/Default.aspx

American Holistic Nurses Association. Publications and products. (2007b). Retrieved November 18, 2007, from www.ahna.org/Resources/Publications/tabid/1218/Default.aspx

Amyotrophic Lateral Sclerosis Association. (2008a). Fighting Lou Gehrig's disease. Diagnosing ALS. Retrieved March 14, 2008, from www.alsa.org/als/diagnosing.cfm?CFID=5940348&CFTOKEN=2f383a7-15c49b95-79284b308c7d-8151e5db14b7

Amyotrophic Lateral Sclerosis Association. (2008b). Fighting Lou Gehrig's disease: Initial symptoms of the disease. Retrieved March 14, 2008, from www.alsa.org/als/symptoms.cfm?CFID=5940348&CFTOKEN=2f383a7-15c49b95-7928-4b30-8c7d-8151e5db14b7

Atkinson, D. (2008). ALS/motor neuron disease, a very important discovery! Retrieved March 14, 2008, from baar.com/als_xlnk.htm

The Ayurvedic Center. (2007). Discovering your ayurvedic constitution. Retrieved November 18, 2007, from www.holheal.com/ayurved3.html

Baker, S.M. (2007). Who ignores individuality fails the patient. *Alternative Therapies in Health and Medicine*, *13*(2), S88-S95.

Bezold, C. (2005). The future of patient-centered care: Scenarios, visions, and audacious goals. *The Journal of Alternative and Complementary Medicine*, *11*(Suppl. 1), 77-84.

Boozang, K.M. (1998). Western medicine opens the door to alternative medicine. *American Journal of Law and Medicine*, *24*(2-3), 185-212.

Boozang, K.M. (2003). National policy on CAM: The White House Commission report. *The Journal of Law, Medicine and Ethics*, *31*(2), 251-261.

Burke, A., Ginzburg, K., Collie, K., Trachtenberg, D., & Muhammad, M. (2005). Exploring the role of complementary and alternative medicine in public health practice and training. *The Journal of Alternative and Complementary Medicine*, *11*(5), 931-936.

Burman, M.E. (2003). Complementary and alternative medicine: Core competencies for family nurse practitioners. *Journal of Nursing Education*, *42*(1), 28-34.

Chez, R.A., & Jonas, W.B. (2005). Challenges and opportunities in achieving healing. *The Journal of Alternative and Complementary Medicine*, *11*(Suppl. 1), 3-6.

Coelho, H.F., Pittler, M.H., & Ernst, E. (2007). An investigation of the contents of complementary and alternative medicine journals. *Alternative Therapies in Health and Medicine*, *13*(4), 40-44.

College of Registered Nurses of British Columbia. (2006). Complementary and alternative health care: The role of the nurse. *Nursing-bc*, *38*(3), 20-22.

Cuellar, N.G., Cahill, B., Ford, J., & Aycock, T. (2003). The development of an educational workshop on complementary and alternative medicine: What every nurse should know. *The Journal of Continuing Education in Nursing*, *34*(3), 128-135.

Cuellar, N.G., Rogers, A.E., & Hisghman, V. (2007). Evidenced based research of complementary and alternative medicine (CAM) for sleep in the community dwelling older adult. *Geriatric Nursing*, *28*(1), 46-52.

Council for Homeopathic Education. Standards. (2008). Retrieved March 14, 2008, from www.chedu.org/standards.html

Dellasega, C., & Morris, D. (1993). The MMSE to assess the cognitive state of elders. *Journal of Neuroscience Nursing*, *25*(3), 147-152.

Earth Clinic. (2008). Supplements and holistic cures: Supplements for Lou Gehrig's disease. Retrieved March 14, 2008, from www.earthclinic.com/CURES/lou_gehrigs_disease.html

Flannery, M.A., Love, M.M., Pearce, K.A., Jingyu, L., & Elder, W.G. (2006). Communication about complementary and alternative medicine: Perspectives of primary care clinicians. *Alternative Therapies in Health and Medicine*, *12*(1), 56-63.

Grzywacz, J.G., Arcury, T.A., Bell, R.A., Lang, W., Suerken, C.K., Smith, S.L., et al. (2006). Ethnic differences in elders' home remedy use: Sociostructural explanations. *American Journal of Health Behavior*, *30*(1), 39-50.

Helms, J.E. (2006). Complementary and alternative therapies: A new frontier for nursing education? *Journal of Nursing Education*, *45*(3), 117-123.

Integrated Healthcare Policy Consortium. (2007). Retrieved November 18, 2007, from ihpc.info/

Integrative Health Institute at Mount Royal. (2007). What is integrative health? Retrieved November 18, 2007, from www.mtroyal.ab.ca/integrativehealth/whatisIH.shtml

Isaacs, L.L. (2007). Evaluating anecdotes and case reports. *Alternative Therapies in Health and Medicine*, *13*(2), 36-38.

The Johrei Institute. (2003). Frequently asked questions. Retrieved November 18, 2007, from http://www.johrei-institute.org/faq.asp#1

Kligler, B. (2004). The role of the optimal healing environment in the care of patients with diabetes mellitus type II. *The Journal of Alternative and Complementary Medicine, 10*(Suppl. 1), 223–229.

Magin, P.J., Adams, J., Heading, G.S., Pond, D.C., & Smith, W. (2006). Complementary and alternative medicine therapies in acne, psoriasis, and atopic eczema: Results of a qualitative study of patients' experiences and perceptions. *The Journal of Alternative and Complementary Medicine, 12*(5), 451–457.

Matthews, A.K., Sellergren, S.A., Huo, D., List, M., & Fleming, G. (2007). Complementary and alternative medicine use among breast cancer survivors. *The Journal of Alternative and Complementary Medicine, 13*(5), 555–562.

Miller, I.W., Bishop, S., Norman, W.H., & Maddever, H. (1985). The modified Hamilton rating scale for depression: reliability and validity. *Psychiatry Research, 14*(2), 131–142.

National Center for Complementary and Alternative Medicine. (2003). Research report: questions and answers about homeopathy. (Publication No. NCCAM D183). NCCAM, National Institutes of Health. Retrieved March 14, 2008, from nccam.nih.gov/health/homeopathy/

National Center for Complementary and Alternative Medicine. (2004). Expanding horizons of health care: strategic plan 2005–2009. (Publication No. NIH 04–5568). U.S. Department of Health and Human Services National Institutes of Health. (2007). Retrieved November 18, 2007, from nccam.nih.gov/about/plans/2005/index.htm

National Center for Complementary and Alternative Medicine. (2007). What is ayurvedic medicine? (Publication No. NCCAM D287). U.S. Department of Health and Human Services National Institutes of Health. (2007). Retrieved November 18, 2007, from nccam.nih.gov/health/ayurveda/

Niasari, M., Kosari, F., & Ahmadi, A. (2007). The effect of wet cupping on serum lipid concentrations of clinically healthy young men: A randomized controlled trial. *The Journal of Alternative and Complementary Medicine, 13*(1), 79–82.

Oguamanam, C. (2006). Biomedical orthodoxy and complementary and alternative medicine: Ethical challenges of integrating medical cultures. *The Journal of Alternative and Complementary Medicine, 12*(5), 577–581.

Robinson, A., Chesters, J., Cooper, S., & McGrail, M. (2007). The PUC-CAM-Q: A new questionnaire for delving into the use of complementary and alternative medicines. *The Journal of Alternative and Complementary Medicine, 13*(2), 207–216.

Sarnat, R.L., Winterstein, J., & Cambron, J.A. (2007). Clinical utilization and cost outcomes from an integrative medicine independent physician association: An additional 3-year update. *Journal of Manipulative and Physiological Therapeutics, 30*(4), 263–269.

Saydah, S.H., & Eberhardt, M.S. (2006). Use of complementary and alternative medicine among adults with chronic diseases: United States 2002. *The Journal of Alternative and Complementary Medicine, 12*(8), 805–812.

Sleath, B., Callahan, L., DeVellis, R.F., & Sloane, P.D. (2005). Patients' perceptions of primary care physicians' participatory decision-making style and communication about complementary and alternative medicine for arthritis. *The Journal of Alternative and Complementary Medicine, 11*(3), 449–453.

Smith, R.A. (2008). David Atkinson Story. Retrieved March 14, 2008, from baar.com/atkinson.htm

Sommers, E., & Porter, K. (2006). Price elasticities for three types of CAM services: Experiences of a Boston public health clinic. *The Journal of Alternative and Complementary Medicine, 12*(1), 85–90.

Spence, D.S., Thompson, E.A., & Barron, S.J. (2005). Homeopathic treatment for chronic disease: A 6-year, university-hospital outpatient observational study. *The Journal of Alternative and Complementary Medicine, 11*(5), 793–798.

Standards and Competencies for the Professional Practice of Homeopathy in North America. (2006). A Report of a Summit Meeting Sponsored by the Council for Homeopathic Education. Retrieved March 14, 2008, from www.chedu.org/2001%20CHE%20Standards%20revised%201106.pdf

Tombaugh, T.N., & McIntyre, N.J. (1992). The Mini-Mental State Examination: A comprehensive review. *Journal of the American Geriatrics Society, 40*(9), 922–935.

Wagner, E.H., Bennett, S.M., Austin, B.T., Greene, S.M., Schaefer, J.K., & Vonkorff, M. (2005). Finding common ground: Patient-centeredness and evidence-based chronic illness care. *The Journal of Alternative and Complementary Medicine, 11*(Suppl. 1), 7–15.

Wu, H.S., Lin, L.C., Wu, S.C., & Lin, J.G. (2007). The psychologic consequences of chronic dyspnea in chronic pulmonary obstruction disease: The effects of acupressure on depression. *The Journal of Alternative and Complementary Medicine, 13*(2), 253–261.

IV

Impact of the System

19

Models of Care

Pamala D. Larsen

INTRODUCTION

As the population age 65 and older increases and the healthcare system sees more individuals with chronic illness, healthcare providers and third party payors are examining how they care for individuals with chronic disease long term. Increasingly we hear about disease management models that have demonstrated better patient outcomes than "usual care." Less well publicized, however, is nursing's role in caring for individuals with chronic disease. For some of us, it has always made sense that chronic care should be nursing's domain, particularly as we are looking at care as opposed to cure.

We continue, as a country, to outspend similar nations in health care. As noted previously in Chapter 1, however, more money does not translate into better patient outcomes or better value for the consumer. A phrase that is often heard today is "value-based" and "value-added," whether it be manufacturing, architecture, engineering, and now health care. What is the value in the health care that the patient is receiving? Robinson (2008) defines value in health care as measured in terms of contributions of health care minus the attendant costs, with both costs and contributions conceptualized broadly (p. 11).

The issues with the healthcare system are not new. The last push for reform and universal healthcare was the Clinton administration's attempt in 1994. When that failed, it was left up to the managed care markets to "control" care and costs. During this Fall 2008 presidential election, health care is front and center as an issue, as it should be. Public and private purchasers of care are tired of absorbing increasing costs. Employers are dropping or reducing healthcare coverage for employees. As enrollment shrinks in these managed care plans, these plans must realize more profit per member since they have less members (Schaeffer, 2007). In addition, Medicare and Medicaid are increasingly in the spotlight, and with the baby boomer generation approaching Medicare age, it's becoming clear that our country will not be able to sustain these programs indefinitely. Clearly, health care is at a crossroads, and at the core of that crossroads, is chronic care. How do we effectively provide quality care to those with chronic conditions?

This chapter provides an overview of a wide variety of models and frameworks that provide care for individuals and families with chronic illness.

Historical Perspectives

In 1983, Diagnosis Related Groups (DRGs) for reimbursement were initiated for all Medicare

459

patients. This was the direct result of trying to find a better way to pay care providers than the retrospective payment system that was in place from 1965 to 1983. Furthermore, healthcare costs were escalating and it seemed that paying care providers prospectively, per diagnosis group, would decrease costs. DRGs were implemented using the International Classification of Diseases, Ninth Revision, Clinical Modifications (ICD-9-CM). ICD-9-CM coding classifies diseases, symptoms, and procedures with individual codes. Although DRGs were used initially only for Medicare patients, now third party payors use the coding as well.

With the advent of DRGs, acute care facilities soon developed clinical pathways or care algorithms for patients with a diagnosis that matched a specific DRG. Patients with heart failure, myocardial infarction, appendectomy, cholecystectomy, stroke, diabetes, and so forth were placed within standard care plans, care maps, clinical pathways, or algorithms (the name varied in each institution) as a way to monitor these patients and make sure they were "on track" for discharge. Because the hospital was to be paid a certain amount of money for that individual with a specific condition, it was critical that patients were treated swiftly and effectively and discharged in a timely manner. Although one would not consider DRGs a disease or illness management model, this change in Medicare 25 or more years ago has influenced how we manage care today.

IMPACT

The direct and indirect costs associated with providing appropriate care for someone with multiple chronic conditions cannot be overstated (see Chapter 1). Fully 23% of Medicare beneficiaries with five or more chronic conditions account for 68% of the program's funding (Anderson, 2005). From a cost perspective alone, the need to provide high quality care efficiently hailed the advent of disease management programs, both formal and informal. These disease management

programs may originate from federal and state agencies as well as in for-profit and not-for-profit companies.

Disease Management Versus Illness Management

The majority of models available today for patient care are disease management models. These models monitor the physiologic markers of disease, the measurement of one's glycosylated hemoglobin (HbA1c), the forced expiratory volume (FEV) of a patient with chronic obstructive pulmonary disease (COPD), the number of medications prescribed to a patient, the number of visits to the healthcare provider, and so forth. However, as this book addresses, looking at the disease, the pathophysiology, and the required medications, is only caring for part of the patient, and, quite frankly, that is the easier part, the measurable part. The illness experience of individuals, the uniqueness of the patient, their living situation, social support, their coping mechanisms and whether they are effective or ineffective, that is the other component of the patient's life that disease management programs do not address.

INTERVENTIONS

During the mid to late 1990s, many disease management companies were formed, with most having the goal of providing cost-effective care to those with chronic conditions. By 1999 there were 200 companies nationwide offering disease management services for such conditions as diabetes, asthma, and heart failure (Bodenheimer, 2003). Most of these programs did not originate within healthcare institutions, but were outsourced to outside firms. Today, fewer of those companies exist or are profitable, primarily because their focus was on one specific disease, when typically the older adult population has multiple chronic conditions. As an example, fewer than one half of the rehospitalizations among patients initially hospitalized with heart failure are actually attributed to the heart failure. The other hospitalizations are related to conditions that predispose to heart failure such as coronary artery disease, hypertension, chronic obstructive pulmonary disease, and so forth (DeBusk, West, Miller, & Taylor, 1999). Disease management companies offered programs that were just that, programs, with neither a systems approach nor an integration of these programs into a healthcare system or institution. In addition, a number of those disease management programs were based on physician specialty practice and not primary care. As we look at older adults, they may have several chronic conditions necessitating going to several different specialty physicians. Therefore, programs based on specialty practice typically did not work.

Most of the literature today looks at disease management models versus illness management models. However, in most studies, the definition of disease management and the components of each program vary, making it hard to compare programs and health outcomes of participants. When performing a meta-analysis or systematic review, it becomes difficult to figure out inclusion criteria for studies, since each program is different. Furthermore, when looking at outcomes, what specific component of the program "makes a difference" in the health outcome or was it the combination of components acting interdependently?

Mattke, Seid, and Ma (2007), in their analysis of disease management programs, suggest in broad terms that disease management refers to a system of coordinated healthcare interventions and communications to help patients address chronic disease and other health conditions. Disease management programs are "big business," with 96% of the top 150 US payers offering some form of disease management service and 83% of more than 500 major US employers using programs to help individuals manage their health (cited in Mattke et al., 2007, p. 670). Revenues associated with these programs have grown significantly from $78 million in 1997 to nearly $1.2 billion in 2005 and projected to top $1.8 billion by the end of 2008 (Mattke et al.). What are the health outcomes of spending $1 to 2 billion a year? Are these programs making a difference in health outcomes, and, if so, are they reducing costs in other areas?

Mattke and colleagues in their review of three evaluations of large scale population-based programs, 10 meta-analyses and 16 systematic reviews covering 317 studies, found consistent evidence of improved processes of care and disease control, but no conclusive support of improved health outcomes. In addition, when the costs of the programs and/or interventions were accounted for and then cost savings subtracted, there was no evidence of a net reduction in medical costs (p. 675–676).

In an effort to define the specifics of disease management programs, the Disease Management Association of America (DMAA) offers the following interpretation. The DMAA, comprising managed care organizations, insurance companies and pharmaceutical companies, suggests the term "population health improvement" model versus the previous term disease management. Key components of the population health improvement model include:

- Population identification strategies and processes
- Comprehensive needs assessments that assess physical, psychological, economic, and environmental needs
- Proactive health promotion programs that increase awareness of the health risks associated with certain personal behaviors and lifestyles
- Patient-centric health management goals and education, which may include primary prevention, behavior modification programs, and support for concordance between the patient and the primary care provider
- Self-management interventions aimed at influencing the targeted population to make behavioral changes
- Routine reporting and feedback loops, which may include communications with patients, physicians, health plans, and ancillary providers

■ Evaluation of clinical, humanistic, and economic outcomes on an ongoing basis with the goal of improving overall population health (DMMA, 2008)

Chronic Care Model

The best known model for providing care to those with chronic disease is the Chronic Care Model (CCM). Work on this model began in the early 1990s with Dr. Edward Wagner, an internist and director of the Seattle-based MacColl Institute for Healthcare Innovation at the Center for Health Studies, Group Health Cooperative. Wagner identified three issues in providing care to those with chronic illness through primary care (Wielawski, 2006).

■ Primary care offices are set up to respond to acute illnesses rather than anticipate and respond proactively to patients' needs (which is what individuals with chronic illness need).
■ Patients with chronic illness are not adequately informed about their conditions and they are not supported in the self-care of their conditions beyond the physician's office.
■ Physicians are too busy to educate and support patients with chronic illness to the degree needed for them to stay healthy (Wielawski, 2006, p. 5).

Wagner's solution was to replace the physician centered office with a structure that supported a team of professionals that collaborate with the patient in his or her care. Early implementation of his model took place with a population of 15,000 diabetic patients at the Group Health Cooperative, a 590,000 member health maintenance organization in Seattle. During 5 years, the percentage of patients with up-to-date screening improved; blood sugar levels and the regularity of monitoring improved; patients reported higher satisfaction with their care; and admission to acute care facilities decreased.

During this period of time in the mid to late 1990s, Wagner and associates partnered with The

Robert Wood Johnson Foundation (RWJ) to further develop the model. The model was refined and published in its current form in 1998. Improving Chronic Illness Care, a national program through RWJ, was launched in 1998 with the Chronic Care Model as its core (Figure 19-1) (Improving Chronic Care, 2007).

The CCM has demonstrated successful disease management outcomes in a number of studies. What follows are representative studies of those outcomes.

Two state-level collaboratives were conducted on diabetes in the state of Washington, with a total of 47 clinic teams covering six different health plans. The majority of the teams demonstrated successful outcomes as evidenced by: 23 teams reporting an increased percentage of patients with HbA1c <8%; 18 teams improved blood pressure readings <140/90 mm Hg; and 19 teams reported changes in the low-density lipoprotein (LDL) cholesterol level (Daniel et al., 2004).

The Bureau of Primary Health Care in North Carolina, using the CCM, partnered with 12 community health centers across the state to improve patient outcomes in diabetes. These clinics typically serve mostly uninsured and underinsured individuals. There was a downward trend in HbA1c values in this population (Wang et al., 2004).

Nutting et al. (2007) examined 30 small, independent primary care practices to determine the association between clinician-reported use of elements of the CCM and diabetic patients' HbA1c levels, lipid levels, and patient self-reported care. Clinician-reported use of elements of the CCM was statistically significant, with lower HbA1c levels and lower ratios of total cholesterol to high-density lipoprotein cholesterol (Nutting et al., 2007).

The Health Disparities Collaboratives of the Health Resources Services Administration (HRSA), using the CCM as a model, executed a pre-intervention and post-intervention study of community health centers focusing on diabetes, hypertension, and asthma (Landon et al., 2007). There were 44 centers in the experimental group and 20 centers in the control group. There were mixed

FIGURE 19-1

The Chronic Care Model

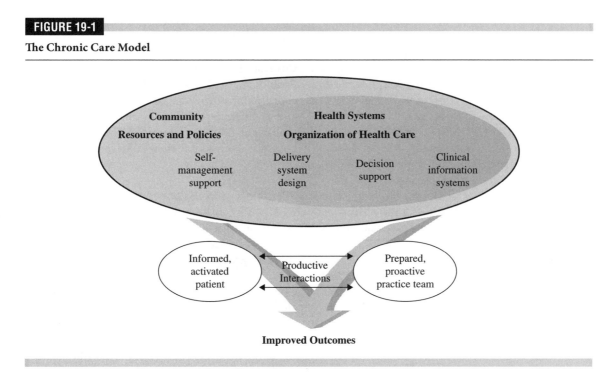

Improved Outcomes

Source: Wagner, E.H. (1998). Chronic disease management: What will it take to improve care for chronic illness? *Effective Clinical Practice, 1,* 2–4.

results, with a 21% increase in the foot examinations for patients with diabetes, a 14% increase in the use of anti-inflammatory medications in asthma, and a 16% increase in the assessment of HbA1c. However, there was no improvement in urgent care or hospitalization for asthma, control of HbA1c, and control of blood pressure in hypertensive patients (p. 921).

Guided Care

Using the CCM as a basis, researchers at Johns Hopkins University, developed a care model designed to improve the quality of life and efficiency of resource utilization for older adults with multiple chronic conditions. Guided Care enhances the use of primary care (versus specialty care) and utilizes the following seven principles of chronic care: disease management; self-management; case management; lifestyle modification; transitional care; caregiver education and support; and geriatric evaluation and management (Boyd et al., 2007, p. 697). What is unique about the Guided Care model is the use of specially trained registered nurses in Guided Care concepts, who, in turn, use a computerized electronic health record (EHR) in working with two to five primary care physicians to meet the needs of 50–60 older adults with multiple comorbidities. The Guided Care Nurse (GCN) is based in the primary care physician's office, and performs eight clinical activities, guided by scientific evidence and the patients' priorities (p. 698). Pilot versions of Guided Care included several of the eight core activities. Currently a cluster-randomized controlled trial (RCT) through Johns Hopkins University is utilizing 8 sites (49 physicians) in the Baltimore-Washington, DC area, with 904 patients in either the experimental group of Guided Care or the control group (usual care) (Boult et al., 2008). Patients eligible for the study were those 65 years old or older and ranking in the upper quartile of risk for using health services during the coming year. The eight clinical activities performed by the GCN include:

Assessment. Initial assessments include medical, functional, cognitive, affective, psychosocial, nutritional, and environmental. Other tools used may include the Geriatric Depression Scale and the CAGE alcoholism scale. The client is also asked what his/her priorities are for improved quality of life.

Planning. The EHR merges the assessment data with evidence-based practice guidelines to create a preliminary Care Guide that manages and monitors the patients' health conditions. The GCN and the primary care physician then personalize the Care Guide with input from the patient and family. The end result is a patient-friendly version of the plan called My Action Plan, which is written in lay language and given to the patient.

Chronic Disease Self-Management (CDSM). The GCN encourages the patient's self-efficacy in the management of his/her chronic conditions. The patient is referred to a free, local 15-hour CDSM course led by trained lay people and supported by the GCN. The program utilized is the one developed by Kate Lorig and associates at Stanford University. In this program, the patient learns how to operationalize his/her Action Plan.

Monitoring. The GCN monitors each patient at least monthly by telephone to address issues promptly. The EHR plays an important role in the monitoring by providing reminders about each patient (Boyd et al., 2007).

Coaching. Motivational interviewing is used to facilitate the patient's participation in care along with reinforcing adherence to the Action Plan (Boyd, 2007, p. 700). The GCNs are trained in motivational interviewing principles and strategies to assist in this process.

Coordinating Transitions Between Sites and Providers of Care. The GCN is the primary coordinator of care for patients in this program, and is thus responsible for the care transitions that occur between home, the emergency room, hospitals, long-term care facilities, and other care settings.

Educating and Supporting Caregivers. The GCN works with family or other unpaid caregivers of the patients to educate and support them. This may include individual or group assistance, support group meetings, or ad hoc telephone consultation (Boyd et al., 2007, p. 701). Accessing Community Resources. Determining appropriate community resources for the patient, such as Meals on Wheels, transportation needs, and so forth are key functions of the GCN. The idea is not to duplicate services, but to utilize the services available in the community.

In April 2008, 6 months into the RCT, data suggest that the Guided Care model provides improved quality of care, reduced medical care costs, and high satisfaction in both the primary care physicians and the GCNs (Boult et al., 2008). Based on these early results, two of the managed care partners in the trial, Kaiser Permanente and Johns Hopkins HealthCare, agreed to continue to pay the costs of the GCNs for an additional year.

Program of All-Inclusive Care for the Elderly (PACE)

Although the Program of All-Inclusive Care for the Elderly (PACE) was not specifically developed for individuals with chronic illness, it is obvious that the majority of older adults accessing this program could have at least one chronic condition. PACE is a capitated benefit authorized by the Balanced Budget Act (BBA) of 1997 that offers comprehensive health care to older adults. PACE is modeled after the successful On Lok Senior Health Services program in San Francisco. The On

Lok model demonstrated successful outcomes in a number of demonstration projects funded through The Centers for Medicare & Medicaid Services (CMS), then known as the Health Care Financing Administration (HCFA), in the 1980s and 1990s.

Participants in PACE must be 55 years of age, live in a PACE service area, and be certified as eligible for nursing home care. For most participants in the program, it allows them to receive services while they continue to live at home. Capitated financing allows care providers to deliver all services that the participants needs, rather than those that are limited under Medicare and Medicaid fee-for-service systems (www.cms.hhs.gov/PACE). PACE becomes the sole source of services for the Medicare and Medicaid eligible enrollees. Currently there are 37 PACE providers located in 19 states.

Mukamel and colleagues (2007) attempted to determine what program characteristics of PACE were associated with the risk-adjusted health outcomes of mortality, functional status, and self-assessed health. The research examined 3042 newly enrolled persons in 23 PACE programs over a 4-year period, 1997 to 2001. There were a number of program characteristics that were significantly associated with better functional outcomes. These included: a medical director who was a trained geriatrician; medical directors who spent time providing direct patient care; programs with effective interdisciplinary teams; teams composed of more aides than professionals; the same ethnicity of participant and team member; and larger and older PACE programs (Mukamel et al., 2007).

Fewer program characteristics were associated with participant self-assessed health outcomes. Higher staffing levels, having more diverse services, and having a match between the ethnicity of the participant and the staff member were associated with higher self-assessed health outcomes (Mukamel et al., 2007, p. 524).

Medicare Health Support Organizations

One of the components of the Medicare Modernization Act (MMA) of 2003 was the Chronic Care Improvement Program in Section 721 P.L. 1080–173.

This program was Medicare's commitment to improving and strengthening the traditional fee-for-service Medicare program. Eight agencies were funded across the United States. The original Phase I pilot programs were phased in between August 1, 2005 and January 16, 2006, and were to operate for three years and be tested through RCTs (CMS, 2005). Since that time, the project has been re-named Medicare Health Support (MHS).

Medicare Health Support Organizations (MHSO):
■ Healthways Maryland and District of Columbia
■ LifeMasters Supported SelfCare Oklahoma
■ Health Dialog Services Corporation Pennsylvania (western region)
■ McKesson Health Solutions, LLC Mississippi
■ Aetna Life Insurance Company Chicago, IL (surrounding area)
■ Cigna Health Support Georgia (northern region)
■ Green Ribbon Health Florida (west-central region)
■ XL Health Corporation Tennessee (selected counties)

This program is seen as a new form of customer service in Medicare. The programs are free and voluntary, and do not change a beneficiary's Medicare coverage or claims processing, or restrict choice of providers or access to care (Foote, 2006). The first of the mandated four Reports to Congress was presented in June 2007. Of note in the report is the fact that the intervention group participants, the Medicare Health Support Organizations (MHSOs), were statistically and substantively different from the nonparticipant populations across demographic, health status, utilization, and payment characteristics. Typically the MHSOs had healthier beneficiaries and lower rates of comorbid conditions than the nonparticipants. Within the first 6 months of operations, the MHSOs have not been successful in recruiting either dual eligible (Medicare/Medicaid) or the most costly beneficiaries to participate (McCall, Cromwell, & Bernard, 2007).

For most participants in the study as of the June 2007 report, there had been 6 months or less of participation in the program; therefore, results were minimal. The June 2007 report noted that there were not any significant differences in quality of care and health outcomes between the experimental or control group (McCall et al., 2007, p. 3). The report also showed that none of the vendors left in the project could meet its performance guarantee of 5% net savings (Mattke, Seid, & Ma, 2007, p. 676). Currently there are five active MHSOs in 2008, with all projects slated to end during 2008 unless re-authorized.

Medical Homes

The American Academy of Pediatrics (AAP) first used the term "medical home" in 1967 to refer to children with special needs. More recently the AAP along with the American Academy of Family Physicians, the American College of Physicians, and the American Osteopathic Association have refined the concept and expanded it to the care of all patients (http://www.commonwealthfund.org/publications). There is widespread agreement that primary care is in crisis. Patients are not satisfied with their care, and purchasers and insurers are disappointed with its cost and quality. The "medical home" attempts to provide comprehensive primary care through stronger physician–patient partnerships.

As defined by the four medical societies, patient-centered medical homes support the following seven principles:

■ Each patient receives care from a personal physician.
■ The personal physician leads a team of providers who are responsible for a patient's ongoing care.
■ The personal physician is responsible for the "whole person."
■ A patient's care is coordinated across the healthcare system and community.

■ Quality and safety are hallmarks of the practice.
■ Enhanced access to care is offered through open scheduling, expanded hours, and new care options such as group visits.
■ The payment structure recognizes the enhanced value provided to patients. (Foubister, 2008)

The National Committee for Quality Assurance (NCQA) developed the Physician Practice Connections Patient-Centered Medical Home standards in parallel with the four medical societies' efforts. The NCQA sees the medical home concept as strengthening the physician–patient relationship and replacing episodic care with coordinated care (www.ncqa.org). The NCQA has nine standards for medical practices to meet that focus on patient access and communication, patient tracking and registry functions, care management, patient self-management support, electronic prescribing, track of patient tests, referral tracking, performance reporting, and improvement and advanced electronic communications. Since 2004, 283 practice sites representing 3,499 physicians have been recognized by the Physician Practice Connections program. However, most of these sites (97%) received this recognition as part of the Bridges to Excellence program, and thus had a financial incentive to provide medical home services in their practices (Foubister, 2008).

There are a number of demonstration projects with the medical home concept that are ongoing. TransforMed, funded by the American Academy of Family Physicians, launched a 24-month project in June of 2006 with 36 family medicine practices across the country. Concepts that have been found to be important include: technology; managing access to care; accessing evidence-based reminders at the point of care; providing patients with the option of group visits, and ensuring that the right people are doing the right jobs (Foubister, 2008).

Medicare will launch a 3-year Medicare Medical Home Demonstration Project in eight states in 2009. It will provide a "care coordination" fee to physicians for managing the care of Medicare patients with multiple chronic conditions.

Self-Management Programs

The term self-management initially appeared in a book by Thomas Creer on the rehabilitation of children with chronic illness (Lorig & Holman, 2003). Creer and colleagues used the concept to indicate that the patient was an active participant in their care. Creer and Holroyd (2006) state that self-management differs from adherence in that "self-management places greater emphasis on the patient's active role in decision-making, both inside and outside the consultation room" (p. 8). Self-management is also seen as different from disease management. Creer and Holroyd view disease management as being more focused on healthcare professionals' algorithms and interventions to standardize care as opposed to self-management, which emphasizes the patients' involvement in defining the problems.

Kate Lorig and colleagues' work at Stanford University has conceptualized best what we know about self-management programs. Her work is based on Corbin and Strauss' framework of medical management, role management, and emotional management. These concepts along with how the chronic condition is perceived by the patient and family are hallmarks of Lorig's work. Lorig's framework for self-management programs includes five core self-management skills: problem solving; decision making; resource utilization, forming of a patient–healthcare provider partnership; and taking action (Lorig & Holman, 2003).

Empirical results of self-management programs have been mixed. What follows are examples of the literature in this area.

Lorig and colleagues (1999) studied 952 patients, 40 years of age and older with a diagnosis of heart disease, lung disease, stroke, or arthritis in a 6-month-long RCT. The Chronic Disease Self-Management Program (CDSMP), the intervention, consisted of seven, weekly 2½-hour sessions on making management choices and achieving success in reaching self-selected goals as opposed to prescribing specific behavior changes (Lorig et al., 1999, p. 7). Outcome measures included health behaviors, health status, and health service utilization. At 6 months, the experimental group demonstrated improvements in weekly minutes of exercise, frequency of cognitive symptom management, communication with physicians, and self-reported health. Participants also had decreased fatigue and disability and less social/role activities limitations with less health distress, fatigue, and disability. There were no differences between the groups in pain/physical discomfort, shortness of breath, or psychological well-being (Lorig et al., 1999, p. 5).

A systematic review (Warsi et al., 2004) and a meta-analysis of self-management education programs (Chodosh et al., 2005) appeared in the literature in 2004 and 2005, respectively. The systematic review searched literature from 1964 to 1999 and reviewed 71 trials. Diabetic patients had reductions in HbA1c levels and improvements in systolic blood pressure, and asthmatic patients experienced fewer attacks. Arthritis self-management education programs were not associated with statistically significant effects. Warsi and colleagues found a large number of limitations with the studies they reviewed. The methods of conducting (i.e., study design) and reporting these trials were suboptimal. There was also evidence of publication bias (Warsi et al., 2004, p. 1648).

Chodosh and colleagues (2005) assessed the effectiveness of self-management programs with a meta-analysis design. Of the 780 studies screened, 53 met the researchers' criteria for inclusion. Self-management interventions led to statistically and clinically significant results of decreased HbA1c (amounting to a decrease of .81%), a decrease of 5 mm Hg in systolic blood pressure, and a decrease of 4.3 mm Hg in diastolic blood pressure. There were no significant results for participants with osteoarthritis in either pain or function. Their conclusion was that the studies had variable quality, making it difficult to analyze, and there was possible publication bias present (pp. 435–436).

In addition, it was not clear what constituted a self-management program.

Other

Although this chapter focuses on models of care for physical chronic illness, there are disease management models that focus on mental illness as well. Badamgarav and colleagues (2003) reviewed the literature to assess the effectiveness of disease management programs in clients with depression. Utilizing 24 depression disease management programs that met the researchers' inclusion criteria, the findings demonstrated that programs had statistically significant results in improvement in depression, clients' satisfaction with treatment, clients' compliance with treatment and adequacy of prescribed treatment (Badamgarav et al., 2003, p. 2088). However, these authors had concerns like others have in that there is no firm definition of a disease management program, and the authors feel they may or may not have included the appropriate studies for their systematic review.

In a unique collaborative effort between diabetes prevention and control programs in Montana and Wyoming and the University of North Dakota,

a field-based approach was used to improve diabetes care in rural primary care practices (Johnson et al., 2005). Forty primary care practices with more than 7000 clients with diabetes participated in a quality improvement project. There were improvements in Montana in rates of HbA1c testing, blood glucose control, LDL cholesterol testing, foot and retinal examinations, and pneumococcal vaccinations, and there were improvements in pneumococcal vaccinations in Wyoming. Primary care practices used preprogrammed reports generated by the Diabetes Quality Care Monitoring System (DQCMS) and technical support from the state quality-improvement coordinators to make changes in their delivery of diabetes care and education.

In a systematic review and meta-analysis of COPD management programs, Peytremann-Bridevaux and colleagues (2008) reviewed nine RCTs, one controlled trial, and three uncontrolled before–after trials (that met their definition of a disease management program). These programs demonstrated modest improvement in exercise capacity, health-related quality of life, and decreased hospital admissions. However, the researchers caution that it is unclear which specific

■ CASE STUDY

Mary Brown is an 80-year-old widow living alone on her farm 5 miles from town in a western rural state. Mrs. Brown's town with a population of 10,000 has a critical access hospital. She lives in the farmhouse that she moved to when she married 60 years ago. She would like to stay there as long as possible, but after her hip replacement surgery last fall, her mobility is not as good as it used to be. She is mildly hypertensive and is on medication. Her type 2 diabetes is under control with diet and medication. She has lots of friends in the community, but her grown children live several states away.

Because of her isolation and age, she might be considered "at risk." She does not live near a PACE service area or an MHSO.

Discussion Questions

1. What are Mrs. Brown's "at risk" variables?
2. What self-management tasks should be initiated with her?
3. What does Mrs. Brown need? What are her potential needs? This is a small community with few resources available. Be creative and develop a model of care for her.

component(s) of the program had the most benefit for the clients. Again, the study struggled with defining and identifying the components of the disease management programs, as each program in the review was slightly different.

The Gatekeeper Program

The Gatekeeper Program was developed in 1978 by Ray Raschko, a social worker at Spokane, Washington's Mental Health Elder Services, to identify at-risk older adults that may have mental health issues. The goal of the Gatekeeper Program is to systematically locate and identify at-risk older adults 60 years and older, living alone, and in need of some type of assistance to maintain their independence. The program's intent is to address the health, social, and emotional issues prevalent in the at-risk older adult population. Gatekeepers are employees of corporations, businesses, and other organizations who, in the course of their daily work activities, come into contact with older adults in the community. Although this is not strictly a program for those with chronic disease, since it is targeting older adults, it is probable that those individuals have chronic disease. Today, there are numerous Gatekeeper Programs nationwide (to locate programs use the Google search engine and type in The Gatekeeper Program).

VNS CHOICE Program

In the early 1990s, New York State explored several options to increase the range of community services available to the older adult population. Managed long-term care (MLTC) is the result of that initiative (Dehm & McCabe, 2007). Visiting Nurse Service (VNS) CHOICE operates under a contract with the New York State Department of Health and is licensed by the state as a managed care organization. The program receives a fixed per-member per-month premium from the state, at a rate that is negotiated with the MLTC plan annually. All covered services, care management, and administrative costs are paid for and managed through this monthly payment. The average VNS CHOICE member is 81 years old, female, and lives with either a family member or alone. Most members speak English, Spanish, or Chinese. The average member has 3.6 chronic illnesses, the most common ones being hypertension, diabetes, osteoarthritis and related disorders, and heart disease. The cornerstone of the VNS CHOICE program is a care management model that links home- and community-based services, acute care, and long term care with the assistance of an interdisciplinary team. Currently the plan covers 9700 individuals with plans to expand the MLTC area (Dehm & McCabe, 2007).

Telephone Disease Management

This diabetes disease management program used the telephone as the source of education in a sample of 1220 individuals in the Medicare + Choice recipients older than age 65 in Ohio, Kentucky, and Indiana (Berg & Wadhwa, 2007). There were 610 intervention group members matched to a control group of the same number of members. The disease management program used a structured, evidence-based telephonic nursing intervention to provide patient education, counseling, and monitoring services. The self-management intervention plan included risk stratification, formal scheduled nurse education sessions, 24-hour access to a nurse counseling and symptom advice telephone line, printed action plans, workbooks, medication compliance and vaccination reminders, physician alerts, and signs and symptoms of complications. The participants in the study were high users of services, with rates of hospitalization of 605 of 1000 in the intervention group and 612 of 1000 in the control group. Emergency room visits were also high with 700 of 1000 in both groups during the baseline period (p. 230). The groups were well matched and could be assumed to be moderately ill to severely ill older adults with diabetes.

The intervention group had significantly lower rates of acute service utilization compared with the control group, 23.8% increase in

EVIDENCE-BASED PRACTICE BOX

Guided care, a new model of care developed from the Chronic Care Model (CCM), is being evaluated in a randomized controlled trial in the Washington DC/Baltimore, Maryland area. Key to this model are specially trained nurses. These guided care nurses (GCNs) perform eight clinical activities in working with older adult clients with multiple chronic illnesses. These activities include: assessing the patient and caregiver in the home, creating an evidence-based care plan, promoting patient self-management, monitoring the patient's conditions monthly, coaching the patient to practice healthy behaviors, coordinating the patient's transitions between sites of and providers of care, educating and supporting the primary caregiver, and facilitating access to community resources.

Of the 13,534 patients screened, 2391 were eligible to participate in the study of which 904 gave informed consent and were cluster-randomized. After 6 months in the program, guided care participants were more likely than the "usual care" control group to rate their care highly, and primary care physicians were more likely to be satisfied with their interactions with the older adults and their families. Conclusions about the effects of guided care on efficiency, effectiveness, timeliness, and technical proficiency of care cannot be made at this time. Similarly, it is too early to tell if guided care has an effect on functional independence, cost of care, and caregiver strain.

Source: Boult, C., Reider, L., Frey, K., Leff, B., Boyd, C.M., Wolff, J.L., et al. (2008). Early effects of "guided care" on the quality of health care for multimorbid older persons: A cluster-randomized controlled trial. *Journal of Gerontology: Medical Sciences, 73A*(3), 321–327.

angiotensin-converting enzyme (ACE) inhibitor use, 13.3% increase in blood glucose regulator use, 11.8% increase in HbA1c testing, 10.3% increase in lipid panel testing, a 26% increase in eye exams, and a 35.5% increase in microalbumin tests (Berg & Wadhwa, 2007, p. 226).

Another study used the telephone for disease management in patients with heart failure (Smith, Hughes-Cromwick, Forkner, & Galbreath, 2008). This study examined the cost-effectiveness of the approach versus the patient outcomes. Adult subjects with documented systolic heart failure or diastolic heart failure (n = 1069) were randomized into one of three study groups: usual care; disease management; and augmented disease management. Subjects in the intervention arms were assigned a disease manager who was an RN and performed patient education and medication management with the patient's primary care provider for the

full 18 months of the study. Subjects in the augmented disease management group also received in-home devices for enhanced self-monitoring. These data were electronically transmitted to the disease manager. Although the program produced statistically significant survival advantages among all patients, analyses of direct and intervention costs showed no cost savings associated with the intervention. It also did not reduce healthcare utilization of the subjects (Smith et al., 2008).

Shared Care

Smith, Allwright, and O'Dowd (2007) completed a systematic review for the Cochrane Database on "shared care." These authors considered "shared care" as the combined management or joint participation of primary care physicians and specialty care physicians in planning the delivery of care for a client. Twenty studies were identified for chronic disease management, with 19 of them being RCTs. The results were mixed. The authors concluded that, at present, there is insufficient evidence to demonstrate significant benefits from shared care, apart from improving prescribing of medications.

OUTCOMES

With any model of care for individuals and families with chronic conditions, an expected outcome is that both the disease and illness experience are managed appropriately. This chapter has demonstrated that there are improved physical outcomes of care with some models of care. However, results seem to be mixed as to whether there are cost savings related to these programs.

What is not "measured" in these models is how these programs or models of care affect the illness experience of the individual and family. Can we say that because an individual with a chronic illness has a lower HbA1c, or has not been hospitalized within the last 6 months, or checks his blood glucose level regularly, has a better quality of life or experiences more life satisfaction, or in the terms of Strauss (1984), is successful at normalizing his/her life? Perhaps in the near future managing the illness experience of the client with chronic illness will be a higher priority.

STUDY QUESTIONS

1. What are the benefits of disease management models of care?
2. Identify the issues involved with a disease management model of care for an older adult.
3. How do we as nurses care for individuals and families and their *illness experience* within a disease management model?
4. After reading about different models of care in this chapter, what do you think should be included in a model of care for an older adult with multiple comorbidities?
5. How do self-management components of care fit within a disease management program?
6. What role does (or should) the advanced practice nurse have in disease management?

INTERNET RESOURCES

Chronic Disease Self-Management Program, Stanford University: patienteducation.stanford.edu/programs/cdsmp.html
Commonwealth Fund: www.commonwealthfund.org
Disease Management Association of America: www.dmaa.org; and *Disease Management*, the official journal of the DMAA: www.liebertpub.com/publication.aspx?pub_id=12
Guided Care: www.guidedcare.org/
Improving Chronic Illness Care: www.improvingchroniccare.org/supported by The Robert Wood Johnson Foundation
Medicare Disease Management Programs: www.dmprograms.com/
PACE provider organizations: http://www.cms.hhs.gov/pace/lppo/List.asp

REFERENCES

Anderson, G. F. (2005). Medicare and chronic conditions [Electronic version]. *New England Journal of Medicine, 353*(3), 305–309.

Badamgarav, E., Weingarten, S.R., Henning, J.M., Knight, K., Hasselblad, V., Gano, A., et al. (2003). Effectiveness of disease management programs in depression: A systematic review [Electronic version]. *American Journal of Psychiatry, 160*(12), p. 2080–2090.

Berg, G.D., & Wadhwa, S. (2007). Health services outcomes for a diabetes disease management program for the elderly [Electronic version]. *Disease Management, 10*(4), 226–234.

Bodenheimer, T. (2003). Interventions to improve chronic care: Evaluating their effectiveness. *Disease Management, 6*(2), 63–71.

Boult, C., Reider, L., Frey, K., Leff, B., Boyd, C.M., Wolff, J.L., et al. (2008). Early effects of "guided care" on the quality of health care for multimorbid older persons: A cluster-randomized controlled trial. *Journal of Gerontology: Medical Sciences, 73A*(3), 321–327.

Boyd, C.M., Boult, C., Shadmi, E., Leff, B., Brager, R. Dunbar, L., et al. (2007). Guided care for multimorbid older adults. *The Gerontologist, 47*(5), 697–704.

Centers for Medicare and Medicaid Services. (2005). The chronic care improvement program. Retrieved on February 20, 2005 from http://www.cms.hhs. gov/CCIP/Downloads/section_721.pdf.

Chodosh, J., Morton, S.C., Mojica, W., Maglione, M., Suttorp, M.J., Hilton, L., et al. (2005). Meta-analysis: Chronic disease self-management programs for older adults [Electronic version]. *Annals of Internal Medicine, 143*, 427–438.

Creer, T., & Holroyd, K.A. (2006). Self-management of chronic conditions: The legacy of Sir William Osler [Electronic version]. *Chronic Illness, 2*, 7–14.

Daniel, D.M., Norman, J., Davis, C., Lee, H., Hindmarsh, M.F., McCulloch, D.K. et al. (2004). A state-level application of the chronic illness breakthrough series: Results from two collaboratives on diabetes in Washington state. *Joint Commission Journal of Quality and Safety, 30*(2), 69–79.

DeBusk, R., West, J., Miller, N., & Taylor, C. (1999). Chronic disease management: Treating the patient with disease(s) vs. treating the disease(s) in the patient. *Archives of Internal Medicine, 159*, 2739–2742.

Dehm, K., & McCabe, S. (2007). Managing care for adults with chronic conditions: The VNS CHOICE Model. *Policy & Practice*, 14–17.

Disease Management Association of America. (2008). Population health: Advancing the Population Health Improvement Model. Retrieved on June 10, 2008 from www.dmaa.org/phi_definition.asp.

Foote, S.M. (2006) Medicare health support: Reinventing chronic care [Electronic version]. *American Heart Hospital Journal, 4*, 39–42.

Foubister, V. (2008). Quality matters: Patient-centered medical homes. *Quality Matters, 28*.

Johnson, E.A., Webb, W.L., McDowall, J.M., Chasson, L.L., Oser, C.S., Grandpre, J.R., et al. (2004). A field-based approach to support improved diabetes care in rural states. *Preventing Chronic Disease* [serial online]. Retrieved on May 20, 2008 from www.cdc.gov/pcd/issues/2005/oct/05_0012.htm

Landon, B.E., Hicks, L.S., O'Malley, A.J., Lieu, T., Keegan, T., McNeil, B.J., et al. (2007). Improving the management of chronic disease at community health centers [Electronic version]. *New England Journal of Medicine, 356*(9), 921–934.

Lorig, K.R., Sobel, D.S., Steward, A.L., Brown, B.W., Bandura, A., Ritter, P., et al. (1999). Evidence suggesting that a chronic disease self-management program can improve health status while reducing hospitalization: A randomized trial. *Medical Care, 37*(1), 5–14.

Lorig, K., & Holman, H.R. (2003). Self-management education: History, definition, outcomes and mechanisms. *Annals of Behavioral Medicine, 26*(1), 1–7.

Mattke, S., Seid, M., & Ma, S. (2007). Evidence for the effect of disease management: Is $1 billion a year a good investment? [Electronic version]. *American Journal of Managed Care, 13*, 670–676.

McCall, N., Cromwell, J., & Bernard, S. (2007). Evaluation of Phase I of Medicare Health Support (Formerly Voluntary Chronic Care Improvement) Pilot Program under Traditional Fee-For-Service Medicare. (2007). Report to Congress, June 2007. Retrieved on June 2, 2008 from http://www.cms. hhs.gov/CCIP/02_Highlights.asp

Improving Chronic Illness Care. (2007). Chronic care model. Retrieved on March 20, 2007 from http://www.improvingchroniccare.org/index.php?p=The_Chronic_Care_Model&s=2

Mukamel, D.B., Peterson, D.R., Temkin-Greener, H., Delavan, R., Gross, D., Kunitz, S.J., et al. (2007). Program characteristics and enrollees' outcomes in the Program of All-Inclusive Care for the Elderly (PACE). *The Milbank Quarterly, 85*(3), 499–531.

Nutting, P.A., Dickinson, W.P., Dickinson, L.M., Nelson, C.C., King, D.K., Crabtree, B.F., et al. (2007). Use of chronic care model elements is associated with higher-quality care for diabetes. [Electronic version] *Annals of Family Medicine, 5*, 14–20.

Peytremann-Bridevaux, I., Staeger, P., Bridevaus, P.O., Ghali, W.A., & Burnand, B. (2008). Effectiveness of chronic obstructive pulmonary diseas.-management programs: Systematic review and meta-analysis [Electronic version]. *The American Journal of Medicine, 121*, 433–443.

Program for All Inclusive Care of the Elderly (PACE). Retrieved on June 3, 2008 from www.cms.hhs.gov/PACE

Robinson, J.C. (2008). Slouching toward value-based health care [Electronic version]. *Health Affairs, 27*(1), 11–12.

Schaefer, L.D. (2007). The new architects of health care reform.[Electronic version]. *Health Affairs, 26*(6), 1557–1559.

Smith, B., Hughes-Cromwick, P.F., Forkner, E., & Galbreath, A.D. (2008). Cost-effectiveness of telephonic disease management in heart failure [Electronic version] *The American Journal of Managed Care, 14*(2), 106–115.

Smith, S.M., Allwright, S., & O'Dowd, T. (2007). Effectiveness of shared care across the interface between primary and specialty care in chronic disease management. *Cochrane Database of Systematic Reviews, 3*, Art. No.: CD004910. DOI: 10.1002/14651858. CD004910.pub2.

Strauss, A., Corbin, J., Fagerhaugh, S., Glaser, B., Maines, D., Suczek, B., & Wiener, C. (1984). *Chronic illness and the quality of life* (2nd ed.). St. Louis: Mosby.

Wagner, E.H. (1998). Chronic disease management: What will it take to improve care for chronic illness?. *Effective Clinical Practice.1*, 2–4.

Wang, A., Wolf, M., Carlyle, R., Wilkerson, J., Porterfield, D., & Reaves, J., (2004). The North Carolina experience with the diabetes health disparities collaboratives [Electronic version]. *Joint Commission Journal on Quality and Safety, 30*(7), 396–404.

Warsi, A., Wang, P.s., LaValley, M., Avorn, J., & Solomon, D.H. (2004). Self-management education programs in chronic disease. A systematic review and methodological critique of the literature [Electronic version]. *Archives of Internal Medicine, 164*(15), 1641–1649.

Wielawski, I.M. (2006). Improving chronic illness care. In S.L. Isaacs & J.R. Knickman (Eds.). *To Improve Health and Health Care, 10, The Robert Wood Johnson Foundation Anthology* (pp. 1–17). Princeton, NJ: Robert Wood Johnson Foundation.

20

Home Health Care

Cynthia S. Jacelon

INTRODUCTION

The home healthcare industry delivers a variety of services to individuals with chronic health problems living in homes within communities. Services can be divided into two types. Skilled healthcare providers, under the direction of a physician's order and supported by third party reimbursement, provide some services. Other services can be termed "supportive community services" (SCS), and include support for instrumental activities of daily living and personal care (Capitman, 2003). Individuals and agencies provide SCS on a fee-for-service basis. It is common that healthcare providers and SCS workers are providing services to the same patient, and often through the same agency. The major focus of this chapter is on the roles of nurses and other skilled healthcare providers in the home.

Home health nurses provide nursing care to patients with acute, chronic, and terminal care needs in the individual's place of residence. The overall goal of care is to enhance quality of life or support patients at the end of life (American Nurses Association, 2008). Home health nurses use holistic strategies to work with patients, families, and informal caregivers to manage disease or disability. They have highly independent practice,

often being the only professional care provider in the home. The specialty of home health nursing differs from other nursing specialties in that care is provided in the patient's home; the duration and frequency of care is dependent upon the care delivery model and the holistic needs of the patient, family, and caregivers; and the nurse must have advanced knowledge of healthcare payment systems and cost containment (ANA, 2008).

History of Home Care

William Rathbone, a wealthy British businessman and philanthropist founded the first district nursing association. The district nursing services combined therapeutic nursing care and education for healthful living practices. Working with Florence Nightingale, he advocated for district nursing throughout England in the mid 1880s (Stanhope & Lancaster, 2006) and founded a visiting nurses training school to ensure that nurses had the necessary knowledge and skills to work successfully in a community setting (Hitchcock, Schubert, & Thomas, 2003).

The visiting nurse model established in England was adapted by the United States as a means of addressing some of the serious public health problems of the late 19th century. Large

American cities faced many challenges associated with increasing numbers of immigrants entering the country. Poverty-stricken communities with congested living conditions quickly gave rise to epidemics of infectious diseases such as tuberculosis, small pox, scarlet fever, typhoid, and typhus (Schoen & Koenig, 1997).

The first visiting nurse associations to provide care in the needy person's home were established in the United States in Buffalo (1885); Philadelphia (1886); and Boston (1886). Charitable activities, supported by the wealthy people, funded both settlement houses and the early visiting nursing associations. One of the early settlement houses in the United States began through the efforts of Lillian Wald and Mary Brewster (Stanhope & Lancaster, 2006).

Lillian Wald and Mary Brewster revolutionized the concept of public health nursing (Hitchcock et al., 2003). Lillian Wald is credited with developing the title, public health nurse, and with that title the focus of nursing care was broadened to encompass the health of individuals and the health, social, and economic needs of the community as a whole. In 1893, Wald and Brewster co-founded the first organized public health nursing agency, New York City's Henry Street Settlement. The settlement house provided a unique combination of social work, nursing, and social activism (Schoen & Koenig, 1997). The focus was public education to improve maternal and child health, communicable disease control, nutrition, and mental health.

The roles of the visiting nurse and public health nurse became more distinct by the late 1920s. Visiting nurses, employed by the private sector and financed by charity and public contributions, clearly were the "hands-on" providers of bedside nursing care in the home setting. Public health nurses, employed primarily by government health departments, focused their attention on promoting health and preventing disease in the broader community. Although their areas of concentration differed, both groups of nurses functioned independently in the delivery of nursing care outside of an institutional setting and shared

the common goal of promoting, maintaining, and restoring health in the community (Hitchcock et al., 2003) (Table 20-1).

Successes achieved by the collective efforts of visiting nurses, public health nurses, and public health services created a shift in the focus of health care in the first half of the 20th century. Successes in teaching hygiene and decreases in immigration reduced the threat of communicable disease. Success in the community combined with advances in technology and hospital care led to changes in the populations served by home health nurses. During the 1930s and 1940s, fewer patients received care from visiting nurses (Reichley, 1999). However, hospitals quickly realized that although they were the providers of acute care, they were also becoming the providers of care for individuals with long-term chronic disorders. As a result, hospitals began searching for ways to control the increasing costs incurred by chronic illness care.

Establishment of New York City's Montefiore Hospital Home Care Program in 1947 provided one alternative to care of patients needing healthcare interventions outside of an acute care setting. The Montefiore Program, entitled a "Hospital Without Walls," created a model of hospital-linked, home-delivered care utilizing the professional services of physicians, nurses, and social workers (Gundersen, 1999). This hospital-based home care model demonstrated significant cost savings over in-hospital care and served as the catalyst for the resurgence of home health care as we know it today (Reichley, 1999). The focus for home care from Montefiore was not only the patient's illness, with its subsequent chronic state, but also their holistic needs. Social workers addressed the patient's social needs and were interested in the patient's family, their overall well-being, and their role in providing for the patient's health care (Lundy & Janes, 2001).

For more than half a century, philanthropists, public charities, and contributions raised by Visiting Nurse Associations (VNA) funded the home care services. In 1966, the federal government began providing for home care services as a benefit of the new legislation known as Medicare. Medicare

TABLE 20-1

Similarities and Differences Between Public Health Nursing and Home Health Nursing

Similarities

Setting	Nursing care is provided to patients in their residences or in a community environment.
Independent nature of practice	Nurses practice independently outside of institutions.
Control and environment	Patient is an active participant in care decisions. Control is shifted to the patient. Environment empowers the patient.
Family-centered care	The family is considered as a unit of care. Family members contribute significantly to patient care.
Broad goals	Public health and home health services strive to promote, maintain, and restore health in the community.

Differences	*Public Health Nursing*	*Home Health Nursing*
Focus of intervention	Population	Individual/family
Caseload acquisition	Case finding in community at large	Referral by physician
Interventions	Continuous	Episodic
Orientation	Wellness	Illness
	Primary prevention	Secondary prevention
		Rehabilitation
		Tertiary prevention
Entry into services	Risk potential	Medical diagnosis
	Social diagnosis	

Source: Hitchcock, J., Schubert, P., & Thomas, S. (Eds.). (2003). *Community health nursing: Caring in action* (2nd ed.) (p. 480). Albany, NY: Delmar. Reprinted with permission of Cengage Learning/Nelson Education.

allowed for the expansion of home care services to many people, particularly the elderly who did not have access to such care. In 1973, the Medicare home care benefit was expanded to include disabled Americans regardless of age. However, home care advocates became increasingly concerned that the narrowness of home care legislation limited services as a means of avoiding the excessive costs of providing the full range of services that many patients needed (Reichley, 1999).

Between 1980 and 1996, the home healthcare industry experienced a 400% increase in Medicare-sponsored home care. During that time period, the number of agencies certified to bill Medicare rose by 200% (Montauk, 1998). This was a direct result of many reimbursement changes

affecting hospitals. In an effort to control the cost of care in acute care hospitals, Congress passed the Social Security Amendments of 1983 to initiate the prospective payment system for inpatient services (Stanhope & Lancaster, 2006). Therefore, federal government shifted reimbursement to a prospective payment system based on diagnosis-related groups (DRGs). With reimbursement for hospital care now predetermined by patient diagnosis, hospitals responded to the significant revenue reductions by decreasing the average length of stay for patients. The direct consequence was shorter hospital stays and increased referrals to home care (Stanhope & Lancaster, 2006).

However, in 1997, Congress targeted home health care as a place to reduce healthcare expenditures. The passage of the Balanced Budget Act of 1997 (BBA) imposed stricter limits on Medicare reimbursement for home care services. The BBA narrowed the definition of those individuals eligible to receive home care services to those individuals who were deemed "home-bound." Under these guidelines, Medicare recipients were no longer eligible for home care if they were able to leave home for any reason other than medical services (Maurer & Smith, 2005). The number of persons eligible for Medicare home care funding declined by 50% between 1997 and 2000 (USDHHS, 2002). Today, the industry continues to provide holistic care in a fiscally restrained environment.

Theoretical Frameworks for Management of Chronic Illness in Home Care

Home care nurses provide intermittent care and rely heavily on the patient's ability to self-manage their health problems. As such, the nurse is in a unique position to apply frameworks for practice that help the nurse work with patients to promote independence. Below, are discussions of mid-range theories that promote patient's self-management of chronic health problems, conceptualize nursing care as based in relationships and coaching, and provide guidelines for collaborative decision making. Also included are models for community-based care of patients with chronic illness and hospice care.

Self-Management and Family Management of Chronic Conditions

The framework for self- and family management of chronic conditions is designed to provide a structure for understanding factors influencing the ability of individuals and their families manage their chronic illness (Grey, Knafl, & McCorkle, 2006; Tanner, 2004) (Figure 20-1). The components of the framework are: self-management; risk and protective factors including condition factors, individual factors, psychosocial characteristics, family factors, and the environment.

Self- and family management of chronic illness is defined as the decisions and activities that individuals make on a daily basis to manage their chronic health problems (Improving Chronic Illness Care, 2007; Grey et al., 2006). For some individuals, particularly those who are older or have cognitive deficits, engaging in self-management will be an ongoing challenge (Tanner, 2004). The concept of self-management extends the responsibility of the individual with the chronic illness beyond the ideas of compliance and adherence to managing an ongoing condition within the context of his or her daily lives In home care it is imperative that the nurse consider both the patient's ability to self-manage and the family's ability to support the individual's self-management (Grey et al., 2006).

The ability of individuals and families to manage their chronic illness is dependent on the severity of the condition, the treatment regimen, the course of the disease, the individual and family characteristics, and the environment in which the individual will manage their disease. (Grey et al., 2006). The severity of the illness from the perspective of the individual with the chronic illness may not be the same as the nurse's perception. The meaning of the condition and the implications for management may be affected by the meaning of the illness to the individual and family. The etiology of the condition, a lifestyle disease such as emphysema as a result of smoking, or a genetically determined disease, will affect the ability for self-management. The implications for the family in these situations may cause guilt, or concern for the susceptibility of other family members. The treatment regimen for a chronic illness may be complex, requiring significant lifestyle adjustment. Individual factors such as the person's age, psychosocial situation, functional ability, the individual's perceived ability to manage the illness, education, and socioeconomic status all contribute to the individual's ability for self-management. Careful assessment by the nurse is imperative in providing care. Once an assessment is complete, the home care nurse is in a position to coach the individual or family in management of their illness.

FIGURE 20-1

Self Management and Family Management Framework

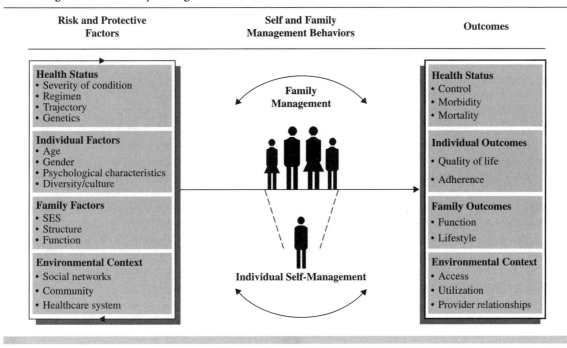

| Risk and Protective Factors | Self and Family Management Behaviors | Outcomes |

Health Status
• Severity of condition
• Regimen
• Trajectory
• Genetics

Individual Factors
• Age
• Gender
• Psychological characteristics
• Diversity/culture

Family Factors
• SES
• Structure
• Function

Environmental Context
• Social networks
• Community
• Healthcare system

Family Management

Individual Self-Management

Health Status
• Control
• Morbidity
• Mortality

Individual Outcomes
• Quality of life
• Adherence

Family Outcomes
• Function
• Lifestyle

Environmental Context
• Access
• Utilization
• Provider relationships

Source: Grey, M., Knafl, K., & McCorkel, R. (2006). A framework for the study of self- and family management of chronic conditions. *Nursing Outlook, 54,* 278–286.

In the model of self-management and family management, outcomes can include improved condition symptoms, and improved individual and family outcomes such as better disease management, improved quality of life, or improved self efficacy (Grey et al., 2006). The main goal of the model is to help the individual improve his or her health, using the broadest definition of health possible. The home-care nurse will want to support the self- and family's self-management, teach them the skills needed to improve health, and coach the individual and family on incorporating those activities into their daily lives.

Coaching as a Technique to Enhance Self-management and Family Management

The home care nurse is in an excellent position to coach the patient and family in the management of the chronic illness. Coaching, or motivational interviewing, is a strategy in which the nurse uses a combination of providing education, collaborative decision making, and empowerment to help the patient manage their health needs (Huffman, 2007). Health coaching has its roots in substance abuse counseling, and has been found to be a relatively short term, successful strategy. Health coaching is a patient-centered approach to care with the focus on health coaching the issues and barriers to self-management.

To employ health coaching, the home health nurse begins with asking the patient about what he or she is the most concerned about. In this way, the nurse can capitalize on the patient's interest in resolving or managing a particular problem. The next step is to validate the patient's feelings about his or her capacity to manage the problem.

CASE STUDY

While walking in the kitchen barefoot, Mr. Shelton, an 82-year-old man, dropped and broke a drinking glass. Subsequently he stepped on a glass sliver that became embedded in a cut on his foot. Because of peripheral neuropathy from poorly controlled type 2 diabetes, Mr. Shelton did not notice the sliver for several days. When he finally asked his wife to look at his foot, she discovered an infected cut with purulent drainage and blackened areas. Topical and systemic antibiotics were not successful in reducing the infection. He was discharged from the hospital after surgical debridement and amputation of his right great toe. The surgeon is concerned that the wound may not heal well, and has ordered home care.

When Mr. Shelton was discharged from the hospital, the home care nurses telephoned and made an appointment for the next day. During the first visit, the nurse introduced herself, and had a long talk with both Mr. and Mrs. Shelton to determine how they had been managing Mr. Shelton's health problems before this hospitalization. When the Sheltons finished their story, the nurse began her assessment of their current situation. She asked about Mr. Shelton's activities, and how he checks his blood glucose and manages his diet. She asked Mr. Shelton about his other health problems. The nurse also asked Mrs. Shelton about her health problems, and her ability and confidence in caring for Mr. Shelton. The nurse asks Mrs. Shelton about food preparation and meal patterns.

As the Sheltons and the nurse form a relationship, the nurse begins to strengthen the Shelton's self-efficacy by positively commenting on how well they have managed to date. She also notes that both Mr. and Mrs. Shelton are shaken by this current health problem. The nurse mentions that the Sheltons seem worried about their continued ability to manage, and their fear that Mr. Shelton will have to go to

a nursing home. Although the nurse does not diminish the seriousness of the situation, she suggests that they look at the wound and talk about what type of care is now needed so that the Sheltons can make an informed decision about their next steps.

As the nurse takes off the dressing to look at the surgical wound, she invites both Mr. and Mrs. Shelton to look at the wound. Mr. Shelton cannot bend his leg to adequately inspect the foot, so the nurse uses a mirror to help him see the wound. Once the nurse redresses the foot, she tells Mrs. Shelton that when she returns in 2 days, the nurse would like Mrs. Shelton to help her with the dressing. Mrs. Shelton comments that the dressing did not seem too complicated, and that the wound did not look as bad as she had feared.

Then, the nurse has Mr. Shelton inspect his other foot and explains that he should look at his feet daily to note any injury and prevent further infections. She also suggests that Mr. Shelton wear socks and shoes at all times to protect his feet. The nurse suggests that Mr. Shelton establish a time each day to look at his feet, and asks his wife to help. Mr. Shelton could do the same for his wife. The nurse suggests that rubbing each other's feet might be a very satisfying activity.

As the nurse completes her assessment of the Sheltons' ability to manage the acute wound problem and the chronic type 2 diabetes, she determines that the Sheltons manage most of their daily activities as a team. They do not understand Mr. Shelton's diabetes, and are anxious about caring for the toe wound. Mr. Shelton had a brother who lost a leg to peripheral vascular disease secondary to diabetes, and the Sheltons are afraid that that might happen to Mr. Shelton.

Mrs. Shelton is willing to change the dressings, but she is worried about her ability to

(Continued)

CASE STUDY (*Continued*)

properly assess the wound. Using the OASIS assessment tool, the nurse determines that the Sheltons need teaching and coaching with management of the toe wound and Mr. Shelton's diabetes. Mr. Shelton might also need some physical therapy for improving balance after the toe amputation. He meets the criteria for being homebound, and the nurse determines the agency can be reimbursed for four skilled nursing visits.

As the end of the visit draws near, the nurse shows Mr. and Mrs. Shelton how to look up information about type 2 diabetes on the Internet. She places bookmarks at the site for the American Diabetes Association and the National Institutes of Health Web sites. As the nurse prepares to end the visit, she makes an appointment for 2 days hence. The Sheltons and the nurse together agree on the following goals: the nurse will telephone the Sheltons the following morning to see how they are doing. Mr. Shelton will inspect his feet each morning. Mrs. Shelton will inspect the area around

the dressing, and both will look at the material available on the two Web sites. The nurse gave the Sheltons her card with a 24-hour response phone number and instructed them to call if they had any concerns.

Discussion Questions

1. What actions would the nurse take to implement the chronic care model of care to help the Sheltons manage Mr. Shelton's health?
2. How might the nurse form relationships to build trust and self-management skills with the Sheltons?
3. Discuss how the use of telehealth might increase the amount of support available to the Sheltons from the home care agency.
4. Suggest ways for the nurse and the physical therapist to effectively collaborate to provide the strongest support for the Sheltons.
5. What outcomes might indicate that the Sheltons were satisfied with and benefited from the home care they received?

Following this, the nurse might help the patient develop solutions to the problem by asking about what strategies the patient has tried in the past, and what strategies he or she might like to try (Huffman, 2007).

Relationship-Based Care

In this model, relationship is the basis of nursing practice (Doane, 2002). Individuals are "viewed as contextual beings who exist in relation with other people and with social, cultural, political, and historical processes" (Doane & Varcoe, 2007, p. 198). Every day nurses engage in relationships with patients, other nurses, and healthcare professionals. This network of relationships forms a web of mutual dependencies (2007, p. 193). Relationship-based care is a model of human

relating that reflects this web of interactions within the context of humanistic values (Hartrick, 1997). In the past, models of nursing care have been based on behavioral models in which the nurse learns a set of communication skills and applies those skills when interacting with patients. This model is unique in that it is based on the recognition of the relational nature and complexity of human experience (p. 524). Rather than enhancing communication between nurse and patient, applying communication techniques may impede communication because the nurse may be focused on performing these techniques, and not be able to be in-caring-human-relation (p. 525). According to this model, "health and healing are promoted through the development of an increasing openness to learning and growth, an increasing capacity to tolerate ambiguity and uncertainty, and an increasing experience of empowerment and choice" (1997, p. 525). For patients with chronic illness, this model of human relation may provide a means for the patient, family, and nurse to grow in relationship with each other as well as the relationship with the chronic illness.

Relationship-based care is not founded on problem identification and resolution, but on responding to the patient in a manner that acknowledges and supports the significance of the chronic illness as the patient experiences it. Nursing action is based on five capacities: (1) initiative, authenticity, and responsiveness; (2) mutuality and synchrony; (3) honoring complexity and ambiguity; (4) intentionality in relating; and (5) re-imaging (Hartrick, 1997, p. 526).

Initiative, authenticity, and responsiveness addresses the nurse's active concern for others (Hartrick, 1997, p. 526). Within this model, these concepts are intertwined. The nurse takes the initiative to engage in relationship with the patient. She or he is authentic, responding to the patient and the situation in a way that is consistent with his or her personality, and showing emotions as they arise. Finally the nurse is responsive to the feelings, needs, and goals of the patient. The nurse is mindful of her presence with the patient and is attentive to the patient with conscious listening.

Concepts of mutuality and synchrony explain the nature of relationships. Mutuality refers to the commonalities experienced by people in relationships. A mutual relationship is a negotiated, collaborative process where patient and nurse both participate, make choices, and act (Doane & Varcoe, 2007, p. 193). These commonalities include shared visions and goals, while acknowledging differences in perspectives. Synchrony describes the rhythms naturally occurring in the relationship including synchrony between internal and external patterns, and periods of silence (Hartrick, 1997, p. 526).

The nurse honors complexity and ambiguity by acknowledging the complexity of human experience. The nurse, in relation with the patient, seeks to uncover the numerous and possibly conflicting elements of the experience. Through this process of discovery, the nurse and patient begin to mutually make connections between seemingly disparate actions, feelings, and events. Through this process, the patient and nurse are able to appreciate the relevance of the experience and make choices regarding the management of the disease process (Hartrick, 1997, p. 526).

Intentionality involves the nurse exploring his or her values and then maintaining consistency between personal values and values in use during professional practice. Each nursing moment is shaped by the actions and intentions of the nurse, the actions and responses of others, and by the contexts within which those interactions occur (Doane & Varcoe, 2007, p. 202). The intent of relational practice is to help patients understand the meaning of their health and healing experiences, and to discover choice and power within the experiences (Hartrick, 1997, p. 527).

Finally, re-imaging is the process of questioning the usual ways of being in the world. Through this process, the nurse can help patients transform their health and healing experiences and enhance their relational capacity (Hartrick, 1997, p. 527).

The nurse who engages in relational nursing practice makes a conscious commitment to act using the values and goals of the nursing profession to attend to each patient's unique context and situation, helping that person grow in health. Difficulty and suffering can provide a vehicle for meaningful relationships and is the base for ethical decision making. In these situations, responsive nursing care creates the space for mutual experience, and for nurse and patient to develop clarity and courage to act in health promoting ways (Doane & Varcoe, 2007, p. 202)

Chronic Care Model of Disease Management

Individuals with chronic disease require a new strategy for health management. The Chronic Care Model (CCM) (Figure 20-2) was developed through a grant from the Robert Wood Johnson Foundation to change the way health care was

FIGURE 20-2

The Chronic Care Model

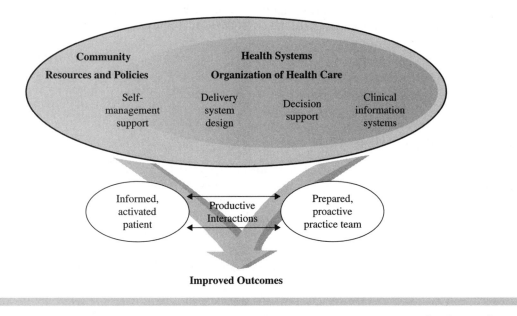

Source: Wagner, E.H. (1998). Chronic disease management: What will it take to improve care for chronic illness? *Effective Clinical Practice, 1*, 2–4.

delivered to individuals with chronic illness (The Chronic Care Model, 2007). The model is designed to support the person with the chronic illness to self-manage their health using appropriate community and healthcare system resources. The home health nurse is in an excellent position to assist the patient in managing his or her own health and chronic illness within this model (see Chapter 19).

Traditionally, the healthcare system in the United States has been focused on providing acute care for acute illness in an episodic manner. Individuals with chronic illness require a proactive approach, combining self-management with effective use of community resources and the healthcare system (The Chronic Care Model, 2007). Care is based on evidence-based protocols that are then tailored to the needs of the individual patient. Common areas of difficulty for self-management

include managing multiple medications, recognizing early warning signs of condition changes, coordinating and appearing for multiple physicians' appointments, understanding the plan of treatment, and coordinating support services (Meckes, 2005).

According to the CCM, healthcare systems need to retool to provide planned visits focused on maintaining wellness. In this model, the patient is recognized as having the central role in managing their health. It is the role of the healthcare providers to support the patient's ability to self-manage their health (CCM, 2007). The nurse can also affect the patient's understanding of the disease process and choices for management. By being in the patient's home, the home care nurse has a unique perspective on the patient's culture, and the meaning of the illness in his or her life.

The home healthcare nurse can play a role in case management, helping the patient navigate complicated interactions with several medical care professionals, and guiding the patient to seek medical care for condition changes in a timely manner. In addition, the nurse can encourage patients to engage with community organizations to help support their self management strategies; these community agencies might include food programs and disease-focused organizations (e.g., The Alzheimer's Association).

Philosophy of Hospice Care

The focus of hospice is the belief that each person has the right to die pain-free and with dignity, and that family members and informal care givers will receive the necessary support to allow people to do so (Organization, 2007). Hospice care is a constellation of services provided with the goal of providing comfort and symptom management at the end of life (Stuart, 2003). Many home healthcare agencies offer hospice services in addition to their regular home care services. Medicare pays for service to hospice patients on a per diem basis. None-the-less, the hospice benefit is underutilized; only 20% of those people eligible use their hospice benefit (Stuart, 2003). In order to be eligible for the hospice benefit, physicians must determine that the patients has fewer than six months to live, patients must forgo treatment that may extend life (see Chapter 22).

INTERVENTIONS

It is anticipated that the need for home care services will increase as the population ages. Because of the unique characteristics required to be a successful home care nurse, the shortage of qualified nurses in home care may be more severe than in other areas of the healthcare system (Ellenbecker, 2004). Home care nurses must possess unique skills including "flexibility, creativity, and innovative approaches to situations and problems in the context of individual and environmental differences and widely varying resource availability" (ANA, 2008, p. 7). According to *Home Health Nursing Scope and Standards of Practice* (ANA, 2008), the nurse best suited to home care practice is the baccalaureate prepared nurse. This is because of his or her broad-based education. Nurses prepared at the associate degree or diploma level are typically members of the home care team. All nurses engaged in home care are expected to advance their ability to meet patient needs in the home care setting. This goal is accomplished by supporting colleagues, structured preceptor programs, clinical experience, and lifelong learning (ANA, 2008). See Table 20-2 for the ANA minimum qualifications for a home care nurse.

Using grounded theory techniques, Neal developed a model of Home Health Nursing Practice (1998). The model outlines three stages of proficiency in home care nursing. At the first level, termed "Dependency," the nurse is typically

TABLE 20-2

Minimum Qualifications of Home Care Nurses

A baccalaureate degree in nursing.
Ability to incorporate communication and motivation skills and principles in the home health setting.
Ability to apply critical thinking to physical, psychosocial, environmental, cultural, family, and safety issues.
Ability to utilize clinical decision-making in applying the nursing process to patients in their places of residence.
Ability to practice as an effective member of an interdisciplinary team.
Competency in applying care-management skills

Source: American Nurses Association. (2008). *Home health nursing: Scope and standards of practice.* Silver Springs, MD: ANA.

new to the setting, overwhelmed by the complexity of the setting, and is dependent on support and assistance from others. As the nurse moves to the second phase, "Moderate dependency," he or she becomes less dependent on others, before finally moving to the phase of "Autonomy," where the nurse achieves confidence, self-assurance, and autonomy in the role of a home health nurse (p. 23). Later, Neal used a triangulated design combining focus groups with one sample of home care nurses and a survey with a second group to test and enhance the model (Neal, 2000).

Cultural Competence

As the older population grows, and diversity of individuals with chronic illness increases, there are persistent trends in usage of home care services. Caucasians are more likely to use formal services than Hispanics, African Americans, and Asian Americans. However, it is difficult to tell if this pattern is a choice of the care recipient or if this trend represents a cultural bias of the care providers who refer individuals to home care (Young, 2003).

Reimbursement in Home Care/Documentation

Skilled services that are reimbursable by third party payers drive the home care industry. The majority of skilled home care services are paid for by health insurance, particularly Medicare and Medicaid. Usually, private insurance companies follow the guidelines set by Medicare. Therefore, changes in Medicare regulations and reimbursement have a major effect on the home healthcare industry.

Medicare establishes regulations that determine who is eligible to receive reimbursable home care services. Accompanying the Medicare funding stream were strict regulations for patient eligibility, home care practice, and reimbursement mechanisms. Although the Medicare home care benefit was designed to extend care to more people, access was difficult because only certain agencies could provide care, and restrictions limited

who was eligible for care, which services patients could receive, and length of service. An additional burden on home care agencies was a complex billing system that often resulted in extensive payment delays.

Agencies adhering to the Medicare Guidelines to receive Medicare and Medicaid payment are classified as "Certified." "Non-certified" home health agencies render home health care privately without consideration of the Medicare Guidelines, and thus receive no payment from Medicare. A home health agency may choose to participate in the Medicare program and can receive payment from Medicare for those patients who meet the eligibility criteria. Agencies choosing not to participate in the Medicare program follow their respective state-established regulations that govern the provision of home care services. However, as a quality measure, private payment agencies often follow the standards of adequate care as established by Medicare.

The need to control Medicare spending began in the mid-1980s as a result of escalating acute care costs. By the mid-1990s, an estimated 10,000 home healthcare agencies had received certification to participate in the Medicare benefit and bill for services (Reichley, 1999). Over a 5-year period, as the number of Medicare-certified home health agencies grew, there was an astronomical rise in Medicare payments. Continuing growth rates of 23–30% per year led to predictions of Medicare home health expenditures reaching 100 billion dollars by the year 2000 (Remington, 2000). To restrain these spiraling costs, governmental controls were set in motion that resulted in a dramatic altering of home care services and led to profound revenue reductions (Grindel-Waggoner, 1999).

The Balanced Budget Act (BBA) of 1997 changed home healthcare reimbursement from a cost-based to a prospective payment system (PPS). The BBA imposed stricter limits on Medicare reimbursement for home care services and narrowed the definition of "home-bound." Patients were no longer eligible for home care if they were able to leave home for any reason other than medical services (Maurer & Smith, 2005). The number of persons eligible for Medicare home care funding declined by 50% between 1997 and 2000 (USDHHS, 2002). Consequently, there was a 45% drop in payments from 1997 through 1999. Unable to continue operations with such profound revenue reductions, approximately 2500 home health agencies closed nationwide by 1999 (Malugani, 1999).

When a patient's care can no longer be billed to Medicare, the agency is responsible for providing advanced notice to the physician and patient, and assist with finding other sources of care. The patient can independently pay the agency. This arrangement provides an alternative to third-party reimbursed care. Since the inception of PPS, many long-term care patients have paid their own bills for care. As Medicare defines its payment criteria, it was never intended to pay for care other than short-term, acute, intermittent, and skilled, so patients needing longer term services require other means to pay for care.

If a home health agency determines that a patient can no longer be served because of costs, discontinuation of care may make the agency at risk for charges of patient abandonment. The definition of abandonment is cessation of services by an agency to a patient who continues to require care and for whom no provision has been made; nor has the patient received proper and timely notice of impending discharge from service.

In the PPS, a specific dollar amount per patient is given to a healthcare professional for delivery of services. The healthcare provider, in turn, becomes the coordinator of the individual's care and assumes responsibility for managing cost, risk, resources, and outcomes of care (Remington, 2000). Reimbursement amounts are determined by clinical assessment of the patient's needs using the mandated assessment tool, Outcome Assessment System and Information Set (OASIS).

OASIS is a 79-item assessment tool designed to establish the national standard for collecting patient outcome data that can be used to evaluate home care services on an industry-wide basis. The form is used to collect a combination of demographic, clinical, and functional patient care data used in calculating Medicare payments to home health agencies.

The actual charges submitted by an agency are determined by the OASIS clinical scoring system, which assigns points to select items in the OASIS data set plus assigns additional points if therapy services are needed. The OASIS scoring system is intended to calculate Medicare payments based on the severity and acuity of the patient's condition, and, in this way, higher payments are provided for sicker patients. There are no limitations on the episodes of care that a patient can receive. The OASIS has been used to measure outcomes from nursing interventions. However, in a recent study, Schneider, Barkauskas, and Keenan (2008) did not find the OASIS sensitive to the effects of home healthcare nursing, as measured by intervention intensity.

The influence of the implementation of the PPS in home health has been more stringent regulations about which services will be reimbursed, and for how long, in some instances. This may well limit access to care for certain vulnerable groups, such as the frail elderly and chronically ill individuals whose care is largely home-based, and people who are HIV positive. Nurses and other healthcare providers must work even more closely with families to determine the kinds of services needed to foster self-care and the optimal timing of these services (Stanhope & Lancaster, 2006).

The individuals who use home care services often have very complex health needs. In a study designed to determine which hospitalized patients were most likely to be referred for home care services, Narsavage and Naylor found that those individuals most likely to be referred had more than one chronic illness [COPD and congestive heart failure (CHF)], were unmarried, needed help with activities of daily living, and had a longer than average hospital stay (2000).

Home Healthcare Agencies

Home care is a unique healthcare service, in that home care practice is by definition in the home of the recipient of care. The living arrangements of the individual receiving care are an important consideration in determining the "goodness of fit" between the patient's needs and the services provided (Hayes, 2002). The home health nurse uses primary, secondary, and tertiary prevention strategies, and they assist patients and families with coordination of community resources. This is accomplished within the community in the home of the patient (ANA, 2008).

Home healthcare practitioners and standards of practice are governed by state and federal legislation. Individual state regulations must be met for basic licensing of all home health agencies. If participation in the Medicare reimbursement program is desired, there are also federal regulations that govern Medicare certification and coverage of services (Conditions of Participation and HHA-11, respectively) that must be met. These federal mandates, along with individual state licensing or certification requirements, help ensure that home healthcare practitioners are qualified to provide their specialized services.

Language of Home Health Care

Several definitions are important in determining eligibility of patients and subsequent reimbursement by the home healthcare agency. Terms are defined by federal Medicare regulations and include the following: homebound, primary services, continuing services, and dependent services.

Federal Medicare regulations include the qualifications of patients for coverage of home health services. The patient must be confined to the home or to an institution that is not a hospital or skilled nursing facility (SNF). Confined to the home does not mean the patient must be bedridden. Homebound, or home confined, is defined as an inability to leave the home normally and that leaving would be taxing and require considerable effort and assistance. When the patient does leave the home, the absences are infrequent and of relatively short duration, or to receive medical care. The patient must be under the care of a physician

and in need of skilled services on an intermittent-visit, not continuous, basis. Intermittent services are provided on visits to the home, with a physician's certifying order for the number of visits from each service to be made during a week or month and for the total duration or number of weeks for the home health services. These skilled services are the primary services and include nursing, physical therapy (PT), speech therapy, and occupational therapy (OT), which must be initiated in conjunction with the patient's receipt of another primary service and may continue even though other service is no longer necessary until the goals for that discipline have been met (Medicare Conditions of Participation, 1996).

Occupational therapy in home health care is considered a continuing service, meaning that the involvement of OT in the patient's care depends on an initial primary service. However, once the primary service of nursing, physical therapy, or speech therapy has been initiated, the occupational therapist can continue working with the patient after the other services are no longer needed, a continuing service.

In addition to primary skilled services, home health aides and social work services are covered as dependent services under Medicare regulations. The patient must require a skilled service to receive a home health aide or social work services, and once the skilled service is no longer required, the home health aide and social work services are not covered. These dependent services can also be continued if OT (a continuing service) is to be provided to the patient.

Home Healthcare Team

The home healthcare team consists of physicians, nurses, physical therapists, occupational therapists, speech therapists, medical social workers, home health aides, and the patient and informal caregivers. Each member of the team possesses a special set of skills that collectively supports a comprehensive approach to assist the patient in meeting his or her care needs.

Effective home care depends on groups of independent practitioners forming teams to provide services for patients. These practitioners have different skill sets, and are not always all from the same agency. The multiple practitioners on the home healthcare team have the knowledge and skills to identify patients' needs and address those needs through management of complex plans of care (Marelli, 1998). Each practitioner must have a strong grasp of the rules and regulations that govern home health care, the ability to pay attention to detail, well-developed interpersonal skills, strong clinical skills, a working knowledge of the changing economics of health care, and the ability to effectively prioritize and time-manage challenging tasks and responsibilities.

Four models of team functioning have been identified: medical, multidisciplinary, interdisciplinary, and transdisciplinary (Mauk, 2007, p. 3). In a medical model team, the physician leader directs all functions of the team. Team members do not meet together, but communicate through the physician. This team configuration is most common in acute care settings where the physician is in daily contact with the patient. This model is not desirable in a home care situation as the patient may not be in contact with the physician; the care providers are in the patient's home, and independent decision making is a hallmark of this type of care.

The second type of team is the multidisciplinary team. In this model, professionals work in parallel. Each provider develops goals for his or her interaction with the patient, and coordination occurs at the supervisory level. The individuals who are providing care rarely communicate directly with each other. This model of care is common in long-term care settings in which a rigid bureaucratic structure exists. Multidisciplinary models also occur in home care settings. However, the nature of home care is that practitioners work independently, and may interact with other professionals on the team only sporadically (Gantert & McWilliams, 2004).

Transdisciplinary teams are found in rehabilitation settings where team members and the patient are in proximity daily. In this model, the patient and primary care provider work as a team with the counsel of all other team members (Mauk, 2007). Individual team members perform the interventions required for the patient while the provider is with the patient. Although this model is effective in rehabilitation settings, the nature of home care does not lend itself to this type of team function. The billing constraints in home care require that professionals perform the interventions within their scope of practice, and does not reimburse for care outside of that scope. This model works best in a capitated payment system, where the agency receives a predetermined amount of money for care regardless of who is providing the care.

The team configuration that is most effective in the home setting is the interdisciplinary team model. In an interdisciplinary team, professionals working with a patient communicate directly with the patient and each other. In this model, the patient is an integral part of the team, and professionals collaborate with the patient to establish goals for care (Mauk, 2007).

Effective interdisciplinary team collaboration has been associated with benefits for both practitioner and patient. These include increased provider autonomy and job satisfaction, and improved patient outcomes and cost containment (Gantert & McWilliams, 2004).

Gantert and McWilliams (2004) identified three dimensions of interaction among interdisciplinary team members: networking, navigating, and aligning. Each dimension occurs along a continuum. The less interactive end of the continuum is representative of a multidisciplinary team, whereas the more interactive end is representative of a more interdisciplinary model. For networking, the continuum ran from isolation to connectedness. As communication among team members increased, so did feelings of connectedness among team members. Navigating had to do with how the team members trusted each other. The more contact team members had with each other, the more trust they exhibited with each other. Finally, the dimension of aligning described the strategies used to determine roles within the team. Team function ranges from the traditional organization hierarchy to a more fluid organization, where team members function autonomously and collaboratively (2004).

Coordination of Care

Care coordination is defined as, services provided to the chronically ill who are at risk for adverse outcomes and expensive care to remedy shortcomings in current health care by:

- Identifying medical, functional, social and emotional needs that increase risk of adverse outcomes and expensive care.
- Addressing those needs through self-care education and optimization of medical treatment.
- Monitoring progress and identifying problems early (Mathmatica Policy Research, 2000).

Home care nurses and agencies are in an excellent position to incorporate the role of care coordinator into the role of the nurse because these high-risk individuals are often being treated by home care nurses. The nurse has a well established relationship with physicians and the local healthcare system, and are in an excellent position to incorporate technology into the plan of care so as to use telehealth strategies to augment care (Meckes, 2005).

Three major care coordination issues have been identified (Feldman, 2004). The first is coordination between the hospital and the homecare agency at discharge from the hospital or at admission to the hospital from the homecare agency. Transitions from one service to another are fraught with opportunities for miscommunication. The second issue for care coordination is strengthening the effectiveness and communication among the members of the interdisciplinary team (Feldman, 2004). The third issue is to improve the effectiveness of interaction between the formal and informal caregivers and to foster self-management (Feldman, 2004). This issue is described in more detail in the following.

The Program of All-Inclusive Care for the Elderly (PACE) provides for older adults with chronic illness, who are eligible for both Medicare and Medicaid, and who are living at home even though they qualify for nursing home care (Young, 2003). Through PACE, interdisciplinary teams assess individuals and provide comprehensive services across settings. By removing the financial barriers to coordination of care, the PACE concept unites the healthcare team around providing long-term care management in the least restrictive setting (2003).

Formal and Informal Caregivers

Unpaid assistance is provided to older individuals and those with chronic illness in at least 22.9 million households (21%) across the United States. By contrast, less than half (41%) of the individuals receiving informal care reported paying for services from professional care providers (National Alliance for Caregiving and AARP, 2004). The National Caregiving Alliance and AARP (NACAARP) counted individuals as caregivers if he or she was older than18 years of age, and performed one of 13 activities for another adult. Table 20-3 lists the 13 caregiving behaviors. Young (2003) reports that 73% of caregivers are women, with an average age of 46, and 64% work outside of the home (see Chapter 9).

In a study conducted at the Visiting Nurse Service of New York, researchers explored the effects of formal and informal caregiving on the recovery of the patient, and the interaction between formal and informal caregivers. The findings identified gaps in the information and training received by informal caregivers (Feldman, 2004, p. 34). (see Chapter 9).

Assessing the ability of unpaid caregivers to support the individual with chronic illness is critical to developing an effective plan of care. Tanner (2004) developed a scale to be used with individuals with chronic health problems to determine the availability of family support. The Tanner Family Support Scale (TFSS) is a 13-item scale that the

---

TABLE 20-3

Informal Caregiver Behaviors

Instrumental Activities of Daily Living

Transportation (82%)
Grocery shopping (75%)
Housework (69%)
Managing finances (64%)
Preparing meals (59%)
Helping with medication (41%)
Managing services (30%)

Activities of Daily Living

Get in and out of a chair or bed (36%)
Dressing (29%)
Bathing or showering (26%)
Toileting (23%)
Eating (18%)
Incontinence (16%)

Source: National Alliance for Caregiving and American Association of Retired Persons. *Caregiving in the US. Executive summary.* Washington DC: Author. Used with permission.

---

individual answers yes or no to such questions as, "My family members do as much as they can to help me with my health problems when I need help" (2004, p. 314).

Often the home healthcare nurse and the recipient of care rely heavily on the informal caregiver. Collaboration and decision-making often involve a triad rather than the usual nurse–patient dyad (Dalton, 2003). However, the nurse must carefully negotiate the relationship to make sure that the recipient of care is not silenced (Dalton, 2003). Dalton (2005) identified three types of decisions commonly made about nursing care to include: program decisions (goals and content of care), operational control decisions (how the plan is implemented), and agenda decisions (timing and frequency of nursing visits and care delivery). Coalitions formed between two of the three parts of the triad can affect all care decisions. Home care nurses should collaborate with both the patient

receiving care and informal caregivers to optimize the benefit of the available professional care. Leff (2004) found that patients demonstrated higher satisfaction with care when they were included in decision-making regarding goals, the plan, who (which disciplines and personnel) will provide care, how often and what time of day visits would occur, the activities occurring during the visit, how care is provided, and who will communicate with the physician (p. 298).

Information Technology and Telehealth

One of the fastest growing areas of home health care is telehealth. Assistive devices in the home have the potential to improve home safety, enhance the independence, and reduce the risk for injury of individuals with chronic illness (Young, 2003). Some individuals, both patients and care providers, are ambivalent about the use of monitoring technology in the home because of the potential invasion of privacy (Percival & Hanson, 2006). At the same time that home technology is exploding, home care is an industry that has embraced that technology from cellular phones and laptop computers to the Internet and telehealth (ANA, 2008). Appropriate use of information technology and telehealth can lead to enhanced quality of care, improved patient and clinician safety, and increased productivity (2007). Meanwhile, the ethical issues of privacy and data protection are significant (Percival & Hanson, 2006).

The American Telemedicine Association (ATA) has defined telemedicine as "the use of medical information exchanged from one site to another via electronic communications to improve patients' health status" (ATA, 2006/2007). Telemedicine may include distance monitoring of an individual's health status, routine consultations with healthcare providers, referrals to specialists for complex problems, and consumer health information sites on the Internet. However, at the present time, a telehealth visit may not be substituted for an in-person visit, and if telemedicine is to be used for a home care patient, the plan of care and the physician's order must specify the expected level of live visits and the expected level of telehome care (Pushkin, 2001).

Guidelines for telehealth programs have been developed, including generic guidelines for all home telehealth applications, interactive home telehealth guidelines, and telemonitoring (Britton, 2003). The generic guidelines should be included in all telehealth programs and include determining patient inclusion criteria, explaining the program and obtaining patient consent, protection of individual's health information, home assessment for appropriateness of the plan, patient/caregiver education, and a plan for performance improvement that includes the patient (2003). In addition, programs using interactive home telehealth should establish procedures to protect the patient's privacy when he or she does not wish to be observed, and the plan of care must be guided by physician order and clearly outline the plan for live and virtual visits. Finally, for programs that use telemonitoring, formal care providers must be adequately trained, and the protocol for monitoring and for action when the patient symptoms deviate from the normal parameters for that patient clearly established (2003).

As the available technology expands, the efficacy of telemedicine and telehealth is being tested. In a study evaluating the effectiveness of a telemedicine intervention for patients with CHF who had recently been discharged from the hospital as opposed to a group of similar patients receiving the usual home care services, researchers found that while the telemedicine intervention reduced the number of nursing visits, home health costs, and improved the patient's self-perceived quality of life, it did not affect the number of re-admissions or visits to the emergency department (Myers, Grant, Lugn, Holbert & Kvedar, 2006). Unexpected findings included a need for ongoing education and support for the patients using the telehealth equipment throughout the treatment period. In addition, several potential research participants declined or withdrew from the study because they were anxious about using the equipment (Myers et al., 2006).

Telehealth is here to stay. In a Cochrane review of controlled clinical trials evaluating the efficacy of telehealth, Murray and colleagues (2005) found that interactive health communication applications (IHCAs) had a positive effect on several aspects of functioning. The review included 3739 patients involved in 24 randomized controlled clinical trials. Across studies, people with chronic illnesses using IHCAs had a better understanding of their health problems, and IHCAs had a positive effect on social support, behavioral, and clinical outcomes. In addition, IHCAs were positively related to improved self-efficacy (2005, p. 1).

Clinical Care Classification (CCC) System

The CCC was developed in 1991 by Saba and colleagues as a way of predicting resource needs and measuring the outcomes of home care (Saba, 1998). Since then, the system has gained credibility through independent research and use in both clinical and educational settings (Table 20-4). The most recent update was in 2004 (Saba, 2004).

The classification system consists of two standardized, interrelated terminologies: one for nursing diagnosis and another for nursing interventions. The two terminologies are classified by 21 care components and organized into four health patterns: health behavioral, functional, physiologic, and psychological, representing a comprehensive approach to patient care (1998). The system was designed, in part, to facilitate computerized patient record-keeping and relating nursing diagnosis and interventions to patient outcomes. It can be incorporated into an existing home healthcare record, and linked to reimbursement software (1998, p. 12). More information on the CCC can be obtained at www.sabacare.com.

The home health industry is challenged to skillfully manage the risk, cost, resources, and outcomes of client care. All agency staff require a thorough education to be familiar with the rules and regulations for agency operations and how each staff member's skills and talents will be used to achieve agency goals. Clinicians need continuing education focused on maximizing the value of provided care. Accurate, thorough patient assessments

TABLE 20-4

CCC System: 21 Care Components by Four Clinical Patterns

Health Behavioral Components
Medication
Safety
Health behavior

Functional Components
Activity
Fluid volume
Nutritional
Self-care
Sensory

Physiologic Components
Cardiac
Respiratory
Metabolic
Physical regulation
Skin integrity
Tissue perfusion
Bowel elimination
Urinary elimination
Life cycle

Psychological Components
Cognitive
Coping
Role relationship
Self-concept

Source: Saba, V.K. Clinical Care Classification (CCC) System. Retrieved from www.sabacare.com/. Used with permission.

and rapid submission of these data are critical for the agency to obtain timely reimbursement.

Home health nurses can promote patients' self-management of their chronic diseases. The nurse can be effective in helping patients and their informal caregivers to maximize the support available to them. Using strategies such as coaching and telemedicine can help patients improve their self-care abilities. Resources such as protocols, care maps, and clinical pathways will become more useful, along with the incentive to explore advanced technologies such as point-of-service computers and telemedicine devices.

OUTCOMES

The desired outcomes for the role that home health care plays in the management of the long-term patient with chronic illness seem initially to be quite apparent. The positive effects of the health care delivered in the home to the patient, as well as the positive effects of the caregiver support mechanisms in order to keep the patient at home and not necessitating institutionalization, are clearly important outcomes. However, the urgency of establishing outcome criteria that are stable and dependable in order to measure outcome attainment is essential to knowing if positive effects are occurring to the advantage of the patient and caregiver or simply because there is no alternative to providing care.

Maurer and Smith (2005) have established nine possible outcome measures for evaluating the outcome attainment judged by changes in the population, the healthcare system within the community, or the environment. The identified outcome measures include (1) knowledge; (2) behaviors, skills; (3) attitudes; (4) emotional well-being; (5) health status (epidemiology); (6) presence of healthcare system services and components; (7) satisfaction or acceptance regarding the program interventions; (8) presence of policy allowing, mandating, and funding; and (9) altered relationship with the physical environment (p. 403).

Evaluating the outcomes of care rendered by any of the disciplines participating in home health care for the first five measures is inclusive in the care itself. The professionals and paraprofessionals who work within the home care teams function within and by delivering care using these first five principles, thereby making their use as measurement variables relatively easy and functional. The last four outcome measures, however, have been a continuous struggle for home health care throughout the 20th and now the 21st centuries. These four measures are unpredictably influenced by the ups and downs of financial support, government regulations, management control in home health itself, and in the institutional care that passes patients on to in-home care.

EVIDENCE-BASED PRACTICE BOX

In a small, randomized, experimental two-group (n = 50), repeated-measures design, Barnason and colleagues evaluated the contribution of a home communication intervention (HCI) to functional and recovery outcomes in patients who had undergone coronary artery bypass grafting (CABG) and were receiving home health care (HHC). The control group received the usual HHC. The experimental group received HHC and HCI. The HCI consisted of the use of the "Health Buddy," a small telehealth device that attaches to the telephone. The Health Buddy is developed and manufactured by Health Hero Network, Redwood City, California (Barnason et al., 2006, p. 228). The device has four buttons to enable the user to respond to information on the screen. The subjects received daily Health Buddy sessions for 12 weeks. Each session included: (1) assessment of recovery and strategies to manage reported symptoms; (2) education on CABG recovery; and (3) positive reinforcement to increase self-efficacy. The Health Buddy intervention was scripted, and provided standardized comments to subjects' responses to information provided. The sessions were generally less than 10 minutes in length.

Outcome measures included the Medical Outcomes Survey (MOS) SF-36, a short measure of physical and psychosocial functioning that was administered before discharge from the hospital to ascertain pre-surgical functioning, at 6 weeks and 3 months postoperatively. In addition, all subjects completed a self-report recovery follow-up tool. HHC use was also monitored. When the subject completed their HHC, the number of visits, type of services, and duration of HHC were provided by the HHC agency.

Data were analyzed using repeated measures analyses of covariance, with number of HHC visits as covariate to determine differences in outcomes between the two groups. The main finding was that intervention group was found to have significantly higher general health functioning as compared to the control group. At the 6-week follow-up, only 33% of the intervention group as compared with 52% of the control group reported lower functioning than their baseline function. At 3 months, 22% of the intervention group as compared with 29% of the control group had physical functioning scores lower than their 6-week scores. The intervention group had earlier rebound scores in both physical and role function (p. 230). The control group had recovered to baseline function at 3 months, whereas the intervention group had improved function over baseline at 3 months (p. 231). This study demonstrates that HCI can be used to augment usual HHC for enhanced outcomes. Further research is needed to determine the appropriate dose of HCI to maximize the benefit while minimizing the burden.

Source: Barnason, S., Zimmerman, L., Nieveen, J., & Hertzog, M. (2006). Impact of a telehealth intervention to augment home healthcare on functional and recovery outcomes of elderly patients undergoing coronary artery bypass grafting. *Heart and Lung, 35*(4), 225–233.

Home Care Satisfaction Measures

In health care, objective measures of patient satisfaction with care are often used as an indicator of positive outcomes. However, in home care, it has been more difficult to measure patient satisfaction with care (Geron Smith, Tennstedt, Jette, Chassler, & Kastern, 2000, 2000). Although some scales of patient satisfaction have been adapted from acute care, few measures have been developed specifically for home care. The Home Care Satisfaction Measure (HCSM) is a 60-item instrument measuring overall satisfaction with home care and satisfaction with five common services (Geron et al., 2000). The HCSM is designed to measure satisfaction with homemaker and home health aide services, case management, home-delivered meal service, and grocery service. The instrument is designed so that each service could be measured separately or the scores summed for an overall measure of satisfaction. The HCSM can be completed in person or by telephone. It is to be noted that the HCSM evaluates patient satisfaction with aspects of home care that are not usually covered by Medicare and private insurance.

With the establishment of capitation payment and agencies learning how best to serve the patient within this system, along with increased Medicare support to both the individual patient and to the caregiver, the desired outcomes of home health care should become more realistic. These outcomes should be more attainable as well. Outcomes evaluation and analysis can demonstrate that the home healthcare process results in appropriate, adequate, and effective patient care.

Positive client outcomes require that home care agencies become aware of the roles that clients, family, and caregivers play before the client is admitted for service. Home care providers, patients, families, and caregivers must enter into partnerships to provide the care needed for the patient. Informal care providers need to know the significance of their roles in the plan of care, and nurses must enlist these informal caregivers to continue to provide care, In turn, the client's family must understand what can be expected from agency services.

Several forces are coming to bear on the need for home care services. As the population ages and individuals survive longer, chronic illness is increasing, and there is a social movement to decrease institutionalization in nursing homes in favor of keeping patients in their own communities. The home care industry is in an excellent position to create partnerships with patients and families to help patients stay in their own environments and manage their chronic illness.

ACKNOWLEDGMENT

The author would like to thank Margaret M. Patton and Gwendolyn F. Foss for their work on this chapter in the sixth edition.

STUDY QUESTIONS

1. What is the goal of home care according to the American Nurses Association?
2. Describe how home care nurses differ in practice from public health nurses.
3. Discuss the definition of homebound and how that definition might affect an individual's ability to go to church regularly and the provision of their health care.
4. Describe the Self and Family Management of Chronic Illness model. How might you apply the model to an individual with type 1 diabetes?
5. Discuss how the home care nurse might use the Chronic Care Model to provide care to a patient with chronic illness.
6. How does including telehealth in the list of interventions affect the delivery of home care?
7. Discuss strategies the home care nurse might use to help a patient and his or her family manage the disease process.
8. What skills does a nurse need to be an affective home care nurse?
9. How can the interdisciplinary team maintain effective communication in the home?
10. Discuss how nurses might use home care outcome measures to improve the healthcare delivery system.

INTERNET RESOURCES

Center for Medicare and Medicaid Services: www.cms.hhs.gov/OASIS/
Home Healthcare Nurses Association: www.hhna.org/
National Association for Home care and Hospice: www.nahc.org/

REFERENCES

American Nurses Association (2008). *Home health nursing: Scope and standards of practice.* Silver Springs, MD: ANA

American Telemedicine Association (2006/2007). American telemedicine association. Retrieved on January 11, 2008, from http://www.americantelemed.org/

Barnason, S., Zimmerman, L., Nieveen, J., & Hertzog, M. (2006). Impact of a telehealth intervention to augment home healthcare on functional and recovery outcomes of elderly patients undergoing coronary artery bypass grafting. *Heart and Lung, 35*(4), 225–233.

Britton, B., (2003). First home telehealth clinical guidelines. *Home Healthcare Nurse, 21*(1), 703–706.

Capitman, J. (2003). Effective coordination of medical and supportive services. *Journal of Aging and Health, 15*(1), 124–164.

Dalton, J. (2003). Development and testing of the theory of collaborative decision-making in nursing practice for triads. *Journal of Advanced Nursing, 50*(1), 22–33.

Dalton, J. (2005). Client-caregiver-nurse coalition formation in decision-making situations during home visits. *Journal of Advanced Nursing, 52*(3), 291–299.

Doane, G. (2002). Beyond behavioral skills to human-involved processes: Relational nursing practice and interpretive pedagogy. *Journal of Nursing Education, 41*(9), 400–404.

Doane, G., & Varcoe, C. (2007). Relational practice and nursing obligations. *Advances in Nursing Science, 30*(3), 192–205.

Ellenbecker, C. (2004). A theoretical model of job retention for home health care nurses. *Journal of Advanced Nursing, 47*(3), 303–310.

Feldman, P. (2004). Penny Feldman on home healthcare quality and research. *Journal for Healthcare Quality, 26*(3), 31–37

Gantert, T., & McWilliams, C. (2004). Interdisciplinary team processes within an in-home service delivery organization. *Home Health Services Quarterly, 23*(3), 1–17.

Geron, S., Smith, K., Tennstedt, S., Jette, A., Chassler, D., & Kastern, L. (2000). The home care satisfaction measure: A client-centered approach to assessing the satisfaction of frail older adults with home care services. *Journal of Gerontology: Social Sciences, 55B*, 5.

Grey, M., Knafl, K., & McCorkel, R. (2006). A framework for the study of self- and family management of chronic conditions. *Nursing Outlook, 54,* 278–286.

Grindel-Waggoner, M. (1999). Home care: A history of caring, a future of challenges. *MedSurg Nursing, 8,* 118–122.

Gundersen, L. (1999). There's no place like home: The home health care alternative. *Annals of Internal Medicine, 131,* 639–640.

Hartrick, G. (1997). Relationship capacity: The foundation for interpersonal nursing practice. *Journal of Advanced Nursing, 26,* 523–528.

Hayes, J. (2002). Living arrangements and health status in later life: A review of recent literature. *Public Health Nursing, 19*(2), 136–151.

Hitchcock, J., Schubert, P., & Thomas, S. (Eds.). (2003). *Community health nursing: Caring in action* (2nd ed.). Albany, NY: Delmar.

Huffman, M. (2007). Health coaching: A new and exciting technique to enhance patient self-management and improve outcomes. *Home Healthcare Nurse, 25*(4), 271–274.

Improving Chronic Care (2007). The chronic care model. Retrieved on January 8, 2008 from www.improvingchroniccare.org/index.php?p=The_Chronic_Care_Model&s=2

Leff, E. (2004). Involving patients in care decisions improves satisfaction: An outcomes based quality improvement project. *Home Healthcare Nurse, 22*(5), 297–301.

Lundy, K., & Janes, S. (2001). *Community health nursing: Caring for the public's health.* Sudbury, MA: Jones & Bartlett.

Malugani, M. (1999). No place like home: Always adaptable, home care faces the future. *Nurseweek, 12*(24), 1–18.

Marelli, T. (1998). *Handbook of home health standards and documentation guidelines for reimbursement.* St. Louis: Mosby.

Mathematica Policy Research (2000). *Best practices in coordinated care: Prepared for health care financing administration.* Retrieved on March 17, 2008 from http://www.mathematica-mpr.com

Mauk, K. (2007). *The specialty practice of rehabilitation: A core curriculum.* Glenview, IL: Association of Rehabilitation Nursing.

Maurer, F., & Smith, C. (2005). *Community public health nursing practice.* St. Louis: Elsevier Saunders.

Meckes, C. (2005). Opportunities in care coordination. *Home Healthcare Nurse, 23*(10), 663–669.

Montauk, S. (1998). Home health care. *American Family Physician, 58,* 1609–1614.

Murray, E., Burns, J., See Tai, S., Lai, R., & Nazareth, I. (2005). Interactive health communication applications for people with chronic disease. Cochrane Database of Systematic Reviews(4), CD004274. DO004271:004210.001002/14751858.CD14004274, publ4651854

Myers, S., Grant, R., Lugn, N., Holbert, B., & Kvedar, J. (2006). Impact of home-based monitoring on the care of patients with congestive heart failure. *Home Health Care Management and Practice, 18*(6), 444–445.

Narsavage, G., & Naylor, M. (2000). Factors associated with referral of elderly individuals with cardiac and pulmonary disorders for home care services following hospital discharge. *Journal of Gerontological Nursing, 26*(5), 14–20.

National Alliance for Caregiving and the American Association of Retired Persons (2004). *Caregiving in the U.S.: Executive Summary.* Washington, D.C.: Author.

National Hospice and Palliative Care Organization (2007). Caring connections. Retrieved on January 14, 2008, from http://www.caringinfo.org/LivingWithAnIllness/Hospice.htm

Neal, L. (1998). *Rehabilitation nursing in the home health setting.* Glenview, IL: Association of Rehabilitation Nurses.

Neal, L. (2000). Validating and refining the Neal theory of home health nursing practice. *Home Health Care Management and Practice, 12*(2), 16–25.

Percival, J. & Hanson, J. (2006). Big brother of brave new world? Telecare and its implications for older people's independence and social inclusions. *Critical Social Policy, 26*(4), 888–909.

Pushkin, D. (2001). Telemedicine: Follow the money. *The Online Journal of Issues in Nursing, 6*(3). Retrieved from www.nursingworld.org/MainMenuCategories/ANA Marketplace/ANAPeriodicals/OJIN/TableofContents/ VolumeTelemedicine.aspx

Reichley, M. (1999). Advances in home care: Then, now and into the future. *Success in Home Care, 3*(6), 10–18.

Remington, L. (2000). PPS is making people run out of excuses for a change. *The Remington report: Business and clinical solutions for home care and post-acute markers.* July/August, 13–15.

Saba, V.K. (1998). Home health care classification system: An overview. *The Online Journal of Issues in Nursing, 3*(2). Retrieved from http://www.nursingworld.org/MainMenuCategories/ANAMarketplace/ANAPeriodicals/OJIN/TableofContents/ Volume72002/No3Sept2002/ArticlesPreviousTopic/HHCCAnOverview.aspx

Saba, V.K. (2004). CCC System Version 2.0. www.sabacare.com/index.html.

Scheneider, J.S., Barkauskas, V., & Keenan, G. (2008). Evaluation of home health care nursing outcomes with OASIS and NOC. *Journal of Nursing Scholarship, 40*(1), 76–82.

Schoen, M., & Koenig, R., (1997). Home health care nursing: Past and present. *Medsurg Nursing, 6*(4), 230–234.

Stanhope, M., & Lancaster, J. (2006). *Foundations of nursing in the community: Community-oriented practice* (2nd ed.). St. Louis: Mosby.

Stuart, B. (2003). Transition management: A new paradigm for home care of the chronically ill near the end of life. *Home Health Care Management & Practice, 15*(2), 126–135.

Tanner, E. (2004). Chronic illness demands for self-management in older adults. *Geriatric Nursing, 25*(5), 313–317.

The Chronic Care Model. (2007). Retrieved on January 18, 2008, from http://www.improvingchroniccare.org

Young, H. (2003). Challenges and solutions for care of frail older adults. *The Online Journal of Issues in Nursing, 8*(2). Retrieved from www.nursingworld.org/MainMenuCategories/ANA Marketplace/ANAPeriodicals/OJIN/TableofContents/Volume82003/Num82002May82031_82003/ OlderAdultsCareSolutions.aspx.

21

Long-Term Care

Kristen L. Mauk and Susan J. Barnes

INTRODUCTION

"One of CDC's highest priorities as the nation's health protection agency is to increase the number of older adults who live longer, high-quality, productive, and independent lives" [Centers for Disease Control and Prevention (CDC) and the Merck Company Foundation, 2007, p. i]. As of 2004, there were 36.3 million people in America older than the age of 65 and by 2030, approximately 71 million persons (20% of the population) will be older than age 65 (CDC and Merck, 2007).

In 2005, approximately 9 million people used long-term care (LTC) services in the United States (Chandra, Smith, & Paul, 2006). The cost of providing health care to persons older than age 65 is three to five times greater than for younger persons. The changing demographics of the baby boomer generation entering the older age group will have a significant impact on the whole of society (Lomastro, 2006).

For many persons, increased age is accompanied by one or more chronic illnesses. Reported health conditions among those in the Health and Retirement Study (National Institute on Aging, 2007) included (in order of frequency): arthritis, hypertension, heart conditions, diabetes, psychological/emotional problems, cancer, chronic

lung disease, and stroke. These chronic conditions represent many of the frequent complaints of older adults as they experience the aging process. The National Interview Health Survey (National Center for Health Statistics, 2007) found that nearly one third of adults older than 75 had fair or poor health. As chronicity increases, there often follows deficits in a person's ability to perform self-care, which can eventually lead to the need for LTC services. According to a document from the AARP (Houser, Fox-Grage, & Gibson, 2006), indicators of the need for LTC services include advanced age, living alone, poverty, less education, not owning a home, and not having a vehicle for transportation. The issue of LTC is sufficiently significant that the 2005 White House Conference on Aging focused on the "booming" dynamics of aging, tackling difficult issues relating to the baby boomer generation entering the older age group. The topics of the conference included promoting dignity, healthy independence, and financial security of older adults (Kaisernetwork, 2005).

LTC is an umbrella term that may refer to a range of services that address the health, personal care, psychoemotional, and social needs of persons with some degree of difficulty in caring for themselves. Although family members may assist those persons with age-related functional decline or those with disabilities, LTC is often needed as time progresses to bridge the gap in care. The ideal LTC services promote independence of the person for as long as possible and allows them to remain at home as appropriate.

The concept of LTC may best be visualized on a continuum. Care needs may be minimal or extensive (Figure 21-1). Long-term care services are offered in a variety of settings, as discussed in greater detail in this chapter. There is a growing trend in community-based services. Often, persons visualize a nursing home setting when they think of LTC, but this setting is used by only a small portion of the population at any given time.

FIGURE 21-1

Long-Term Care Continuum in Terms of Intensity

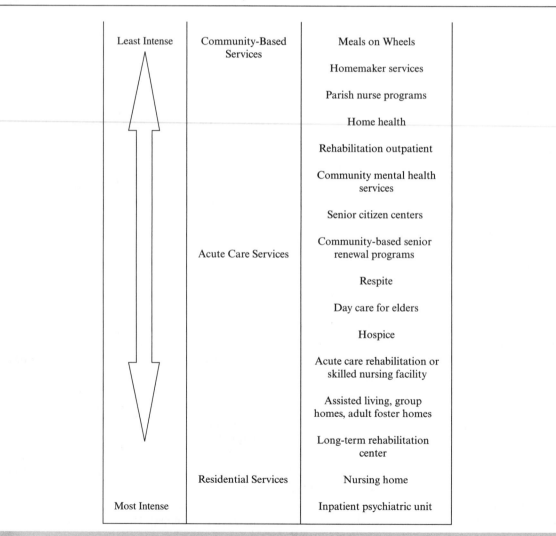

In between these two ends of the spectrum—independence with minimal assistance at home and skilled care in the nursing home—are many alternatives and options.

Historical Perspectives

Caring for a client with complex health needs over a long period continues to be a challenge for the healthcare system. Throughout history, consideration given to the quality of care for older adults is seen as a reflection of societal values (Koop & Schaeffer, 1976). In societies with more fluid resources, vulnerable populations such as the frail elderly or individuals with chronic illness are better cared for because of the availability of assistance with health care (Kalisch & Kalisch, 2004). History has demonstrated that in societies under the strain caused by famine, war, or social upheaval, the vulnerable may not be able to survive because of malnutrition, lack of health care, and the lack of ability of the family unit to provide support (Kalisch & Kalisch, 2004).

A review of LTC in the United States reveals several significant events in the last century that have led to our current system of providing care. Prior to the 20th century, older adults in the United States were usually cared for within extended family units (DeSpelder & Strickland, 2002). Those without family to care for them might have gone to a facility supported by a religious organization or by charitable citizens, such as a poor house or almshouse. Changes in medical care altered hospital stays and allowed LTC to evolve, with group rest homes and private charitable homes providing care for chronically ill, dependent persons. Because life expectancies continued to increase, the demand for LTC accompanied that increase (Lekan-Rutledge, 1997). Political response came in the form of the enactment of the Social Security Act in 1932, which provided services for the elderly and chronically ill. In 1951, the first White House Conference on Aging was held. The first conference (now held every 10 years) focused on issues that affected the quality of life of the aged person.

Title XVIII of the Social Security Act, which passed in 1965 and was a part of the Great Society of President Lyndon B. Johnson, provided medical insurance for the elderly (Medicare) and further involved the federal government in health care [Centers for Medicare and Medicaid Services (CMS), 2004b]. At the same time, in 1965, public policy was altered by the enactment of the Older Americans Act, which established aging networks throughout the states and funded community-based health services. Medicare opened the door for the government to dictate regulations and set the standard for care in formal caregiving settings. Evolution of the system included a recent restructuring of the Health Care Financing Authority into the Centers for Medicare and Medicaid Services with the emphasis on improving the overall process of coordinating care of complex illness in the context of managed care (White House Conference on Aging, 2004).

Part of the Social Security Amendments of 1965 was Title XIX, Medicaid, to provide medical and health-related services for individuals and families with low incomes. Medicaid, a cooperative work between each state and the federal government, is the largest source of funds for services to the poor. Each state establishes its own eligibility standards, sets the rate of payment for services, and administers its own program (CMS, 2005). Further changes in LTC were accomplished by Title XX of the Social Security Act Amendments, which made in-home services for medically indigent more widely available. In 1972, legislation was established that paid for intermediate care. The Omnibus Reconciliation Act, passed in 1987, included the Nursing Home Reform Act, which established high quality of care as a goal, along with the preservation of residents' rights in LTC facilities. Among the changes included was the requirement that comprehensive assessments of all nursing home residents were to be done to determine functional, cognitive, and affective levels of the residents and to be used in planning care. In addition, more specific requirements for nursing, medical, and psychosocial services were designed to attain and maintain the highest possible mental and physical functional statuses by focusing on outcomes (such as incontinence, immobility, pressure sores). Resident rights were also clearly defined (Harrington, Carrillo, & Crawford, 2004). Organizations such as the National Association for Home Care & Hospice and others (Kempthorne, 2004) have seen the need for continued work on health policy in this area and have made long-term care a high priority on their legislative agenda.

As our culture has evolved over the last 50 years, the family structure has been modified by the increasing number of women who work outside the home and are unavailable to care for aging parents (Lekan-Rutledge, 1997; Wagner, 2006; Gaugler & Teaster, 2006). Current cultural values have made it less common for extended families to live together. The Hispanic and Asian cultures often include extended families, with several generations living in the same household or nearby, which makes it possible for family members to look after the interests of vulnerable elder members and limits the need for formal LTC services (Leininger, 2002). In many cultures, the concept of the "double caregiver" adds enormous stress to women who both work and provide care for a family and ailing parents (Remennick, 2001). However, current US values emphasize single-family dwellings, dual-income families, and transient life-styles, which have led to families no longer residing in the same area but geographically separated by great distance. This culturally driven environment has created a high demand for services from an already inefficient LTC care system.

The Continuum of Care

Community-Based Long-Term Care

The premise of community-based long-term care is to provide seamless, comprehensive programs to facilitate aging in place (Willging, 2006). There is a variety of services available within the LTC continuum. Current trends advocate using a case management approach to coordinate services and to ensure that individuals receive services in an efficient, timely fashion. Case management promotes aging in place with chronic illness, trying to keep a person in the home setting for a long as possible. The LTC system may be confusing to clients and families, but case managers can help to arrange and coordinate services such as Meals on Wheels, medical care, home health aides, and companion services. For older adults, the role of the geriatric care manager is an emerging one. Professional geriatric care managers (PGCMs) help families care for their older relatives while promoting independence. The National Association of Professional Geriatric Care Managers (2007, paragraph 1) lists services that families might expect with a PGCM as follows:

- Conduct care-planning assessments to identify problems and to provide solutions.
- Screen, arrange, and monitor in-home help or other services.
- Provide short- or long-term assistance for caregivers living near or far away.
- Review financial, legal, or medical issues and offer referrals to geriatric specialists.
- Provide crisis intervention.
- Act as a liaison to families at a distance, overseeing care, and quickly alerting families to problems.
- Assist with moving an older person to or from a retirement complex, assisted care home, or nursing home.
- Provide consumer education and advocacy.
- Offer counseling and support.

Related services for the frail elder or individual with chronic illness could also include legal services, adult protective services, area councils on aging, ombudsman programs, senior centers, and elder advocacy groups. Older adults with chronic illnesses that are rehabilitative may receive assistance with recovery through Medicare, which pays for inpatient and limited outpatient therapies ordered by a physician. Respite care for family members who care for loved ones with chronic illness and disability is also a community-based service.

The Program of All-Inclusive Care for the Elderly (PACE) is another community-based alternative that promotes aging in place (Beeber, 2005). This program is an evidence-based model of care whose services are often covered by Medicare and Medicaid. The National PACE Association (2007) stated that the average user is 80 years old, and preliminary studies suggest that involvement in a PACE program may slow functional decline for older adults. "One key to the PACE model is the combining of dollars from different funding streams in order to deliver a comprehensive set of services focused on the health and well-being of the individual" (National PACE Association, 2007, p. 1). The number of states with participating organizations has increased to 22 in the last few years. Those currently enrolled include: California, Colorado, Florida, Hawaii, Illinois, Kansas, Maryland, Massachusetts, Michigan, Missouri, New Mexico, New York, Ohio, Oregon, Pennsylvania, Rhode Island, South Carolina, Tennessee, Texas, Virginia, Washington, and Wisconsin. Continuing evaluation of this program in terms of cost benefit to the funding agencies may make it available on a wider scale.

Residential Long-Term Care Settings

LTC facilities are formal, organized agencies that provide care for persons unable to live alone because of physical or other problems, but who do not require hospitalization. Persons living in LTC are not called patients, but residents, as the LTC setting is their home. The three most common types of residential LTC facilities are group homes, assisted-living centers, and nursing homes. Many retirement communities combine independent living facilities and assisted living facilities, although these represent two different levels of care. Those living independently in a retirement community may do so because of declining health caused by chronic illness, safety factors, frailty, and the need for socialization. The decision to move from

one's own home to a community living situation is difficult, and often involves the advice of family members who are concerned about the older adult's ability to live alone safely. Long-term care residents are a vulnerable population who tend to have more chronic illnesses and may require advocacy from health or social professionals.

Group Homes. Group homes are also referred to as personal care homes, foster homes, domiciliary care homes, board and care homes, and congregate care homes. The philosophy embraces a home environment with a limited number of residents who share common characteristics in needing assistance with such things as activities of daily living, shopping, cleaning, and medication management. Much like a boarding house, the owner of the home provides services such as meals, laundry and cleaning, medication management, and assuring a safe environment. These homes are licensed by the state. This type of care is most appropriate for those with uncomplicated medical problems. Payment for group homes can be private, although in some states, it may be covered by welfare.

Assisted-Living Centers. Persons in assisted living are those who require some type of help with activities of daily living. According to the 2006 Overview of Assisted Living, nearly 70% of assisted living residents required help with bathing, about 46% needed help with dressing, and about one fourth of residents needed assistance with other tasks such as toileting, transferring, and eating. More than 90% of persons required assistance with housekeeping and 86% needed help with medication (National Center for Assisted Living, 2006). Assisted living has taken over approximately 15% of what was previously the nursing home population (Kinosian, Stallard, & Wieland, 2007).

Because Medicare, Medicaid, and the VA do not pay for assisted living, the cost for this living arrangement and services are paid for out of pocket. Assisted living centers may be found as free-standing facilities, as part of retirement communities, or attached to nursing homes to allow for smoother transition of care for those expected to need skilled nursing in the future.

The National Center for Assisted Living has summarized the characteristics of the United States's 36,000 assisted living centers (2006). The typical profile of a resident in assisted living is an 86-year-old woman who is ambulatory but needs help with at least two activities of daily living. Residents' average age in 2006 was 85 years and the average length of stay was 27 months. One third of these residents die, another third move into nursing homes, and the remaining third go to other living situations. From these statistics, it is evident that although today's older adults value their independence, the frailties that accompany old age make it necessary for more than 900,000 people in the United States to have some assistance with everyday activities.

Although assisted living facilities are accountable to a board of directors and may employ an RN consultant, the care is generally provided by aides, with LPNs used regularly to supervise daily services. Assisted living facilities provide autonomy for older adults, allowing them to live in a safe, home-like environment adapted for those with physical challenges. Assisted living provides personal space in the form of apartments or suites, and also provides meals through community dining as well as transportation and social activities.

CASE STUDY

Mr. Jones

Mr. Jones is an 88-year-old widower who has lived alone for 8 years after his wife of 58 years died of cancer. For most of their lives, Mr. and Mrs. Jones lived in the same neighborhood and in the same house where they raised their two children. During the majority of those years, Mr. Jones was an active senior and had many lifelong friends with whom he spent time. He played on the senior bowling league and attended lunch and bingo at the local senior center. Mr. Jones's health status was stable and he reported his health as excellent, despite having a history of controlled hypertension, high cholesterol, and arthritis. However, during the last 8 years, Mr. Jones began to experience the effects of chronic illnesses, including having a bilateral knee replacement due to pain and decreased mobility from arthritis, and taking more medications to control his high blood pressure and lower his cholesterol. With advanced age, Mr. Jones found that these conditions slowly progressed, and he also developed diabetes and Parkinson's disease,

decreasing his ability to take care of himself. Mr. Jones' children live over 1,000 miles away and after a fall and hip fracture during one visit over the holidays, they suggested that their father explore the possibility of going to an assisted living facility. Having successfully completed outpatient rehabilitation after a hip arthroplasty following his fracture, he wanted to remain at home. His children insisted that he should be where he could receive help managing medications and have someone to assist him with tasks that had become difficult, such as cleaning and transportation to doctor's visits. Mr. Jones was no longer able to bowl or drive, making him socially isolated and lonely. Mr. Jones' children began to make arrangements for him to enter an assisted living unit within a long-term care facility so that when further health decline occurred, he would not have to move to another place.

Mr. Jones was absolutely opposed to leaving the home he had shared with his wife, and then remained in after her death. He did not want to be in an "institution" as he called it. He said he would rather die. He expressed deep

(Continued)

CASE STUDY (*Continued*)

resentment toward his children for suggesting this arrangement and exhibited signs of depression including withdrawal and poor appetite. When his daughter insisted that he take a tour of the place they had found that might suit his needs, Mr. Jones was unhappy, but finally agreed to "check it out." During his tour of the facility, the staff was warm and friendly. Mr. Jones even found that an old friend, Joe Stark, from the bowling team had recently moved into the facility as well, for health reasons similar to those of Mr. Jones. Joe said the place was "pretty nice" and that "they treat you real good." Mr. Jones's mood brightened after talking with Joe. He observed that the residents seemed to be happy, there were many active older adults walking around, and the surroundings were pleasant and clean. The apartment he would have gave him privacy (and had its own kitchenette, refrigerator, and large bathroom), but also allowed the staff to check on him. There were meals served in a nice dining room with linen table cloths and a formal menu, and there was a library, big screen TV, pool table, and exercise room available to him. A barber shop was on the premises and transportation to doctor's office and shopping was available for a nominal charge. Mr. Jones and his children met with the activity director and the director of nursing,

who assured him that there were many residents just like Mr. Jones who called this facility their home. After the visit to the assisted living facility, Mr. Jones told his children that perhaps it was time for him to consider moving to a place like that, and so the arrangements were made. The assisted living staff was alerted to Mr. Jones' fears and hesitation and made an extra effort to make him feel at home and encouraged him to be involved in activities as much as possible. The quality of Mr. Jones' life improved significantly through socialization and activities in his new environment. His adjustment to a change in living situation was facilitated by the attitudes of his children, the staff, and other residents.

Discussion Questions

1. What factors prompted Mr. Jones's children to encourage him to consider other living arrangement?
2. From the information in this chapter, was moving to an assisted living facility a prudent choice for Mr. Jones? Why or why not?
3. What problems and issues with adaptation to his new home is Mr. Jones likely to face?
4. What interventions might be helpful to assist with his adjustment?

Skilled Nursing Facilities or Nursing Homes. Nursing home is a term used to refer to a facility that has either skilled nursing services (SNFs) and/ or intermediate care. Nursing homes are LTC facilities for chronically ill, medically frail, and disabled persons. The level of care may be described as residential, long-term, nonemergent, or custodial care. A number of facilities may include an intermediate care or rehabilitation unit for individuals who need assistance in increasing self-care abilities.

The majority of such agencies are "for profit." Exceptions are agencies generally associated with churches or other nonprofit organizations such as the US Department of Veterans Affairs. The Veterans Health Administration (VHA) predicted that the number of veterans older than age 85 will double in the next decade and that the VHA-enrolled veterans in this oldest old age group will increase seven times, resulting in a 22–25% increase in both nursing home and community-based services. The VHA currently uses 90% of its

LTC resources on nursing home care. For veterans, age and marital status were found to be significant predictors of the use of LTC services (Kinosian, Stallard, & Wieland, 2007).

Agencies that receive income from the Centers for Medicare and Medicaid Services (CMS) are required to meet minimum state and federal standards. Standards address items such as: nutritional and fluid intake; provision of social interaction and activities; and support services such as physical therapy, rehabilitation therapy, housekeeping, and laundry services. There is a continued concern by those employed in LTC settings that facility structure and staffing are often based on minimal standards that contain costs instead of considering first what is desirable or needed for the client. However, as the baby boomer generation ages, it is expected that its interest in this issue will influence the creation of higher standards, and quality of care may improve in LTC facilities.

Approximately 5% of the elderly population resides in nursing homes in the United States, and 28% pay for their own care (CMS, 2004b). Care in nursing homes may be funded by the individual (self-pay), insurance, Medicare (with limits), or Medicaid. To be eligible for Medicaid payment for residential care, the client must have limited assets with which to pay for the services required. Often an LTC resident will enter a nursing home, paying for services until their estate is spent down, and then Medicaid pays for care until the client's death (AARP, 2002).

Much of the care provided in the traditional nursing home setting is considered custodial care. Rehabilitative services are provided for those who have the capacity to regain function. Because the institutionalized individual may require a great deal of help with the physical aspects of care, such as bathing, dressing, eating, and space maintenance, the cognitive needs (emotional, psychological, and spiritual) may be considered less important. Activity programs are sometimes geared only toward one segment of the facility population. Care in LTC settings should include not only appropriate physical care, but also appropriate cognitive stimulation.

Long-Term Care Recipients—A Vulnerable Population

Vulnerable individuals are those who are at increased risk for loss of autonomy, loss of self-will, injustice, loss of privacy, and increased risk for abuse. A vulnerable adult is defined as an individual who is either being mistreated or is in danger of mistreatment and who because of age and/or disability is unable to protect him/herself (Teaster, 2002). A vulnerable individual can be described as one who has been judged by someone to be a nonperson. Examples of vulnerable persons in LTC may include those with physical or mental or emotional problems, the elderly, those with dementia, and those who have been in prison. In a culture that values youth, energy, strength, and work ability, many devalue an elder or one with a chronic illness. The National Adult Protective Services Association (National Association of Adult Protective Services Administrators, 2005) estimated that between 500,000 and 5,000,000 older adults and other vulnerable adults in America are abused, neglected, or taken advantage of in some way. Laws and practices differ between states in the areas of abuse, neglect, and protective services. Ultimately, it is the care providers and administrators in LTC who are responsible for maintaining an environment that supports the unique personhood of the client and protects the vulnerable.

Many individuals requiring LTC have already lost some autonomy and self-will because of illnesses that affect the individual's ability to make decisions or carry out intentional behavior. Vulnerability is of special concern in these individuals. Decisions must be made for them regarding many aspects of life, such as eating, bathing, medication administration, socialization, and exercising religious practices. Some persons may benefit from the services of a guardian, discussed later in this chapter.

PROBLEMS AND ISSUES IN LONG-TERM CARE

There are a number of issues in LTC, ranging from overall system breakdown to individual treatment issues for clients in the system. The issues mentioned in this chapter are not an exhaustive list, but can be considered an introduction to current problems.

Provision of Care

Along the continuum of LTC, problems in the provision of care include organization of services and access to care, gaps in public policy, funding, staffing, and standards. Specific issues vary within individual states or communities. It is imperative that the professional nurse involved in LTC is cognizant of the local and state issues that affect delivery and quality of LTC services. Being a political activist in order to further the issues of the recipients of LTC is also important.

Organization of Services

It was not surprising that the second most important resolution that came from the most recent White House Conference On Aging was the need for a more comprehensive and well-coordinated LTC strategy (Lomastro, 2006). In community-based LTC, the array of services in a given community may not be organized according to any hierarchy. Each specialized service, such as home care, elder daycare, hospice, or nutrition programs, was most likely begun in response to a specific need or business opportunity in the community. It is often necessary for a program of LTC to be pieced together from a number of different organizations to meet one client's needs. This is especially true for those who are community-dwelling residents.

Partial help with this problem comes from the United Way, a nonprofit service-based agency. The United Way publishes a resource book in larger cities that describes community programs and services. This resource book assists clients, family, and care providers in identifying appropriate services, phone numbers, and eligibility requirements. Many times, individuals with chronic illness and their families are not aware that when they are involved with one system (such as a

nursing home), they have access to other services (such as hospice). This publication can be obtained by calling the local United Way office. A list of all local United Way offices in the United States can be obtained online at http://www.unitedway.org. The United Way also operates in many other countries, collaborating with a number of agencies to promote community services.

Individuals with chronic illnesses often view access to the LTC system as complicated and overwhelming. Those with chronic illnesses and their families may have a limited amount of energy to invest in problem solving and identifying the best options. Oftentimes, access to the LTC system is controlled by gatekeepers who have minimal training and experience with complex medical conditions. Rules may be seen as arbitrary, and appear to exclude the very individuals intended to benefit from programs.

With the utilization of more case management for individuals with chronic illness, whether through the local or federal VA, state health and human services divisions, or private insurance companies, some progress is being made in assisting community-dwelling individuals to more effectively access LTC services. However, for most clients and families, access to the LTC system remains confusing and complex.

Gaps in Public Policy

Related to organization of LTC services are the gaps in policy. Despite the creation of significant public policy, as discussed in the historical overview, no overall umbrella of comprehensive care exists. There are many individuals who fall outside of policy parameters and cannot benefit from services (Komisar, Feder, & Kasper, 2005). Pharmaceutical costs, extended home health care, and rehabilitative services are problematic for many in LTC. As a result, clients either self-pay, if possible, or go without services or medications. With the implementation of Medicare Part D prescription drug plans, certain persons will be eligible for a discount on medication costs with a prescription benefit card. Consumers may have to pay a monthly fee, and/or a deductible or co-insurance, depending on the plan chosen. However, the plan is complicated for a lay person to follow, and the most cost-effective plan to join may change with the type of medications a person takes. Users choose a plan based on whether or not that plan covers their particular prescriptions, how much it costs, and whether or not their pharmacy participates (CMS, 2008). There is also a gap in coverage in Medicare Part D plans, resulting in the consumer having to cover all medication expenses out-of-pocket while in the gap. Although catastrophic coverage is good for some with exceptionally high medications costs, it is unclear how much savings over time will benefit the average consumer of these plans.

Funding

Gaps in service and public policy are both related to funding issues. Billions of dollars were spent by state and federal agencies to pay for nursing home care in 2002 (Harrington, Carillo, & Crawford, 2004). Medicaid alone spent 94.5 billion dollars on LTC services in 2005 (Houser, Fox-Grage, & Gibson, 2006). In addition, approximately 28% of residents in nursing homes and other residential care facilities pay privately for their care (CMS, 2004a). Many persons may be dual eligible for both Medicare and Medicaid. Although these persons do not generally report difficulty obtaining medical care, 58% of those who need LTC report their needs as being unmet. This problem has led to additional consequences such as falls (Komisar, Feder, & Kasper, 2005). Private insurance and nonprofit organizations also provide services for those in need of LTC. However, beyond the nursing home setting, piecing together a comprehensive LTC program for a frail elder with comorbidities who wishes to remain in the community is challenging. Certification for eligibility for certain benefits, such as extended home care, is strict. Recertification is often difficult and for a limited amount of time only.

Resources, whether private or public, are limited. Community-dwelling elders may be eligible for Medicare to pay for certain services, such as home health care, but only as long as some rehabilitation progress can be documented. Once progress stops, and the condition is considered chronic, the individual may have to pay privately for rehabilitative and home services. For individuals who have lived through the Great Depression, World War II, and other historical events that have required genuine frugality, spending nearly $100 to pay for less than an hour of a home visit from an agency RN is not a viable option. Many older adults from working class backgrounds do without needed care rather than pay privately. One study found that the greater the use of paid home care in a state, the less likely persons were to report unmet need (Komisar, Feder, & Kasper, 2005). This suggests that state policies can make a difference in the health care of their citizens.

It is important to consider the entitlement to care that older adults and those with chronic illness possess because of Social Security programs. These programs were designed to provide some comfort and security to the older individual. One view is that society has an obligation to provide for those in need, particularly the elderly, because of the labor and service that they have provided (Tobin & Salisbury, 1999). Another view is that society is obligated to provide care for frail and chronically ill elders because of the sanctity of all human life, and not simply because of work undertaken during the adult life. Philosophical origins play an important part not only in the establishment and continuation of programs, but also in setting standards for ongoing programs.

Another alternative offered by Medicare is the Social Managed Care Plan. However, there are only four plans in the following states: Kaiser Permanente (Portland, OR), Scan (Long Beach, CA), Elderplan (Brooklyn, NY), and Health Plan of Nevada (Las Vegas, NV). Medicare describes these plans thus:

> A Social Managed Care Plan is an organization that provides the full range of Medicare benefits offered by standard Managed Care Plan's plus additional services which include care

coordination, prescription drug benefits, chronic care benefits covering short term nursing home care, a full range of home and community based services such as homemaker, personal care services, adult day care, respite care, and medical transportation. Other services that may be provided include eyeglasses, hearing aids, and dental benefits. These plans offer the full range of medical benefits that are offered by standard Managed Care Plan's plus chronic care/extended care services. Membership offers other health benefits that are not provided through Medicare alone or most other senior health plans (Medicare, 2007).

Alternative financing for LTC needs to be explored. Although both PACE (mentioned previously in this chapter) and social managed care plans offer alternatives to nursing homes and promote aging in place, it is evident that their scope and availability is significantly limited. Other alternatives that have been proposed to decrease the funding gap include efforts at the state level. In Idaho, the governor had a comprehensive vision of a carefully restructured workforce and social infrastructure to deliver health care to seniors using community-based care services (Kempthorne, 2004). In Arkansas, research revealed a need to expand health services because of unmet needs, suggesting policy recommendations to improve access to community-based care (Stewart, Felix, Dockter, Perry, & Morgan, 2006). In addition, a couple of strategies to fund LTC costs have arisen from the financial sector: reverse mortgages and life settlement. Both concepts focus on helping an individual liquidate assets (for example, a home or life insurance policy) to provide cash to privately pay to enter or remain in a facility (Feaster, 2006). It is only in the last decade that using one's life insurance as a financial tool to obtain relatively quick cash has been considered. However, individuals considering this option should consult with a financial adviser.

Staffing

Health care agencies that receive Medicare and Medicaid funding are licensed by each state or are accredited by a recognized accrediting agency. Each agency must meet requirements in staffing. Two main issues in staffing are the training of the staff member and the staff-to-client ratio.

Standards for required staff training are often minimal. For example, medication aides working in an assisted-living center may be required to attend a 6-week training course, yet the medication regimens for the assisted-living center clientele may be extremely complex. For proper medication management, much more time is required to educate a person on the pharmacologic effects of medications, side effects, and complications. Although assisted-living centers are required to have an RN available, that one RN may act as a consultant for multiple centers under the same ownership umbrella. The actual individual who "supervises" the medication aides may be an LPN who works a 40-hour week.

Qualifications for a home manager in an assisted-living center are minimal and may be as little as attending a state-sponsored seminar lasting 2 weeks or less, with yearly continuing education. The majority of staff working in such facilities may be minimally trained personnel, and client safety is a legitimate concern.

Staffing challenges in providing home health care are also significant. State requirements vary for home health aides, but no training program is more than 8–12 weeks in length. Often, aides are trained and then expected to work independently, with little supervision. In LTC settings, staff morale may often be low.

Staffing in nursing homes is a continuing issue. There is conclusive evidence that a positive relationship exists between nursing staffing and quality of nursing home care. Fewer RN and nursing assistant hours are associated with quality-of-care deficiencies (Harrington, Zimmerman, Karon, Robinson, & Beutel, 2000; Arling, Kane, Mueller, Bershadsky, & Degenholtz, 2007). Aides who provide most of the care in LTC settings may make about $9 per hour and have few benefits. The turnover rate can be as high as 40–100% in some facilities because of poor wages, lack of benefits, and working conditions (Service Employees International Union, 2007). High turnover rates have been associated with poor quality care (Castle, Engber, & Men, 2007). Recruitment and retention of qualified nursing assistants is an ongoing problem. Creating an environment that promotes teamwork, addresses care-related stressors, promotes positive communication, reduces paperwork inefficiencies and staffing shortages, and has high organizational morale have shown to increase job satisfaction and commitment to the organization, but there are many other factors to consider in the complex process of staff turnover in these settings (Sikorska-Simmons, 2006; Arling, Kane, Mueller, Bershadsky, & Degenholtz, 2007; Donoghue & Castle, 2006; Cherry, Ashcraft, & Owen, 2007). The decreasing level of RN staffing is also of growing concern, and yet reimbursements and prospective payments have been reduced in some cases, making it impossible to increase the number of RNs in residential facilities.

To complicate this situation, there is a projected shortage of healthcare professionals. Half of the registered nurse workforce is at least 45 years old. It is estimated that by 2020 there will be a shortage of between 380,000 and 1,000,000 RNs because of a number of significant factors including the population growth, retirement of nurses in the current workforce, and the lack of faculty to educate willing students in nursing programs (American Association of Colleges of Nursing, 2007a). Currently, less than 1% of RNs are certified in geriatrics, yet Congress facilitated a recent cut in spending for geriatric education.

Standards

Residential and community-based LTC facilities that accept government payments are regulated by federal and state mandates. Agencies and institutions in LTC that receive outside funding are required to meet certain standards and undergo regular inspection (Harrington et al., 2003).

Requirements change frequently. Part of the responsibility of both the administrator and the director of nursing of an LTC facility is to be aware of and implement changes that are necessary as a result of new state and federal requirements. In home health agencies, the number and type of visits that can be reimbursed by insurance or Medicare are limited. If evidence in regard to why the visits were made and what health-related goal was achieved is unclear, the payer may bill the agency back for those services, which can be financially devastating to an organization.

Nursing homes undergo an initial survey to become certified and then undergo inspection at least every 15 months (CMS, 2004b). State surveyors evaluate both process and outcomes of nursing home care in several areas (Table 21-1). Tags are assigned depending on the severity of the violation. If deficiencies are found, follow-up surveys may be conducted. If care is so poor that residents are deemed to be in danger, facilities can be fined large amounts of money, be prohibited from admitting any residents, and even be closed for violations. Agencies must demonstrate that the staff meets educational requirements, that residents are being given adequate care, and that documentation is appropriate. Requirements vary for various types of agencies and are complicated. Most states post the results of surveys on a public Web site, where family members can access information and compare facilities when making decisions about placing loved ones into LTC.

Standards address issues such as nursing hours per client, nursing assessments, care plans, accidents, number of pressure sores, use of physical restraints, nutrition, use of certain medications, and housekeeping services. In addition, facilities are to provide care for residents in a manner that maintains dignity and respect by providing grooming, appropriate dress, and promotion of independence in dining; allowing private space and property; and interacting respectfully. For example, nursing staff must not perform any invasive assessment or task in a public area, but should take the resident to his room for procedures such as listening to lung sounds or checking a glucometer reading.

TABLE 21-1

Nursing Home Quality Indicators

Domain	Quality Indicator	Resident Risk Category
Accidents	Incidence of new fractures	
	Prevalence of falls	
Behavior/emotional patterns	Prevalence of behavior symptoms affecting others	High risk
	Prevalence of symptoms of depression	Low risk
	Prevalence of symptoms of depression without antidepressant therapy	
Clinical management	Use of 9 or more medications	
Cognitive patterns	Incidence of cognitive impairment	
Elimination/ incontinence	Prevalence of bladder or bowel incontinence	High risk
	Prevalence of occasional or frequent bladder or bowel incontinence without a toileting plan	Low risk
	Prevalence of indwelling catheter	
	Prevalence of fecal impaction	
Infection control	Prevalence of urinary tract infections	
Nutrition/eating	Prevalence of weight loss	
	Prevalence of tube feeding	
	Prevalence of dehydration	
Physical functioning	Prevalence of bedfast residents	
	Incidence of decline in late-loss ADLs	
	Incidence of decline in range of motion	
Psychotropic drug use	Prevalence of antipsychotic use, in absence of psychotic or related conditions	High risk
	Prevalence of antianxiety/hypnotic use	Low risk
	Prevalence of hypnotic use more than two times in last week	
Quality of life	Presence of daily physical restraints	
	Presence of little or no activity	
Skin care	Prevalence of stage 1–4 ulcers	High risk
		Low risk

Source: From Nursing Home Quality Indicators Development Group, Center for Health Systems Research and Analysis (Marnard, 2002).

Harrington and colleagues (2004) points out that quality of care provided in nursing homes has long been a matter of great concern to consumers, professionals, and policy makers. If the regulation and inspection process is ignored, LTC residents may suffer. Examples of system failures can be found at both the local and state levels. Deficiency reports are readily available online through the CMS. The RN is at times required to act as an advocate for the residents and to ensure compliance with minimal standards.

Ethical Issues in Long-Term Care

Individuals who are chronically ill or who are frail are a vulnerable population who are often at the mercy of the caregivers in the LTC system. Healthcare professionals in LTC should have a solid understanding of the ethics involved in this type of care. Principles upon which decisions should be made include: autonomy, nonmaleficence, beneficence, and justice (Beauchamp, 2001; Jonsen, 2007). The manner in which these principles are executed in the professional nurse–client relationship can make a visible difference in the quality of life of the LTC resident. Some of the more common ethical issues are discussed herein.

Client Autonomy Versus Dependence

One principle of critical importance in LTC is autonomy. Healthcare professionals and caregivers should observe the particularly essential rule of bioethics: respect the autonomy of persons (Jonsen, 2007). Autonomy is sometimes misapplied or ignored (Kane, Freeman, Chaplan, Asashar, & Uru-Wong, 1990). It is possible for an individual to gradually lose increments of their autonomy because of limitations imposed by sensory deprivation, immobility, weakness, and cognitive impairment (Mezey, Mitty, & Ramsey, 1997). Research suggests that even frail elderly who are homebound have a greater sense of person control than those in nursing homes (Crain, 2001), making those living in facilities at greater risk for loss of decision-making and independence. Frail older women who perceived their health as good and who had positive social support tended to feel more independent than other persons in the same age cohort who did not have those factors. "Older people fear the prospect of dependency and, therefore, an essential health outcome is maintenance of functional independence" (Schank & Lough, 1990, p. 680). Loss of autonomy and development of excess disability is a problem for many LTC clients.

Excess Disability

Excess disability is an inability to perform an activity that is not usually associated with the impairment. It suggests a dependence of a client on a caregiver to perform a task the client has the ability to perform (Dawson, Wells & Kline, 1993). This type of "disability" is a significant problem in the LTC setting. Depression, learned helplessness, perception of locus of control, and the sick role contribute to the development of excess disability (Salisbury, 1999). Caregivers may be unintentional contributors to excess disability. Providing unnecessary assistance or an inappropriate type of assistance can contribute to residents' dependency. "Factors influencing excess disability include: a desire of the caregiver to be helpful; lack of knowledge and skill of the caregiver; and lack of time and staff" (Remsburg & Carson, 2006, p. 584). An example of excess disability is dressing assistance provided to nursing home residents. Aides often do the dressing activities for residents in order to save time, instead of allowing the residents to perform the activity at their own pace (Beck et al., 1997). This action moves the resident toward unnecessary and unwanted dependence.

Custodial Care

Using basic ethical principles, an issue arises whether providing minimal physical care for those with chronic illness is acceptable versus providing more comprehensive care extending beyond custodial physical care. This is particularly challenging in a residential LTC environment. As a result of regulation, funding, and staffing patterns for Medicare/Medicaid residential facilities, the goal inadvertently becomes custodial care.

Physical issues of the resident are important, but those issues should not be the only focus. Mental health needs should also be considered in the chronically ill and elderly populations. With limited attention to these needs, the client is at risk of suffering boredom, anxiety, and, consequently, depression. In 2004, persons age 65 and older accounted for 16% of suicide death, although they comprised only 12% of the entire population at that time [National Institute of Mental Health (NIMH), 2008]. Suicide rates of non-Hispanic white men over age 85 are the highest in the nation (Shalala, 2000). Appropriate referral is a responsibility of the nurse who detects symptoms of emotional difficulties. Signs of depression include feeling nervous, empty, guilty, tired, restless, irritable, and unloved, and that life is not worth living. Physical symptoms associated with mental health problems include eating more or less than normal, sleep disturbances, headaches, stomachaches, and an increase in chronic pain (Varcarolis, 2002). The risk of depression in the elderly increases with the presence of chronic illness and a loss of physical function (NIMH, 2008). If symptoms of depression are present in an LTC client, services are available to provide assistance.

End-of-Life Decision Making

Difficult and complex decisions at end of life are an inherent component of LTC. Many older adults lack the resources, or lack knowledge of the available resources, that could help with decision-making at end of life. All older adults should be encouraged to have advance directives. Making one's wishes known in the event of terminal illness or incapacity is essential to preserving autonomy for the older adult.

In many states, an older person can make his wishes known by completing a document such as Five Wishes, which can be downloaded from the internet at http://www.agingwithdignity.org/5wishes.html. The Five Wishes program, sponsored by Aging with Dignity, is unique from other Living Will declarations, in that it addresses all aspects of the person's life: emotional spiritual, personal, and medical (Aging with Dignity, 2007). This document is legally recognized in 40 states, and allows the person to use their own lay language to express their end of life desires. Five Wishes documents the following information for the older adult's family and doctors (Aging with Dignity, 2007):

- Which person should make healthcare decisions.
- The kind of medical treatment the person wants and does not want.
- How comfortable the person wishes to be made.

- How the person wants others to treat him.
- What the person wants his loved ones to know.

Cultural and religious beliefs play an important part in end-of-life decision-making. There are some religions that dictate that everything should be done to preserve life and others that support allowing natural death. For example, African Americans are generally opposed to placing a loved one in a nursing home, preferring family members to die at home. Healthcare professionals should familiarize themselves with the major traditions and practices of their clients so that culturally appropriate care can be provided.

In a study of older community-dwelling adults (with a mean of 80.7 years of age), a durable power of attorney for health care had been completed by 60.8% of respondents before death. However, a startling finding of this research was that persons with lower levels of cognitive functioning were less likely to have completed an advanced directive than those older adults with higher cognitive functioning (McGuire, Rao, Anderson, & Ford, 2007). This research underscores the need for healthcare professionals to address advance directives with persons while they are capable of expressing their end-of-life wishes.

Abuse and Neglect of Vulnerable Adults

The incidence of abuse and neglect of vulnerable adults is difficult to estimate. In 2000, 472,813 cases of abuse were reported, with 4857 of those cases being substantiated (Teaster, 2002). The National Adult Protective Services Association (National Association of Adult Protective Service Administrators, 2005) estimated that anywhere between half a million and five million elders and other vulnerable adults in the United States were in some way victims of abuse. It is believed that cases of abuse, neglect, or exploitation are grossly under-reported because of fear, intimidation, lack of sound research, or other factors. Nursing home residents are particularly vulnerable to being victims of abuse (Lindbloom, Brandt, Hough, & Meadows, 2007).

Abuse can be categorized as domestic or institutional. Within these categories, physical, sexual, and emotional/psychological abuse may occur as well as neglect, self neglect, abandonment, and financial exploitation. Because of longer life expectancies for those with chronic illness, it is very likely that the incidence of abuse will increase (Teaster, 2002). The individual with chronic illness, if cognitively competent, may be hesitant to discuss the mistreatment because fearing the loss of the relationship or other reprisal by the perpetrator. If the individual is not capable of expressing information regarding the abuse, identification may be by forensic evidence. Fulmer (1999) discusses three main types of abuse: physical abuse, neglect, and exploitation.

Physical abuse is the actual assault of an individual, and evidence exists with the presence of unexplained bruises, fractures, cuts, or burns in various stages of healing. Sexual abuse also falls within this category. The victim of such treatment is in danger and requires immediate advocacy. Physical abuse often escalates from neglect or other forms of abuse. Perpetrators often share similar characteristics such as lack of social support, history of being an abuse victim, and mental or emotional problems.

Neglect is defined as the lack of provision of basic necessities, such as food, water, and medical care. Neglect may be evidenced by poor hygiene, malnutrition or dehydration, pressure ulcers, and reports of being left in an unsafe condition or being left without resources to obtain necessary medications. Neglect can take place because of willful intention or because home management has become overwhelming to the client's aging spouse or family. This type of abuse may be seen more frequently in homes where the caregiver lacks the knowledge or resources to provide care. Neglect can include self neglect, which is defined as an individual losing the will or the ability to properly care for himself. Abandonment is the extreme form of neglect.

The third type of elder abuse, exploitation, is defined as the use of an elder's resources without knowledge or consent for the gain of another. Signs of elder exploitation include the disappearance of monetary resources or the "taking over" of personal belongings without permission or consent (Fulmer, 1999). Financial abuse in the form of fraud or deception may also be considered exploitation and may come through family members who borrow money with no intention to repay it, or from mail fraud schemes that attempt to cheat persons out of money by promising prizes and rewards.

Each state has a Department of Adult Protective Services (APS) the purpose of which is to protect the rights and health of older people and people with disabilities who are in danger of being mistreated or neglected, unable to protect themselves, and have no one to assist them. APS is responsible for receiving the report of abuse, investigating the report, assessing the individual's risk, developing and implementing case plans, service monitoring, and evaluation. Some agencies may provide more in depth services including housing, medical care, social support, and economic and legal services (National Association of Adult Protective Services Administrators, 2005). Healthcare professionals and paraprofessionals such as RNs, physicians, nurse aides, and homemaker aides are mandated by law to report suspected adult or elder abuse.

INTERVENTIONS

Theoretical Framework for Practice

Using a theoretical framework to plan and implement nursing care in an LTC setting helps the nurse to avoid doing things simply "because they have always been done that way." Nurses draw from the sciences and use physiologic theory, pharmacologic theory, and theories of communication, change, caring, grief and bereavement, and ethics. A theoretical framework is used to explain or guide one's practice. Mid-range theories are those defined as specific to particular caregiving situations and that have measurable outcomes.

Theoretical frameworks give direction in the choice of interventions so that nursing care is tailored to each client.

Several middle-range frameworks are appropriate for LTC. One example is "The Needs-Driven Dementia-Compromised Behavior Model." It can assist the care professional in understanding how to better interact with dementia clients (Algase et al., 1996). This model hypothesizes that problematic behaviors in dementia clients are a result of needs that, when identified, can be addressed by the care provider, thereby avoiding a crisis. Such frameworks are helpful in assisting the care provider in solving problems encountered in the clinical area when dealing with LTC clients (Peterson & Bredow, 2004; Mitty & Flores, 2007a).

Admission and Assessment in the Long-Term Care Setting

Admission to a nursing home for any individual can be very distressing. From the individual's perspective, the move to a nursing home or even assisted living away from their home may symbolize the reality of the loss of health, autonomy, economic power, productivity, and independence. Adjustment to such facilities may evoke a mix of emotions. The stress of going into a facility in which one is surrounded by strangers can be difficult. In addition, the individual must adjust to schedules determined by others, instead of following routines established throughout a lifetime. In many nursing homes, eating and bathing schedules are relatively fixed. Although not ideal, the resident is often the one who must change expectations to make allowance for the workload of the nursing home staff.

The decision to move to a nursing home is usually made after much consideration by the client and family. The transition may be made more smoothly when the client retains as much participation in the process as possible. The client should be encouraged to have input into choosing the facility and in planning the move. Retention of personal items gives the elder a better sense of self in the new facility. The predictability of the move, the reason for the move, and the degree of control the elder client retains in the decision-making process all affect the outcome (Reinardy, 1995).

Admission to a nursing home may be one of the most traumatic life transitions. The nurse needs to assist in making the adjustment of the client to the facility as smooth as possible. The client experiencing psychological and emotional difficulty during the admission and transition into any LTC facility needs support from the attending nursing staff. The use of therapeutic communication techniques by the staff in addition to spending adequate time with a transitioning resident can make a difference in the level of anxiety and stress experienced. If indicated, the nurse should initiate a referral for the resident to be seen by mental health services. These services are generally an underused resource for elders.

Accessing community-based LTC services may seem a natural and necessary transition for an elder needing help with either rehabilitation or assistance with other aspects of care. For others, accessing services may create significant emotional turmoil. Once a frail elder can no longer stay in the community environment, the individual and family may decide that a move to another environment that provides needed services is necessary (see the case study of Mr. Jones). For those who can afford assisted living, this option may be less emotionally traumatic. Individuals feel they have retained a great deal of autonomy while paying for the services that they can no longer perform, such as food preparation, laundry, housekeeping, and medication management.

An accurate assessment of the client is the critical beginning for the client's experience in the LTC system. During the admission process to a LTC facility, the care provider will complete a battery of paperwork that documents the client's condition and reason for admission. In residential nursing homes, this assessment is important because of the potential to enhance health, as opposed to the creation of excess disability (Dawson, Wells & Kline, 1993). It is imperative that the admission process not be limited to completing paperwork but include gaining insight into the client to provide individualized care. The information that the nurse gathers during the admission process is the basis for appropriate care planning activities. There are several tools available that assist in admission assessment of the physical, functional, psychological, and social status of the LTC client (Sehy & Williams, 1999).

The Minimum Data Set (MDS) for Resident Assessment and Care Screening was developed for use by nursing homes in response to the Nursing Home Reform Legislation of 1987. The MDS provides extensive data about individual clients, but it also makes possible the establishment of a nationwide database regarding nursing home residents. Information requested by the MDS covers the areas of the resident's functional, medical, cognitive, and affective status at the time of admission and periodically thereafter (Sehy & Williams, 1999). This type of information also helps in tracking the improvement or decline of a resident over time, and whether or not quality indicators for care are being met. In the initial or follow-up assessment, the assessment protocol summarizes vulnerable aspects of the client's life that may require special care planning, interventions, and reporting of progress or problems in the resident's chart. The reliability of the information obtained varies with the knowledge that evaluators are able to obtain about the client.

Beginning in 2006, the MDS 3.0, an update and revised version of MDS 2.0, is being evaluated by constituents. This revision to the MDS (CMS, 2007a) had the following broad goals:

To make the MDS more clinically relevant, while still achieving the federal payment mandates and quality initiatives

To improve ease of use and efficiency

To integrate selected standard scales

To elicit resident voice by introducing interview questions

Other assessment tools are available and can provide more specific or multidimensional information. Tools can help the nurse determine functioning in cognitive, communication, behavioral, and social support domains. Other instruments measure vision, personality, depression, affect, comorbidity, and quality of life (Teresi & Evans, 1997). Examples of individual tools that are readily available in the literature include the Katz Index of Activities of Daily Living (Katz et al., 1970), Older American Resources and Services (OARS) (Duke University, 1978), the Beck Depression Rating Scale (Beck et al., 1979), and the Arthritis Impact Measurement Scale (AIMS) (Meenan, 1985).

A helpful Web site with a list of more than 30 assessment tools that can be downloaded for immediate use is www.consultGeriRN.org. For each assessment tool in the *Try This* series from the AACN/Hartford Foundation, explanation of the tool by an expert, validity and reliability information, the tool itself, and how to use it are succinctly provided.

Preservation of Autonomy of the Person

Healthcare professionals dealing with clients in LTC have special responsibilities in protecting and preserving their clients' autonomy (American Nurses Association, 2004; Mysak, 1997). The concept of autonomy is rooted in the idea of self-rule and independent decision-making. There is a great deal of discussion related to autonomy and personal rights.

Autonomy

The role of the nurse in providing LTC along the continuum of care is to preserve the autonomy of the client. At the same time, the client must be protected from harm. Balancing these issues is not always easy. It is imperative that the care provider not assume that because an individual has lost some physical autonomy, such as requiring personal assistance with daily hygiene, that the individual has given up his or her autonomy or is incapable of making his own decisions. Promotion of autonomy is accomplished by allowing the individual to make as many decisions as possible. In decisions that can impact health or health care, the nurse must provide the appropriate information to enable the client to make an informed decision. To more fully understand the concept of autonomy, the caregiver is encouraged to think about autonomy from the client's perspective when making caregiving decisions.

An individual's decision-making capacity may change during chronic illness and frailty (Mezey, Mitty & Ramsey, 1997). The law in some states defines the line of authority for decision making when competence is in question. In cases where the person has been legally deemed unable to make his own decisions, the designated family member or legal guardian must be informed of all important aspects of the persons' life and is responsible for making decisions that are in the person's best interest, that is, on his behalf or at his behest. When a person has lost some degree of autonomy, the nurse must also act in a judicious way that protects the individual from harm or exploitation.

It is also possible for someone who has legally lost autonomy (been declared incompetent) to continue to participate in the decision-making process. For example, a person with early stage dementia may have a legal guardian who is ultimately responsible for decision-making in the person's best interest. However, as much as the person is able, the guardian would involve the person in the decision-making process, seeking input and finding out the wishes of the person prior to taking any action.

Decision-making or autonomy can be viewed on a continuum. An example of this might be when a person with advanced dementia decides to walk the halls. Autonomous decision-making in a small way is appropriate as long as other principles, such as the client's safety and the safety of others, is considered. It is the nurse's responsibility to recognize an individual's capacity for autonomy and preserve that capacity as much as possible (Mezey, Mitty &

Ramsey, 1997; Roberto et al., 1997). Sometimes, the nurse must compromise what he or she perceives to be the best treatment in order to incorporate client preferences. An example would be a client's bathing twice a week as opposed to more frequent bathing. In that case, the nurse might alter other interactions, such as frequency of spot baths or application of lotion to ensure skin integrity, while respecting the autonomy of the client.

Guardianship

One of the ways in which the healthcare system provides for those who are unable to make informed decisions for themselves because of a cognitive or other health problem is to appoint a legal guardian. The responsibility of the guardian is to ensure safety and quality care for the person and to make decisions in the person's best interest. The guardian may be a family member, a friend, or a healthcare professional appointed by the court. In complex cases involving large estates, difficult family relationships, or divorce, the court may choose to appoint a professional guardian or person who will assist in making legal decisions for the incompetent person. The appointment of a guardian by the court usually follows the legal determination of incapacity. The person who has been declared by the court to be an incapacitated person is then no longer able to make any type of contractual decision independently. The guardian of the person is responsible to the court for getting to know the person sufficiently to be able to make decisions in his best interest, provides documentation to the court as needed on the status of the person, and may be responsible for a variety of tasks ranging from healthcare advocacy to managing finances to assuring that daily care needs are being met.

Guardianship guidelines vary from state to state and even from county to county within states. There is no established fee for these services, and guardians may be paid a small fee monthly, or a significant hourly fee as a consultant if additional services such as case management is also being provided, if there are funds from the estate to cover such costs. These arrangements are generally agreed upon through the court as part of the legal guardian's acceptance of this responsibility.

There is some controversy as to the methods and process used for legal provisions for guardianship and assessment of a person's capacity. A tri-state study (Moye, Butz, Marson, & Wood, 2007) found that the quality of written clinical evidence to establish the need for guardianship was significantly lacking and that key information about the individual's values, preferences, and wishes were rarely documented. Persons were rarely present at the hearing. Functional assessments of persons during the evaluation of the need for guardianship should be routinely used. An assessment template that incorporates six assessment domains of interest to the court is recommended. The areas that should be addressed according to one such model include: medical condition, cognition, functional abilities, values, risk for injury and supervision needed, and ways to enhance capacity (Moye et al., 2007). Continued communication between clinical and legal team members is needed to protect the rights of vulnerable persons.

Nurses and social workers often make excellent guardians, as they are able to professionally address these areas and provide a holistic approach to care for the incapacitated person. Some court systems develop a rapport with certain professionals who act as guardians and will request their appointment in cases such as for older adults with dementia who reside in LTC facilities. To preserve the autonomy of persons as long as possible, guardians should encourage as much participation as possible in decision-making, while keeping in mind the goal of safety and quality care for the incapacitated person.

Enablement

Enablement of the client is one way of improving care for the cognitively impaired individual (Dawson, Wells & Kline, 1993). This perspective focuses on how the disease affects the client's abilities to carry out day-to-day activities. The purpose of this nursing intervention is to determine the client's existing abilities and to enhance those abilities. Three areas of human behavior considered by this approach are self-care, social interaction, and interpretive abilities. This approach specifically targets the prevention of excess disability in the client. In the area of self-care, when the client is having difficulty achieving purposeful behaviors, certain nursing interventions have been identified that can assist the caregiver in enhancing the client's abilities. These include object cueing, touch, direct physical assistance, and verbal prompting (Dawson, Wells & Kline, 1993). When a client with dementia loses many of the skills required for daily activity, there is the possibility of retention of some significant skill or pleasure, such as a music-related activity or game playing. The nurse should help preserve those abilities as much as possible by providing opportunities for their expression (Beatty, 1999; Greiner et al., 1997).

Abuse in the home or in a residential facility is an extreme threat to the autonomy of the client. If the nurse providing care is the first one to observe signs and symptoms of mistreatment, reporting these observations to Adult Protective Services (or other public agency, as designated in the particular state) is required by law (Fulmer, 1999). In the home, the home healthcare nurse may be the one in a position to discover abuse and act as the primary advocate to prevent further abuse. The nurse may work with various agencies to ensure that appropriate intervention is made. Because elder mistreatment is often subtle, the nurse must be persistent in reporting signs until action is taken. If abuse or neglect of the community-based client is profound, a move to residential care may be indicated.

Advocacy: The Role of the Ombudsman

The LTC ombudsman is an advocate charged with the protection of the rights of all residents in LTC. The purpose of this role is to enhance quality of life for LTC residents and do the following

(National Long Term Care Ombudsman Resource Center, 2008, p. 1):

- Advocate for residents' rights and quality care
- Educate consumers and providers
- Resolve residents' complaints
- Provide information to the public

The LTC ombudsman is a person hired by a state LTC service agency under the auspices of the state or local health department or the statewide aging services. Volunteers who report to the ombudsman supervisor may do many of the actual investigations. The contact information for the ombudsman should be posted inconspicuously in each LTC facility. Complaints may come from the LTC resident, concerned family, or caregivers. Findings must be reported to the client and/or family, and the ombudsman is responsible for achieving an equitable settlement between the resident and the LTC facility. The role of the ombudsman is founded in ethical principles and is implemented on behalf of the vulnerable client. Updates on the organizational activities contacts can be found at http://www.ltcombudsman.org.

Nursing Care

Nursing care is the primary service provided by residential LTC facilities. The further one progresses along the LTC continuum, the more intense are the nursing care needs. According to a study of nursing homes done in 1996, the Agency for Health Care Policy and Research listed the most frequently occurring conditions for nursing home residents younger than age 65 as seizures, hypertension, stroke, diabetes, and dementia. For those older than 65 years of age, the most common conditions were dementia, heart disease, hypertension, arthritis, and stroke. It is notable that the majority of nursing home residents experience chronic conditions such as these. Thus nursing care in LTC settings is much more complex than it has been in the past and requires greater knowledge and expertise on the part of the nursing

staff to manage comorbidities and provide a high quality of care to all residents.

Care that nurses provide in LTC facilities should be holistic and multidimensional. Eight percent of patients in home care and 85% in LTC settings are over age 65 (Mezey, Stierele, Huba, & Esterson, 2007). Because most persons in LTC settings are older, nurses would benefit from education in gerontology. The Geriatric Nursing Education Consortium (GNEC, 2007) is a training system, similar to ELNEC discussed later in this chapter, which has compiled essential information to be taught within the senior year of baccalaureate programs. This national initiative of the American Association of Colleges of Nursing (AACN) with funding from the Hartford Foundation uses a train the trainer approach in which faculty members attend an intensive educational workshop to receive information on how to integrate and teach gerontology within the nursing curriculum. Six regional faculty development institutes are being held from 2007 to 2009 in various parts of the country. By developing champions at schools and college of nursing throughout the United States, it is hoped that the care of the older adult will improve.

Pain Management

The science of pain management has advanced significantly over the last two decades (Celia, 2000). It is important for the nurse in LTC to adequately assess pain and to provide adequate treatment of that pain (Ferrell & Coyle, 2001). Of particular importance is assessing clients' suffering from the pain associated with arthritis, osteoporosis, or neuralgia. A great deal of information is available on appropriate pain management strategies, and the nurse dealing with such clients should access this body of literature. When implementing pain management strategies in the LTC setting, follow-up is critical. Pain relief varies for many reasons, and pain may not be relieved by a method that was previously successful for the client. When pain is chronic and affects the ability of the client to function, current treatment strategies include routine regular administration of medication to manage the pain. Breakthrough pain, or pain experienced intermittently when a client is on routine pain medication, is then treated with "as needed" medication. Addiction is not generally considered to be a major problem for elders suffering from chronic pain, but tolerance can be problematic.

For individuals unable to verbally express pain, its presence is noted in other ways. Evidence of pain may include facial expression (grimacing), body position, bracing, guarding, and rubbing of the painful body part. Alternative methods of dealing with pain should be considered. Massage, heat, cold, and support mechanisms such as knee or back braces may be helpful. The quality of life of the LTC client can be greatly affected by pain. With current advances in pharmacology and treatment, most pain can be managed effectively.

Disease Prevention/Health Promotion

Although it may be impossible to prevent some of the chronic diseases seen in the LTC population, others are certainly preventable to a large degree. An important preventive health measure provided along the LTC continuum is the provision of flu and pneumonia vaccines to clients. A vaccination program in residential facilities is essential; in such settings, infections such as influenza can spread rapidly and cause deaths among the frail elderly. These types of infections may affect a number of residents at one time, and place a difficult burden on staff to deal with a number of acutely ill clients. Admission of clients to acute care settings in such circumstances is not unreasonable to ensure that all clients receive adequate nursing care during an outbreak of illness.

Certain screenings are recommended for older adults and can be helpful with early identification and treatment initiation. Screenings that are recommended by the US Preventive Services Task Force (USPSTF) and *Healthy People 2010* for older adults with chronic illness include: nutrition,

tobacco, safety, immunizations, depression, alcohol abuse, lipids, hypertension, osteoporosis, vision and hearing, breast cancer, and colorectal cancer. Each of these screenings is rated as beneficial and supported by at least fair evidence that health outcomes and benefits outweigh the screening risk (Nelson, 2006).

Several key areas are considered standard for health promotion in older adults. These include exercise, not smoking, maintaining a healthy weight, social support, medication adherence, a safe environment, and activities that strengthen cognition and memory (Hardin, 2006). One study of assisted living residents found that "social support is a key variable in bolstering residents' psychological well-being" (Cummings, 2002, p. 300). Thus health promotion, even for those with existing chronic illness, emphasizes the same important strategies, ones which healthcare professionals should encourage in LTC residents.

Cognitive Impairment

Individuals in LTC may suffer cognitive impairment from a variety of pathologic processes. These processes may be either acute or chronic. Individuals with cognitive impairment caused by irreversible causes such as closed head injuries, stroke, or dementia from a number of pathologic processes such as Alzheimer's disease, Pick's disease, Lewy body disease, often need special assistance to manage activities of daily living. Individuals in LTC who have cognitive impairment caused by an acute condition (delirium) need to receive immediate intervention to reverse the cause of the impairment before permanent disability or death results.

The first and foremost consideration in dealing with cognitively impaired individuals is the determination of whether the cognitive impairment is caused by delirium or dementia. Even an individual who has a diagnosis of dementia may experience a sudden change in cognition with an acute cause. Appropriate evaluation of the condition can prevent unnecessary suffering or death.

Delirium is an acute condition brought on by one or more conditions that have altered brain functioning. The chief symptoms include sudden disturbance in consciousness and/or cognition. The underlying condition can be a single factor or a combination of conditions, which include but are not limited to fever, infection, allergic reaction, malnutrition, vitamin deficiency, drug toxicity (over the counter or prescription), drug interactions, food supplement toxicity, hyper- or hypoglycemia, and hypoxia. The underlying condition can be life-threatening and must be corrected or the incident may result in death. If the nurse providing care in the LTC setting determines that a client is suffering from delirium, it may be necessary to arrange transportation to an acute care facility where appropriate emergent care can be provided. In addition to these physiologic processes, cognitive impairment can be brought about by psychosocial factors such as depression, change in health brought on by aging or disease, or change in location such as a move from a long time home to live with another family member or a move to an institutionalized setting. The nurse assessing the patient should consider these possibilities in order to provide appropriate interventions.

Because of the physiologic changes that occur with aging, the signs of delirium in a frail elder may develop over a period of days as a subclinical condition worsens to a crisis point. In addition, in a patient who has a complicated medication regimen, symptoms of increased confusion may initially be mild. The astute nurse will make the appropriate observations to detect delirium even when the symptoms are subtle. In a client population with fluctuating cognition, such as at many residential facilities, detection of delirium becomes more challenging.

Dementia differs from delirium in that the condition is chronic and the underlying pathologic process is progressive and irreversible. It is estimated that 13% of individuals older than age 65, and 42% percent of those 85 and older, suffer from Alzheimer's disease or a related dementia (Alzheimer's Association, 2007). In addition, it is estimated that between 40 and 80% of those living in nursing homes have a cognitive impairment (CDC, 2006).

Dementia is defined as the development of multiple cognitive deficits manifested by memory impairment and other problems, such as aphasia (inability to speak), apraxia (loss of ability to use familiar objects or carry out purposeful movements not caused by loss of sensory ability), and agnosia (loss of ability to determine the significance of sensory input, such as recognition of a familiar face or voice) (American Psychiatric Association, 2000). Primary dementias have no cure, and although a large investment is being made in drugs that could affect the progression of disease, outcomes of pharmacologic interventions have shown varying levels of success.

It is estimated that as much as 70% of dementia care is delivered in the home by a family caregiver. In the community LTC setting, the role of the nurse is to support the family caregiver with problem solving or identifying resources such as respite care, adult day care, or the local chapter of the Alzheimer's Association. The nurse may play a key role in the decision-making that takes place when caregiving for a demented loved one is negatively affecting the health of the spousal caregiver (Maas et al., 2004). When caregiving becomes overwhelming at home, the decision to place the individual with dementia in a residential facility is appropriate.

Periodic evaluation of individuals with chronic cognitive changes is necessary so that decline can be detected and care strategies adjusted. Many nurses working in the LTC setting rely on intuitive detection of cognitive changes, but this method can be improved by the inclusion of an objective measure of cognition such as the Mini Mental Status Exam (MMSE) (Folstein, Folstein & McHugh, 1975), the Dementia Rating Scale (Alexopoulos & Mattis, 1991), the Blessed Dementia Scale (Blessed, Tomlinson & Roth, 1968), or the Cognition Assessment (Barnes, 2002). Use of one or more of these instruments can provide data by which to track changes in cognitive functioning.

Nursing interventions that deal with dementia generally address one or more of three symptom domains: cognitive, functional, and/or behavioral. All clients with dementia demonstrate functional difficulties, whereas only some demonstrate behavioral problems. Dealing with individuals suffering from permanent cognitive impairment takes patience and understanding. It is important that the caregiver not lose sight of the client perspective. It is more important to validate the client's personhood rather than to insist that he or she achieve "reality orientation." The client may find comfort in some behavior, such as carrying a doll, and this behavior, although not grounded in immediate reality, is grounded in the reality of a universal human behavior regarding caring for others, specifically infants. An evidence-based practice approach should be used in structuring care and the environment in LTC facilities responsible for patients with dementia. This assures that the patient benefits from the latest research findings regarding best practice in dementia care.

The nurse needs to work closely with the activity director to meet the needs of the clients and to find appropriate and enjoyable activities for those with dementia. The activity director is responsible for providing activities for residents; individuals at different stages of dementia enjoy different types of activities. Those with mild dementia may still enjoy activities requiring personal interaction and following rules such as games or group singing. Those with more advanced dementia may enjoy more isolated activities such as the opportunity to fold laundry or a task related to food preparation.

Many nursing homes and even some assisted-living centers have special care units for dementia clients. The environment in such settings allows for safe wandering. Ideally, the staff has received training specific to caring for clients with dementia. The units are generally set up with consideration

CASE STUDY

Mrs. McFarlain

Mrs. McFarlain is an 80-year-old woman who resides in an Alzheimer's special care unit that is part of a nursing home. She spends much of her time wandering the halls mumbling to herself and sometimes singing. A new nurse's aide, Mary, tries to get Mrs. McFarlain more involved in group activities such as playing games and doing art projects, but Mrs. McFarlain's behavior becomes agitated at these attempts. The RN supervisor who is orienting Mary, the nurse's assistant, explains that Mrs. McFarlain was a music teacher who gave private piano and voice lessons to students for more than 50 years of her life. She preferred solitary activities then and now, and music was very important to her. Because her behavior is not a danger to herself or others, she does not want or need to be redirected, and it is best for her reality to be validated by allowing her to continue this behavior as long as she is content. Mary also learned that Mrs. McFarlain enjoyed reminiscence in combination with music therapy, and this was a more appropriate activity for her than group games or art. Mary learned that it is best to individualize residents' care by being informed about their history and preferences.

Discussion Questions

1. Why might Mary not recognize Mrs. McFarlain's behavior as appropriate for her?
2. What indicates that Mrs. McFarlain's actions are not related to a progressive new problem?
3. Describe what types of music therapy might be most appropriate for Mrs. McFarlain.

given to lighting, color, noise levels, congregate areas, and room set-ups. Such considerations are used to make the environment more pleasant for the residents. Again, an evidence-based practice approach will ensure that the latest research findings are incorporated into the caring regimen.

Risk Reduction and Safety

One of the most important functions of the nurse in an LTC setting is to reduce risk and ensure client safety. In a community setting, part of the home assessment includes a thorough examination of the environment to detect possible hazards and correct them. The most obvious hazards include throw rugs, electrical cords strung across traffic areas, stairs (especially those without handrails), loose tiles in the shower, slick flooring, small pets, and similar environmental conditions. In residential settings, the nurse has similar responsibilities to ensure client safety. Facilities should provide a safe environment with adaptations for those with chronic health problems that would place them at higher risk for injuries or falls.

Nurse researcher Audrey Nelson (2006) has led some pioneering work in safe patient handling and linking organized safety programs to positive outcomes for both patients and staff. Researchers found that implementing a safe patient-handling program in a LTC through the VA system resulted in better quality of patient care for residents. Safe-handling programs include four key interventions: appropriate patient-handling equipment and devices, assessment protocols, safe lifting policies, and patient lift teams. Key areas of change for residents after implementation of the program included: improved physical functioning, decreased sedentary states of residents, less deterioration in activities of daily living, decreased fall rate, and increased wakeful states in the mornings (Nelson, Collins, Siddharthan, Matz, & Waters, 2008).

Another important safety consideration is the use of restraints. Falls are a significant problem in LTC, and of persons who fall, 20–30% suffer significant injuries such as hip fractures (Cowley, Deibold, Gross, Hardin-Fanning, 2006). Originally restraints were thought to prevent injury to clients and were applied to ensure patient safety through limiting movement. Research has demonstrated, however, that restraints do the opposite and are likely to cause injury (Lekan-Rutledge, 1997). Both physical and chemical restraints in LTC facilities are now strictly regulated. The most current reports regarding restraint use are available online (CMS, 2004a).

Exercise has emerged as the "most effective factor in reducing the risk of falls and injuries from falls" (Mitty & Flores, 2007b, p. 349). All LTC facilities should have an exercise plan and program available to residents. The ideal environment for LTC residents is restraint-free, with environmental and staffing accommodations made to meet the needs of each resident and promote optimum physical functioning through exercise, adequate nutrition, and safety.

Palliative and Hospice Care

Palliative care is defined as "an approach that improves the quality of life of patients and their families facing the problem associated with life-threatening illness, through the prevention and relief of suffering by means of early identification and impeccable assessment and treatment of pain and other problems, physical, psychosocial and spiritual" (World Health Organization, 2008, paragraph 1). The goals of this care are not curative, but for comfort. It is both a philosophy of care as well as a treatment system, and not necessarily just for those considered terminally ill. In palliation, physiologic needs are met and aggressive measures are taken for pain relief. A holistic view of the client should be maintained, and the personhood of the client is of primary consideration in this type of nursing care. Palliative care may be used in conjunction with life-prolonging care. For adults, the WHO (2008, paragraph 2) stated the following about palliative care:

- Provides relief from pain and other distressing symptoms;
- affirms life and regards dying as a normal process;
- intends neither to hasten or postpone death;
- integrates the psychological and spiritual aspects of patient care;
- offers a support system to help patients live as actively as possible until death;
- offers a support system to help the family cope during the patients illness and in their own bereavement;
- uses a team approach to address the needs of patients and their families, including bereavement counseling, if indicated;
- will enhance quality of life, and may also positively influence the course of illness;
- is applicable early in the course of illness, in conjunction with other therapies that are intended to prolong life, such as chemotherapy or radiation therapy, and includes those investigations needed to better understand and manage distressing clinical complications.

One can see from the preceding information that there is a difference between palliative and hospice care. A person with chronic illness may benefit from palliative care services and yet not qualify for hospice. Hospice is a type of palliative care and is usually delivered in the home by a team of trained professionals who address the needs of the patient and the entire family. Hospice is covered under Medicare Part A and pays for most of the needed services for the terminally ill. However, Medicare will not pay for curative treatment in hospice. The general requirement for Medicare reimbursement for hospice service is that a physician must certify that patient probably has 6 months or less to live (CMS, 2007b). Determination of the terminal phase of an illness is sometimes difficult, and patients may improve during that 6-month period of time. Patients must be re-certified by their physician as terminal in order to continue receiving hospice services. Hospice teams do come into nursing homes to augment and oversee comfort care. In the terminal phase of life, appropriate care

includes pain relief, comfort, and emotional and spiritual support for the client and family (Tarzian, 2000). The client and family can be referred for grief counseling related to the experience of incurable illness (Ferrell & Coyle, 2001). Death is a natural part of life, and the nurse should be prepared to facilitate the client's end-of-life transition and provide support to the family survivors (DeSpelder & Strickland, 1996). Once hospice services are begun for community-dwelling elders, other LTC services may not be allowed by reimbursement policy.

The End of Life Nursing Education Consortium (ELNEC) has made enormous strides in providing core information to nurses interested in end-of-life care. This project began in 2000 with a grant from The Robert Wood Johnson Foundation and has provided specialized education and curricula to more than 4000 nurses representing all 50 states, using a train the trainer approach (AACN, 2007b). During the next decade, it is expected that knowledge on palliative and end-of-life care will continue to increase and that this treatment methodology will advance (see Chapter 22).

Research in Long-Term Care

The science of caring for those who have chronic illness is changing rapidly. Andersen and Horvath (2004) reported that 85% of seniors and 45% of the working adult population have at least one chronic illness. This growing burden of care for long-term health problems accounts for 78% of the nation's healthcare spending. Research in LTC settings is essential if the complex problems of clients are to be addressed appropriately (Baldwin & Nail, 2000). Research often begins with clinical observations of problems or recurring events that require solutions. A number of nurse researchers have focused research programs dealing with chronic illness and issues related to the nursing home experience (e.g., Cornelia Beck, Jeanne Kaiser-Jones, and Terri Fulmer). Nurses in a clinical role should take the opportunity to define a problem and propose a solution. A novice researcher may partner with a more experienced researcher to develop an idea into a researchable question. Regional research organizations such as the Southern Nursing Research Society, the Midwest Nursing Research Society, and local chapters of Sigma Theta Tau, are available to provide assistance.

OUTCOMES

Desired outcomes for LTC clients are as multifaceted as the clients (see case study on Mrs. McFarlain). Simple medical models are rarely sufficient to state desired outcomes for those with complicated chronic medical conditions (Mold, 1995). It is not sufficient to consider the quality of life based on absence of sickness, but one must consider the overall well-being of the client. Many frail older adults with multiple chronic health problems continue to perceive their health as good, provided they have strong social support (Schank & Lough, 1990).

Outcomes will vary along the LTC continuum. For community-based clients, the overall outcome may be to remain in their homes as long as possible. Interventions to support that outcome may include client and family teaching on medication management, safety issues, or wound care. Rehabilitation may be a desired outcome for a community-based client following hospitalization.

For the resident in an LTC facility, outcomes are different and may include a reduction in the exacerbations of a chronic illness such as congestive heart failure. A client in the rehabilitative area of the facility may have as an outcome to live independently again. Outcomes for others may be to function at the highest potential with the limitations imposed by the chronic illness. A decrease in pain and/or nausea might be an appropriate outcome for an individual in palliative care. Living each day with optimal quality of life is an outcome for most clients in LTC. Nurses can empower even frail older persons to obtain better outcome by good listening skills, working with them to identify the meaning of frailty to each person, and identifying positive coping and self-care solutions (Hage & Lorensen, 2005).

EVIDENCE-BASED PRACTICE BOX

These researchers conducted a project in nine different senior centers in Connecticut using a variety of investigators, administrators, senior members, and staff. A fall prevention program based on the Yale Frailty and Injury Cooperative Studies of Intervention Trials (Yale FICSIT) was used. The results indicated that the project reached a small portion of the total members [457 (4%) of 7000 members]. Lessons learned from the challenges of implementing a fall-risk management program included the need to tailor the intervention to Senior Centers, delineate authority and responsibility, environmental issues such as lack of space and geographic dispersion of participants, engaging the senior center membership, addressing cultural differences, and initiating change. In this article, researchers provided strategies they used to address each of these challenges, including using simple prevention messages and photographs for fall prevention, obtaining administrative support and buy-in, making programming convenient for seniors and staff, using focus groups and kick-off events to recruit interest in the older adult membership, and making materials available in the native language of the participants. This article provides some insight into the challenges and solutions to integrating fall prevention programs into Senior Centers in the community.

Source: Baker, D.I., Gottschalk, M. & Bianco, L.M. (2007). Step by step: Integrating evidence-based fall-risk management into senior centers. *The Gerontologist, 47*(4), 548–554.

STUDY QUESTIONS

1. How is long-term care defined?
2. Describe the major settings in which long-term care is provided, giving a specific example of each in your local community.
3. What are some of the precipitating factors for an individual to access the long-term care system?
4. What are the major problems facing both caregivers and clients in today's long-term care continuum?
5. What individuals are considered vulnerable populations?
6. There are a number of issues in long-term care today. What are the most essential issues for the federal government to address first?
7. Discuss the ethical principle of autonomy when constructing an appropriate plan of care for a long-term care recipient.
8. Discuss the principle of autonomy in relationship to the community-dwelling client versus the person in a residential facility.
9. Analyze nursing interventions that would most likely support the goals of an ideal long-term care system.

INTERNET RESOURCES

Across the States 2006: Profiles of Long-Term Care and Independent Living: assets.aarp.org/rgcenter/health/d18763_2006_ats.pdf

American Association of Homes and Services for the Aging: www2.aahsa.org/

Geriatric Nursing Education Project: www.aacn.nche.edu/gnec.htm

Hartford Institute for Geriatric Nursing: www.consultGeriRn.org

Long-term care planning tool from CMS: www.medicare.gov/LTCPlanning/Include/DataSection/Questions/SearchCriteria.asp?version=default&browser=IE%7C6%7CWinXP&language=English&defaultstatus=0&pagelist=Home

Medicare and You, 2008. Center for Medicare and Medicaid Services publication: www.medicare.gov/Publications/Pubs/pdf/10050.pdf

Long-term Care Ombudsman: www.ltcombudsman.org

Medicare Hospice Benefits: www.medicare.gov/publications/pubs/pdf/02154.pdf

National Gerontological Nursing Association: https://www.ngna.org/

National Association of Professional Geriatric Care Managers: www.caremanager.org/

National Center for Assisted Living: www.ncal.org/about/index.cfm

National Hospice and Palliative Care Organization: www.nho.org

Practicing physician education in geriatrics: www.gericareonline.net

REFERENCES

AARP. (2002). Understanding Long-term Health Care. Retrieved from www.aarp.org/research/health/privinsurance/fs7r_ltc.html

Aging with Dignity. (2007). Five wishes 2007 edition. Retrieved January 14, 2008, from www.agingwithdignity.org/fw2007.html.

Alexopoulos, G.S., & Mattis, S. (1991). Diagnosing cognitive dysfunction in the elderly: Primary screening tests. *Geriatrics, 46*(12), 33–38, 43–44.

Algase, D., Beck, C., Kolanowski, A., Whall, A., Berent, S., Richards, K., et al. (1996). Need-driven dementia-compromised behavior: An alternative view of disruptive behavior. *American Journal of Alzheimer's' Disease, 11*(6), 10–19.

Alzheimer's Association. (2007). Alzheimer's disease facts and figures. Retrieved from www.alz.org/national/documents/report_alzfactsfigures2007.pdf

American Association of College of Nursing. (2007a). Nursing shortage. Retrieved January 4, 2008, from www.aacn.nche.edu/Media/FactSheets/Nursing-Shortage.htm.

American Association of College of Nursing. (2007b). ELNEC Fact sheet. Retrieved January 11, 2008 from www.aacn.nche.edu/ELNEC/about.htm.

American Psychiatric Association. (2000). *Diagnostic and statistical manual IV-TR*. Arlington, VA: American Psychiatric Association.

Andersen, G., & Horvath, J. (2004). The growing burden of chronic disease in America. *Public Health Reports, 119*, 263–270.

Arling, G., Kane, R., L., Mueller, C., Bershadsky, J. & Degenholtz, H.B. (2007). Nursing effort and quality of care for nursing home residents. *The Gerontologist, 47*(1), 672–682.

Baldwin, K.M., & Nail, L.M. (2000). Opportunities and challenges in clinical nursing research. *Journal of Nursing Scholarship, 32*(2), 163–166.

Barnes, S.J. (2002) Cognition assessment in elders with dementia: testing with developmental tasks. Presentation at Southern Nursing Research Society Annual Meeting, February 8, 2002, San Antonio, Texas.

Beatty, W. (1999). Preserved cognitive skills in dementia: Implications for geriatric medicine. *Oklahoma State Medical Association, Reprint, 92*(1).

Beauchamp, T.L. (2001). *Principles of biomedical ethics* (5th ed.). New York: Oxford University Press.

Beck, A.T., Rush, A.J., Shaw, B.F., & Emery, G. (1979). *Cognitive therapy of depression*. New York: Guilford.

Beck, C., Heacock, P., Mercer, S.O., Walls, R.C., Rapp, C.G., Vogelpohl, T.S. (1997). Improving dressing behavior in cognitively impaired nursing home residents. *Nursing Research, 46*(3), 126–132.

Beeber, A.C. (2005). Knowing the whole story: A qualitative description of enrollment in a program of all-inclusive care for the elderly (PACE). Doctoral dissertation: Author.

Blessed, B., Tomlinson, B., & Roth, M. (1968). The association between quantitative measures of dementia and of degenerative changes in the cerebral gray matter of elderly subjects. *British Journal of Psychiatry, 114*, 797–811.

Castle, N.G., Engberg, J., & Men, A. (2007). Nursing home staff turnover: Impact on nursing home compare quality measures. *The Gerontologist, 47*(1), 650–661.

Celia, B. (2000). Age and gender differences in pain management following coronary artery bypass surgery. *Journal of Gerontological Nursing, 26*(5), 7–13.

Centers for Disease Control and Prevention (CDC) and the Merck Company Foundation. (2007). *The state of aging and health in America, 2007*. Whitehouse Station, NJ: The Merck Company Foundation.

Centers for Medicare and Medicaid Services. (2000). *Medicare 2000: 35 years of improving Americans' health and security: Profiles of Medicare beneficiaries*. Washington, DC: U.S. Government Printing Office.

Centers for Medicare and Medicaid Services. (2005). Medicaid at a Glance 2005. Retrieved from www.cms.hhs.gov/MedicaidGenInfo/Downloads/MedicaidAtAGlance2005.pdf

Centers for Medicare and Medicaid Services. (2007a). MDS 3.0. Retrieved from www.cms.hhs.gov/NursingHomeQualityInits/25_NHQIMDS30.asp#TopOfPage

Centers for Medicare and Medicaid Services. (2007b). Medicare hospice benefits. Retrieved from www.medicare.gov/publications/pubs/pdf/02154.pdf

Centers for Medicare and Medicaid Services. (2008). Medicare and you 2008. Retrieved from www.medicare.gov/Publications/Pubs/pdf/10050.pdf.

Centers for Medicare and Medicaid Services. (2004a). Restraint reduction newsletter. Retrieved from http:www.hcfa.gov

Centers for Medicare and Medicaid Services. (2004b). State operations manual. Retrieved from www.cms.hhs.gov

Chandra, A., Smith, L.A., & Paul, D.P. (2006). What do consumers and healthcare providers in West Virginia think of long-term care? *Healthcare and Public Policy, 84*(3), 33–38.

Cherry, B., Ashcraft, A., & Owne, D. (2007). Perceptions of job satisfaction and the regulatory environment among nurse aides and charge nurses in long-term care. *Geriatric Nursing, 28*(3), 183–192.

Cowley, J., Diebold, C., Gross, J. C., & Hardin-Fanning, F. (2006). Management of common problems.

In K.L. Mauk (Ed.) *Gerontological Nursing: Competencies for Care,* (pp. 475–560). Sudbury, MA: Jones & Bartlett.

Crain, M. (2001). Control beliefs of the frail elderly. *Case Management Journals, 3*(1), 42 – 46.

Cummings, S. (2002). Predictors of psychological well-being among assisted-living residents. *Health & Social Work, 27*(4), 293–302.

Dawson, P., Wells, D., & Kline, K. (1993). *Enhancing the abilities of persons with Alzheimer's and related dementias: A nursing perspective.* New York: Springer.

DeSpelder, L.A., & Strickland, A.L. (2002). *The last dance: Encountering death and dying* (6th ed.) Boston: McGraw Hill.

Donoghue, C., & Castle, N.G. (2006). Voluntary and involuntary nursing turnover. *Research on Aging, 28*(4), 454–472.

Duke University Center for the Study of Aging and Human Development (1978). *Multidimensional functional assessment: The OARS methodology.* Durham, NC: Duke University.

Feaster, M. (2006). Financing LTC with life insurance. *Provider,* November, 39–40.

Ferrell, B., & Coyle, N. (2004). *Textbook of palliative nursing.* Oxford: Oxford University Press.

Folstein, M.R., Folstein, S.E., & McHugh, P.R. (1975). Mini-mental state: A practical method for grading the cognitive state of patients for the clinician. *Journal of Psychiatric Research, 12,* 189–198.

Fulmer, T.T. (1999). Elder mistreatment. In J.T. Stone, J.F. Wyman, & S.A. Salisbury (Eds.). *Clinical gerontological nursing: A guide to advanced practice* (2nd ed.), (pp. 665–674). Philadelphia: Saunders.

Gaugler, J.E. & Teaster, P. (2006). The family caregiving career: Implications for community-based long-term care practice and policy. *Journal of Aging & Social Policy, 18*(3–4), 141–145.

Geriatric Nursing Education Consortium. (2007). AACN Hartford-sponsored faculty development project: Enhancing gerontology in senior-level undergraduate courses. Retrieved January 12, 2008 from www.aacn.nche.edu/gnec.html

Grady, P. (2000). Prologue from the director, National Institute of Nursing Research. www.ninr.nih.gov/NR/rdonlyres/3583868E-6766-4439-AEA8-67738086C2D7/0/Strategic Prologue.pdf

Greiner, F., English, S., Dean, K., Olson, K.A., Winn, P. & Beatty, W.W. (1997). Expression of game-related and generic knowledge by dementia patients who retain skill at playing dominoes. *Neurology, 49,* 518–523.

Hage, A.M., & Lorensen, M. (2005). A philosophical analysis of the concept empowerment: the fundament of an education-programme to the frail elderly. *Nursing Philosophy, 6,* 235–246.

Hardin, S. (2006). Promoting quality of life. In K.L. Mauk (Ed.) *Gerontological Nursing: Competencies for Care,* (pp. 703–733). Sudbury, MA: Jones & Bartlett.

Harrington, C., Carrillo, H., & Crawford, C.S. (2004). Nursing facilities, staffing, residents, and facility deficiencies, 1997 through 2003. Retrieved from http://www.nccnhr.org/uploads/CHStateData04.pdf

Harrington, C., Zimmerman, D., Karon, S.L., Robinson, J. & Beutel, P. (2000). Nursing home staffing and its relationship to deficiencies. *The Journals of Gerontology Series B: Psychological Sciences and Social Sciences 55:* S278–S287.

Houser, A., Fox-Grage, W., & Gibson, M. J. (2006). Across the states: Profiles of long-term care and independent living. Retrieved on January 8, 2008 from assets.aarp.org/rgcenter/health/d18763_2006_ats.pdf

Jonsen, A.R. (2007). A history of bioethics as discipline and discourse. In N.S. Jecker, A.R. Jonsen, & R.A. Pearlman (Eds.). *Bioethics: An introduction to the history, methods, and practice,* (pp. 3–16) Sudbury, MA: Jones & Bartlett.

Kaisernetwork. (2005). The 2005 Whitehouse conference on aging. Retrieved from www.kaisernetwork.org/health_cast/hcast_index.cfm?display=detail&hc=1612

Kalisch, P.A., & Kalisch, B.J. (2004). *American nursing: A history* (4th ed.). Philadelphia: Lippincott Williams & Wilkins.

Kane, R., Freeman, I.C., Caplan, A.L., Aroskar, M.A., & Urv-Wong, E.K. (1990). Everyday autonomy in nursing homes. *Generations, 14*(Suppl), 69–71.

Katz, S., Downs, T.D., Cash, H.R., & Grotz, R.C. (1970). Progress in development of the index of ADL. *The Gerontologist, 10,* 20–30.

Kempthorne, D. (2004). State efforts toward creating a national policy on healthy aging and long-term care. *Caring, 23*(1), 52–56.

Kinosian, B., Stallard, E., & Wieland, D. (2007). Projected use of long-term care services by enrolled veterans. *The Gerontologist, 47*(3), 356–364.

Komisar, H.L., Feder, J., & Kasper, J.D. (2005). Unmet long-term care needs: An analysis of Medicare-Medicaid dual eligibles. *Inquiry, 42*(2), 171–182.

Koop, C.E., & Schaeffer, F. (1976). *Whatever happened to the human race?* Old Tappan, NJ: Fleming H. Revell.

Leininger, M. (2002). Culture care theory: A major contribution to advance transcultural nursing and practices. *Journal of Transcultural Nursing, 13*(3), 189–192.

Lekan-Rutledge, D. (1997). Gerontological nursing in long-term care facilities. In M. Matteson, E. McConnell, & A. Linton (Eds.). *Gerontological nursing: Concepts and practice* (2nd ed.), (pp. 930–960). Philadelphia: Saunders.

Lindbloom, E.J., Brandt, J., Hough, L. D., & Meadows, S. E. (2007). Elder mistreatment in the nursing home: A systematic review. *Journal of the American Medical Director's Association, 8*(9), 610–116.

Lomastro, J.A. (2006). The White House conference on aging: A positive view. *Nursing Homes: Long Term Care Management, 55*(1), 14–16, 18.

Maas, M.L., Reed, D., Park, M., Specht, J.P., Schutte, D., Kelley, L.S. et al. (2004). Outcomes of family involvement in care interventions for caregivers of individuals with dementia. *Nursing Research, 53*(2), 76–86.

Marnard, B. (2002). *Nursing home quality indicators.* Washington, DC: AARP.

McGuire, L.C., Rao, J.K., Anderson, L.A., & Ford, E.S. (2007). Completion of a durable power of attorney for health care: What does cognition have to do with it? *The Gerontologist, 47*(4), 457–467.

Medicare. (2007). Nursing homes: Alternatives to nursing homes. Retrieved from www.medicare.gov/Nursing/Alternatives/SHMO.asp

Meenan, R.F. (1985). New approaches to outcome assessment: The AIMS questionnaire for arthritis. *Advances in Internal Medicine, 31*, 167–185.

Mezey, M., Stierele, L.J., Huba, G.J., & Esterson, J. (2007). Ensuring competence of specialty nurses in care of older adults. *Geriatric Nursing, 28*(6S), 9–14.

Mezey, M., Mitty, I., & Ramsey, G. (1997). Assessment of decision making capacity: Nursing's role. *Journal of Gerontological Nursing, 23*(3), 28–34.

Mitty, E. & Flores, S. (2007a). Assisted living nursing practice: The language of dementia: Theories and interventions. *Geriatric Nursing, 28*(5), 283–288.

Mitty, E. & Flores, S. (2007b). Fall prevention in assisted living: Assessment and strategies. *Geriatric Nursing, 28*(6), 349–357.

Mold, J.W. (1995). An alternative conceptualization of health and health care: Its implications for geriatrics and gerontology. *Educational Gerontology, 21*, 85–101.

Moye, J., Butz, S.W., Marson, D.C., & Wood, E. (2007). A conceptual model and assessment template for capacity evaluation in adult guardianship. *The Gerontologist, 47*(5), 591–603.

Moye, J., Wood, S., Edelstein, B., Armesto, J.C., Bower, E.H., Harrison, J.A., & Wood, E. (2007). Clinical evidence in guardianship of older adults is inadequate: Findings from a tri-state study. *The Gerontologist, 47*(5), 604–612.

Mysak, S. (1997). Strategies for promoting ethical decision making. *Journal of Gerontological Nursing, 23*(1), 25–31.

National Association of Adult Protective Services Administrators (2005). Retrieved from www.apsnetwork.org/

National Association of Professional Geriatric Care Managers. (2007). What can a PGCM do for me? Retrieved on December 30, 2007 from www.caremanager.org/displaycommon.cfm?an=1&subarticlenbr=87

National Center for Assisted Living. (2006). Assisted living resident profile. Retrieved on December 30, 2007 from www.ncal.org/about/resident.cfm

National Center for Health Statistics. (2007). National Health Interview Survey. Retrieved from www.cdc.gov/nchs/nhis.htm

National Center for Health Statistics. (2006). *Health, United States 2006 with chartbook on trends in the health of Americans.* Hyattsville, MD: NCHS.

National Long Term Care Ombudsman Resource Center (2008). What does an ombudsman do? Retrieved from www.ltcombudsman.org/ombpublic/49_151_855.cfm

National Institute on Aging. (2007). Growing older in America: The Health and Retirement Study. Retrieved from http://www.nia.nih.gov/NR/rdonlyres/D164FE6C-C6E0-4E78-B27F-7E8D8C0F-FEE5/0/HRS_Text_WEB.pdf

National Institute of Mental Health (NIMH). (2008). Older adults: Depression and suicide facts. Retrieved from www.nimh.nih.gov/health/publications/older-adults-depression-and-suicide-facts.shtml#how-common

National PACE Association (2007). About us. Retrieved from www.npaonline.org/website/article.asp?id=5

Nelson, A., Collins, J., Siddharthan, K., Matz, M., & Waters, T. (2008). Link between safe patient handling and patient outcomes in long-term care. *Rehabilitation Nursing, 33*(1), 33–43.

Nelson, A. (Ed.) (2006). *Safe patient handling and movement: A practical guide for health care professionals.* New York, NY: Springer Publishing Company.

Nelson, J.M. (2006). Identifying and preventing common risk factors in the elderly. In K.L. Mauk (Ed.) *Gerontological Nursing: Competencies for Care,* (pp. 357–388). Sudbury, MA: Jones & Bartlett.

Peterson, S.J., & Bredow, T.S. (2004). *Middle range theories: Application to nursing research.* Philadelphia: Lippincott, Williams and Wilkins.

Reinardy, J.R. (1995). Relocation to a new environment: Decisional control and the move to a nursing home. *Health & Social Work, 20*(1), 31–38.

Remennick, L.I. (2001). All my life is one big nursing home: Russian immigrant women in Israel speak about double caregiver stress. *Women's Studies International Forum, 24*(6), 685–700.

Remsburg, R. & Carson, B. (2006). Rehabilitation. In Lubkin, I. & Larsen, P. (Eds.) *Chronic illness: Impact and interventions,* (pp. 579–616). Sudbury, MA: Jones & Bartlett.

Roberto, D.A., Wacler, R.R., Jewell, M.A., & Rickard, M. (1997). Resident rights: Knowledge of and implementation by nursing staff in long term care facilities. *Journal of Gerontological Nursing, 23*(12), 32–37.

Salisbury, S.A. (1999). Iatrogenesis. In J. T. Stone, J. F. Wyman, & S. A. Salisbury (Eds.). *Clinical gerontological nursing: A guide to advanced practice* (2nd ed.), (pp. 369–383). Philadelphia: Saunders.

Schank, M.J., & Lough, M.A. (1990). Profile: Frail elderly women, maintaining independence. *Journal of Advanced Nursing, 15,* 674–682.

Sehy, Y. B., & Williams, M. P. (1999). Functional Assessment. In W. C. Chenitz, J. Takano Smith, & S. A. Salisbury (Eds.). *Clinical gerontological nursing: A guide to advanced practice* (2nd ed.), (pp. 175–199). Philadelphia: Saunders.

Service Employees International Union. (2007). Workforce shortages. Retrieved on January 4, 2008 from http://www.seiu.org/longterm/issues/workforce_shortage.cfm

Shalala, D. (2000). Message from Donna E. Shalala, Secretary of Health and Human Services. Retrieved from www.surgeongeneral.gov/Library/MentalHealth/home.html

Sikorska-Simmons, E. (2006). Innovations in long-term care: Organizational culture and work-related attitudes among staff in assisted living. *Journal of Gerontological Nursing, 32*(2), 19–27.

Stewart, M.K., Felix, H., Dockter, N., Perry, D.M., & Morgan, J.R. (2006). Program and policy issues affecting home and community-based long-term care use: Findings from a qualitative study. *Home Health Care Services Quarterly, 25*(3–4), 107–127.

Tarzian, A.J. (2000). Caring for dying patients who have air hunger. *Journal of Nursing Scholarship, 32*(2), 137–143.

Teaster, P.B. (2002). *A response to the abuse of vulnerable adults: The 2000 survey of state adult protective services.* Washington, DC: The National Center on Elder Abuse.

Teresi, J.A., & Evans, D.A. (1997). Cognitive assessment measures for chronic care populations. In J.A. Teresi, M.P. Lawton, D. Holmes, & M. Ory (Eds.). *Measurement in elderly chronic care populations,* (pp. 1–23). New York: Springer.

Tobin, P., & Salisbury, S. (1999). Legal planning issues. In J. T. Stone, J. F. Wyman, & Salisbury, S.A. (Eds.). *Clinical gerontological nursing: A guide to advanced practice* (2nd ed.), (pp. 31–44). Philadelphia: Saunders.

Varcarolis, E.M. (2002). *Foundation of psychiatric mental health nursing: A clinical approach.* Philadelphia: Saunders.

Wagner, D.L. (2006). Families, work, and an aging population: Developing a formula that works for the workers. *Journal of Aging & Social Policy, 18*(3–4), 115–125.

White House Conference on Aging. (2004). Retrieved from www.whitehouse.gov

Willging, P. (2006). Get ready for community-based long-term care. *Long Term Living, 55*(3), 20, 22–23.

World Health Organization. (2008). WHO definition of palliative care. Retrieved from www.who.int/cancer/palliative/definition/en/

22

Palliative Care

Barbara M. Raudonis

The art of living well and dying well are one.

Epicurus

INTRODUCTION

The aging American population will eventually experience one or more chronic illnesses with which they will live with for years before death (Morrison & Meier, 2004). Four chronic diseases—heart disease, cancer, cerebrovascular disease, and chronic respiratory disease—are the leading causes of death for older adults (Centers for Disease Control and Prevention, 2007). These chronic diseases share protracted illness trajectories that include phases of decline resulting in progressively advanced disease and disability. Individuals who have illness trajectories such as those in chronic disease can benefit from palliative care. In reality many aging adults experience several chronic illnesses simultaneously, which demand complex care and often overwhelm both the elder and their family members. A conceptual framework published by Nolan and Mock (2004) entitled *Integrity of the Person: A Conceptual Framework for End-of-Life-Care* addresses the complexity of needs, interventions, and processes needed to provide palliative care.

The framework is organized around the core concept of the integrity of the human person and

the relationship of the healthcare professional to the patient. It builds on the earlier work of Pellegrino (1990). The framework involves relationships among the following components: External Factors—the integrity of the health professional, organizational culture, and healthcare resources; Internal Factors—spiritual domain, psychological domain, physical domain, functional domain, and community culture and family. Completing the framework are patient care goals and outcomes of care. Although end of life appears to be a prominent part of the framework, Nolan and Mock (2004) use the Institute of Medicine's (IOM's) definition of end of life that extends further up the illness trajectory to include "the period of time during which an individual copes with declining health from an ultimately terminal illness—from a serious though perhaps chronic illness or from the frailties associated with advanced age even if death is not clearly imminent" (Lunney, Foley, Smith, & Gelband, 2003, p. 22).

The multidimensional nature of the framework provides a structure for future research related to the factors that influence the integrity of the person, patient care goals, and outcomes of care. In essence this framework summarizes the major points about palliative care discussed throughout this chapter. In addition, it provides a foundation to passionately go forward in clinical practice, teaching, and research to build the science and the care to relieve suffering and improve quality of life.

Historical Perspectives

Palliative care grew out of the hospice movement. Hospice is both a philosophy of care and an organized form of healthcare delivery. The Latin origin of the word *hospes* relates to hospitality. During the Middle Ages, pilgrims to the Holy Lands stopped at way stations for food, water, and respite. These way stations (hospices) were also centers of refuge for poor, sick, and dying people.

Dame Cicely Saunders is considered the founder of the modern hospice movement. Educated as a nurse, social worker, and physician, she founded St. Christopher's Hospice in Sydenham England in 1967. St. Christopher's Hospice was the first research and teaching hospice, and was known for several innovations including pain and symptom management, a holistic approach to care, home care, family support throughout the illness, and bereavement follow-up (Lattanzi-Licht, Mahoney, & Miller, 1998). The services provided by St. Christopher's Hospice evolved over time to meet the needs of patients and families. Services include in-patient care, home care, and a day center. In the United Kingdom, hospice and palliative day care is the fastest growing (but least researched) component of palliative care services (Hearn & Myers, 2001). Hospice and palliative day care is a complex service with the goal of improving the quality of life of terminally ill persons through a variety of programs in an individualized, flexible, and nonmedical environment (Hearn & Myers, 2001). In the United Kingdom, no eligibility criteria related to prognosis exists. Therefore, patients are admitted earlier in their illness trajectory. Earlier admission enables them to participate in activities such as arts and craft projects and outings. The traditional services offered include a review of symptom control and medications, respite for relatives and friends, companionship of people with similar

problems, opportunities to talk to others without hurting family or friends, counseling and support, and help with personal hygiene (Haywood House, 1996; St. Christopher's Hospice, 1996). St. Christopher's Hospice continues to serve as a prototype for hospice and palliative care throughout the world. However, Dame Saunders cautions not to clone St. Christopher's but to refine the principles of hospice and palliative care within the cultural context of the needs of the individuals served.

Two years after the opening of St. Christopher's Hospice, Dr. Elisabeth Kubler-Ross's book *On Death and Dying* (1969) was published. One of the outcomes of her seminal work was the identification of the stages of dying. More importantly, her work initiated a national dialogue recognizing the needs of the dying.

Florence S. Wald, a nurse and pioneer in the hospice movement in the United States, strengthened her vision for improving the quality of life for terminally ill persons during a visit to St. Christopher's Hospice. She conducted a needs assessment for hospice care in Connecticut. In 1974 the first hospice program in the United States was established in Branford, Connecticut. At that time, the Connecticut Hospice was only a home-care program (no in-patient beds) and became a model of care for the entire United States. As services evolved, inpatient beds were added and Connecticut Hospice became the first independent hospice inpatient facility in the country (Lattanzi-Licht et al., 1998). Wald's work for the next 30 years led the way in translating the English hospice philosophy and models of care into the American hospice movement. She is considered the "mother of hospice and palliative nursing care in the United States" by the Hospice and Palliative Nurses Association and Foundation. She became the first recipient of the Hospice and Palliative Nurses Association Leading the Way Award in January 2004 (Hospice and Palliative Nurses Association, 2005).

The National Hospice and Palliative Care Organization (NHPCO) (2007) estimated there were 4500 operational hospice programs throughout the United States in 2006. An estimated 1.3 million patients were served by these programs. These figures illustrate the enormous growth and progress in hospice care in the United States since 1974. The majority of hospice patients, 74.1%, died at home (NHPCO, 2007), whereas approximately 50% of the general population die in acute care hospitals (Teno, 2004). These numbers suggest that hospice care is still a "best kept secret."

In the 1990s two reports, the *Study to Understand Prognosis and Preferences for Outcomes and Risks of Treatments* (SUPPORT) (1995) and the IOM report, *Approaching Death: Improving Care at the End of Life* (Field & Cassel, 1997) ignited a concern regarding the status of end-of-life care in the United States. As a result improving end-of-life care was placed on the national healthcare agenda.

SUPPORT Study

The landmark SUPPORT study (SUPPORT Principal Investigators, 1995) was funded by The Robert Wood Johnson Foundation for $29 million to study the process of dying in five American major teaching hospitals. The study involved approximately 9000 participants with diagnoses such as heart failure (HF), chronic obstructive pulmonary disease (COPD), colon, lung cancer, and liver failure. Findings included that more than 50% of patients had serious pain the last 3 days of life. In addition, there was poor communication between doctors and patients about their goals of care. There was substantial emotional suffering of patients, families, and professionals. Thirty-one percent of the families lost most of their life savings. The findings from this study sparked a groundswell of initiatives in research, education, and practice, with the goal of changing the culture of death and dying in the United States.

IOM Report

The second landmark study was the IOM's Committee on Care at the End of Life report,

Approaching Death: Improving Care at the End of Life (Field & Cassel, 1997). The committee found four broad deficiencies in the care of persons with life-threatening and incurable illnesses. Deficiencies included:

▪ Too many people suffer needlessly at the end of life both from errors of omission—when caregivers fail to provide palliative and support care known to be —and from errors of commission—when caregivers do what is known to be ineffective and even harmful.

▪ Legal, organizational, and economic obstacles conspire to obstruct reliably excellent care at the end of life.

▪ The education and training of physicians and other healthcare professionals fails to provide them with the knowledge, skills, and attitudes required to care well for the dying patient.

▪ Current knowledge and understanding are inadequate to guide and support the consistent practice of evidence-based medicine at the end of life (pp. 264–265).

Healthcare professionals, patients, families, health plan administrators, agency administrators, and policymakers must work together to change attitudes, policies, and actions in order to surmount the deficiencies in palliative care (Field & Cassel, 1997). The report concluded with optimism that a "vigorous societal commitment . . . would motivate and sustain individual and collective efforts to create a humane care system that people can trust to serve them well as they die" (Field & Cassel, 1997, p. 13).

Clinical Practice Guidelines for Palliative Care

The landmark studies, the SUPPORT study and the IOM report, recognized the need to integrate palliative care into health care for all individuals with chronic, debilitating, and life-limiting illnesses. This need resulted in the National Consensus Project for Quality Palliative

Care (NCPQPC) and the establishment of Clinical Practice Guidelines (National Consensus Project for Quality Palliative Care, 2004).

The Clinical Practice Guidelines promote consistent high standards for palliative care. In addition, individual providers regardless of setting can use the guidelines to provide palliative approaches in their daily clinical practice across the health care continuum (NCPQPC, 2004). The National Institutes of Health (NIH) recognized the need to evaluate the current science regarding end-of-life care and convened a State-of-the-Science Conference on Improving End-of- Life Care in December 2004.

Clinical Specialty of Palliative Care

Palliative care is the broad term used to describe the care provided by an interdisciplinary team consisting of physicians, nurses, social workers, chaplains, and other healthcare professionals. Palliative medicine is a medical specialty practiced by physicians (Derek, Hanks, Cherny, & Calman, 2004).

Palliative Medicine

On October 6, 2006, the American Board of Medical Specialties (ABMS) announced the addition of a new subspecialty certificate in Hospice and Palliative Medicine. Historically this was the first time that 10 ABMS Member Boards collaborated in the offering of certification in one specific area. The first certification examination will be offered in October, 2008 (American Board of Medical Specialties, 2006). This recognition as a subspecialty was the result of the diligent collaboration of the American Academy of Hospice and Palliative Medicine (AAHPM) and the American Board of Hospice and Palliative Medicine (ABHPM). The United States now joins members of the international community such as Great Britain, Ireland, Australia, and Canada in formally recognizing palliative medicine as a subspecialty (von Guten & Lupu, 2004).

The AAHPM's mission can be succinctly summarized in the organization's tag-line: "Advancing

the Science of Comfort....Affirming the Art of Caring" (AAHPM, 2008). Celebrating its 20th anniversary in 2008, the organization currently has 3300 members, which include physicians and other medical professionals. The ABHPM defined Palliative Medicine in 2000 as:

> ...the medical discipline of the broad therapeutic model known as palliative care. This discipline and model of care are devoted to achieve the best possible quality of life of the patient and family throughout the course of a life-threatening illness through the relief of suffering and the control of symptoms. Such relief requires the comprehensive assessment and interdisciplinary team management of the physical, psychological, social, and spiritual needs of patients and their families. Palliative medicine helps the patient and family face the prospect of death assured that comfort will be a priority, values and decisions will be respected, spiritual and psychological needs will be addressed, practical support will be available, and opportunities will exist for growth and resolution (von Gunten, Ferris, Portenoy, & Glajchen, 2001).

Palliative Care Nursing

Palliative care nursing parallels the continuing development of the art and science of palliative care. Individuals and families experiencing life-limiting progressive illness are the focus of the nurse's evidenced based physical, emotional psychosocial, and spiritual or existential care (Hospice and Palliative Nurses Association & American Nurses Association, 2007). Coyle (2006) describes the distinctive features of palliative care nursing as "a whole person" philosophy of care. This care is provided across the lifespan, in different care settings, and throughout the illness trajectory and the patient's death and the family's bereavement. A nurse's individual relationship with the patient and family is a critical part of the healing relationship. This healing relationship together with scientific knowledge (effective pain and symptom management) and clinical skills (addressing the emotion, psychosocial, spiritual needs and cultural values) is the essence of palliative care nursing, setting the specialty apart from other nursing specialty areas (Coyle, 2006, pp. 6–7). As a philosophy of care and therapeutic approach, palliative care can be practiced by all nurses (Coyle, 2006).

Professional Associations Related to Hospice and Palliative Nursing

The Alliance for Excellence in Hospice and Palliative Nursing (AEHPN) includes the National Board for Certification of Hospice and Palliative Nurses (NBCHPN), the Hospice and Palliative Nurses Association (HPNA), and the Hospice and Palliative Nurses Foundation (HPNF). The mission of the Alliance is to "serve as the unified voice in hospice and palliative nursing to integrate and coordinate end of life care with other members of the interdisciplinary team, to act as a visionary for specialty trending nursing issues, to be a primary resource fostering excellence in hospice and palliative nursing, and to advance end of life care for the benefit of the public at large" (AEHPN, 2004).

The NBCHPN offers four certification examinations: the advanced practice nurse (APN), the registered nurse (RN), licensed practical/vocational nurse (LPN/LVN), and nursing assistant (NA). Role-delineation studies were conducted to support the original certification examinations for each of the respective levels of nursing practice. The role delineation studies are repeated periodically to ensure that the certification examinations match the reality of clinical practice. Hospice and Palliative Nursing is the only nursing specialty that offers certification at all levels of practice.

The Hospice Nurses Association formed in 1987 to serve the networking and support needs of nurses caring for terminally patients and their families who were receiving hospice care. In 1998 the name of the organization was changed to the Hospice and Palliative Nurses Association (HPNA) to reflect the needs of nurses working in palliative care settings outside of the realm of hospice agencies. HPNA is now the largest professional nursing organization dedicated to care of those with life-threatening and terminal illness.

The HPNF was incorporated in 1998 to: (1) support research and education in end-of-life care; and (2) to strive to meet the strategic goals of the HPNA. The Foundation believes that evidenced-based-practice is the key to quality care for people with life-limiting and terminal illness. HPNF is a source for funding research and supporting education related to hospice and palliative care to both individuals and groups. In recognition of nursing's lack of a "cohesive commitment to palliative care nursing research" (Ferrell & Grant, 2006) and the lack of scientific knowledge to support clinical decisions, the HPNA Research Committee was given the charge to develop a research agenda that could guide nurse researchers in developing programs of research in palliative nursing and the HPNF in funding those programs (D.J. Sutermaster, personal communication, January 30, 2008).

Differentiating Hospice Care and Palliative Care

It is critical to differentiate between hospice care and palliative care in the context of clinical practice. The terms hospice and palliative care are frequently used interchangeably. Palliative care is a broader concept and includes the entire continuum of care. Hospice care is palliative care, but not all palliative care is hospice care.

Hospice is a specific type of palliative care, and in the United States it is generally considered a philosophy or program of care rather than a building of bricks and mortar. Hospice programs provide state-of-the-art palliative care and supportive services to dying persons and their families. This comprehensive care is available 24 hours a day, every day of the year in community-based settings, patients' homes, and facility-based care settings. A medically directed interdisciplinary team (clients, family members, professionals, and volunteers) provide physical, psychosocial, and spiritual care

CASE STUDY

Casey, Part I

Casey is a 70-year-old man who resides in an apartment with his 63-year-old wife. They have been married for 45 years. Casey has a 10-year history of Parkinson's disease. He has osteoarthritis in his back, coronary artery disease, hypertension, and dry macular degeneration in his left eye. His medications have kept him stable and able to enjoy his daily life. He is able to perform all of his own activities of daily living. The Parkinson's disease continues to progress slowly and requires him to use a cane.

Spontaneously one day he developed severe, acute pain in his right shoulder. His wife took him to an orthopedic surgeon to have the shoulder evaluated. The diagnosis was a torn rotator cuff. The surgeon explained that if they were going to perform surgery they needed to do it soon. Then Casey's wife explained the comorbidities: Parkinson's disease and coronary artery disease. It was then explained that rehabilitation after the surgical repair would be intense and painful. Casey's wife was very concerned that he would not have the stamina for the rehab, and that he might develop pneumonia after surgery and would experience intense pain.

The decision was made to confer with Casey's neurologist and cardiologist. Casey was still able to perform his own activities of daily living but his eating was more awkward since he was right-handed. Pain was controlled with extra strength Tylenol. The final decision was to forgo the surgical repair. The risk–benefit ratio was not worth it, and the cardiologist and the neurologist agreed.

Three months later Casey had full range of motion in his right shoulder without any pain. The tear had spontaneously healed.

Discussion Questions

1. Would you describe this situation as palliative care? If so, why? If not, why not?
2. What would have been your recommended plan of care for Casey?

Casey, Part II

Over the next 2 years Casey and his wife noticed that he was experiencing more difficulty walking. Pain from the osteoarthritis in his back limited the length of their outside walks. Casey had to stop frequently to rest. Over time his stamina and gait also declined. His neurologist increased the doses of his Parkinson's medications. Late one fall, Casey asked his wife if she thought his oldest daughter and son-in-law would come to celebrate Christmas, because he thought this would be his last one. His wife perked up and immediately asked, "Are you feeling ok?" He responded, "I'm ok, but I'm just weaker than last year."

Casey got his wish that Christmas—all those he invited were present and they enjoyed the celebration of this time together. No further critical incidents occurred until the following October. After one of his quarterly visits, Casey's neurologist took his wife aside and told her to prepare for coming changes. The doctor felt that Casey was at a tipping point, and increased dosage of the medications would not be effective. She suggested that Casey review his goals of care.

In December, Casey's ankles were very swollen so his cardiologist prescribed a more potent diuretic. A cascade of events followed: an extensive diuretic response, confusion, and inability to walk. These events all occurred around Christmas, so efforts to get a hospital bed and other equipment were difficult. His daughter was able to come and help care

(Continued)

▮ CASE STUDY (*Continued*)

for him. Home health care and an evaluation by physical therapy were ordered. Casey did not like the hospital bed or the wheelchair but accepted them, since his legs were no longer carrying the weight of his six-foot body.

Casey and his wife had completed their advance directives and living wills years ago. They knew hospice care was their choice. A month later the decision was made to enroll Casey in hospice home care. This choice would also provide his wife with support in caring for Casey. He was enrolled in hospice and died 26 days later at home with his wife, daughter, and son-in-law at his bedside. Although we are never prepared for the final goodbye, his wife found peace and comfort in the fulfillment of Casey's last wishes: he wanted to die at home with her present. Before and after Casey's

death there was minimal stress-related decision making because Casey, his wife, and family had discussed his wishes, documented them, and chose the healthcare providers that would support them along this final journey.

Discussion Questions

1. Discuss the indications that Casey was transitioning from palliative care to hospice care?
2. How would you have responded to Casey's request to celebrate Christmas at home?
3. What did the neurologist mean that Casey was at a "tipping point"?
4. Based on this case study how would you describe the differences between palliative and hospice care?

during the final phase of an illness, the process of imminently dying, and the period of bereavement (National Consensus Project, 2004). In hospice care the dying person and the family are the unit of care. Client and family values direct the care. However, the current Medicare hospice benefit eligibility criteria for hospice services include a terminal diagnosis and a 6-month prognosis. In addition, it requires that clients discontinue curative or life-prolonging treatments to access comprehensive hospice care (Lynn, 2001). There are three outcomes of hospice care: self-determined life closure; safe and comfortable dying, and effective grieving (National Hospice Organization Standards and Accreditation Committee, 1997). Humane, holistic, comprehensive plans of care involving an interdisciplinary healthcare team are critical to maintain quality of life for the person and family making the transition to end of life. In the United States hospice is the gold standard for end-of-life care (Billings, 1998).

One of the first definitions of palliative care accepted throughout the world was developed by

the World Health Organization (WHO) (1990). Subsequent definitions have been developed or refined by the National Hospice and Palliative Care Organization (NHPCO), IOM, and other professionals providing palliative care (Table 22-1). As the number of palliative care programs continue to grow, differentiating between hospice and palliative care is necessary for consumers and healthcare providers.

Although it appears that hospice and palliative care have much in common, there are two major distinctions. First, palliative care permits life-prolonging therapies. Secondly, palliative care is integrated throughout the course of a chronic, progressive, and incurable disease, from diagnosis through death, rather than only during the final 6 months of life. The chronic illness experience of clients and their families demonstrate the need for comprehensive palliative care earlier in the disease trajectory (Portenoy, 1998).

In response to the need for broadening the scope of palliative care, the Last Acts Palliative

---

TABLE 22-1

Definitions of Palliative Care with Distinctions from Hospice Care

World Health Organization (WHO)

The active total care of clients whose disease is not responsive to curative treatment. Control of pain, of other symptoms, and of psychological, social, and spiritual problems is paramount. The goal of palliative care is achievement of the best quality of life for clients and families. It affirms life and regards dying as a normal process. Palliative care neither hastens nor postpones death. It emphasizes relief from spiritual aspects of client care and offers a support system to help the family cope during the client's illness and in their own bereavement.

National Hospice and Palliative Care Organization (NHPCO)

The treatment that enhances comfort and improves the quality of an individual's life during the last phase of life. No specific therapy is excluded from consideration. The test of palliative care lies in the agreement between the individual, physician(s), primary caregiver, and the hospice team that the expected outcome is relief from distressing symptoms, the easing of pain, and/or enhancing the quality of life. The decision to intervene with active palliative care is based on an ability to meet the stated goals rather than affect the underlying disease. An individual's needs must continue to be assessed and all treatment options explored and evaluated in the context of the individual's values and symptoms. The individual's choices and decisions regarding care are paramount and must be followed.

Institute of Medicine (IOM)

Palliative care seeks to prevent, relieve, reduce, or soothe the symptoms of disease or disorder without effecting a cure (Field & Cassel, 1997).

Distinctions Between Hospice and Palliative Care

The Center to Advance Palliative Care (CAPC) developed a Web site for patients and their families (www.getpalliativecare.org). The Web site states that: Palliative care is not the same as hospice care. Palliative care may be provided at any time during a person's illness, even from the time of diagnosis. And, it may be given at the same time as curative treatment. Hospice care always provides palliative care. However, it is focused on terminally ill patients—people who no longer seek treatments to cure them and who are expected to live for about 6 months or less.

Sources: Center to Advance Palliative Care. Resources for patients and families. Retrieved on February 1, 2008 from http://getpalliativecare.org; Field, M.J., & Cassel, C.K. (Eds.). (1997). *Approaching death: Improving care at the end of life.* Committee on Care at the End of Life, Division of Health Care Services, Institute of Medicine. Washington, DC: National Academy Press; National Hospice and Palliative Care Organization (NHPCO). Retrieved on January 28, 2008 from http://www.nhpco.org; WHO (World Health Organization). (1990). *Cancer pain relief and palliative care.* WHO Technical Report Series 804 (p.11).Geneva: WHO.

Care Task Force reformulated palliative care to include all persons with serious or life-threatening illness. The Last Acts Palliative Care Task Force developed five palliative care precepts or principles of care (Table 22-2). Integration of these precepts into clinical practice enables clinicians to provide a continuum of care otherwise unavailable to clients with advancing illness and their families (Cumming & Okun, 2004).

Palliative Care and Chronic Illness

According to Curtin and Lubkin (1995), chronic illness is never completely cured and it involves the "total human environment for supportive care and self-care, maintenance of function and prevention of further disability" (pp. 6–7). Symptoms may increase or decrease during phases of stability, exacerbation, remission, and eventually death (Corbin, 2001).

TABLE 22-2

Precepts of Palliative Care

1. Respecting patient goals, preferences, and choices
2. Providing comprehensive caring
3. Utilizing the strengths of interdisciplinary resources
4. Acknowledging and addressing caregiver concerns
5. Building systems and mechanisms of support

Source: Lomax, K.J., & Scanlon, C. (1997). *Precepts of palliative care.* Princeton, NJ: The Robert Wood Johnson Foundation.

Palliative care seeks to treat, reduce, or prevent symptoms of diseases, relieve suffering, and improve the patient and family's quality of life without affecting a cure. It is not restricted to dying hospice patients (Field & Cassel, 1997). The principles of palliative care extend to broader populations that could benefit from holistic, comprehensive plans of care involving interdisciplinary healthcare teams from the time of diagnosis and throughout the disease processes and illness trajectory.

According to Charles von Guten (2001), palliative care is interdisciplinary care that focuses on relief of suffering and improving quality of life. This simple definition illustrates the fit between chronic illness and palliative care. Based on the preceding description, it is clear that persons with chronic illness would benefit from palliative care.

PROBLEMS AND BARRIERS RELATED TO PALLIATIVE CARE

Barriers to palliative care exist for numerous reasons. The major underlying resistance to palliative care stems from a medical philosophy that emphasizes cure and prolongation of life over the quality of life and relief of suffering (Morrison & Meier, 2004). Insurance reimbursement also forces consumer choice between cure and comfort care. Regular Medicare only reimburses for curative treatment, leaving the Medicare hospice benefit

to cover comfort care (Fisher, Wennberg, Stukel, Gottlieb, Lucas, & Pinder, 2003).

The SUPPORT study (1995) findings identified several problems related to palliative care. Patient suffering included dying in pain with a severe symptom burden. Poor communication among patients, families, and their physicians led to undesired resuscitation efforts and extensive use of hospital resources.

Communication is a core skill of palliative care. However, many clinicians are uncomfortable sharing bad news and poor prognoses. Recent studies suggest that "patient-centered" interviews are associated with improved levels of satisfaction on the part of patients and their families (Dowsett et al., 2000; Steinhauser et al., 2000).

The IOM (Field & Cassel, 1997) study, *Approaching Death: Improving Care at the End of Life*, revealed a critical need for improvement in the education and training of healthcare professionals in palliative and end-of-life care. Healthcare professionals have traditionally received inadequate education and training in the safe and effective management of pain and other symptoms. They also lack the skills and confidence to address the psychological, social, and spiritual aspects of care (Sullivan, Lakoma, & Block, 2003).

Nursing curricula and textbooks were found to be deficient in palliative and end-of-life content and clinical learning opportunities. If nurses are not taught that their professional role includes providing quality palliative and end-of-life care, then they cannot practice it (Ferrell, Virani, & Grant, 1999). In response to these identified needs, resources for teaching palliative care nursing to students and practicing nurses have been and continue to be developed and disseminated. Essential nursing competencies in end-of-life care were proposed and disseminated by the American Association of Colleges of Nursing (AACN) in the document entitled "Peaceful Death" (American Association of Colleges of Nursing, 1998). Matzo and Sherman (2001, 2006) used the AACN competencies as the framework for their nursing textbook entitled *Palliative Care Nursing: Quality*

Care to the End of Life. Ferrell and Coyle (2001, 2006) wrote a comprehensive volume entitled the *Textbook of Palliative Nursing.* An indication that the science of palliative care continues to grow is that these two textbooks are both in their second editions. Recognizing the special needs of older adults, Matzo and Sherman also authored a textbook entitled *Gerontologic Palliative Care Nursing* (2004). Morrison and Meier, two expert palliative care physicians, authored the textbook, *Geriatric Palliative Care* (2003).

Prognostication in chronic, debilitating, and life-threatening illness presents a major challenge for healthcare professionals and is a barrier to adequate palliative care (Christakis & Lamont, 2000). Our current healthcare system forces patients and families to choose between curative treatment and comfort care. However, there is growing recognition that palliative care is needed from diagnosis through the process of dying (Foley, 2001). Reiterating von Guten's (1999) definition of palliative care: interdisciplinary care focused on the relief of suffering and improving quality of life, removes any burden of prognostication and the requirement of a terminal diagnosis.

The public's lack of understanding related to the options available to dying patients and their families results in delayed access to hospice and palliative care services (Field & Cassel, 1997). Surveys consistently indicate patients prefer to die at home. However, in 2003, for all Americans who died: approximately 25% died at home; 25% died in a nursing facility, and approximately 50% of the deaths occurred in a hospital. In comparison 74.1% of hospice patients died at a place that was currently their "home" (private residence, nursing home, or other residential facility), but not in an acute care hospital setting (NHPCO, 2007). Consumers' and communities' lack of understanding of what comprehensive palliative care programs offer, and poor communication about patient and family preferences and denial of death, all impede timely referrals to palliative care services [End of Life Nursing Education Consortium (ELNEC) Curriculum, Module 1, 2005].

Family Caregiving: Burden

In palliative care, the client and family are the unit of care. Family caregivers provide supportive care throughout the chronic illness trajectory, in all care settings, and for all types of needs (McMillan, 2004). The caregiver's burden is increasing significantly as more complex health care moves into the home setting. Evidence is growing that extended service as a caregiver can negatively impact the physical, social, and emotional well-being of caregivers (Pinquart & Sorenson, 2003). Some caregivers experience sustained stress related to highly stressful times of caregiving, and this negatively impacts their bereavement process (Schultz et al., 2003; Schultz, Newsom, Fleissner, DeCamp, & Nieboer, 1997).

Successful intervention studies have been carried out with caregivers of clients with Alzheimer's disease, but little has been done with caregivers of hospice and palliative care clients. The NIH Consensus Statement on Improving End of Life Care (2004) concluded that more randomized clinical trials examining decreasing caregiver burden are needed. Studies are needed to determine which caregivers are at greatest risk for distress and specific interventions that are most likely to relieve the distress (see Chapter 9, on family caregiving).

Although these barriers seem overwhelming, progress has been made since the release of the two seminal reports (SUPPORT and IOM) brought to the forefront the unfavorable conditions of dying persons in the United States to the national healthcare agenda.

■ INTERVENTIONS

The IOM report made seven recommendations (see Table 22-3) to resolve the four identified areas of deficiency in palliative and end-of-life care. Change is occurring in part because of the increased involvement of healthcare consumers of the 21st century in the issues related to quality of care, quality of life, advance care planning, and the burdens of caregiving (Berry, 2004).

Approximately 100 articles have been published based on the findings of the SUPPORT study. Implications of the data for future reform suggest that improved, individual, patient-level decision-making may not be the most effective strategy for improving end-or-life care. The SUPPORT investigators recommend system-level innovations and quality improvement in routine care as potentially effective strategies for change (Lynn et al., 2000).

Interventions for palliative care must relate to the domains of its science and practice. Researchers (Emanuel & Emanuel, 1998; Steinhauser et al., 2000; and Teno, 2001) and professional organizations such as the National Hospice and Palliative Care Organization (2006) and the American Geriatrics Society (Lynn, 1997) have published standards of care as well as philosophical or conceptual frameworks describing proposed domains of end-of-life care (Ferrell, 2004).

A major advancement of the science and practice of palliative care occurred with the release of the Clinical Practice Guidelines by the National Consensus Project for Quality Palliative Care (NCPQPC) (2004). Groups that participated in the NCPQPC were the American Academy of Hospice

---

TABLE 22-3

Recommendations from the IOM Committee on Care at the End of Life

1. People with advanced, potentially fatal illnesses and those close to them should be able to expect and receive reliable, skillful, and supportive care.
2. Physicians, nurses, social workers, and other health professionals must commit themselves to improving care for dying patients and to using existing knowledge effectively to prevent and relieve pain and other symptoms.
3. Because many deficiencies in care reflect system problems, policymakers, consumer groups, and purchases of health care should work with healthcare providers and researchers to:

    a. strengthen methods for measuring the quality of life and other outcomes of care for dying patients and those close to them;

    b. develop better tools and strategies for improving the quality of care and holding healthcare organizations accountable for care at the end of life;

    c. revise mechanisms for financing care so that they encourage rather than impede good end-of-life care and sustain rather than frustrate coordinated systems of excellent care; and

    d. reform drug prescription laws, burdensome regulations, and state medical board policies and practices that impede effective use of opioids to relieve pain and suffering.

4. Educators and other healthcare professionals should initiate changes in undergraduate, graduate, and continuing education to ensure that practitioners have the relevant attitudes, knowledge, and skills to care well for dying patients.
5. Palliative care should become, if not a medical specialty, at least a defined area of expertise, education, and research.
6. The nation's research establishment should define and implement priorities for strengthening the knowledge base for end-of-life care.
7. A continuing public discussion is essential to develop a better understanding of the modern experience of dying, the options available to dying patients and families, and the obligations of communities to those approaching death.

Source: Field, M.J., & Cassel, C.K. (Eds.). (1997). *Approaching death: Improving care at the end of life.* Committee on Care at the End of Life, Division of Health Care Services, Institute of Medicine (pp. 270–271). Washington, DC: National Academy Press.

and Palliative Medicine, the Center to Advance Palliative Care, the Hospice and Palliative Nurses Association, the Last Acts Partnership, and the National Hospice and Palliative Care Organization. The purpose of the NCPQPC was to establish Clinical Practice Guidelines that promoted care that was consistent and high quality, and guided the development and structure of new and existing palliative care services. The 2-year consensus process involved the review of 2000 articles from the literature, 31 consensus documents and standards, and peer review by 200 experts in the field (Ferrell, 2004). The purposes of the Clinical Practice Guidelines for Quality Palliative Care are to:

- Facilitate the development and continuing improvement of clinical palliative care programs providing care to patients and families with life-threatening or debilitating illness.
- Establish uniformly accepted definitions of the essential elements in palliative care that promote quality, consistency, and reliability of these services.
- Establish national goals for access to quality palliative care.
- Foster performance measurement and quality improvement initiatives in palliative care services (Ferrell, 2004, p. 30).

Recognizing a need for clarity in the definitions of key concepts or domains of end-of-life care and a framework for advancing research and practice, the NCP developed the following domains.

- Domain 1: Structure and processes of care
- Domain 2: Physical aspects of care
- Domain 3: Psychological and psychiatric aspects of care
- Domain 4: Social aspects of care
- Domain 5: Spiritual, religious, and existential aspects of care
- Domain 6: Cultural aspects of care
- Domain 7: Care of the imminently dying patient
- Domain 8: Ethical and legal aspects of care

Determining Goals of Care

These domains identified by the NCPQPC guide decision-making regarding research, practice, and policy. Each domain is an area for an intervention for improving end-of-life care and meeting the needs of palliative care patients and families. Palliative care interventions logically flow from goals of care. Therefore, the first step in palliative care is to establish the goals of care (Morrison & Meier, 2004). In the context of chronic, debilitating, and life-threatening illness, realistic and attainable goals of care that relieve pain and other symptoms, improve quality of life, limit the burden of care, enhance personal relationships, and provide a sense of control are crucial to the dying person and their families (Steinhauser et al., 2000; Singer, Martin, & Kelner, 1999).

Healthcare professionals must work with clients and their families to establish appropriate goals of care. Using open-ended and probing questions may be helpful when interviewing the client (Morrison & Meier, 2004). Examples of possible questions are: "What makes live worth living for you?" "Given the severity of your illness, what are the most important things for you to achieve?" "What are your most important hopes?" "What are your biggest fears?" and "What would you consider to be a fate worse than death?" (Quill, 2000).

Goals of care are dynamic across the trajectory of a disease (EPEC Project, 2004; Quill, 2000). Meier, Back, and Morrison (2001) describe some of the warning signs of ineffective or contradictory goals as: frequent or lengthy hospitalizations, physician feelings of frustration, anger or powerlessness, and feelings of caregiver burden.

Assessment and Treatment of Symptoms

A core principle of palliative care is comprehensive care that includes the relief of pain and other symptoms (Steinhauser et al., 2000). Effective symptom management begins with a thorough assessment. Research findings support the practice of routine and standardized symptom assessment with validated instruments (Morrison & Meier, 2004). Benefits attributed to routine assessments include identification of overlooked or unreported symptoms (Bookbinder et al., 1996; Manfredi et al., 2000). Dissemination and increased use of the same validated instruments will facilitate the comparison of findings across practice settings and research studies. The Center to Advance Palliative Care (www.capc.org) and Brown University's Center for Gerontology and Health Care Research provide access to clinically useful instruments through their respective Web sites. Brown's Web site features a tool kit of instruments to measure end-of-life care (www.chcr.brown.edu/pcoc/tool-kit.htm).

The nursing assessment of clients who are receiving palliative care is the same as a standard nursing assessment. However, the palliative care assessment focuses on enhancing the client's quality of life. Ferrell's (1995) quality of life framework is useful in organizing the assessment according to four domains: physical, psychological, social, and spiritual well-being. Based on the changing needs of clients and families across the trajectory of the chronic illness, quality of life should be assessed four times: (1) at the time of diagnosis; (2) treatment, post-treatment; (3) long term survival or terminal phase; and (4) active dying. A comprehensive assessment serves as the foundation for goal-setting, developing a plan of care, implementing interventions, and evaluating the outcomes and effectiveness of care (Glass, Cluxton, & Rancour, 2001).

The prevalence and symptom burden for clients at the end of life is high. According to the NIH State of the Science Consensus Statement on Improving End-of-Life Care (2004), assessment and management of symptoms have been studied most thoroughly in clients with cancer. Clients with other life-limiting illnesses, such as congestive heart failure, have their own challenges. Regardless of the diagnosis, there are symptoms common to advanced disease (see Chapter 17). These common symptoms include anorexia and cachexia, anxiety, constipation, depression, delirium, dyspnea, nausea, and pain (Morrison & Meier, 2004). It is beyond the scope of this chapter to describe in detail the assessment and management recommendations for these symptoms; however, there are numerous resources in the literature with specific protocols and interventions. [Examples include the AGS Panel on Persistent Pain in Older Persons (2002); Block (2000); Casarett & Inouye (2001); Luce & Luce (2001); and Strasser & Bruera (2002).]

Palliative care is needed across the lifespan, and assessments and interventions should be tailored to the specific population served. Often the literature categorizes adults as a homogenous group needing palliative care. Experts in gerontology, however, are calling for recognition of the unique palliative care needs of older adults (Cassel, 2003). Amella (2003) described the common goal of helping clients experience the best quality of life as the touchstone for collaboration between geriatric and palliative care nurse specialists. Symptoms of illness and dying may appear differently, for longer periods, and in greater numbers in older adults (Amella, 2003). Pain, confusion, dyspnea, fatigue, satiety and anorexia, gastrointestinal distress, infection and fever and fears and depression are symptoms that can present differently in older adults.

At the other end of the lifespan, initiatives are underway that address palliative care in children. In 2003, the IOM released its report, *When Children Die: Improving Palliative and End-of-Life Care for Children and Their Families* (Field & Behrman, *2003*). The report identified challenges that can be used to focus efforts and resources to improve palliative care for children and their families (see Table 22-4). Many palliative care textbooks are now including chapters addressing pediatric palliative care (Ferrell & Coyle, 2006).

Advance Directives

Following the establishment of the goals of care, the next logical intervention is the completion of

TABLE 22-4

Four Basic Challenges to Improve Pediatric Palliative Care

1. Children should have care that is focused on their special needs and the needs of their families.
2. Health plans should make it easier for children and families to get palliative care.
3. Healthcare professionals should be trained to give palliative care to children.
4. Researchers should find out more about what care works best for children.

Source: Field, M.J., & Behrman, R.E. (Eds.). (2003). *When children die: Improving palliative and end-of-life care for children and their families.* Washington, DC: National Academy Press.

advance directives. Goals of care reflect the values, beliefs, and culture of the person with a serious, life-threatening illness. Numerous studies (Miles, Koepp, & Weber, 1996) report that most people do not have advance directives and that the documents that do exist are ineffective in improving communication between clients and their physicians (Morrison & Meier, 2004). Other authors report that advance directives are ineffective related to the decision-making relative to cardiopulmonary resuscitation (Teno et al., 1997). Morrison and Meier (2004) suggest that as the number of advance directives increase, more consumers and healthcare professionals will become familiar with the documents, thus improving their effectiveness.

However, current literature suggests that the focus of advanced care planning should shift to determine an acceptable quality of life and goals of care (Fried, Bradley, Towle, & Allore, 2002; Meier & Morrison, 2002). This type of discussion is the crucial element, not the mere completion of the forms. Consumers and healthcare professionals can use a variety of resources such as the *Caring Conversations Program* developed through the Center for Practical Bioethics. Workbooks can be purchased that help families discuss their

values and wishes regarding medical treatment if they cannot speak for themselves. More information is available at www.practicalbioethics.org It is also important to be aware of your state's required documents and process for the completion of advance directives. The process and forms vary from state to state. The names of the documents may also vary. The basic two forms are: (1) Power of Attorney for Health Care (this document appoints an agent or proxy who becomes the decision-maker when the person can no longer do so) and (2) Directive to Physician (Living Will) (this document gives direction to a physician regarding what type of care/procedures are wanted or not wanted—for example, artificial nutrition, hydration, or mechanical ventilation—if the individual cannot speak for him/herself.

Psychosocial, Spiritual, and Bereavement Needs

Psychosocial, spiritual, and bereavement care are key components of palliative care. Professional and accrediting bodies such as Joint Commission on Accreditation of Hospital Organizations (JCAHO) requires documentation of spiritual assessments of patients. Members of interdisciplinary palliative care teams assess and intervene to meet the spiritual and psychosocial needs of clients and their families. Bereavement support is part of the follow-up after an individual dies. Research demonstrates that family members with spiritual and psychological distress are more likely to experience an extended or complicated grief and bereavement process (McClain, Rosenfield, & Breitbart, 2003).

Acknowledgement of spiritual distress, alone, can be an intervention. However, a common language and mutual comfort must be present for a meaningful exchange to occur (Chochinov, 2004). Helping clients die with dignity is a basic tenet of palliative care. Empirical work with dying clients found that the paradigm of dignity, which includes matters of spirituality, meaning, purpose, and other psychosocial issues related to dying, was acceptable language and topics for discussion

(Chochinov et al., 2004). This work is adding to the growing empirical evidence that palliative care is more than symptom management and must include the spiritual, psychosocial, and existential concerns.

Chochinov's research team developed a Dignity Model (2004), which serves as the basis for the psychotherapeutic intervention, Dignity Therapy. The phase I data from this work is undergoing analysis at the present time. Those results will be the basis for a randomized clinical trial which will "attempt to further establish the efficacy of this approach to addressing suffering, distress, or paucity of meaning and purpose in patients nearing death" (Chochinov et al., 2004, p. 140).

Culture and Palliative Care

Culture is a defining component of the human experience. Each individual's culture provides the sense of security, belonging, and guidelines regarding how to live and die [End of Life Nursing Education Consortium (ELNEC), 2005]. Cultural diversity refers to differences between people based on shared teachings, beliefs, customs, language, and so forth, which influence both an individual's and family's response to illness, treatment, death, and bereavement (Showalter, 1998). Despite the enormous differences among individuals, an understanding of common cultural characteristics is helpful in providing culturally sensitive and effective care (Kemp, 1999). It is beyond the scope of this chapter to describe all the cultural perspectives of individual populations regarding dying, death, and bereavement. However, it is important to be aware of the principles of culturally sensitive care to provide quality palliative care for clients and their families. Table 22-5 outlines 10 principles of culturally sensitive care originally developed by the Council on Social Work Education (CSWE) Faculty Development Institute, 2001, as cited in Sherman (2004).

An example of the cultural beliefs of Hispanic Americans (Latinos) that may impact palliative

---

TABLE 22-5

Principles of Culturally Sensitive Care

Healthcare providers should:

1. Be knowledgeable about cultural values and attitudes
2. Attend to diverse communication styles
3. Ask the patient for his/her preferences for decision-making early in the care process
4. Recognize cultural differences and varying comfort levels with regard to personal space, eye contact, touch, time orientation, learning styles, and conversation styles
5. Use a cultural guide from the palliative care patient's ethnic or religious background
6. Get to know the community, its people, and its resources available for social support
7. Create a culturally friendly physical environment (e.g., decorate facilities with artwork or pictures valued by the cultural groups to whom care is most commonly provided.
8. Determine the acceptability of patients; being physically examined by a practitioner of a different gender.
9. Advocate for availability of services, accessibility in terms of cost and location, and acceptability of services that are compatible with cultural values and practices of the person served.
10. Conduct a self-assessment of the healthcare provider's own beliefs about illness and death

Source: Adapted from Council on Social Work Education (CSWE) Faculty Development Institute, 2001 as cited in Sherman, D.W. (2004). Cultural and spiritual backgrounds of older adults. In M.L. Matzo & D.W. Sherman (Eds.) *Gerontologic palliative care nursing* (p. 11). St. Louis: Mosby.

care for this population follows. Hispanics from Mexico, Puerto Rico, and Central and South America all have distinct cultures. However, many non-Hispanics use the frequently shared language (Spanish) or religion (Catholicism) to group these clients together.

Sullivan (2001) identified Latino views regarding end-of-life care using focus groups as the method of data collection. The focus groups were conducted in Latino communities. The Latino participants believed: they could not communicate effectively with healthcare providers due to language barriers; and they did not understand the concept of informed consent even with the use of interpreters. Latinos believe it is the responsibility of the family to care for their relatives and not send them away to nursing homes. Consequently, these participants did not want to die in nursing homes. Most of the participants were unaware of hospice services or had inaccurate information. Religious beliefs, primarily reliance on God, and fatalism were critical components of their decision-making regarding end-of-life care. Racial discrimination and cultural insensitivity were perceived by many of the participants.

Several beliefs in the Hispanic culture can influence the experience of palliative care for individuals. Many Hispanic families will assume the responsibility of caring for their dying member at home based on their belief in strong family support, including extended family members. The dying member is protected from the prognosis. A major challenge to thorough pain assessment in palliative care is the reluctance of Hispanics to acknowledge, report, or describe pain. Stoicism is highly regarded. However, moaning is acceptable but cannot serve as a valid indicator of the severity of pain (Kemp, 1999). Although death is an adversity, funerals are an integral part of family life, lasting several days. They hold a belief in the afterlife. The Day of the Dead is celebrated in November on the same day that All Souls Day is celebrated in the Catholic religion. Day of the Dead is a day of celebration with special foods and decorating of the graves.

Education for Healthcare Professionals

The American Association of Colleges of Nursing (AACN) and City of Hope National Medical Center received major funding from The Robert Wood Johnson Foundation for the development and dissemination of the ELNEC Curriculum. Versions for baccalaureate, graduate, continuing education/in-service, pediatric, oncology, and geriatric nurses and nurse educators have been developed with Train-the-Trainer methodology utilized. A quarterly newsletter "ELNEC Connections" is sent to all ELNEC trainers. The newsletter provides updates, ongoing resources, and project ideas from the ELNEC staff as well as trainers throughout the country. Collegial sharing is in the spirit of improving and disseminating the science and art of palliative care nursing. One of the outcomes of the project was the award-winning series of palliative care articles that ran every other month in the *American Journal of Nursing* from August 2004 through December 2006 and included 17 articles.

Physicians have a parallel program to ELNEC: The EPEC Project, Education on Palliative and End of Life Care. However, the mission is to educate ALL healthcare professionals on the essential clinical competencies in palliative care. Conferences using the Train-the-Trainer methodology are also used. In addition, the entire curriculum is now available on-line (see www.epec.net). Another useful resource for healthcare professionals is the End of Life/Palliative Education Resource Center found at www.eperc.mcw.edu. Its purpose is advancing end-of-life care through an on-line community of educational scholars. Case studies, presentations, and articles are a few of the resources available.

Research

The continued evolution of palliative care to meet the needs of an aging population rests in part on research. These needs include interventions to manage the symptoms and distress of chronic illness. However, the knowledge base to support symptom management, communication, and decision-making skills and models for the delivery of palliative care are inadequate. The National Palliative Care Research Center (NPCRC) (refer to www.npcrc.org) was developed in direct response to this need and consistent recommendations from multiple IOM reports and the National Institute of Health's State of the Science Conferences on End-of-Life Care (2004) for the development of a prioritized research agenda, researchers committed to palliative care research, as well as a developing new generation of palliative care researchers. NPCRC's initial funding of research grant proposals occurred in 2007. The NPCRC is located in New York City, and receives direction and technical assistance from the Mount Sinai School of Medicine. It also works closely with the Center to Advance Palliative Care.

The National Hospice and Palliative Care Organization (NHPCO) developed a Research Agenda in 2004 to guide researchers in developing the scientific knowledge to support hospice and palliative care. The broad topics include improving access to hospice and palliative care, improving the quality of hospice and palliative care, and improving the conduct of research in hospice and palliative care.

Goldstein and Morrison (2005) called for a new research agenda for geriatric palliative care. Their premise, based on the NIH (National Institutes of Health, 2004) and IOM (Field & Cassel, 1997; Cleeland, 2001) reports, was that the evidence base for palliative care in older adults is sparse. Adults 75 years or older, with comorbidities, and noncancer diagnoses have repeatedly been excluded from palliative care research. Their proposed research agenda for palliative care in geriatrics includes the following: (1) establishing the prevalence of symptoms in patients with chronic disease, (2) evaluating the association between symptom treatment and outcomes, (3) increasing the evidence base for symptom treatment, (4) understanding patients' psychological/spiritual well-being and quality of life, (5) elucidating sources of caregiver burden, (6) reevaluating service delivery, (7) adapting research methodologies specifically for palliative care, and (8) increasing the number of geriatricians trained in palliative care research (2005, p. 1594).

As we build the science supporting the practice of palliative care, the question becomes whether the research, education, and clinical interventions already funded to improve care for individuals with life-limiting or terminal illnesses were effective. Measuring the effectiveness of palliative care is a challenge that requires both prospective and retrospective studies (Steinhauser, 2004). Four challenges exist related to outcome measurement in palliative care:

1. End of life is a complex multidimensional experience in which understanding of the interrelatedness of domains is unclear.
2. The period "end of life" is ill-defined.
3. Both patient and family are the unit of care, yet little is known about the correlations between the trajectories of their experiences.
4. Patients, the primary focus of care, are often unable to communicate in their last days or weeks, rendering their subjective experience unable to be evaluated (Steinhauser, 2004, p. 33).

Palliative Care and Genomics

The sequence of the human genome was completed in April 2003. Advances in technology now allow the exploration of genetic material ranging from genetic screening to genomic-based therapies (Conley & Tinkle, 2007). The genetic risk for many diseases, such as Huntington disease, can be determined, but there is no cure yet available (Heitkemper & Bond, 2003). How does this apply to hospice and palliative care? This discussion focuses on three connections between palliative care and genomics: pharmacogenomics, family history, and nurse competencies in genetics and genomics. (See Table 22-6 for definitions of terms used in this section.)

Pharmacogenetics (role of inheritance in the individual variation in drug response) has converged with knowledge from the sequencing of the

TABLE 22-6

Definition of Terms Related to Genetics and Genomics

Allele—An alternative form of a gene.

Genetics—The study of individual genes and their impact on relatively rare single gene disorders (Guttmacher & Collins, 2002).

Genomics—The study of the functions and interactions of all the genes in the genome, including their interactions with environmental factors (Guttmacher & Collins, 2002).

Genotype—A person's genetic makeup as reflected by his or her DNA sequence.

Pharmacogenetics—The study of genetic factors that influence an organism's reaction to a drug (Howe & Eggert, 2007).

Pharmacogenomics—The study of how an individual's genetic inheritance affects the body's response to drugs (Howe & Eggert, 2007).

Phenotype—The clinical presentation or expression of specific gene or genes, environmental factors, or both (Guttmacher & Collins, 2002).

human genome resulting in pharmacogenomics (effect of DNA sequencing on the effect of a drug; science combining pharmacology and genomics) (Weinshilboum, 2003). Medications are a major intervention for symptom management in palliative care. It is important that physicians and nurses, including those in palliative, care understand the impact of genotypic variation on the therapeutic effect and adverse effects of medications. The cytochrome P450 system is an example. A specific cytochrome enzyme, CYP2D6, converts codeine to morphine. Genotypic variants of the CYP2D6 enzyme in 5–10% of the population results in too little or no CYP2D6 enzyme produced. Therefore, these individuals cannot change codeine into morphine and have little or no analgesic relief with codeine or codeine-derivative medications (e.g., hydrocodone, oxycodone, ethylmorphine, and dihydrocodeine) (Howe & Eggert, 2007; Meyer, 2000; Prows, 2004).

Scientists discovered genetic variations in the gene that plays a major role in an individual's initial sensitivity to warfarin treatment (Schwarz et al., 2008). Members of the NIH Pharmacogenetics Research Network found that these variations explain why some patients require a higher or lower dose to reach the therapeutic benefit of the drug. The Food and Drug Administration (FDA) now recommends genetic testing to assist in the

quick and precise determination of optimal warfarin doses. These are just two examples that illustrate the impact of pharmacogenomics in providing safe and effective care regardless of the trajectory of their illness.

In palliative care, the patient and the family are the unit of care. However, what is the impact of a family's health history? Is the patient who is receiving palliative care worried about an illness that may be transmitted to other family members? Are family members concerned that they may be carriers for an incurable disease? The US Surgeon General spearheaded the Family History Initiative. Family history is the best inexpensive, noninvasive genetic test available (http://familyhistory.hhs.gov). Many diseases "run in" families. Detailed family histories allow individuals at risk to be identified and to implement disease-prevention strategies. Patterns of inheritance may be sources of guilt in persons with advanced disease or concerns of bereaved individuals. The current palliative literature does not yet discuss these types of concerns.

Finally, what is the role of palliative care for individuals diagnosed with genetic diseases? How can palliative care providers help those diagnosed with the genotype for a terminal disease that is not yet expressed? Huntington's disease is such an example. These individuals would benefit from the support of palliative care.

The Hospice and Palliative Nurses Association along with 48 other professional nursing organizations have endorsed the Genetic and Genomic Nursing Competencies (http://www.genome.gov/17517037). Regardless of specialty and setting, all nurses need to understand that all diseases have a genetic and genomic component. Patients and their families may turn to the nurse seeking genetic and genomic information involved in the prevention, screening, diagnostics, prognostics, and selection of and effectiveness of treatment. Within the context of hospice and palliative care, requests for this information may occur during bereavement, and thus add another layer of complexity to the grief process. The following are two examples of the competencies relevant to the preceding discussion.

Domain: Professional Responsibility
■ Incorporate genetic and genomic technologies and information into registered nurse practice

Domain: Professional Practice
■ Demonstrates an understanding of genetics/genomics to health, prevention, selection of treatment, monitoring of treatment effectiveness. (Consensus Panel, 2006)

It may have seemed strange to some readers to find a section of this chapter related to genomics and palliative acre. Palliative care is not practiced in a vacuum. We must be aware of the advances in science that impact the health of our patients and their families prior to their interactions with us. The advances in the science of comfort and the art of caring must converge to improve the quality of life for those with life-limiting or terminal illness.

OUTCOMES

Outcomes research in palliative care continues to develop. There is consensus about the broad domains related to end of life: physical or psychosocial symptoms, social relationships, spiritual or philosophical beliefs, hopes, expectation and meaning, satisfaction, economic considerations, and caregiver and family experiences. Quality of life is also considered an outcome, but quality of life needs a clearer definition and consistent measurement in order to strengthen the relationship.

The Center to Advance Palliative Care (CAPC) has identified major outcomes of palliative care (www.capc.org). They include: (1) relief of pain and other distressing symptoms; (2) clear communication and decision-making regarding goals of care and development of treatment plans; (3) completion of life-prolonging or curative treatments; and (4) increased patient and family satisfaction; and (5) ease of referral to appropriate care settings to achieve the goals of care, resulting in reduced hospital and intensive care unit (ICU) length of stay and cost. The next steps in palliative care are to develop the science, the care delivery systems, and the instruments to deliver and evaluate the outcomes of quality palliative care.

Morrison (2005) eloquently described the progress of the palliative care movement in the United States as well as the next steps that need to be taken to continue to meet the needs of an aging population.

As we look at the growth and development of the field of palliative care in the United States, we have moved from recognition of a public health crisis (poor quality of life for patients with serious illness and their families), to identifying the system and care gaps that result in this compromised quality of life (inadequate assessment and treatment of pain and other symptoms, disjointed and unclear goals of care, poor transition management), to developing interventions (palliative care education at all levels of professional training, creation of hospital-based palliative care teams) to address these care and system gaps. What is now needed is comprehensive and rigorous research to evaluate the effect of well-delineated and generalizable palliative care structures and process on important clinical and utilization outcomes to guide the further development of the field (Morrison, 2005, p. 14).

EVIDENCE-BASED PRACTICE BOX

This study compared the effects of a nurse-led intervention focused on specific nurse strategies as compared with usual care in a randomized clinical trial of 406 minority adults in Harlem, New York. During the 12-month study, bilingual nurses counseled patients on diet, medication adherence, and self-management through an initial visit and regularly scheduled follow-up telephone calls. The majority of the patients (45%) were classified as New York Heart Association (NYHA) Class IV heart failure. Outcome measures were hospitalization and self-reported functioning at 12 months. At the study's end, the nurse-managed patients had fewer hospitalizations and better functioning than the "usual care" patients.

Source: Sisk, J., Hebert, P., Horowitz, C., MaLguhlin, M., Wang, J., & Chassin, M. (2006). Effects of nurse management on the quality of heart failure care in minority communities. *Annals of Internal Medicine, 145,* 273–283.

STUDY QUESTIONS

1. Discuss the differences in the definitions of palliative care listed in Table 22-1.
2. Describe how the goals of care might differ for an 85-year-old man diagnosed with heart failure (HF) at the time of diagnosis and goals of care in an advanced stage of the illness.
3. Explain the statement: hospice care is palliative care but not all palliative care is hospice care.
4. Differentiate between hospice and palliative care.
5. List the domains of end-of-life care developed by the National Consensus Project.
6. Identify barriers to palliative care for an individual with a serious, life-limiting illness.
7. Identify the components of Ferrell's framework/model for quality of life.
8. What is your vision of palliative care?
9. Discuss how stoicism may impact palliative care for a Latino grandmother?
10. List three online resources to use to continue your education in palliative care.
11. Go online and find support information appropriate for the family caregiver of a palliative care patient.
12. Describe how you could you use *Integrity of the Person: A Conceptual Framework for End-of-Life Care* as an organizing framework in your clinical practice.
13. Identify two nurse competencies in genetics and genomics.
14. Discuss how pharmacogenomics can help relieve the pain for future patients receiving hospice care.
15. How would palliative care assist a man diagnosed with Huntington's disease?
16. Discuss your vision for integrating genomics into palliative care.

INTERNET RESOURCES

American Association of Colleges of Nursing, End-of-Life Care: www.aacn.nche.edu/elnec
American Pain Society: www.ampainsoc.org
Edmonton Regional Palliative Care Program: www.palliative.org
Education in Palliative and End-of-Life Care: www.epec.net
Hospice and Palliative Nurses Association: www.hpna.org
National Consensus Project: www.nationalconsensusproject.org
National Guideline Clearing House: www.guideline.org
National Hospice and Palliative Care Organization: www.nhpco.org
National Palliative Care Research Center: www.npcrc.org
Oncology Nursing Society: www.ons.org
Pain Resource Center: prc.coh.org
Palliative Care: www.getpalliativecare.org
Toolkit of Instruments to Measure End of Life Care (TIME): www.chcr.brown.edu/pcoc/toolkit.htm

REFERENCES

AGS Panel on Persistent Pain in Older Persons. (2002). The management of persistent pain in older persons. *Journal of the American Geriatrics Society, 50*(Suppl.), S205–S224.

Alliance for Excellence in Hospice and Palliative Nursing (AEHPN)(2004). *Mission statement.* Retrieved on March 1, 2008 from Hospice and Palliative Nurses Association www.hpna.org

Amella, E.J. (2003). Geriatrics and palliative care: Collaboration for quality of life until death. *Journal of Hospice and Palliative Nursing, 5*(1), 40–48.

American Academy of Hospice and Palliative Medicine (AAHPM) *About AAHPM.* Retrieved on January 30, 2008 from www.aahpm.org/about/index.html

American Association of Colleges of Nursing. (1998). *Peaceful death: Recommended competencies and curricular guidelines for end-of-life nursing care.* Retrieved on August 25, 2007 from www.aacn.nche.edi/Publications/deathfin.htm

American Board of Medical Specialties (ABMS) (2006). *News Release: ABMS Establishes New Subspecialty Certificate in Hospice and Palliative Care.* Retrieved on February 1, 2008 from www.abms.org.

Berry, P.H. (2004). Promoting quality of life during the dying process. In M.L.Matzo & D.W. Sherman (Eds.). *Gerontologic palliative care nursing* (pp. 1–2). St. Louis: Mosby.

Billings, J.A. (1998). What is palliative care? *Journal of Palliative Medicine, 1*(1), 73–81.

Block, S.D. (2000). Assessing and managing depression in the terminally ill patient. *Annals of Internal Medicine, 132*(3), 209–218.

Bookbinder, M., Coyle, N., Kiss, M., Goldstein, M.L., Holritz, K., Thaler, H. et al. (1996). Implementing national standards for cancer pain management: Program model and evaluation. *Journal of Pain and Symptom Management, 12,* 334–347.

Casarett, D.J., & Inouye. S.K. (2001). Diagnosis and management of delirium near the end of life. *Annals of Internal Medicine, 135,* 32–40.

Cassel. C.K. (2003). Foreword. In R. S. Morrison, & D. E. Meier (Eds.). *Geriatric palliative medicine* (pp. vii–ix). Oxford, UK: Oxford University Press.

Centers for Disease Control and Prevention, National Center for Health Statistics. (2007). *National vital statistics report, 55*(19).

Chochinov, H.M. (2004). Interventions to enhance the spiritual aspects of dying. *National Institutes of Health state-of–the science conference on improving end-of-life care program & abstracts.* Bethesda, MD: U.S. Department of Health and Human Services, National Institutes of Health.

Chochinov, H.M., Hack, T., Hassard, T., Kristjanson, L.J., McClement, S., & Harlos, M. (2004). Dignity and psychotherapeutic considerations in end-of-life care. *Journal of Palliative Care, 20*(3), 134–142.

Cleeland, C.S. (2001). Cross-cutting research issues. A research agenda for reducing distress of patients with cancer. In K. Foley & H. Gelband (Eds.), *Improving Palliative Care for Cancer* (pp. 233–274). Washington, DC: National Institute of Medicine.

Christakis, N., & Lamont, E.B. (2000). Extend and determinants of error in doctors' prognoses in terminally ill patients: Prospective cohort study. *British Medical Journal, 320,* 469–473.

Conley, Y. P., & Tinkle, M. B. (2007). The future of genomic nursing research. *Journal of Nursing Scholarship, 39*(2), 17–24.

Consensus Panel. (2006). *Essential nursing competencies and curricula guidelines for genetics and genomics.* Washington, DC: American Nurses Association.

Corbin, J. (2001). Introduction and overview: Chronic illness and nursing. In R. Hyman & J. Corbin (eds.), *Chronic illness: Research and theory for nursing practice* (pp. 1–15). New York: Springer.

Council on Social Work Education (CSWE) Faculty Development Institute, 2001 as cited in Sherman, D.W. (2004). Cultural and spiritual backgrounds of older adults. In M.L. Matzo & D.W. Sherman (Eds.) *Gerontologic palliative care nursing* (p. 11). St. Louis: Mosby.

Coyle, N. (2006). Introduction to palliative nursing care. In B.R. Ferrell & N. Coyle (Eds.). *Textbook of palliative nursing* (2nd ed.) (pp. 5–11). Oxford, UK: Oxford University Press.

Cumming, K.T., & Okun, S.N. (2004). Community-based palliative care for older adults. In M.L. Matzo, & D. W. Sherman (Eds.). *Gerontologic palliative care nursing* (pp. 52–65). St. Louis: Mosby.

Curtin, M., & Lubkin, I. (1995). What is chronicity? In I. Lubkin (Ed.), *Chronic illness: Impact and interventions* (3rd ed.) (pp. 3–25). Sudbury, MA: Jones & Bartlett.

Derek, D., Hanks, G., Cherny, N., & Calman, K. (2004). Introduction. In D. Doyle, G. Hanks, N. Cherny, & K. Calman (Eds.). *Oxford textbook of palliative medicine* (3rd ed.) (pp. 1–4). Oxford, UK: Oxford University Press.

Dowsett, S.M., Saul, J.L., Buttow, P.N., Dunn, S.M., Boyer, M.J., Findlow, R. & Dunsmore, J. (2000). Communication styles in the cancer consultation: Preferences for a patient-centered approach. *Psychoncology, 9,* 147–156.

Emanuel, E.J., & Emanuel, L.L. (1998). The promise of a good death. *Lancet, 351*(Suppl. 2), SII21–SII29.

End of Life Nursing Education Consortium (ELNEC) (2005). *Module 1: Nursing at the end of life.* American Association of Colleges of Nursing and City of Hope National Medical Center.

End of Life Nursing Education Consortium (ELNEC). (2005). *Module 5: Cultural considerations in EOL care.* American Association of Colleges of Nursing and City of Hope National Medical Center.Washington, DC: Author

EPEC Project. (2004). Education on palliative and end-of-life care. Retrieved on May 25, 2004 from www.epec.net

Ferrell, B.R. (2004). Overview of the domains of variables relevant to end-of-life care. *National Institutes of Health state-of–the science conference on improving end-of-life care program & abstracts.* Bethesda, MD: U.S. Department of Health and Human Services, National Institutes of Health.

Ferrell, B.R., & Coyle, N. (2001). *Textbook of palliative nursing.* New York: Oxford University Press.

Ferrell, B.R., & Coyle, N. (2006). *Textbook of palliative nursing* (2nd ed.). New York: Oxford University Press.

Ferrell, B.R., & Grant, M. (2006). Nursing research. In B.R. Ferrell & N. Coyle (Eds.). *Textbook of palliative nursing* (2nd ed., pp. 1093–1105). New York: Oxford University Press.

Ferrell, B., Virani, R., & Grant, M. (1999). Analysis of end-of-life content in nursing textbooks. *Oncology Nursing Forum, 26*(5), 869–876.

Ferrell, B.R. (1995). The impact of pain on quality of life: A decade of research. *Nursing Clinics of North America, 30,* 609–624.

Field, M.J., & Behrman, R.E. (Eds.). (2003). *When children die: Improving palliative and end-of-life care for children and their families.* Washington, DC: National Academy Press.

Field, M.J., & Cassel, C.K. (Eds.). (1997). *Approaching death: Improving care at the end of life.* Committee on Care at the End of Life, Division of Health Care Services, Institute of Medicine. Washington, DC: National Academy Press.

Fisher, E.S., Wennberg, D.E., Stukel, T.A., Gottlieb, D.J., Lucas, F.L., & Pinder, E.L. (2003). The implications of regional variations in Medicare spending: Health outcomes and satisfaction with care. *Annals of Internal Medicine, 138,* 288–298.

Foley, K. (2001). Preface. In K.M. Foley & H. Gelband (Eds.). *Improving palliative care for cancer* (pp. xi-xii). Washington, DC: National Academy Press.

Fried, T.R., Bradley, E.H., Towle, V. R., & Allore, H. (2002). Understanding the treatment preferences of seriously ill patients. *New England Journal of Medicine, 346*, 1061–1066.

Glass, E., Cluxton, D., & Rancour, P. (2001). Principles of patient and family assessment. In B.R. Ferrell & N. Coyle (Eds.) *Textbook of palliative nursing.* New York: Oxford University Press.

Goldstein, N.E., & Morrison, R.S. (2005). The intersection between geriatrics and palliative care: A call for a new research agenda. *Journal of the American Geriatrics Society, 53*, 1593–1598.

Haywood House. (1996). *Day care at Haywood House, City Hospital* (pamphlet). Nottingham, England: Author.

Hearn, J., & Myers, K. (2001). *Palliative day care in practice.* New York: Oxford University Press.

Heitkemper, M.M., & Bond, E. F. (2003). State of nursing science: On the edge. *Biological Research for Nursing, 4*(3), 151–162; Discussion 163–164, 170.

Hospice and Palliative Nurses Association & American Nurses Association, (2007). *Scope and standards of hospice and palliative nursing practice.* Washington, DC: Author.

Hospice and Palliative Nurses Association (2005). Florence Wald. Retrieved on January 5, 2005 from http://www.hpna.org/FlorenceWald_home.asp

Howe, L.A., & Eggert, J. (2007). Influence of pharmacogenomics on disease and symptom management. Retrieved on March 2, 2008 from journal. hsmc.org/ijnidd

Kemp, C. (1999). *Terminal illness: A guide to nursing care* (2nd ed.). Philadelphia: Lippincott.

Kubler-Ross, E. (1969). *On death and dying.* New York: Macmillan.

Lattanzi-Licht, M., Mahoney, J.J., & Miller, G.W. (1998). *The hospice choice: In pursuit of a peaceful death.* New York: Simon & Schuster.

Lomax, K.K., & Scanlon, C. (1997). *Precepts of palliative care* (Last Acts Task Force on Palliative Care). Princeton, NJ: The Robert Wood Johnson Foundation/Last Acts.

Luce, J.M., & Luce, J.A. (2001). Perspective on care at the close of life: Management of dyspnea in patients with far-advanced lung disease: "Once I lose it, it's kind of hard to catch it…" *JAMA, 285*, 1331–1337.

Lunney, J.R., Foley, K.M., Smith, T.J., & Gelband, H. (2003). *Describing death in America: What we need to know.* Washington DC: National Academy Press.

Lynn, J. (1997). Measuring quality of care at the end of life: A statement of principles. *Journal of the American Geriatrics Society, 45*, 526–527.

Lynn, J. (2001). Serving patients who may die soon and their families: The role of hospice and other services. *JAMA, 285*, 925–932.

Lynn, J. et al. (2000). Rethinking fundamental assumptions: SUPPORT's implications for future reform. *Journal of the American Geriatrics Society, 48*(5), S214–S221.

Manfredi, P.L., Morrison, R.S., Morris, J., Goldhirsch, S.L., Carter, J.M., & Meier, D.E. (2000). Palliative care consultations: How do they impact the care of hospitalized patients? *Journal of Pain and Symptom Management, 20*, 166–173.

Matzo, M.L., & Sherman, D.W. (Eds.). (2004). *Gerontologic palliative care nursing.* St. Louis: Mosby.

Matzo, M.L., & Sherman, D.W. (Eds.). (2001). *Palliative care nursing: Quality care at the end of life.* New York: Springer.

Matzo, M.L., & Sherman, D.W. (2006). *Palliative care nursing: Quality care at the end of life* (2nd ed.). New York: Springer.

McClain, C.S., Rosenfield, B., & Breitbart, W. (2003). Effect of spiritual well-being on end-of-life despair in terminally ill cancer patients. *Lancet, 361*, 1603–1607.

McMillan, S.C. (2004). Interventions to facilitate family caregiving. *National Institutes of Health state-of-the science conference on improving end-of-life care program & abstracts.* Bethesda, MD: U.S. Department of Health and Human Services, National Institutes of Health.

Meier, D.E., & Morrison, R.S. (2002). Autonomy reconsidered. *New England Journal of Medicine, 346*, 1087–1089.

Meier, D.E., Back, A.L., & Morrison, R.S. (2001). The inner life of physicians and care of the seriously ill. *JAMA, 286*, 3007–3014.

Meyer, U.A. (2000). Pharmacogenetics and adverse drug reaction. *Lancet, 356*(b), 1667–1671.

Miles, S.H., Koepp, R., & Weber, E.P. (1996). Advance end-of-life treatment planning: A research review. *Archives of Internal Medicine, 156*, 1062–1068.

Morrison, R. S. (2005). Palliative care outcomes research: The next steps. *Journal of Palliative Medicine, 8*(1), 13–16.

Morrison, R. S., & Meier, D.E. (2004). Palliative care. *New England Journal of Medicine, 350,* 2582–2590.

Morrison, R..S., & Meier, D. E. (Eds.). (2003). *Geriatric palliative care.* New York: Oxford University Press.

National Consensus Project (NCP) for Quality Palliative Care. (2004). *Clinical practice guidelines for quality palliative care.* Retrieved on September 24, 2007 from www.nationalconsensusproject.org

National Hospice and Palliative Care Organization. (2007). *Hospice facts and figures.* Retrieved on February 1, 2008 from www.nhpco.org

National Hospice and Palliative Care Organization (2006). *Standards of Practice for Hospice Programs,* Arlington, VA: Author.

National Hospice and Palliative Care Organization. (2004). *Research agenda,* Arlington, VA: Author. Retrieved on February 20, 2008 from www.NHPCO.org/files/public/2004_Research_Agenda_May04.doc

National Hospice Organization Standards and Accreditation Committee. (1997). *A pathway for patients and families facing terminal illness.* Arlington, VA: Author.

National Institutes of Health. (2004). *National Institutes of Health State-of-the Conference Statement: Improving End-of-Life Care.* Washington, DC: Author. Retrieved on November 10, 2007 from consensus.nih.gov/PREVIOUSSTATEMENTS.htm

Nolan, M. T., & Mock, V. (2004). A conceptual framework for end-of-life care: A reconsideration of factors influencing the integrity of the human person. *Journal of Professional Nursing, 20*(6), 351–360.

Pellegrino, E. (1990). The relationship of autonomy and integrity in medical ethics. *Bulletin of PAHO, 24,* 361–371.

Pinquart, M., & Sorenson, D. (2003). Differences between caregivers and noncaregivers in psychological health and physical health: A meta-analysis. *Psychology and Aging, 18*(250–257).

Portenoy, R.K. (1998). Defining palliative care. *Newsletter*: Department of Pain Medicine and Palliative Care, *1*(2). Beth Israel Medical Center, New York.

Prows, C.A. (2004). Medication selection by genotype. *American Journal of Nursing, 104*(5), 60–70.

Quill, T.E. (2000). Perspectives on care at the end of life: Initiating end-of-life discussions with seriously ill patients: addressing the "elephant in the room." *JAMA, 284,* 2502–2507.

Schulz, R., Mendelsohn, A.B., Haley, W.E., Mahoney, D., Allen, R., Zhang, S. et al. (2003). End of life care and the effects of bereavement among family caregivers of persons with dementia, *New England Journal of Medicine, 349,* 1936–1942.

Schulz, R. Newsom, J. T., Fleissner, K., DeCamp, A.R. & Nieboer, A.P. (1997). The effects of bereavement after family caregiving. *Aging and Mental Health. 1,* 269–282.

Schwarz, U. I., Ritchie, M.D., Bradford, Y., Li, C., Dudek, S.M., Fry-Anderson, et al. (2008). Genetic determinants of response to warfarin during initial anticoagulation. *New England Journal of Medicine, 358,* 999–1008.

Sherman, D.W. (2004). Cultural and spiritual backgrounds of older adults. In M.L. Matzo & D.W. Sherman (Eds.). *Gerontologic palliative care nursing* (p. 11). St. Louis: Mosby.

Showalter, S. (1998). Looking through different eyes: Beyond cultural diversity. In K. Doka & J. Davidson (Eds.), *Living with grief when illness is prolonged* (pp. 71–82). Washington, DC. Hospice Foundation of America.

Singer, P.A., Martin, D.K., & Kelner, M. (1999).Quality end-of-life care: Patients' perspectives. *JAMA, 281,* 163–168.

Sisk, J., Hebert, P., Horowitz, C., McLaughlin, M., Wang, J., & Chassin, M. (2006). Effects of nurse management on the quality of heart failure care in minority communities. *Annals of Internal Medicine, 145,* 273–283.

St. Christopher's Hospice. (1996). *St. Christopher's Hospice Day Center* (Handout). Sydenham, England: Author.

Standards and Accreditation Committee. (1999). *Hospice standards of practice.* Arlington, VA: Hospice and Palliative Care Organization.

Steinhauser, K.E., (2004). Measuring outcomes prospectively. *National Institutes of Health state-of-the science conference on improving end-of-life care program & abstracts.* Bethesda, MD: U.S. Department of Health and Human Services, National Institutes of Health.

Steinhauser, K.E., Christakis, N.A., Clipp, E.C., McNeilly, L., & Tulsky, J.A. (2000). Factors considered important at the end of life by patients, family, physicians, and other care providers. *JAMA, 284,* 2476–2482.

Strasser, F, & Bruera, E.D. (2002). Update on anorexia and cachexia. *Hematology and Oncology Clinics of North America, 16,* 589–617.

Sullivan, A.M., Lakoma, M.D., & Block, S.D. (2003). The status of medical education in end-of-life care: A national report. *Journal of General Internal Medicine, 18,* 685–695.

Sullivan, M.C. (2001). Lost in translation: How Latinos view end-of-life care. *Plastic Surgery Nursing, 21*(2), 90–91.

SUPPORT Principal Investigators. (1995). A controlled trial to improve care for seriously ill, hospitalized patients: The study to understand prognoses and preferences for outcomes and risks of treatments (SUPPORT). *JAMA, 274,* 1591–1598.

Teno, J.M. (2004). Brown Atlas of Dying. Brown University Center for Gerontology and Health Care Research. Retrieved on February 1, 2008 from www.chcr.brown.edu/dying

Teno, J. (2001). Quality of care and quality indicators for lives ended by cancer. In K.M. Foley & H. Gelband (Eds.). *Improving palliative care for cancer.* Washington, DC: National Academy Press.

Teno, J., Lynn, J., Wenger, N., Phillips, R.S., Murphy, D.P., Connors, A.F., et al. (1997). Advance directives for seriously ill hospitalize patients: Effectiveness with the patient self-determination act and the SUPPORT intervention. *Journal of the American Geriatrics Society, 45,* 500–507.

von Guten, C.F. & Lupu, D. (2004). Recognizing palliative medicine as a subspecialty: What does it mean for oncology? *The Journal of Supportive Oncology, 2*(2), 166–174.

von Guten, C.F., Ferris, F.D., Portenoy, R.K., Glajchen, M. (Eds.). (2001). *Manual: How to Establish a Palliative Care Program,* New York: NY: Center to Advance Palliative Care.

von Guten, C., & Romer, A.L. (1999). Designing and sustaining a palliative care and home hospice program: An interview with Charles von Guten. *Innovations in end-of-life care, 1*(5).

Weinshilboum, R. (2003). Inheritance and drug response. *New England Journal of Medicine, 348*(5), 529–537.

World Health Organization. (1990). *Cancer pain relief and palliative care* (Technical Report Series 804) (p. 11). Geneva, Switzerland: World Health Organization.

23

Politics and Policy

Betty Smith-Campbell

You can't ignore politics, no matter how much you'd like to.

Molly Ivins

INTRODUCTION

Chronic disease represents a global challenge that accounts for 60% of global deaths, with an estimated increase to greater than 66% by 2020 (World Health Organization, 2005). In the United States, chronic illness and disabling conditions are major public health problems. More than 90 million Americans live with a chronic illness and 7 of 10 die of a chronic illness (National Center for Chronic Disease, 2005). Approximately 33% or 57 million of working-aged Americans live with at least one chronic condition (Tu, 2004). One aspect of providing and improving the care of individuals with chronic illness is to understand how policy influences the care and life of individuals with chronic conditions.

Nurses have described caring not only as the essence of nursing (Benner & Wrubel, 1989; Watson, 1988) but essential if culturally appropriate care is to be provided to our clients (Kavanagh & Knowlden, 2004). Most nurses who care for individuals with chronic illnesses would agree

that caring is a part of their professional practice and perhaps the most important part; yet caring is often viewed only at the individual level (Smith-Campbell, 1999). It is important for nurses to understand how practice and thus the care our patients receive is influenced by policy. To be involved in the caring process, system factors, including political, social, cultural, and economic factors, must be incorporated into the nursing process to impact clients and nursing practice. For example, policy affects the availability of health insurance for persons with chronic illness. In the United States, health care is not a right; therefore, the government is not obligated to provide health insurance to everyone. Some policy initiatives have been very successful; for example, the elderly and those with the most severe disabilities have hospitalization coverage. Because of policy gaps, however, those same individuals who receive excellent hospital coverage may not be able to receive home care, or obtain needed medical equipment or nursing home care. To have an impact on nursing practice and the types of services available to clients with chronic conditions, nurses must be able to (1) assess and understand current health policies, (2) evaluate the strengths and weaknesses of healthcare policies, and then (3) act to implement or change healthcare policy to improve care for clients with chronic illnesses and conditions.

Policy Defined

To better understand how policy influences the care of clients and nursing practice, a definition of policy is needed. Policy has been defined as the "choices society, segments of society, or organizations make regarding its goals and priorities and the ways it will allocate its resources to attain those goals" (Mason, Leavitt, & Chaffee, 2007, p. 3). Public policy was defined by Milio (1989) "as a guide to government action, whether by legislation, executive order or regulatory mandate" (p. 316). Social and health policies are included within the context of public policy. Social policy pertains to governmental action that promotes the welfare of the public. For example, the Family Medical Leave Act was passed to promote the welfare of families by allowing parents the right to care for sick children or elderly parents without losing their jobs.

Governmental action that promotes the health of citizens is considered health policy. Examples of federal legislation include Medicare and funding to support research related to chronic diseases such as Alzheimer's disease, arthritis, and diabetes. Local examples include city or county governments restricting smoking in public buildings. State and local boards of health have policies that monitor water quality and provide minimum safety requirements for nursing homes and day care centers. Regulatory agencies also affect public health policy. State boards of nursing set specific regulations that define who can practice nursing within their state.

Beyond public policy there are also institutional and organization policies that affect individuals with chronic conditions. Institutional policies govern the workplace (Mason et al., 2007). Such policies establish the way an institution is operated, its goals and mission, and thus influence how the institution will treat its employees and how employees will work. For example, if a goal of a business is to have a diverse work force, policies

may be incorporated to assist employees who have physical or mental disabilities. Rules governing, and positions taken by organizations, are considered to be organizational policies. For example, organizational governing rules may include a nonsmoking rule during all official business meetings or have a policy that requests members not to use strong perfumes to protect members who are sensitive to strong odors.

Policy is never static but is continuously influenced by cultural, political, and financial factors in the environment (Chopoorian, 1986). Policy development and implementation is often not logical, rational, or orderly, and can be influenced during any part of the process. It is important to note that all policies reflect current societal values, beliefs, and attitudes and are shaped by politics (Mason et al., 2007).

Private and governmental policies have developed a multitude of programs that have benefited millions of Americans. The majority of citizens in the United States receive excellent acute care through private insurance paid by their employers. The population with severe disabilities and the very poor receive some healthcare services. Individuals and their families with present or past military service receive a broad range of healthcare services, including acute care, home care, and long-term care. Quality standards are being implemented throughout our healthcare system based on national policy; persons with disabilities have equal access to employment, buildings, and transportation. As a nation, there is much of which to be proud regarding our policies, yet many problems remain.

PROBLEMS AND ISSUES

The aging population has been recognized as a "demographic time bomb." The first of the baby boomers turned 60 in 2006, and will reach age 65 in 2011, greatly increasing the number of individuals with chronic diseases. The current cost to the US economy for treatment and lost productivity caused by chronic illness is more than $1.3 trillion per year, and this is expected to rise to $5.7 trillion by 2050 (DeVol et al., 2007). However, healthcare policymakers have taken few decisive steps to restructure healthcare financing and delivery systems to accommodate the expanding number of vulnerable populations, including individuals with chronic illness and disability (Navarro, 2004).

US Health Care: A System in Trouble

The United States is the only industrialized nation in the world in which health care is not considered a right. This cultural value has directed both past and current public policy decisions regarding health. Historically, the value of individual choice has been predominant. There has been a strong cultural belief that if one works hard enough, one should be able to support one's self and one's family, implying that one should then be able to afford health care (Bellah, Madsen, Sullivan, Swidler, & Tipton, 1985). In addition, current health policy is guided by society's value that a competitive market is the best way to provide healthcare services. Allowing the market to provide the majority of healthcare services has left policy makers with only the ability to "fix" problems in the healthcare system. Policy makers, with the approval of society, have agreed that some segments of the population need assistance, such as the elderly, the very poor, and the disabled. This "fixing" of the problem has led to separate programs for the elderly and disabled (Medicare), the poor (Medicaid), and uninsured children (SCHIP—State Children's Health Insurance Program). Policy makers have also agreed to reward, through healthcare coverage, those who have provided service to the nation, those in the military and veterans, leading to another separate healthcare system (Veterans Affairs). This mix of private and public healthcare coverage has given us one of the most fragmented and complex healthcare systems in the world. To better understand this fragmented and complex system, an overview of key policies, healthcare system programs, and their limitations are discussed.

Health Insurance

Although declining, the preponderance of health care in the United States is financed through private insurance, and the majority (59.7%) of US residents younger than the age of 65 obtain health insurance through their employers (DeNavas-Walt, Proctor, & Smith, 2007). It is important to note that the goal, and thus the policy, of private US health insurance companies is to generate revenue. This is accomplished through risk rating—the practice of setting premiums and other terms of the policies, according to age, sex, occupation, health status, and health risks of policyholders. Ideally, insuring large numbers of persons spreads the risk. This philosophy may work in large companies (or governments) with thousands of employees/citizens, but the majority of businesses in the United States are small and their risks of needed health care are not spread over a large group of individuals. For insurance companies to make money, they need to enroll healthy individuals and limit the enrollment of those with high healthcare expenses.

Rising costs have become a major problem for insured people with chronic conditions. The percentage of individuals with chronic illness with private insurance who spent more than 5% of their income on out-of-pocket expenses grew from 28% in 2001 to 42% in just 2 years (Tu, 2004).

Traditional or Conventional Insurance

In the past the most common type of insurance provided was a traditional fee-for-service plan. The numbers of traditional or conventional plans have declined dramatically from 73% in 1988 to just 3% in 2007 (Kaiser Family Foundation [KFF], 2004; Kaiser Family Foundation & Health Research and Education Trust [KFF-HRET], 2007). Traditional health insurance plans generally allow the insured to choose their healthcare provider, and the healthcare provider is able to make most healthcare decisions with little oversight by the insurance company. A majority of covered services are for acute care services, such as hospitalization, medication, and medical equipment, with little or no emphasis on prevention, health maintenance, or supportive healthcare services. This type of coverage limits the services needed to prevent chronic conditions and provide the long-term care services needed to support individuals with disabilities and chronic illnesses.

Another major problem under the traditional fee-for-service plan has been the lack of control on service use and thus cost. Healthcare providers have little incentive to control cost, and the more services they provide, the more income they generate. Therefore, insurance premiums increase to cover rising services. Rising insurance costs have become a major issue for employers, who pay for most of the insurance premiums. As the cost of providing insurance continues to rise above inflation, employers often look for less costly options to provide coverage for their employees. One solution for employers is to look at managed care organizations.

Managed Care Organizations

Originally, managed care organizations (MCOs) were defined as healthcare delivery systems with a capitated financing mechanism. Currently, MCO generally refers to any non–fee-for-service plan that attempts to contain costs and manage care (KFF, 2004). Types of MCOs include health maintenance organizations (HMOs), preferred provider organizations (PPOs), and point of service (POS) plans. Of those insured through an employer, there has been an inverse relationship in growth with MCOs and traditional health plans. Although the percentage of individuals who have traditional health plans has decreased, the percentage of persons with MCOs has risen dramatically, from 27% in 1988 to 91% in 2003 (KFF, 2004; KFF & HRET, 2007). With the resurgence of MCOs in the 1990s, many were hopeful that there would be a system to actually manage care. It was hoped that MCOs would promote health and assist in preventing disease, with a final goal of reducing costs. Managed

care organizations could help eliminate inappropriate overutilization of services and also offer advantages in setting standard protocols by providing preventive healthcare services. Unfortunately, most experts agree that the main system change MCOs, especially HMOs, have emphasized is that of controlling costs. Currently, MCOs have had some limited success, yet costs remain out of control and continue to rise. The majority of covered workers (57%) in 2007 were enrolled in a PPO, with an average monthly premium of $386 for single coverage ($4638 annually). The average premium for a family with a PPO policy was $1037 monthly, or $12,443 annually (KFF & HRET, 2007).

Consumer Directed Health Plans

Recently politicians and employers have been advocating health savings accounts (HSAs), which are a component of consumer-directed health plans (CDHPs) or high-deductible health plans (HDHPs). HSAs have been found to have lower premiums but higher deductibles and out-of-pocket spending limits. In 2005, "deductibles were, on average, nearly six times greater than those for employers' traditional plans" (Government Accounting Office, 2006, p. 5).

CDHPs or HDHPs are insurance plans where financial incentives or disincentives are provided for the consumer or person to become more involved with purchasing their healthcare services. To enroll in an HSA, a consumer must be in an HDHP that meets certain requirements. In 2006, these plans required a deductible of at least $1050 for single and $2100 for family coverage, with many plans having higher deductibles. Out-of-pocket costs were limited to $5250 for single and $10,500 for family coverage (Hoffman & Tolbert, 2006). Supporters of these plans believe they will help individuals become more aware of their healthcare needs and, therefore, influence their decisions related to cost and quality of services. Opponents are concerned that individuals will not seek out preventive or needed healthcare services because of high cost. Research studies found enrollees of

CDHPs are less satisfied with their plan; spend significantly more of their income on out-of-pocket expenses; and often avoid, skip, or delay health care because of costs. People in these healthcare plans were also more aware of the cost of their care and considered the cost of care when deciding to use healthcare services when compared to enrollees of other plans (Fronstin & Collins, 2006). The results of these and other studies suggest that CDHP/HSA negatively affect people with low incomes and those with chronic illnesses.

Medicare

Medicare was implemented in 1965 through the federal act, Title XVIII of the Social Security Act—Health Insurance for the Aged and Disabled (Pulcine & Hart, 2007). Medicare is an insurance program that serves more than 43 million Americans [Centers for Medicare & Medicaid Services (CMS), 2007a], and 7 million individuals younger than the age of 65 who have long-term disabilities (Neuman, 2006). Before the enactment of Medicare, 50% of the elderly did not have health insurance (Vladeck & King, 1997).

Medicare includes four parts:

- Part A. Hospital Insurance: Covers inpatient hospital services, skilled nursing facility care, hospice care, and home health care (coverage is limited to a set number of days, and a deductible is required). Individuals are automatically enrolled at age 65. Part A does not include long-term care.
- Part B. Supplemental Medical Insurance: Individuals must apply to the program and pay a monthly premium. Services include healthcare professional services, including physicians, advanced practice nurses, and other providers; outpatient care; durable medical equipment; and ambulance services. Part B does not include long-term care.
- Part C. Medicare Advantage: Provides care through managed care plans and includes Part A, B, and C benefits.

- Part D. Prescription Drug Benefit: A voluntary benefit, provided by insurance plans with individuals paying about 25% of the premium and the government paying 75% (Feldstein, 2007).

Medicare services seem comprehensive and clearly defined; yet, as with all health insurance programs, when assessing how a policy is implemented, either through specific laws or administrative regulatory policy, services are often found to be neither comprehensive nor clearly defined. For example, to receive home health care through Medicare, an individual must meet each of the following requirements: (1) be confined to his or her home; (2) have a physician prescribe treatment; (3) need intermittent skilled nursing care, physical therapy, or speech therapy; and (4) receive services from a certified home health agency participating in Medicare (US Department of Health, 2007). Therefore, if a nurse practitioner's diabetic client with a history of congestive heart failure needed skilled nursing care for leg ulcers, the client would first have to be referred to a physician. Second, if the client could leave his or her home to obtain groceries from the store across the street but could not physically tolerate the half-hour bus ride to the practitioner's office, the client would technically be ineligible to receive home health services through Medicare.

Part D was part of landmark Medicare reform in 2003 with the passage of the Medicare Prescription Drug, Improvement, and Modernization Act of 2003. This law created a subsidized prescription drug benefit for all older adults starting in 2006. In 2007 the national average monthly premium was $27.35 (CMS, 2007a; CMS, 2007c). In addition to a premium, individuals must also pay part of the cost of the prescriptions, including a copayment or coinsurance.

There are several concerns with this new prescription drug program. If beneficiaries have drug expenses that total $2250, coverage is discontinued until they reach drug expenses of $5100. This has been called the *doughnut hole* (Families USA,

2006). At the same time that Medicare beneficiaries do not receive drug benefits, they must continue to pay their monthly premiums. A study by Joyce, Goldman, Karaca-Mandic, and Zheng, (2007) found that capping drug benefits affected many patients with chronic illness, with higher rates of discontinued medications and patients less likely to resume drug therapy even after coverage resumes.

Under the new Modernization Act, disease management initiatives were implemented. In 2004, the administrator for CMS (2004) announced that by the end of (that) year, several Medicare chronic care projects would be launched. It was hoped that increased coordination of care for Medicare beneficiaries would demonstrate healthcare quality and positive outcomes as well as significant cost savings. Outcomes of these new programs are being assessed, but such programs have the potential to positively influence the quality of care particularly for individuals with chronic illnesses.

Medicare has greatly improved access to health care for both older Americans and the disabled. The Medicare Prescription Drug, Improvement, and Modernization Act of 2003 continues to have an immense impact on the US healthcare system. As the baby boomers grow in number and add to the number of individuals with chronic illness and disabilities, many are concerned that with no cost containment measures in the Modernization Act, there will not be enough funds to assist everyone who is currently eligible. Many issues still need to be addressed. Some of the questions include: How will the government be able to afford clients' needed medication without cost controls? How will Medicare beneficiaries be able to afford the rising cost of Medicare B premiums? Will Medicare beneficiaries be able to afford the rising cost of medication, even with the discount drug card? As Feldstein (2007) clearly states: "The currently projected long-run growth rates of Medicare are not sustainable under current financing arrangements" (p. 99). These and other issues related to accessibility and affordability will continue to be debated, and with every new legislative session, new policies will be developed and enacted.

Medicaid

Medicaid was an amendment to the Social Security Act in 1965 and was implemented in 1966. Title XIX of the Social Security Act, Medicaid was established to provide health insurance to low-income families with dependents. Individual states define the program, and it is jointly funded by federal and state governments. Because coverage by Medicaid is administered at the state level, coverage varies from state to state, and there are vast disparities regarding who is eligible (Rowland & Tallon, 2004). To receive matching federal dollars, the state program must offer certain basic medical services, including inpatient and outpatient hospital care and physician and family nurse practitioner services.

Many individuals are dually eligible for Medicare and Medicaid. Services for persons covered by both programs will first be paid by Medicare, with the difference paid by Medicaid, up to each state's limit (CMS, 2005). Medicaid will cover additional services such as long-term nursing facility care, prescription drugs, eyeglasses, and hearing aids. Medicaid also covers those with disabilities and the elderly who are enrolled in Medicare but have incomes below a certain level. This limited coverage for low-income Medicare beneficiaries assists with premiums, deductibles, and coinsurance.

More than 50 million people receive essential healthcare services through Medicaid, with this number including 13 million older adults and persons with disabilities (Rowland, 2005). Although only 16% of Medicaid enrollees are disabled, these enrollees account for 43% of Medicaid expenditures. Over all, Medicaid pays one in five of all US healthcare dollars. Medicaid also pays for 60% of all nursing home residents, and this is viewed as an excessive financial burden on the government, especially as the population ages and the need increases. These costs, in turn, influence the need for more revenue, typically provided through tax dollars, to be generated to fund the program,. With society's reluctance to increase taxes, the future of both Medicaid and Medicare is uncertain.

SCHIP: State Children's Health Insurance Program

The Balanced Budget Act (BBA) of 1997 expanded health insurance coverage to children through the new State Child Health Insurance Program (SCHIP). SCHIP was created to help states cover uninsured children who do not meet Medicaid eligibility requirements (Kaiser Commission on Medicaid and the Uninsured, 2007). Similar to Medicaid, SCHIP is administered through states, and the type of program offered varies by state. Until 2005, SCHIP and Medicaid helped decrease, over the last decade, the rate of uninsured children by one third. In the last several years as employer coverage has declined, the rate of children uninsured has risen. SCHIP was renewed in 2007, but not at a budget level to cover the number of children currently in the program nor the increasing number of children who remain uninsured. Without health insurance, children often do not receive care to prevent chronic conditions or illnesses such as complications from diseases that could have been prevented by immunizations (i.e., hepatitis) or disabilities created because of lack of treatment (i.e., hearing loss from otitis media).

Federal Initiatives

Federal laws and regulatory policies have had and will continue to have an enormous impact on health, especially those who are the most vulnerable—that includes individuals with chronic conditions. The BBA of 1997 and the Medicare Prescription Drug, Improvement, and Modernization Act of 2003 had a huge impact on federal spending related to health care. Every year policy is developed or modified that impacts clients with chronic illnesses. With presidential

elections occurring in 2008 and a new president in the White House in 2009, it is the expectation of many that major policy changes will be made that affect the care we give as nurses and the services provided to our clients.

Affordability, Accessibility, and Policy and Quality Issues

Affordability

In the early 1990s, when it seemed that healthcare reform was a possibility, the American Nurses Association (ANA) (2005) campaigned for affordable, accessible, and quality health care. In 2005, they renewed their commitment to the *Health Care Agenda* campaign. The ANA, as well as many other organizations and consumer groups, continue to support change in the healthcare system, but true reform has never occurred and many Americans continue to lack affordable, accessible, quality health care. The very poor may be eligible for insurance through Medicaid, but obtaining coverage may be cumbersome and demeaning, with coverage varying from state to state. For persons with low to moderate incomes, or persons with a mild disability who may be able to work, affordable health insurance may not be available or affordable.

In 2005, 20% of the US population younger than 65 years of age stated they were uninsured at sometime in the preceding 12 months (Centers for Disease Control and Prevention, 2007). The majority (60%) of this uninsured population were young adults 18–44 years of age, but "more than one-fifth of the uninsured were 45–64 years of age, a time in life when chronic illness becomes more prevalent" (p. 94). The reason individuals most often gave for not having health insurance was their inability to afford coverage. Persons with low incomes are more often uninsured, and persons who have disabilities live disproportionately in families with low incomes and no insurance. Individuals with disabilities who do not have health insurance face great challenges. Of the disabled without insurance, more than two thirds (69%) state they have no regular doctor; 67% go without needed equipment such as wheelchairs and hearing aids; 60% skip doses, split pills, or do not fill prescriptions because of cost; and 66% postpone needed care because of cost (Hanson, Neuman, & Voris, 2003). Uninsured individuals with chronic illness are not only less likely to receive appropriate care than the insured, but have worse clinical outcomes (Institute of Medicine, 2002; Schwartz, 2007). Similar problems also occur for the disabled who have only Medicare coverage. Even with broad Medicare coverage, more than 20% said a doctor would not accept their insurance, twice the rate reported by those with traditional insurance (Hanson et al., 2003).

Americans with incomes above the poverty level who lose access to employer-based coverage include older adults and individuals with chronic illness. These individuals have difficulty obtaining quality insurance at reasonable rates. Before enactment of the Health Insurance Portability and Accountability Act (HIPAA) of 1997, if an insured person lost her or his insurance for some reason, such as losing a job, new insurance could be denied for preexisting conditions, including chronic illnesses. Today, with HIPAA in effect, if a person has been insured for the preceding 12 months, a new insurance company cannot refuse to cover the person and cannot impose preexisting conditions or a waiting period before coverage. The law explicitly states that genetic information shall not be considered a preexisting condition (US Department of Labor, 2007b). One limitation of HIPAA is that neither a previous employer nor a new employer has an obligation to cover any part of the new insurance premiums. Often, an individual who loses insurance is no longer included in a group insurance plan, causing the premiums to be very high. In 2007, the average premium for families was $12,106 and for some, deductibles could be as high as $5,000 (eHealthInsurance, 2007; KFF & HRET, 2007). These rates may even be higher if they included individuals or family members that had one or more chronic illness.

Accessibility

Healthcare accessibility continues to be an issue for many. One problem for those who live in a rural community is geographic accessibility. Individuals with common chronic conditions who live in rural communities often have limited access to healthcare services, especially to needed specialty services. They may have access to basic healthcare services, but getting long-term, consistent care for chronic conditions is difficult. Accessibility may be a problem in urban areas as well. Individuals may find that there are not healthcare providers in their communities that will accept them as patients if they have Medicare or Medicaid. One major reason providers often limit their number of patients with Medicare or Medicaid is the federal policy that sets a specific rate on which the provider is reimbursed, reducing the income of the healthcare provider. There are also clearly documented cases where individuals, even with health insurance, were told they could no longer make appointments with their physician. Examples include insured farmers and ranchers who were unable to pay their out-of-pocket expenses, leading to unpaid medical bills and their medical provider no longer seeing them because of this past debt. This has occurred even in rural communities where families have had longstanding relationships with their healthcare provider (Lottero, Pryor, Rukavina, Prottas, & Knudson, 2007). This access issue is not only a problem for individuals with chronic illnesses, but often prevents individuals and family members from seeking health care to prevent such illnesses.

Currently, the greatest policy issue is that health care is not a right in the United States. The number of individuals and families who are either uninsured or underinsured continues to grow. There are a multitude of reports that have documented that the uninsured or underinsured: (1) are less likely to have a usual source of care outside the emergency room; (2) often go without screenings and preventive care; (3) often delay or forgo needed medical care; (4) are sicker and die earlier than those who have insurance; and (5) pay more for their care. This lack of access places a higher burden on those with chronic illness. Although the United States spends more on health care per person than any other developed nation, we have more access problems than comparable countries. In Great Britain, Canada, and The Netherlands, individuals state they rarely forgo needed medical care because of cost; yet in the United States, 42% of those with chronic diseases "had skipped medications, not seen a doctor when sick, or forgone recommended care in the past year because of costs" (Thorpe, Howard, & Galactionova, 2007). More than 84% of individuals who are considered high users of the emergency room have chronic conditions (Peppe, Mays, Chang, Becker, & DiJulio, 2007).

Policy and Quality Issues

As chronic illness rates rise, one issue individuals and organizations have become concerned about is quality. In 2007, a group of patients, providers, community organizations, business and labor groups, and health policy experts joined together to form the *Partnership to Fight Chronic Disease* (PFCD). This organization is committed to raising awareness on the number one cause of death, disability, and rising healthcare costs in the United States: rising rates of preventable and treatable chronic diseases. One of their goals to "Encourage and reward continuous advances in clinical practice and research that improve the quality of care for those with prevalent and costly chronic diseases" (PFCD, 2007). This organization as well as specific organizations such as the American Heart Association, American Lung Association, United Cerebral Palsy, and many other organizations work to implement and modify policy to impact the quality of life for those with chronic illnesses.

The Medicare Modernization Act of 2003 approved voluntary demonstration projects called chronic care improvement programs (CCIP), later changed to Medicare Health Support. The goal of this policy is to improve the quality of care and life for people living with multiple chronic illnesses,

primarily outside of traditional healthcare institutions (CMS, 2007b). The first of these programs began in 2005, and the results and possible extension of this policy remain in the policy evaluation phase.

Policies That Impact Quality of Life

Social Security Income for the Disabled. Income influences the quality of life for all individuals, including those with chronic illnesses. The US government, under the Social Security Administration (SSA), has two financial assistance programs for the disabled: the Social Security Disability Insurance (SSDI) program and the Supplemental Security Income (SSI) program. The medical requirements are the same for both programs. The SSDI program is based on prior work under Social Security. Disability, as defined by governmental policy, is based on the inability to work. A person can be defined as disabled if unable to do any kind of work, and the disability is expected to last for at least a year or is expected to result in death (SSA, 2007). After receiving SSDI for 2 years, an individual is automatically enrolled in Medicare Part A.

The SSI program provides financial assistance to both adults and children with limited incomes who meet the governmental definition of disabled, persons who have worked in the United States and are age 65 or older, and individuals who are blind. SSI disability payments are made on the basis of financial need and are not based on prior work. Low-income persons receiving SSI disability payments are frequently eligible for Medicaid and the food stamp program (SSA, 2007). Children younger than 18 years of age may receive income from SSI if they are disabled and come from a home with a limited income, or if their parent (or a survivor/spouse of a parent) is collecting retirement or disability benefits. Benefits will continue after the age of 18, only if the child remains classified as disabled.

For a child to be considered disabled, the physical and/or mental condition must result in a severe and marked functional limitation. Under the Personal Responsibility and Work Opportunity Reconciliation Act 1996, also known as the welfare reform bill, a child no longer needs an individual assessment to be classified as disabled. Under this law, if a child's disability is included in SSA's listed disability categories, the government will begin making immediate payments.

The Americans with Disabilities Act. The Americans with Disabilities Act (ADA) was passed in 1990 and affects the quality of life of millions of Americans. Former US Attorney General Janet Reno, in celebrating ADA's tenth year anniversary in 2000, commented that the ADA had made a difference in the lives of many individuals, although more needs to done [US Department of Justice (DOJ), 2000]. To receive protection provided by the ADA, a person must have a disability or have a relationship or association with an individual with a disability. The ADA definition of disabled is less restrictive than that of the SSDI or SSI programs. A disabled person, as defined by the ADA, is someone who has a physical or mental impairment that substantially limits one or more major life activities (DOJ, 2006). The ADA gives individuals with disabilities the right to equal opportunity to employment, restricts questions a potential employer can ask regarding disability, and requires employers to make reasonable accommodations for a person's known physical or mental limitations. This Act is seen as a victory for the disabled, but limits still exist. Provisions of this law restrict its implementation to businesses with 15 or more employees. This policy significantly impacts individual's accessibility, and thus their quality of life, to housing, healthcare institutions, government offices, and places of employment.

The Family and Medical Leave Act. The Family and Medical Leave Act (FMLA), effective in 1993, enables individuals to have time to care for themselves and/or family members who are ill. This is an especially important act for family members with chronic illnesses that may need to take long periods of time off of work to care for a loved one. The Act entitles employees of companies of more than 50 employees up to 12 work weeks of unpaid leave during any 12-month period for one or more of the following reasons: (1) for the birth and care of the newborn child of an employee; (2) for placement with the employee of a child for adoption or foster care; (3) to care for an immediate family member (spouse, child, or parent) with a serious health condition; or (4) to take medical leave when the employee is unable to work because of a serious health condition (US Department of Labor, 2007a). Before enactment of FMLA, many US employees were unable to leave work when they or their families had a major health need, for fear of losing their jobs. The limitations of this act are that the leave may be unpaid and does not affect companies with less than 50 employees.

The Older Americans Act (OAA). Passed in 1965 and amended in 2000 and again in 2006, the OAA established the Administration on Aging (AOA), which was created to organize, coordinate, and provide community-based services and opportunities for older Americans and their families (AOA, 2007). The 2000 amendments maintained many of the original objectives of the program and established the National Family Caregiver Support Program (NFCSP). The AOA awards funds to state units on aging, which then distribute funds to Area Agencies on Aging (AAA). The services of AAAs include:

- Access services: information and assistance; outreach; transportation; case management
- In-home services: homemaker/home health aides; personal care; visiting and telephone reassurance; chore and supportive services
- Community services: congregate meals; senior center activities; adult day care; ombudsman services; abuse prevention; legal services; employment counseling; health promotion
- Caregiver services: respite; adult day care; counseling, and education

The 2006 amendments included:

- Enhanced federal, state, and local coordination of long-term care services provided in home and community-based settings;
- Support for state and community planning to address the long-term care needs of the baby boom generation;
- Greater focus on prevention and treatment of mental disorders;
- Outreach and service to a broader universe of family caregivers under the National Family Caregiver Support Program; and
- Increased focus on civic engagement and volunteerism.

Public policy has greatly influenced the US healthcare system. Basic health services are provided to the majority of US senior citizens and the severely disabled, but, as discussed, the health system is fragmented and complex. Initiating changes in current policies can benefit individuals with chronic illness, but to do so requires political action.

INTERVENTIONS: POLITICS, A CARING ACTION

Each of us is just one personal injustice away from being involved in politics.

(Dodd, 2004, p. 19)

Public and private policies reflect societal values, beliefs, and attitudes and are shaped by politics (Mason et al., 2007). To influence and change policy requires more than a one-time intervention. It requires continued, caring nursing action, which includes being politically active (Smith-Campbell, 1999). Being active in politics allows nurses the ability to shape policy that influences the care individuals with chronic illness receive, and gives nurses an opportunity to partner with clients to meet common goals. Helping clients with chronic conditions and their families understand the political process and the power of politics can empower them to work to change the injustices experienced in the healthcare system.

Politics is often viewed negatively, yet politics is a neutral term that has been defined as influencing (Mason et al., 2007). The reason politics is seen as negative is that influencing often means that individuals differ on what policy should or should not be implemented. These differences can arise from conflicting value and belief systems that elicit strong emotional responses, which are often viewed as negative. As a process, politics is neither negative nor positive but aims to influence the decisions of others and wield control over situations and events, usually in attempts to control scarce resources.

As healthcare providers for individuals with chronic illness, it is imperative that we recognize the need to intervene on policy issues for our patients/clients—because it does affect their health. Can an individual get health insurance with a chronic illness—even if they can pay for it? Will their health insurance cover their medications? Will Medicare or Medicaid provide needed healthcare services for those with chronic illnesses? Does the public health system have enough funding to educate the public on ways to prevent chronic illnesses? These are just a few policy issues affecting those with chronic illness in which interventions may be required. Such interventions or caring action involves influencing policy or becoming politically active.

Stages of Influencing Policy

Agenda Setting

One conceptual model to influence policy uses a staged system approach. Hanley and Falk (2007) and Milio (1989) summarize four stages in which policy can be influenced: (1) agenda setting, (2) legislation/regulation of policy, (3) program implementation, and (4) program evaluation. Identifying a societal problem and bringing it to the attention of government is agenda setting. Most national policy agenda setting begins with congressional members or comes from the office of the President. The personal values and beliefs of public officials and the values and desires of their constituents influence governmental officials in determining new agenda items or attempting to change agenda items. Agendas may be pushed to the forefront, at local, state, or national levels, because of a single injustice or tragedy. Before the organization Mothers Against Drunk Driving (MADD) existed, most of the American populace viewed drinking and driving as normal; yet, drunk drivers were causing death and disabling individuals across the nation. Because one mother felt passionate about the injustice of her child being killed by a drunk driver, a new advocacy organization was formed and MADD chapters that fight drinking and driving now exist everywhere. Policies, as well as national values, have changed regarding drinking and driving, all because one woman became passionate about an injustice (Dodd, 2004). MADD was successful because the political climate was ripe for change.

As conditions in society change or there is a shift in values and beliefs, new agenda items take on more importance. Recently such issues have been and continue to be: healthcare coverage for all, illegal immigration, and the Iraq war. Agenda setting can also be influenced by other factors such as publication of research findings. Based on an IOM report on errors in the healthcare system, patients, families, and legislators continue to ask questions about the quality of health care received (Kohn, Corrigan, & Donaldson, 2000). This report continues to impact health care through new and modified Medicare policies. Once an agenda becomes recognized, governmental officials begin to legislate programs and develop and/or change policy to correct problems identified in agenda setting.

Legislation and Regulation

Legislation and regulation are formal responses to problems identified in agenda setting (Milstead, 2008). There are many ways to influence the process of legislation and regulation. This can be done directly with legislators themselves, but other players may impact the legislative process. These

groups include legislative staff persons, regulatory agency personnel, interest groups, research, media, and constituents (Hanley & Falk, 2007). The process of how a bill becomes law at the national level is outlined in Figure 23-1. The process is similar at the state level, with the endpoint being the governor of the state. The key players not only influence the form of the final bill, but can also have an impact on the bill's continuation or abandonment at any time during the process. Broad language is used to write laws for flexibility and adaptability of their application over time. Once a bill becomes law, it is the responsibility of administrative agencies to write regulations based on the approved law. Examples include State Boards of Nursing implementing nurse practice acts or Centers for Medicare & Medicaid Services writing specific rules on the reimbursement of a medical procedure.

Individuals and stakeholders can also influence the development of regulations. At the national level, a draft of specific regulations must be posted in the Federal Register (www.gpoaccess.gov/fr), and public comment is taken. The administrative agency then reviews the comments and may make changes to the final rules and regulations. Once approved by an executive level agency, the regulations go into effect. After regulations are approved, programs are then established or past programs are modified, based on the new regulations.

Program Implementation

Program implementation occurs when programs are initiated to achieve goals written in either legislation policy or regulation (Milstead, 2008). As in the earlier discussion of policy and the healthcare system, program implementation can have both positive and negative effects. Positive examples include mandating access to public buildings and transportation for the disabled, and national programs that provide funding to the disabled for health insurance and living expenses, as well as nursing home care to those with limited incomes. In turn, other programs have been cut to help balance the budget.

FIGURE 23-1

How a Bill Becomes Law (Federal Level)

Opportunity to Politically Influence

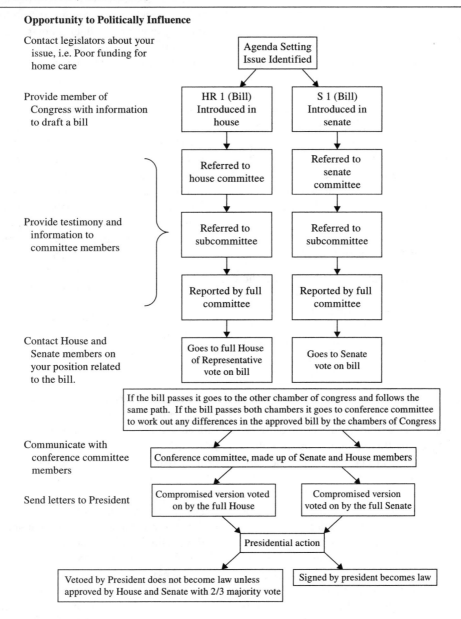

Contact legislators about your issue, i.e. Poor funding for home care

Provide member of Congress with information to draft a bill

Provide testimony and information to committee members

Contact House and Senate members on your position related to the bill.

Communicate with conference committee members

Send letters to President

Agenda Setting
Issue Identified

HR 1 (Bill)
Introduced in house

S 1 (Bill)
Introduced in senate

Referred to house committee

Referred to senate committee

Referred to subcommittee

Referred to subcommittee

Reported by full committee

Reported by full committee

Goes to full House of Representative vote on bill

Goes to Senate vote on bill

If the bill passes it goes to the other chamber of congress and follows the same path. If the bill passes both chambers it goes to conference committee to work out any differences in the approved bill by the chambers of Congress

Conference committee, made up of Senate and House members

Compromised version voted on by the full House

Compromised version voted on by the full Senate

Presidential action

Vetoed by President does not become law unless approved by House and Senate with 2/3 majority vote

Signed by president becomes law

It is possible to influence program implementation and encourage the need for program evaluation when problems are seen within the program.

Program Evaluation

In this stage, programs are evaluated to determine if the original policy goals and objectives were met (Hanley & Falk, 2007). For example, across the nation both national and state policies have attempted to deinstitutionalize the mentally ill. Although the program goals to decrease the number of mentally ill that are institutionalized have been successful, the problem of adequate community services have led many with chronic mental illness to become homeless or housed within the criminal justice system.

Nursing Interventions—Action Steps

To affect public policy, nurses need to learn the skills necessary to influence policy makers at all stages of policy development. These skills can also be taught to clients with chronic conditions and their families so they, too, can be empowered to change the system on their own behalf.

Communication

Vance (1985) identified communication, collectivity, and collegiality as the three components of political influence. Skillful communication can be very influential in the political process. Nurses usually are expert one-to-one communicators, but to affect policy, nurses must broaden their communication skills. The first step of communication is listening and learning. It is essential to learn about the political process. Knowing how a bill becomes law is one way of learning about the political process (Figure 23-1). It is also important to identify the key players at different steps in the process. Knowing when a bill is in committee and the chairperson and committee membership is important information so that one can then attempt to apply influence. In addition to directly trying to influence public policy makers,

indirect influence is also a strategy. Communicating with congressional/executive staff members, the media, and constituents also can influence policy makers. Knowing who you are trying to influence and how you want to influence their actions are key factors. Once you have determined that, there are several communication strategies that can influence policy makers:

- Send your message and/or position by mail, letter, fax sheet, e-mail, or telegram. In small states you will probably be able to contact your legislator directly; in larger states or at the national level you call either talk with a staff person or leave a short message. It is important to note that since the Anthrax attack, email, fax or phone calls are probably the best way to communicate with legislators. In addition, many elected or policy leaders have their own Web site in which there is usually a mechanism to send a message.
- Write letters to your newspaper editor; talk on the radio/TV.
- Visit your legislator and/or their staff (Table 23-1).
- Testify at public hearings.
- Vote and get others to vote.

Building relationships with legislators before controversial issues occur can give you an edge in influencing others. There are several ways to build relationships or friendships with legislators before critical issues. One way is to assist an individual who is running for office. Help with the campaign, hand out flyers, answer phones, or hold a fundraising event in your home. A nurse activist who holds a national governmental appointment states, "Money is the mother's milk of politics. Give it early, and if you don't have it, raise it" (Dodd, 2004, p. 19). Campaigns require money, and providing such assistance to the candidate of your choice then opens the door to your influence once the candidate is elected. This does not mean that money buys votes, but it does provide access. If a legislator has limited time and has to choose to see someone who gave him or her money or another who did not, most likely the

TABLE 23-1

Guidelines for Meeting with Policy Makers or Their Staff

1. Make an appointment. Be on time.
2. Always introduce yourself, even if this is your third or fourth meeting. State that you are a registered nurse, or if a client is speaking, have that person share the nature of the chronic condition he or she or the family member has.
3. Begin on a positive note. Thank the legislator for seeing you and then get down to business. Clearly identify the issue you want to discuss; if it is a specific bill, state its number, its title, your position, and what you want the legislator to do.
4. Depending on the time allotted, give examples and facts to illustrate your position. Most importantly, share client stories.
5. Remain positive; keep the atmosphere open and friendly. The purpose of the meeting is to exchange ideas and keep the lines of communication open. Do not engage in threats or ask for the impossible.
6. Be prepared to answer questions. If you do not know the answer, say so, but state that you will get more information, and then follow through.
7. Always leave written literature on the subject (position paper, outline of your key points, etc.) and contact information (business card).
8. Follow up your visit with a thank-you note.
9. Send copies of your written comments or a summary of your meeting to the organization(s) with which you are working.

Source: Capital Advantage. (2007). Visiting Capitol Hill. Retrieved on December 15, 2007 from www.congress.org; United Cerebral Palsy. (2007). Advocacy tools. Retrieved on December 17, 2007 from www.ucp.org

legislator will choose the person who assisted the campaign financially. This access gives the person, the nurse, the client, or family member the opportunity to share their position and influence the legislator. Political activists would probably agree that although money provides access, constituents can also make a difference with their time (i.e., campaigning, writing letters, or calling legislators on issues). Legislators pay attention to those who vote and to those who communicate with them.

Collectivity

Collectivity is critical to the development of political influence and is built on a foundation of networking, coalition building, and collaboration (Vance, 1985). One of the first steps in advocacy is finding mentors that can assist in developing needed skills (Leavitt, Chaffee, & Vance, 2007). Mentors can assist in learning about the policy process as well as provide access to key stakeholders. Working to change policy at any level

of government requires group action and collaboration. The American Nurses Association, which speaks for more than 2.8 million nurses, has testified on many key issues relevant to nursing and the patients they serve, including healthcare reform, Medicare funding, and funding for nursing educational programs.

National and state professional and community organizations also work for policy initiatives that impact their organization or members of their organization. The American Heart Association has specific legislative goals related to heart disease and stroke. They work with individuals and groups in policy initiatives, including help in finding your local legislator, how and when to write your legislator, as well as keeping the public informed about policy issues that impact their stated goals. Professional and community organizations, especially at the local level, can provide great mentoring opportunities. These organizations are often looking for individuals to help with their advocacy strategies and may often help in the development of those skills.

CASE STUDY

As a nurse who works in a heart failure clinic, you recognize the importance of preventing and reducing heart disease. Lately you have seen younger patients being diagnosed with health failure related to lifestyle behaviors such as obesity and smoking. You have also noted that many of these individuals have not sought out health care prior to their diagnosis of heart failure because they lack health insurance.

Discussion Questions

1. What national and statewide advocacy organization might be able to mentor/assist you in advocacy efforts to reduce heart disease and stroke risks?
2. If your state had a bill pending to ban smoking in all public buildings, who would you contact to support passage of the bill?
3. Who are the potential stakeholders related to a state-wide smoking ban and what strategies would you utilize to influence them?

Personal connections can be another important strategy in moving a critical issue. Consider the nursing student whose mother is a legislator on a health committee discussing reimbursement for healthcare providers. Working with the student nurse, providing education and support to the student to testify in front of the mother's committee, could have a major impact on the direction an issue takes. Networking is key, because sometimes success comes down to having just one important personal connection (Leavitt, Cohen, & Mason, 2007).

Networking with client groups can also be helpful. Having clients communicate with legislators about how they or their families have been or will be affected by legislation is an important strategy to influence policy makers. Working with groups that have been active in advocacy can provide a novice political advocate needed assistance and support. Advocacy groups such as the American Association of People with Disabilities (2007) can help professionals or families of the disabled provide testimony at public hearings.

Collegiality

Central to the political process is collegiality, a spirit of cooperation and solidarity with associates (Vance, 1985). To be a political activist and risk taker requires support from colleagues. It is helpful to work with others with an attitude of mutual respect and shared convictions. Sometimes diverse groups can work together on a mutual issue, even if they are opponents on other issues. Disassociating the emotional context of working with opponents is key. As stated earlier, politics is neither negative nor positive, but each side often has different values and beliefs. Working in solidarity with a group provides support during conflict and can assist in an important factor in political influencing—not taking it personally. As a professional, it is important to address your specific issue and not personally attack those who oppose you. Address only the issue, even if others personally attack you. Eleanor Roosevelt once said, "No one can make you feel inferior without your permission." Often, this is easier said than done. Influencing policy changes requires patience, perseverance, and compromise. Working with those who share similar values, beliefs, and convictions will be of great assistance when working for change.

The strategies discussed in this section emphasize influencing policy at the national level. These same strategies can also be used to influence local and state policy, as well as policy makers in work and community organizations. It is vital that nurses become political, or they risk being excluded from important decisions that affect nursing practice or the care their patients with chronic illness receive.

Becoming a political person can be an overwhelming experience as you realize you cannot change a whole system alone. As a beginning political activist—start by voting. Next, choose an issue about which you feel passionate (e.g., the inability of your chronically ill clients to get long-term home care). Educate yourself on the issue, and join others who are interested in the issue. Communicate your position to the key players. Know that your cause is just, and be proud of the political influence you, your clients, and your colleagues can accomplish.

OUTCOMES

Through public policy, society has made choices to assist many Americans. There are policies to care for the elderly and severely disabled through Medicare, provide health insurance to the poor through Medicaid, and ensure access for the disabled with the ADA. Society's belief in the market system and individual rights has left many with inadequate or absent health care. Because health care is not a right in the United States, there is no "system"' of health care. The system in place is complex, fragmented, and difficult to use, especially for vulnerable populations such as the chronically ill, the disabled, and the elderly. Changes can be made to improve the system. The profession of nursing and clients with chronic illness and their families can influence change through political action. It will take time and perseverance, but as Marian Wright Edema, founder and president of the Children's Defense Fund, states, "We must not, in trying to think about how we can make a big difference, ignore the small daily differences we can make which, over time, add up to big differences that we often cannot see."

EVIDENCE-BASED PRACTICE BOX

The evidence clearly shows that health policy impacts the health of individuals. Policies that increase the number of insured increase the health of individuals:

- A 12-year study of more than 7000 Americans demonstrates that individuals without health insurance experience a dramatic improvement in their subsequent health trends when they become eligible for Medicare at age 65 (McWilliams et al., 2007).
- The uninsured are less likely to get screened for cancer, more likely to be diagnosed with an advanced stage of the disease, and less likely to survive that diagnosis than their privately insured counterparts (Ward et al., 2007).
- Uninsured individuals with a new chronic condition reported receiving less medical care and poorer health status than those with insurance (Hadley, 2007).

STUDY QUESTIONS

1. Describe the trends of chronic illness and how these trends are significant in relation to health policy.
2. Differentiate between Medicare and Medicaid.
3. Identify the major social issues affecting health policy for the individual with chronic illness.
4. How does the current US healthcare system affect those with chronic illness?
5. Explain how a bill becomes law.
6. Identify the three components of political influence, and explain each.
7. What are the first steps in which you will engage to become politically active?

INTERNET RESOURCES

How to find and communicate with legislators and stakeholders:
■ National leaders and issues: www.congress.org
■ Federal Legislative link site: http://thomas.loc.gov/

How to write to the media (info and samples):
■ Kansas Health Consumer Coalition: www.kshealthconsumer.com/media.htm
■ Fairness and Accuracy in Reporting: www.fair.org/activism/communicate.html

Policy/political resources
■ Health System Change policy analysis site: www.hschange.org/
■ Summary of national political news: www.politicalinsider.com/
■ State policy and politics: www.stateline.org/live/

Government Web sites:
■ Centers for Medicare and Medicaid Services (CMS): www.cms.hhs.gov
■ Department of Veterans Affairs: www.va.gov
■ Executive Offices and Executive Departments: ww.loc.gov/rr/news/fedgov.html
■ Social Security Administration—Disability benefits: www.ssa.gov
■ US House of Representatives: www.house.gov/
■ US Senate: www.senate.gov/

Advocacy or other relevant Web sites:
■ American Association of Homes and Services for the Aging: www.aahsa.org
■ American Association of People with Disabilities: www.aapd.com
■ American Heart Association: www.americanheart.org (click on advocacy)
■ American Nurse's Association-legislative newsletter: www.capitolupdate.org/newsletter/
■ Consortium for Citizens with Disabilities: www.c-c-d.org
■ Families USA http://www.familiesusa.org/
■ National Alliance for Caregiving: www.caregiving.org
■ National Citizen's Coalition for Nursing Home Reform: www.nccnhr.org/
■ National Respite Coalition: www.archrespite.org/NRC.htm
■ Partnership to fight chronic disease: www.fightchronicdisease.org/
■ Preventing Chronic Disease Journal: www.cdc.gov/pcd/
■ Understanding Disabilities, Creating Opportunities: www.ucp.org
■ WHO—World Health Organization-Chronic Disease and Health Promotion: www.who.int/chp/en/

REFERENCES

Administration on Aging. (2007). Older Americans Act. Retrieved on December 13, 2007, from www.aoa.gov/

American Association of People with Disabilities. (2007). AAPD policy positions & activities. Retrieved December 15, 2007, from www.aapd.com

American Nurses Association. (2005). Health care agenda 2005. Retrieved on November 1, 2007 from www.nursingworld.org

Bellah, R.N., Madsen, R., Sullivan, W.M., Swidler, A., & Tipton, S.M. (1985). *Habits of the heart: Individualism and commitment in American life*. New York: Harper & Row.

Benner, P., & Wrubel, J. (1989). *The primacy of caring*. Menlo Park, CA: Addison-Wesley.

Capital Advantage. (2007). Visiting Capitol Hill. Retrieved on December 15, 2007 from www.congress.org

Centers for Disease Control. (2007). Health, United States, 2007. Retrieved on December 4, 2007 from www.cdc.gov/nchs/

Centers for Medicare & Medicaid Services. (2004). Medicare awards for programs to improve care of beneficiaries with chronic illnesses. Retrieved on November 1, 2007 from www.cms.hhs.gov/

Centers for Medicare and Medicaid Services. (2005). Medicaid at-a-glance 2005 a Medicaid information source. *Publication No. CMS-11024–05.* Retrieved on November 1, 2007 from www.cms.hhs.gov

Centers for Medicare & Medicaid Services. (2007a). Medicare coverage–general information–overview. Retrieved on October 31, 2007, from www.cms.hhs.gov/MedicareGenInfo/

Centers for Medicare & Medicaid Services. (2007b). Medicare health support–overview. Retrieved on December 17, 2007, from www.cms.hhs.gov/CCIP/

Centers for Medicare & Medicaid Services. (2007c). Your guide to Medicare prescription drug coverage. *CMS Pub. No. 11109,* from www.medicare.gov/Publications/Pubs/pdf/11109.pdf

Chopoorian, T.J. (1986). Reconceptualizing the environment. In P. Moccia (Ed.). *New approaches to theory development* (pp. 39–54). New York: National League of Nursing.

DeNavas-Walt, C., Proctor, B.D., & Smith, J. (2007). Income, poverty, and health insurance coverage in the United States: 2006. Retrieved on October 30, 2007 from www.census.gov

DeVol, R., Bedroussian, A., Charuworn, A., Chatterjee, A., Kim, I.K., Kim, S., et al. (2007). An unhealthy America: The economic burden of chronic disease: charting a new course to save lives and increase productivity and economic growth. Retrieved on October 30, 2007 from www.milkeninstitute.org

Dodd, C. J. (2004). Making the political process work. In C. Harrington & C.L. Estes (Eds.). *Health policy crisis and reform in the U.S. Health care delivery system* (4th ed.)(pp. 18–28). Sudbury, MA: Jones & Bartlett.

eHealthInsurance. (2007). 3 easy steps to health insurance. Retrieved December 4, 2007 from www.ehealthinsurance.com

Families USA. (2006). Coverage through the "doughnut hole" grows scarcer in 2007. Retrieved on November 1, 2007 from www.familiesusa.org

Feldstein, P.J. (2007). *Health policy issues: An economic perspective* (4th ed.). Chicago: Health Administration Press.

Fronstin, P., & Collins, S.R. (2006). The 2nd annual EBRI/commonwealth fund consumerism in health care survey, 2006: Early experience with high-deductible and consumer-driven health plans. Retrieved on January 16, 2008 from www.cmwf.org/

Government Accounting Office. (2006). Consumer-directed health plans early enrollee experiences with health savings accounts and eligible health plans. *GAO-06–798.* Retrieved October 31, 2007 from www.gao.gov

Hadley, J. (2007). Insurance coverage, medical care use, and short-term health changes following an unintentional injury or the onset of a chronic condition. *JAMA, 297*(10), 1073–1084.

Hanley, B., & Falk, N.L. (2007). Policy development and analysis: Understanding the process. In D. J. Mason, J.K. Leavitt & M.W. Chaffee (Eds.), *Policy & politics in nursing and health care* (5th ed.) (pp. 75–93). St. Louis: Saunders Elsevier.

Hanson, K., Neuman, T., & Voris, M. (2003). Understanding the health-care needs and experiences of people with disabilities: Findings from a 2003 survey. Retrieved on December 4, 2007 from www.kff.org

Hoffman, C., & Tolbert, J. (2006). Health savings accounts and high deductible health plans: Are they an option for low-income families? Publication Number 7568. Retrieved on January 16, 2008 from www.kff.org/uninsured/7568.cfm

Institute of Medicine. (2002). *Care without coverage: Too little, too late.* Washington, D.C: National Academy Press.

Joyce, G.F., Goldman, D.P., Karaca-Mandic, P., & Zheng, Y. (2007). Pharmacy benefit caps and the chronically ill. *Health Affairs, 26*(5), 1333–1344.

Kaiser Commission on Medicaid and the Uninsured. (2007). Health coverage of children: The role of Medicaid and SCHIP. Retrieved on November 1, 2007 from www.kff.org/uninsured

Kaiser Family Foundation. (2004). Trends and indicators in the changing health care marketplace, 2004 update. Retrieved on September 13, 2004 from www.kff.org/

Kaiser Family Foundation, Health Research and Education Trust. (2007). Employer health benefits: 2007 annual survey. Retrieved October 31, 2007 from www.kff.org/insurance/

Kavanagh, K. H., & Knowlden, V. (2004). *Many voices: Toward caring culture in healthcare and healing.* Madison, WI: University of Wisconsin Press.

Kohn, L.T., Corrigan, J.M., & Donaldson, M.S. (2000). *To err is human: Building a safer health system.* Washington, DC: National Academy Press.

Leavitt, J.K., Chaffee, M.W., & Vance, C. (2007). Learning the ropes of policy, politics, and advocacy. In D.J. Mason, J.K. Leavitt & M.W. Chaffee (Eds.), *Policy & politics in nursing and health care* (pp. 34–36). St. Louis, MO: Elsevier.

Leavitt, J.K., Cohen, S.S., & Mason, D.J. (2007). Policy analysis and strategies. In D.J. Mason, J.K. Leavitt & M.W. Chaffee (Eds.), *Policy & politics in nursing and health care* (pp. 94–109). St. Louis, MO: Elsevier.

Lottero, B., Pryor, C., Rukavina, M., Prottas, J., & Knudson, A. (2007). Issue brief 2007: Health insurance survey of farm and ranch operators. No. 1. Retrieved on December 14, 2007 from www.accessproject.org

Mason, D.J., Leavitt, J.K., & Chaffee, M.W. (2007). Policy and politics: A framework for action. In D.J. Mason, J.K. Leavitt & M.W. Chaffee (Eds.). *Policy & politics in nursing and health care* (5th ed.). St. Louis: Saunders Elsevier.

McWilliams, J.M., Meara, E., Zaslavsky, A.M., & Ayanian, J.Z. (2007). Health of previously uninsured adults after acquiring Medicare coverage. *JAMA, 298*(24), 2886–2894.

Milio, N. (1989). Developing nursing leadership in health policy. *Journal of Professional Nursing, 5*, 315–321.

Milstead, J.A. (2008). *Health policy and politics: A nurse's guide* (3rd ed.). Sudbury, MA: Jones & Bartlett.

National Center for Chronic Disease Prevention and Health Promotion. (2005). Chronic disease overview. Retrieved on October 30, 2007 from www.cdc.gov/nccdphp/overview.htm

Navarro, V. (2004). Why congress did not enact health care reform. In C. Harrington & C.L. Estes (Eds.). *Health policy crisis and reform in the U.S. Health care delivery system* (4th ed.) (pp. 36–40). Sudbury, MA: Jones & Bartlett.

Neuman, T. (2006). Medicare 101. Retrieved on October 31, 2007 from www.kaiseredu.org

Partnership to Fight Chronic Disease. (2007). About the PFCD. Retrieved on December 17, 2007 from www.fightchronicdisease.org.

Peppe, E.M., Mays, J.W., Chang, H.C., Becker, E., & DiJulio, B. (2007). Characteristics of frequent emergency department users. Publication Number: 7696. Retrieved on October 31, 2007 from http://www.kff.org

Pulcine, J.A., & Hart, M.A. (2007). Financing health care in the United States. In D.J. Mason, J.K. Leavitt & M.W. Chaffee (Eds.), *Policy & politics in nursing and health care* (5th ed.) (pp. 384–408). St. Louis: Saunders Elsevier.

Rowland, D. (2005). Medicaid: The basics. Retrieved on November 1, 2007, from www.kaiseredu.org/

Rowland, D., & Tallon, J.R. (2004). Medicaid: Lessons from a decade. In C. Harrington & C.L. Estes (Eds.). *Health policy crisis and reform in the U.S. Health care delivery system* (4th ed.). Sudbury, MA: Jones & Bartlett.

Schwartz, K. (2007). Survey spotlight on uninsured parents: How a lack of coverage affects parents and their families. Retrieved on December 4, 2007 from www.kff.org.

Smith-Campbell, B. (1999). A case study on expanding the concept of caring from individuals to communities. *Public Health Nursing, 16*, 405–411.

Social Security Administration. (2007). Social security handbook. Retrieved on December 14, 2007 from www.socialsecurity.gov

Thorpe, K.E., Howard, D.H., & Galactionova, K. (2007). International survey: U.S. Adults most likely to report medical errors and skip needed care due to costs. Retrieved on December 17, 2007 from www.commonwealthfund.org/

Tu, H.T. (2004). Rising health costs, medical debt and chronic conditions. Retrieved on October 30, 2007 from www.hschange.org

U.S. Department of Health and Human Services. (2007). Your Medicare coverage. Retrieved on November 1, 2007 from www.medicare.gov/

U.S. Department of Justice. (2000). Enforcing the ADA: Looking back on a decade of progress. Retrieved on December 13, 2007 from www.usdoj.gov/

U.S. Department of Justice. (2006). Americans with disabilities act. Retrieved on December 14, 2007 from www.usdoj.gov

U.S. Department of Labor. (2007a). Fact sheet #28: The family and medical leave act of 1993. Retrieved on December 14, 2007 from www.dol.gov

U.S. Department of Labor. (2007b). Frequently asked questions about portability of health coverage and HIPAA. Retrieved on December 4, 2007 from www.dol.gov

United Cerebral Palsy. (2007). Advocacy tools. Retrieved on December 17, 2007 from www.ucp.org

Vance, C. (1985). Politics: A humanistic process. In D.J. Mason, S.W. Talbott & J.K. Leavitt (Eds.), *Policy and politics for nurses* (pp. 104–118). Philadelphia: WB Saunders.

Vladeck, B.C., & King, K.M. (1997). Medicare at 30: Preparing for the future. In C. Harrington & C.L. Estes (Eds.), *Health policy and nursing* (pp. 319–326). Sudbury, MA: Jones & Bartlett.

Ward, E., Halpern, M., Schrag, N., Cokkinides, V., DeSantis, C., Bandi, P., et al. (2007). Association of insurance with cancer care utilization and outcomes. *CA: A Cancer Journal for Clinicians, article doi: 10.3322/CA.2007.0011,* Retrieved on January 3, 2008 from http://caonline.amcancersoc.org/cgi/content/full/CA.2007.0011v1

Watson, J. (1988). *Nursing: Human science and human care a theory of nursing.* New York: National League of Nursing.

World Health Organization. (2005). Preventing chronic diseases: A vital investment: WHO global report. Retrieved on October 30, 2007 from www.who.int/chp/chronic_disease_report/contents/en/index.html

24

Rehabilitation

Kristen L. Mauk

INTRODUCTION

"Rehabilitation refers to services and programs designed to assist individuals who have experienced a trauma or illness that results in impairment that creates a loss of function (physical, psychological, social, or vocational)" (Remsburg & Carson, 2006, p. 579). Rehabilitation is also an approach to care in which persons with chronic illness and disability are "made able" again (Pryor, 2002).

Rehabilitation assists individuals with long-term health alterations to regain independence and adapt to changes that have occurred as a result of deviations in their health status. A popular rehabilitation saying is that "rehabilitation begins day one" and thus should be considered as part of the overall plan of care for most acute illness episodes and throughout the duration of most chronic illnesses.

The primary goal of rehabilitation is to achieve the highest level of independence possible for the client. This goal is highly individualized. For example, a person with a mild stroke may have the goal to walk again and resume gainful employment at the same job he held previously. Another person with a high-level spinal injury may realistically have a different goal of being able to be

mobile independently with the use of a mechanically adapted wheelchair such as a sip'n puff chair. Both persons have achievable goals, but ones that are based upon their capacity and functional limitations that have resulted from illness or injury.

The goals of rehabilitation may be summarized with a few concepts: restoring or maximizing the level of function, facilitating independence, preventing complications, and promoting quality of life. Rehabilitation typically involves an interdisciplinary team of professionals working toward a common goal. The client and family are considered the most important team members. Professional team members may include physicians, nurses, therapists, social workers, vocational counselors, nutritionists, orthotists, prosthetists, and chaplains. Additional professionals may be consulted to help meet the unique needs of the individual.

Rehabilitation is commonly associated with certain disorders or illnesses in which therapeutic interventions have been shown to be effective. These include health alterations such as stroke, spinal cord injury, traumatic or other brain injury, neurologic diseases (such as Parkinson's disease, multiple sclerosis, Guillain-Barré syndrome); orthopedic problems such as arthritis, fractures or joint replacements; and less commonly, burns, cancer, or respiratory disorders. In each of these conditions, persons can be assisted to regain maximal functioning that may have been altered because of a disease process, injury, or congenital defect.

One of the foci of the rehabilitation process is community reintegration or re-entry, sometimes referred to as resocialization. This is a process by which individuals are reintegrated into society after a life-altering health condition or situation changes their previous roles and abilities. Within a rehabilitation setting, reintegration is an ongoing goal. Rehabilitation professionals work with the disabled client or individual with chronic illness and their family to help them re-enter the community in which they may have to accomplish significant adjustments to adapt to changes that have occurred in every area of their life. Often this process involves the client re-learning how to do self-care with activities of daily living (ADLs) such as bathing, grooming, toileting, eating, and dressing. Rehabilitation is a hopeful process that encourages individuals to maximize their strengths while making positive adaptations to their limitations.

Definitions

Rehabilitation

A number of terms specific to rehabilitation need to be defined before relating them to chronic illness. Many professionals have defined rehabilitation (see Table 24-1), and some common themes among these definitions should be considered. Concepts include the complex, dynamic interactions among the individual, the disease or health condition, and the environment. Most definitions relate to rehabilitation: assisting an individual with a limitation to attain his/her maximal independence and function. For example, the Institute of Medicine (IOM) defines rehabilitation as "the process by which physical, sensory or mental capacities are restored or developed. . . . Rehabilitation strives to reverse what has been called the disabling process, and may therefore be called the enabling process" (Brandt & Pope, 1997, pp. 12–13).

The Royal Hospital for Neuro-disability and the Institute for Neuropalliative Rehabilitation

(2007) suggests that definitions of rehabilitation could be classified into those related to either structure, process, or outcome, and that perhaps no one definition is all-encompassing. They provide an alternate definition for rehabilitation: the planned withdrawal of support.

The National Cancer Institute (2007) defines rehabilitation as "a process to restore mental and/ or physical abilities lost to injury or disease, in order to function in a normal or near-normal way" (p. 1). In addition, various aspects of rehabilitation services such as rehabilitation therapies and community rehabilitation may have more specific definitions related to their particular disciplines.

Rehabilitation Nursing

Rehabilitation is a continuous process and clients rehabilitate themselves through the influence of the comprehensive approach to care provided by the rehabilitation nurse. Rehabilitation nurses are leaders who specialize in assisting individuals affected by chronic illness and disability to maximize their health through health restoration, maintenance, and promotion (Association of Rehabilitation Nurses, 2007a). The Association of Rehabilitation Nurses (ARN) (2008) defines rehabilitation nursing as "the diagnosis and treatment of human responses of individuals and groups to actual or potential health problems related to altered functional ability and lifestyle" (p. 13).

General information for rehabilitation nurses and advanced rehabilitation nurses are included in Standards and Scope of Rehabilitation Nursing Practice (2000) and Scope and Standards of Advanced Clinical Practice in Rehabilitation Nursing (1996). Because the growth of the specialty of rehabilitation nursing, there are many subspecialties associated with this field. The ARN has developed role descriptions of each of the emerging areas in which rehabilitation nurses work.

Restorative Care

"The purpose of restorative care is to actively assist individuals in long-term care settings to maintain

TABLE 24-1

Definitions of Rehabilitation

Source	Definition
Rusk (1965)	Ultimate restoration of a disabled person to his or her maximum capacity: physical, emotional, and vocational
Dittmar (1989)	The process by which an individual's movement toward health is facilitated
Hickey (1992)	A dynamic process by which a person achieves optimal physical, emotional, psychological, social, and vocational potential and maintains dignity and self-respect in a life that is as independent and self-fulfilling as possible
National Council on Rehabilitation (1994)	Restoration of the handicapped to the fullest physical, mental, social, vocational, and economic usefulness of which they are capable
Institute of Medicine, Brandt & Pope (1997)	The process by which physical, sensory, or mental capacities are restored or developed. This is achieved not only through functional change in the person, such as strengthening injured limbs, but also through changes in the physical and social environments, such as making buildings accessible to wheelchairs. Rehabilitation strives to reverse what has been called the disabling process, and may therefore be called the enabling process.
Commission on Accreditation of Rehabilitation Facilities CARF (2000)	The process of providing those comprehensive services deemed appropriate to the needs of persons with disabilities in a coordinated manner in a program or service designed to achieve objectives of improved health, welfare, and realization of the person's maximum physical, social, psychological, and vocational potential for useful and productive activity

their highest level of function and to assist residents in retaining the gains made during formal therapy" (Remsburg & Carson, 2006, p. 580). Restorative care differs from rehabilitation in that it does not include activities directed by therapists, but emphasizes nursing interventions that promote adaptation, comfort, and safety within a long-term care setting (CMS, 2002). Restorative care focuses on maximizing an individual's abilities, helping to rebuild self-esteem, and to achieve appropriate goals (Resnick & Remsburg, 2004; Nadash & Feldman, 2003; Resnick & Fleishall, 2002). Restorative care often focuses on assisting individuals with ADLs as well as walking and mobility exercises, transferring, amputation/prosthesis care, and communication. Self-care skills, such as management of one's diabetes, ostomy care, or medication set-up and administration, are also emphasized (Remsburg, 2004). Restorative care, although conceptually similar to rehabilitation,

is most appropriate for those individuals who either have already reached their maximal functional level and need to maintain that function, or for those who are not appropriate candidates for intensive rehabilitation services.

Vocational Rehabilitation

Vocational rehabilitation assists the disabled individual to return to gainful employment and focus on financial independence through programs specifically designed for this purpose (Lysaght, 2004; Kielkofner et al., 2004; O'Neill, Zuger, Fields, Fraser, & Pruce, 2004; Targett, Wehman, & Young, 2004). The federal government requires each state to have an office of vocational rehabilitation to provide these services for people with disabilities, and provides funding and support to integrate clients into the work community (Parker & Neal-Boylan, 2007).

Rehabilitation Models and Classification Systems

Models are used to help explain, guide, or direct practice or processes. Rehabilitation models can aid in understanding how chronic conditions and disability develop and progress, or how they can be managed. There are several major classification systems used to document rehabilitation processes and outcomes (WHO, 1980; Brandt & Pope, 1997; WHO, 2002). These include the Functional Limitations System (FLS), the Enabling–Disabling Model, and the WHO International Classification of Functioning, Disability, and Health (ICF).

The IOM recommends the use of the Enabling–Disabling Process Model, whereas the WHO recommends the use of the ICF to help standardize and effectively communicate information about diagnoses, care, and treatment. The model used may depend largely on the facility and their preferences and choices. The use of standard terminology within these models can help facilitate communication, but rehabilitation professionals must be thoroughly familiar with the chosen model and understand the terminology within it.

The Enabling–Disabling Process

The Enabling–Disabling Process was developed at the IOM in 1997 as a framework for professional rehabilitation practice. It emphasizes the uniqueness of each individual client by revising the Disability in America model (IOM, 1991). A committee of professionals enhanced the 1991 IOM model "to show more clearly how biological, environmental (physical and social), and lifestyle/behavioral factors are involved in reversing the disabling process, i.e., rehabilitation, or the enabling process" (Brandt & Pope, 1997, p. 13). In the new Enabling–Disabling Process, "disability does not appear in this model since it is not inherent in the individual but, rather, a function of the interaction of the individual and the environment" (Brandt & Pope, 1997, p. 11). Disability is seen as a product of the interaction of an individual with the environment. The model

posits that rehabilitation depends largely upon the individual and his or her unique characteristics, and that the disabling process may even be reversed with appropriate rehabilitation interventions (Lutz & Bowers, 2003). The basic concepts of the model include pathology, impairment, functional limitation, disability, and society limitation (Brandt & Pope, 1997). Table 24-2 provides a summary of the concepts of the Enabling–Disabling Process.

Enabling America, the overall work, urged rehabilitation professionals to adopt a new framework that better described the rehabilitation process (Brandt & Pope, 1997). Since its introduction, however, the Enabling–Disabling Model has not received the recognition or use within healthcare professions that was probably hoped for by the IOM. A search of several notable scholarly databases over the last 10 years revealed few articles written by rehabilitation professionals in healthcare professions that mentioned this process or used it as a framework for research.

International Classification of Functioning, Disability, and Health

In 1980, the World Health Organization (WHO) developed a classification system that was widely used for years internationally. The WHO originally defined impairment as a loss related to structure and function; a disability was related to a loss of ability to perform an activity, and a handicap was a disadvantage for a person related to the environment.

The new International Classification of Functioning, Disability, and Health (ICF) is the WHO's framework for measuring health and disability at both individual and population levels. "ICF is a classification of health and health related domains that describe body functions and structures, activities and participation. The domains are classified from body, individual and societal perspectives" (WHO, 2007, p. 1). The International Classification of Functioning, Disability, and Health provides a shift in viewing disability as gradually becoming a part of the majority of person's lives over time. It provides a holistic look at the process of disability related to

Concepts of the Enabling–Disabling Process

Pathophysiology	Impairment	Functional Limitation	Disability	Societal Limitation
Interruption of or interference with normal physiologic and developmental processes or structures	Loss and/ or abnormality of cognition, and emotional, physiologic, or anatomic structure or function, including all losses or abnormalities, not just those attributable to the initial pathophysiology	Restriction or lack of ability to perform an action in the manner or within a range consistent with the purpose of an organ or organ system	Inability or limitation in performing tasks, activities, and roles to levels expected within physical and social contexts	Restriction, attributable to social policy or barriers (structural or attitudinal), that limits fulfillment of roles or denies access to services and opportunities that are associated with full participation in society

		Level of Impact		
Cells and Tissues	Organs and Organ Systems	Function of the Organ and Organ System	Individual	Society
Structural or functional	Structural or functional	Action or activity performance or organ or organ system	Task performance by person in physical, social contexts	Societal attributes relevant to individuals with disabilities

		Patient Example		
Lacunar infarct of the cerebellum (right hemisphere) related to microvascular changes associated with chronic hypertension	Neuromotor function of the brain	Left hemiparesis or difficulty with spatial–perceptual tasks, difficulty sequencing, memory deficits	Deficits in ambulation, self-care, shopping, work	Lack of adaptations in the work environment that would enable person to continue employment

Source: Whyte, J. (1998). Enabling America: A report from the Institute of Medicine on rehabilitation science and engineering. *Archives of Physical Medicine and Rehabilitation, 79*(11), 1477–1480. Reprinted with permission from Elsevier.

health, considering all aspects, not just the medical or physical (WHO, 2007). The four major sections of the classification document are body functions (by system and including mental health), body structures (by system), activities and participation (such as learning, communication, self-care, community involvement), and environmental factors (such as products, technology, attitudes, service and policy) (ICF, 2007). Table 24-3 provides an overview of ICF.

Other models that can guide rehabilitation practice have emerged from rehabilitation nursing scientists. These middle-range theories are not classification systems for general rehabilitation, but they may provide insight and direction about specific processes or phenomenon. An example of an area in which several new frameworks or models have arisen is in stroke rehabilitation and recovery. Secrest and colleagues (Secrest & Zeller, 2007; Secrest & Thomas, 1999) have explored the relationship of continuity and discontinuity following stroke. They continue to publish about the relationship of this phenomenon with functional ability, depression, and quality of life. Their work resulted in the development of a tool

to measure themes common to the post-stroke experience such as control, connection with others, and independence (Secrest & Zeller, 2003).

Mauk (Easton, 2001; Mauk, 2006) developed a model from grounded theory that identified six phases of post-stroke recovery that may help guide practice and interventions. She found that stroke survivors journey through a predictable pattern, with certain variables influencing the ease of adaptation after stroke. Other rehabilitation nurse scientists have explored the experience of caregivers of stroke survivors (Pierce, Steiner, Hicks, & Holzaepfel, 2004; Pierce et al., 2006; Hartke & King, 2002). Each of these examples suggest that although large, general models and classification systems are necessary and helpful, more manageable models, frameworks, and instruments are also needed to better reflect the unique experiences in rehabilitation and to guide practice.

Historical Perspectives

Rehabilitation as a specialty within first, medicine, and then nursing, was slow to develop (see

---

TABLE 24-3

Concepts of the International Classification of Functioning, Disability, and Health

	Major Concepts		
Health Condition	*Impairment*	*Activity Limitation*	*Participation Restriction*
Diseases, disorders, and injuries, e.g., leprosy, diabetes, spinal cord injury	Problems in body function or structure such as a significant deviation or loss, e.g., anxiety, paralysis, loss of sensation of extremities	Problems in body function or structure such as a significant deviation or loss, e.g., anxiety, paralysis, loss of sensation of extremities	Problems an individual may experience in involvement in life situations, e.g., unable to attend social events, unable to use public transportation to get to church, unable to perform job functions
	Example		
Spinal cord injury	Paralysis	Incapable of using public transportation	Unable to attend religious activities

Source: WHO. (2002). Towards a common language for functioning, disability and health ICF. Retrieved from http://www3.who.int/icf/icftemplate.cfm?myurl=beginners.html&mytitle=Beginner%27s%20Guide

TABLE 24-4

Historical Events and Legislative Initiatives Affecting Rehabilitation

Date	Event/Initiative	Purpose
1910	"Studies of Invalid Occupation"	Published by nurse Susan Tracy; beginning of occupational therapy
1917	American Red Cross Institute for Crippled and Disabled Men personnel	Created to provide vocational training for wounded military
1918	Smith-Sears Legislation (PL 65-178)	Authorized Federal Board for Vocational Education to administer a national vocational rehabilitation service to disabled veterans of World War I
1920	Smith-Fess Legislation (PL 66-236)	Provided vocational rehabilitation services to people disabled in industry and otherwise
1930	Veteran's Administration (VA)	Created by Executive Order 5398 to care for those with service-related disabilities, signed by President Herbert Hoover. At this time there were 54 hospitals, 4.7 million living veterans.
1935	Social Security Act (PL 74-271)	Provided permanent authorization for the civilian vocational rehabilitation program
1938	American Academy of Physical Medicine	Organization formed; physical medicine and rehabilitation emerges as a specialty
1941	First comprehensive book on physical medicine and rehabilitation	Written by Frank Krusen, MD
1942	Sister Kenny Institute	Institute and Sister Kenny's research led to the development of the profession of physical therapy and provided support for physiatry as a specialty.
1943	Welsh-Clark Legislation (PL 78-16)	Provided vocational rehabilitation for disabled veterans of World War II
1943	United Nations Rehabilitation Administration	Organization established with representatives from 44 countries to plan care for disabled WWII veterans
1946	Department of Medicine and Surgery	A department within the VA established to provide medical care for veterans; succeeded in 1989 by the Veterans Health Services and Research Administration, renamed the Veterans Health Administration in 1991
1947	Bellevue Medical Rehabilitation Services	First US rehabilitation program, established by Howard Rusk, MD
1947	American Board of Physical Medicine and Rehabilitation specialty	Board formed, and rehabilitation becomes a board-certified
1954	Hill-Burton Act (PL 83-565)	Provided greater financial support, research and demonstration grants, state agency expansion and grants to expand rehabilitation facilities
1958	Rehabilitation Medicine	H. Rusk and colleagues publish a rehabilitation text.
1965	Vocational Rehabilitation Act (PL 89-333)	Expanded and improved vocational rehabilitation services
1973	Rehabilitation Act (PL 93-112)	Expanded services to the more severely handicapped by giving them priority; affirmative action in employment and nondiscrimination in facilities
1974	Association of Rehabilitation Nurses	Organization formed; rehabilitation nursing emerges as a specialty
1975	Education for All Handicapped Act (PL 94-142)	Provided for a free appropriate education for handicapped children in the least restrictive setting possible
1975	National Housing Act Amendments (PL 94-173)	Provided for the removal of barriers in federally supported housing; established Office of Independent Living for disabled people in Department of Housing and Urban Development

(Continued)

TABLE 24-4

Historical Events and Legislative Initiatives Affecting Rehabilitation (*Continued*)

Date	Event/Initiative	Purpose
1975	*Rehabilitation Nursing*	First issue published
1981	Rehabilitation Nursing: Concepts and Practice—A Core Curriculum	First core curriculum of rehabilitation nursing published
1982	Tax Equity and Fiscal Responsibility Act (TEFRA)	Originally designed to be a bridge from the old fee-for-service system to the DRG system; free-standing rehabilitation hospitals reimbursed based on reasonable costs (with limits)
1984	Diagnosis-Related Groupings (DRGs)	Established to decrease Medicare payments through the establishment of a prospective payment system for acute care
1989	Omnibus Budget Reconciliation Act (OBRA)	Contained legislation on nursing home reform; required standards for nursing assistant education and certification; required Health Care Financing Administration (HCFA) to develop a standardized assessment instrument and move to from a fee-for-service system to a prospective payment system
1989	Department of Veteran's Affairs	VA becomes the 14th department in the President's Cabinet.
1990	Americans with Disabilities Act	Americans with Disabilities Act (PL 101-336);established a clear discrimination on the basis of disability
1997	Balanced Budget Act (BBA)	Enacted to restructure Medicare Part A reimbursement methods; mandated a prospective payment reimbursement system for rehabilitation hospitals and units
1999	Balanced Budget Act Amendment	Provided adjustments to PPS for skilled nursing facilities
2001	PPS for Inpatient Rehabilitation Facilities	PPS mandated by the 1997 BBA phase-in begins
2001	New Freedom Initiative	President George W. Bush launches a nationwide effort to remove barriers to community living for people of all ages with disabilities and long-term illnesses; goals of the initiative include increasing access to assistive technologies, expanding educational opportunities, and promoting full access to community life.
2003	PPS for Inpatient Rehabilitation Facilities	Phase-in complete; Case-mix groups (CMGs) are used as the basis for reimbursement.
2004	CMS modifies criteria used to classify inpatient rehabilitation facilities (IRF)	Phase-in begins for "75% rule." By 2007, 75% of population treated in the facility must match one or more specified medical conditions.

Sources: Adapted from Larsen, P. (1998). "Rehabilitation." In I. Lubkin & P. Larsen (Eds.), *Chronic illness: Impact and interventions* (4th ed.), p. 534; Easton, K. (1999). *Gerontological rehabilitation nursing* (pp. 32, 41). Philadelphia: WB Saunders; Kelly, P. (1999). Reimbursement mechanisms. In A.S. Luggen, & S. Meiner (Eds.), *NGNA core curriculum for gerontological nursing* (pp. 185–186). St. Louis: Mosby; Blake, D., & Scott, D. (1996). Employment of persons with disabilities. *Physical Medicine and Rehabilitation* (p. 182). Philadelphia: WB Saunders; Department of Veterans Affairs. (2000). Facts about the Department of Veterans Affairs. Available on-line at http://www.va.gov/press rel/FSVA2000.htm

Table 24-4). A general apathy toward the poor, disabled, disenfranchised, and elderly prevailed in European countries and the United States. England was the first developed country to pass legislation in

The Poor Relief Act to provide assistance to the poor and disabled (Edwards, 2007).

There was some interest in rehabilitation in the 1800s, mainly with regard to helping "crippled" children (Edwards, 1992). In the 1900s, society began to focus more on the needs of persons with physical limitations. Susan Tracy, a nurse and teacher, helped to develop the discipline of occupational therapy. The first medical social service department was established at Bellevue Hospital in New York City, and Lillian Wald began the first visiting nursing service (Easton, 1999).

The World Wars provided an impetus for the growth of rehabilitation. The number of American soldiers wounded in World War I led to the establishment of a national rehabilitation program for veterans. It is interesting to note that rehabilitation services at this time were not generally available to the public. With the discovery of sulfa drugs and antibiotics, those injured in World War II had a much greater chance of survival. So, the numerous veterans of World War II coming home with multiple trauma, amputations, traumatic brain injuries, and spinal cord injuries necessitated a more comprehensive rehabilitation program. During this time, Dr. Howard Rusk (1965) emerged as both a pioneer and champion for rehabilitation, believing that these therapeutic services should be available not just to veterans, but to the entire world population. He demonstrated to the military powers through his personal assistance with the rehabilitation of those whom other medical professionals deemed a lost cause, that rather than convalescence, rehabilitation could promote recovery (Kottke, Stillwell, & Lehmann, 1990). Rusk showed that disabled persons could still be productive members of society and enjoy a good quality of life. As technology continued to explode in the 1940s, the number of civilians with industry and motor vehicle injuries increased, leading to a need for rehabilitation to address continuing disability. In 1947, Dr. Rusk established the first hospital-based medical rehabilitation services for civilians (Edwards, 2007).

The American Academy of Physical Medicine and Rehabilitation was established in 1938, and rehabilitation medicine was recognized as a board-certified specialty in 1947. In 1974, the Association of Rehabilitation Nurses was created, recognizing rehabilitation as a nursing specialty.

As societies continue to pursue medical and technologic advances that allow persons with extreme levels of physical disability to live longer, rehabilitation has become a specialty in demand. In the civilian population, more persons are living with disabilities, as first responders are better equipped to aid survival of serious injury. However, the need to address continuing adjustment to disability remains. In addition, as life expectancy in developed countries increases, chronic illness rates also rise, providing additional opportunities for rehabilitation professionals to enhance quality of life for those aging with disability or acquiring it with age.

For soldiers, the types of weapons used in the wars in Iraq and Afghanistan have resulted in poly-traumatic injuries never seen before. Rehabilitation professionals are being called upon to address multiple injuries that may include a combination of multiple traumatic amputations, burns, internal organ and, soft-tissue damage from explosive forces, brain and spinal injuries, as well as post-traumatic stress.

Public Policy and Rehabilitation

There are several ways in which rehabilitation services may be paid for. These include Medicare, Medicaid, workers' compensation, private insurance, and social security disability benefits. Rehabilitation professionals should be familiar with these types of reimbursement and what is covered under the client's insurance provider. Case managers and social workers are team members who may be excellent resources regarding payment for rehabilitation.

Medicare

Medicare is a federal social insurance program that provides care for persons over the age of 65 and for certain younger persons with disabilities [Centers for Medicare & Medicaid Services (CMS), 2005a; Beam & O'Hare, 2003]. Medicare Part A is the hospital insurance, providing funds for hospital care, skilled nursing, hospice, and home health care. Medicare Part A covers up to 100 days in a skilled nursing facility (after a hospitalization that lasts for at least 3 days), but not long-term or custodial care. Part A also covers home healthcare services including nursing and therapies when ordered by a physician for a home-bound patient. Medicare Part B covers medically necessary services as well as some preventive services, with a monthly charge. Part B also has a deductible of $135 in addition to the monthly premium before Medicare pays its portion. The standard premium is $96.34 in 2008 (CMS, 2007). Part B covers 80% of the costs of physician services, and other services including physical and occupational therapy, durable medical equipment, and prosthetics and orthotics. Many services that a rehabilitation client may need are not covered under Medicare. For example, Medicare does not cover dental work, eye or hearing exams, routine foot care, or nursing home care. Medicare Part C, referred to as the Medicare Advantage Plan, is a combination of Parts A and B, and functions much like a PPO or HMO using managed care (Doherty, 2004; Emmer & Allendorf, 2004; Stuart, 2004). Medicare Part D (CMS, 2007) is a new prescription drug plan in which private companies issue plans through Medicare. Part D is available for anyone with Medicare regardless of income. Costs vary greatly within this plan.

Rehabilitation facilities and hospitals, collectively called inpatient rehabilitation facilities (IRFs) currently receive reimbursement using a Prospective Payment System (PPS) through the Social Security Act (CMS, 2007a). The IRF PPS uses information from the Uniform Data System for Medical Rehabilitation (UDSmr), better known as the Functional Independence Measure (FIM) tool, "to classify patients into distinct groups based on clinical characteristics and expected resource needs. Separate payments are calculated for each group, including the application of case and facility level adjustments" (CMS, 2007a, paragraph 2). Codes are assigned to case-mix groups (CMGs), and Medicare pays a specific amount per discharge.

Since 2004, Medicare has been phasing in new rules for IRFs. The case-mix classifications for 2008 will use the same as those for 2007. Common medical conditions covered under the IRF rule include stroke, brain injury, spinal cord injury, amputation, multiple trauma, neurologic disorders, cardiac and pulmonary conditions, osteoarthritis, rheumatoid arthritis, pain syndrome, and certain joint replacements (Federal Register, 2007).

Medicare limits the amount it pays for physical, occupational, and speech therapy services. In 2007, the limit for outpatient physical therapy and speech therapy combined was $1,780 and for occupational therapy was $1780. There is a $131 deductible for Part B Medicare, after which Medicare pays 80% and the individual pays 20% up to the set limits for medically necessary therapies. There are some allowable exceptions to this rule, and appropriate documentation by the provider is essential.

Medicaid

Medicaid is a state-run program in concert with the federal government that is the largest source of medical care payments for persons with low income and resources. In 2007, President Bush introduced a plan to place new restrictions on the rehabilitative services (called the rehab option) allowed through Medicaid, to save the federal budget $2.29 billion over 5 years. Nearly 75% of persons receiving rehab services under Medicaid were those with mental health needs, and they were responsible for 79% of the rehab option spending (Kaiser Commission, 2007). Currently 47 states provide some type of mental or physical health services under the rehab option.

Establishing Medicaid is a complex process that varies between states (Santerre, 2002). Although each state sets standards for its own programs, the federal government provides broad guidelines for those who may qualify under categorically needy, medically needy, and special groups (such as some persons with disabilities). States must provide long-term care for persons who are Medicaid eligible. State Medicaid programs offer a variety of services within a variety of settings. Services that are provided relative to rehabilitation for the categorically needy include: hospitalization, lab and X-rays, nursing facilities for those age 21 and older, physician and some nurse practitioner services, medical-surgical dental needs, and home health (CMS, 2005).

Workers' Compensation

Workers' compensation is a state income support program. To be eligible, the injury or condition must be work-related. Benefits are usually calculated as a percentage of the employee's weekly earnings at the time the injury occurred. There are restrictions placed by each state on the maximum amount of benefits, often two thirds of the gross salary (Deutsch & Dean-Baar, 2007). The types of benefits may range from temporary partial or total disability to permanent partial or total disability, or death. Some states have a maximum benefit period and some may require a waiting period. Disabled workers may be compensated through spousal benefits (in case of death), medical and rehabilitation expense coverage, and lost wages (Kiselica, Sibson, & Green-McKenzie, 2004). Current workers' compensation programs are more restrictive than they once were, and limit physician choice and eligibility, provide lower benefits, and use managed care to for cost containment (D'Andrea & Meyer, 2004).

Private Insurance

Most private insurances pay for at least some rehabilitative services. There is generally a deductible and often a co-pay, which may be higher if the provider is not within the network of providers supplied by the insurance company. In the case where the person has private insurance and Medicare as a secondary payor, much of the therapy services may be covered, provided there is sufficient and ongoing documentation of medical necessity and progress toward goals. Private insurance may also provide disability income insurance, accidental death and dismemberment insurance, or other benefits.

Social Security Disability Income

Social Security Disability Income (SSDI) was established in 1956 as part of the Social Security Disability Act of 1954. This is a federally administered disability insurance program for those who meet the strict definition of disability under Social Security. The criteria for disability is threefold: (1) the person cannot do the same work he or she did before; (2) it is determined that the person cannot adapt to other work because of the existing medical condition; and (3) the disability has lasted for at least one year, or is expected to result in death (Social Security Online, 2007). The person must also have worked and paid into the Social Security program before the disability. SSDI is paid as a monthly benefit.

Supplemental Security Income (SSI) may provide disability benefits for persons who have not worked long enough to receive SSDI. The SSI program pays benefits to disabled adults and children with limited income and resources, or certain older persons with severely limited income. Persons may receive a monthly check, and the SSI program also helps individuals to access Medicare benefits and take advantage of other possible assistance through the federal government. Qualifying for the program is based on income and resources (Social Security Online, 2007).

Disability Benefits for Veterans

The Department of Veterans Affairs (DVA), often called the VA, provides a number of benefits for veterans. "Disability compensation is a benefit paid to a veteran because of injuries or diseases that happened while on active duty, or were made worse by active military service. It is also paid to certain veterans disabled from VA health care" (DVA, 2007a). These benefits are tax free and may include a monthly stipend (ranging from $115 to $2471), priority medical care through the VA, clothing and housing allowances (to make accommodations), adaptive equipment, and various grants as needed. The VA also provides vocational rehabilitation by maintaining working relationships with many businesses to employ veterans with physical and mental or emotional disabilities. Consultation is available in many areas including employment, assistive technology, case management, work site and job analysis, and help in addressing ADA compliance issues (DVA, 2007b).

Vocational Rehabilitation

Vocational rehabilitation is an important part of the rehabilitation process, carrying heavier weight for those of working age and certain racial–ethnic groups for whom work is part of personal identify and reputation. In 1918, Congress passed the Smith-Sears Act to assist with national vocational rehabilitation services to veterans who served in World War I. In 1920, The Smith-Fess Act made vocational rehabilitation services available for all persons with disabilities, not just those with war-related injuries (Buchanan, 1996). More significant legislation was enacted when The Rehabilitation Act of 1973 provided funds to support state vocational rehabilitation programs. The Rehabilitation Services Administration (RSA) of the US Department of Education coordinates vocational rehabilitation services. The RSA stated that it "oversees grant programs that help individuals with physical or mental disabilities to obtain employment and live more independently through the provision of such supports as counseling, medical and psychological services, job training and other individualized services" (p. 1). This is accomplished through dispensing funds to state grant programs to assist them with finding work-related services or programs for persons with disabilities, particularly the severely disabled. The RSA is the Congressionally appointed federal agency charged with implementing the various titles associated with The Rehabilitation Act of 1973. This agency acts as a resource for information and a leader in advocating at all levels for national programs that help to remove barriers for persons with disabilities (RSA, 2007).

The services provided in vocational rehabilitation are many, but generally include personal counseling, mental and physical health services, and assistance with vocational placement and job training (Lysaght, 2004; Kielkofner et al., 2004; O'Neill, Zuger, Fields, Fraser, & Pruce, 2004; Targett, Wehman, & Young, 2004). In addition, the RSA helps administer projects with specific groups of persons such as migrant and seasonal farm workers, American Indians, older adults, and the visually impaired. One principle of vocational rehabilitation is that informed consumer choice will promote enhanced employment outcomes. For vocational rehabilitation to be truly effective and enhance quality of life for the person with mental disabilities, the agency and counselors must work closely with the employer and the client to find the working environment suited to that individual (Inman, McGurk, & Chadwick, 2007; Morgan, 2007). Employment outcomes are most frequently used as the measure of the success of vocational rehabilitation for those with disabilities (Kosciulek, 2007). More research is needed to explore the factors related to positive outcomes of vocational rehabilitation.

Vocational rehabilitation may not be a goal for all rehabilitation clients. Many older adults requiring rehabilitation services are retired, and employment is not a goal. However, for those younger persons with functional limitations or mental health impairments, work may be directly related to their sense of self and identify within their culture. For these persons, vocational rehabilitation plays an important part in the comprehensive rehabilitation process, and the vocational rehabilitation counselor will be an essential team member.

Americans with Disabilities Act

The Americans with Disabilities Act enacted in 1990 guarantees individuals with physical disabilities equal access to public accommodations related to transportation, education, and employment. Employment discrimination of qualified applicants due to disabilities is prohibited by

TABLE 24-5	
Americans with Disabilities Act	
Title 1: Employment	Employers cannot discriminate against a qualified disabled job applicant or employee in any manner related to employment and benefits.
	Employers must make their existing facilities accessible and usable by individuals with disabilities.
	Accommodations in all aspects of job attainment and performance are required in order to place individuals on an equal plane with the nondisabled.
Title 2: Public Services	Qualified disabled individuals must have access to all services and programs provided by state or local governments. Public rail transportation must be made accessible to disabled individuals and supplemented with paratransit.
Title 3: Public Accommodations Services Operated by Private Entities	Virtually every entity open to the public must now be made accessible to the disabled. A study is to be conducted concerning accessibility of the over-the-road transportation.
Title 4: Telecommunications Relay	Telephone companies are required to furnish telecommunication devices to enable hearing- and speech-impaired individuals to communicate by wire or radio.

Source: Reprinted from Watson, P. (1990). The Americans with Disabilities Act: More rights for people with disabilities. *Rehabilitation Nursing, 15,* 326. Published by the Association of Rehabilitation Nurses, 4700 W. Lake Avenue, Glenview, IL 60025-1485. Copyright © 1990 by the Association of Rehabilitation Nurses. Used with permission.

this law (US Equal Employment Opportunity Commission, 2006). Although the Rehabilitation Act of 1973 and its amendments also were concerned accessibility to buildings whose organizations received federal financial assistance, the ADA requires private organizations to also comply with accessibility and employment laws. The concept of reasonable accommodation was introduced, requiring employers to make those accommodations within reason that may be necessary for a person with disability. Table 24-5 provides a summary of the ADA related to the four major areas it addresses: employment, public services, public accommodations services by practice entities, and telecommunications relay.

REHABILIATION ISSUES AND CHALLENGES

Rehabilitation services provided by an interdisciplinary team within a variety of settings suggest several possible challenges for providers. These include the rising costs of care, caregiver burden, inequities among those with disabilities, the negative image of disability, the changing composition of the disabled population, ethical issues, providing culturally competent care, and professional and informal caregiver issues.

Rising Care Costs

It is estimated that more than 49 million Americans have some type of long-term condition or disability. More than 34 million persons were limited in their daily activities because of chronic health conditions (US Census Bureau, 2004). Forty-two million (17%) persons were uninsured and 32 million (13%) received Medicaid assistance. Of those uninsured, the major reason cited was cost. About 10.7 million (5%) adults were unable to work because of health-related problems. Persons with less education and who were poor, were less likely to be able to work because of health problems (Adams, Dey & Vickerie, 2007). The American government spends about $200 billion a year on assistance for persons with disabilities (Council of State Administrators of Vocational Rehabilitation, 2004–2005). Given these statistics, major challenges for rehabilitation professionals are to assist persons to attain and regain their health and become productive, working members of society, and to explore other means of providing access to health care.

Caregiver Burden

Because an event requiring rehabilitation happens to the entire family and community, not just the client, it is important to address the needs of caregivers throughout the rehabilitation process and/or chronic illness trajectory. Family members comprise the vast majority (72%) of paid and unpaid caregivers of older persons with functional limitations from chronic disease, with adult caregivers (42%) and spouses (25%) bearing the largest burden of care (Shirey & Summer, 2000). The caregiver's ability to cope with the care demands is influenced by a variety of factors including the type and severity illness, the length of quality of recovery, social support, inherent caregiver factors, and coping ability. This may hold true for both formal and informal caregivers (Bushnik, Wright, & Brudsall, 2007). For example, the caregiver spouse of a person with uncomplicated coronary bypass surgery may be able to meet care demands over a limited period of rehabilitation, whereas the older spouse caregiver of a stroke survivor with severe aphasia and functional deficits may be facing years of care, giving burden that is often overwhelming.

Caregiver burden, the effects of caregiving-related stress on family members or other care providers, has been associated with a number of health problems in the caregiver. Emotional distress, anxiety, depression, decreased quality of life, hypertension, lowered immune function, and increased mortality are among the concerns noted by researchers of caregivers (King, Hartke & Denby, 2007; Ski & O'Connell, 2007; Anderson, Linto, & Stewart-Wynne, 1995; Canam & Acorn, 1999; Brouwer et al., 2004; das Chagas Medeiros, Ferraz & Quaresma, 2000; Grunfeld et al., 2004; Hughes et al., 1999; Kolanowski, Fick, Waller, &

Shea, 2004; Lieberman & Fisher, 1995; Mills, Yu, Ziegler, Patterson, & Grant, 1999; Schulz & Beach, 1999; Shaw et al., 1999; Weitzenkamp et al., 1997; Wu et al., 1999). There is sufficient research over the last decade to demonstrate that the burden of caregiving over time can have a deleterious effect on the health of the family caregiver.

The caregiver burden is thought to be greater when more care is required. Recent research suggested that although education and training programs have some effect on caregiver stress levels, the benefit is short term and caregivers are likely to need ongoing involvement from care professionals to help maintain their own health (Draper et al., 2007; King, Hartke, & Denby, 2007; Halm, Treat-Jacobson, Lindquist, & Savik, 2007). Assessment of caregiver burden should be included in the rehabilitation plan of care (see Chapter 9). Early identification and interventions related to managing caregiver stress may result in better outcomes for the entire family, and appropriate discharge planning and follow-up are an important part of the process.

Inequities Among Disabled Americans

According to the Centers for Disease Control and Prevention (CDC) (2007d), "there are continuing disparities in the burden of illness and death experienced by blacks or African Americans, Hispanics or Latinos, American Indians and Alaska Natives, and Native Hawaiian and Other Pacific Islanders, compared to the US population as a whole" (p. 1). The groups experiencing the most disparity are the ones predicted to grow at a faster rate than the general population. This is especially true of the Hispanic group, with minorities accounting for about 90% of the predicted population growth by 2050 (Minority Business Development Agency, 1999).

The National Health Interview Survey (NHIS) of 2005 "is a household, multistage probability sample survey conducted annually by interviewers of the US Census Bureau for the CDC's National Center for Health Statistics. In 2005, household interviews were completed for 98,649 persons living in 38,509 households, reflecting a household response rate of 86.5%." (Adams et al., 2007, p. 8). The survey looked at multiple factors including respondent-assessed health status, functional ability, healthcare access, and healthcare insurance coverage as well as others. The data revealed several inequities among disabled Americans, similar to the National Organization on Disability (NOD) survey (2004).

The NHIS survey showed that 3.8 (2%) million adults need help with ADLs and 7.8 million (4%) need assistance with IADLs (instrumental activities of daily living such as shopping or household chores). The need for assistance dramatically increases with age, with 10% of those older than 75 years requiring assistance with ADLs and 19% needing help with IADLs (Adams et al., 2007; Fried, Bradley, Williams, & Tinetti, 2001). It is estimated that in 2004, 34% of the noninstitutionalized American population older than age 65 had activity limitations caused by chronic health conditions (Adams et al., 2007). Add to that those older adults who reside in long-term care facilities, and there is a significant number of older adults whose daily lives are affected by chronic illness.

Many persons in minority groups experience a double jeopardy or double minority status when they acquire disability. Caucasians and Asians were more likely to report excellent health than African Americans. Hispanic persons younger than age 65 (34%) were more than 2.5 times as likely as non-Hispanics (14%) in the same age cohort to be uninsured. Both older age and poverty are factors that are associated with poorer health status and increased disability. The poor elderly were three to four times more likely to need assistance with ADLs and IADLs than those who were not poor (Adams et al., 2007).

The survey from the National Organization on Disability (NOD) revealed significant differences among groups within the United States related to the factors of employment, income, education, socialization, religious involvement, access to health care, and transportation (National Organization of Disability, 2004). The NOD/Harris survey examined participation gaps between able-bodied and disabled Americans in 10 life areas. Only 35% of disabled Americans reported working full- or part-time compared with 78% of nondisabled Americans. Three times as many disabled Americans live in households with a total income of less than $15,000. Twenty-two percent of disabled Americans reported experiencing job discrimination. Persons with disabilities were less likely to attend church services, dine out, and socialize than nondisabled persons.

In America, the groups considered vulnerable populations (in which disparities in access to health care and transportation are often most prominent) include some minority groups, children, the elderly, the poor, those living in rural areas, and the mentally ill (US Department of Health and Human Services, 2003; Reichard, Sacco, & Turnbull, 2004; Havercamp, Scandlin, & Roth, 2004). Prisoners are also a vulnerable group. The National Health and Nutrition Examination Survey (NHANES III) indicated that non-Hispanic blacks and Mexican-Americans generally report more disability than nonminorities, with minority women reporting more disability than men (Ostchega et al., 2000). American Indians have the highest disability rate (25%) of any other ethnic group. The most common types of self-reported disabilities include spinal cord injury, complications from diabetes, blindness, difficulty with ambulation, traumatic brain injury, deafness or hardness of hearing, orthopedic conditions, and mental health problems (Lomay & Hinkebein, 2006). Additional research is needed with these high-risk minority groups to understand these healthcare disparities to develop strategies to address them.

Stigma of Disability

Although much progress has been made on a national policy level toward dispelling the negative image and stigma associated with disability through modifying rehabilitation models (WHO,

2002; Brandt & Pope, 1997), many persons with disabilities still report feelings of negative reactions from others regarding their differences. The disability could be something as relatively invisible as a hearing aid worn by an adolescent (Kent & Smith, 2006) to obvious employment discrimination for a person with mental illness (Stuart, 2006; Lloyd & Waghorn, 2007). One study found that a positive factor such as exercise done by a person with a physical disability may undermine the negative impressions that some persons have and fight the stigma of disability (Arbour, Latimer, Ginis, & Jung, 2007).

Changes made in today's rehabilitation models portray disability on a continuum, with a prominent factor being the environment. In a classic work by Zola (1982), the author toured a 65-acre utopia in The Netherlands as a professional visitor. The village was designed for those with disabilities who did not fit well into other existing societies, with complete and full accessibility, environmental adaptation, and removal of barriers. Each of the 400 members of the village had to contribute to their self-crafted society. However, in such an environment, persons functioned well and without stigma, because their situation was the new norm. Zola found himself feeling out of place, although able-bodied, suggesting that the environment is a key factor in perception of disability (see Chapter 3).

Persons with disabilities who have helped to change the perception of the public include role models in the arts, science, politics, and sports. Marla Runyon (Olympic runner), the late actor/director Christopher Reeve, actor Michael J. Fox, scientist Stephen Hawking, and Senator Max Cleland are just a few examples of such role models. Runyon is legally blind, yet participated as an Olympic runner in the 2000 games in Sydney, Australia. Christopher Reeve, the actor best known for his role as Superman, was a high-level, ventilator-dependent quadriplegic. Reeve continued to act and direct movies throughout his life and, along with his late wife, Dana, helped establish services for those with spinal cord injuries.

Michael J. Fox, actor, experienced early onset Parkinson's disease and has been a crusader for research in that area. Stephen Hawking, noted physicist and prolific author, was diagnosed with motor neuron disease (amyotrophic lateral sclerosis, ALS) at a relatively young age and yet has continued to work. Even after he was completely paralyzed by his disease, he continued to write with the use of technology and his blink reflex. Cleland, a triple amputee, was a United States senator and director of the Department of Veterans Affairs. These individuals may seem remarkable because of their accomplishments; however, there are thousands of other "everyday" citizens with disabilities who are productive members and make significant contributions to society. Their stories are the untold ones.

Ethical and Legal Issues

Rehabilitation professionals are often in positions that require difficult decision-making. Masters-Farrell (2006) states that the "conflict occurs when a choice must be made between two equal possibilities" (p. 590) and that an ethical dilemma is present when a situation forces one to evaluate and choose between two equally unattractive choices. For example, take the situation of a nonterminal rehabilitation client who had just told the nurse that he did not wish to be resuscitated if he should "code," but the paperwork for advance directives had not yet been completed, signed, or placed on the chart, and the nurse found him minutes later without a pulse or respirations. Although she must call the code team in this situation, the nurse is in conflict because she has intimate knowledge that this was action was contrary to the client's wishes.

Beauchamp and Childress (2001), in their classic medical text on principles of biomedical ethics, emphasize the four cornerstone principles of respect for autonomy: nonmaleficence, beneficence, and justice. These principles play into many aspects of rehabilitation practice and programming. Common ethical (and often legal) issues that pertain particularly to rehabilitation clients may include the following (Masters-Farrell, 2007; Kirschner, Stocking, Wagner, Foye, & Siegler, 2001; Ellis & Hartley, 2004):

- Withholding or withdrawing treatment
- Determining competence in decision-making
- Do not resuscitate orders
- Use of physical or chemical restraints
- Genetic screening
- Organ donation
- Guardianship
- Research on human subjects
- Disagreement between family members about treatment options
- Use of complementary and alternative medical treatments
- Advance directives (life-prolonging declarations, living wills, durable power of attorney)
- Informed consent
- Estate planning
- Determining legal death or brain death
- Substance abuse
- Confidentiality
- Defining quality of life
- Self-termination or assisted suicide
- Abuse of the vulnerable
- Allocation of resources and insurance coverage
- End-of-life decisions
- Long-term care placement

Ethics committees are becoming more popular in acute care hospitals and even retirement communities to assist in difficult decision-making (Hogstel, Curry, Walker, & Burns, 2004; Johnson, 2004; Hughes, 2004; Nelson, 2004). Ellis and Hartley (2004) view the ethics committee as an interdisciplinary group of healthcare professionals that is specifically established to address ethical dilemmas that occurred in a particular setting. Persons serving on an ethics committee may include physicians, nurses, advanced practice nurses, social workers, therapists, pastoral care personnel, members of the community, and an ethicist. The benefits of an ethics committee include allowing many perspectives to be discussed, providing a forum for communication, fostering development of related policies, promoting awareness of existing and potential issues, and focusing on the patient (Masters-Farrell, 2007). Some disadvantages include the potential for inefficiency and political influence, and lack of time for participation.

Cultural Competency

Cultural sensitivity involves an awareness and consideration of a group's beliefs, values, communication styles, language, and behavior. Providing culturally sensitive rehabilitation care will be an even greater challenge in the future, with the changing demographics and increasing minority elderly population (Niemeier, Burnett, & Whitaker, 2003). How clients and families perceive disability and participate in rehabilitation is heavily influenced by cultural norms and expectations (Campinha-Bacote, 2001). The first step in becoming culturally sensitive is to know one's own self. Although some generalizations will be discussed here related to the major ethnic–racial groups, professionals should avoid stereotyping and seek individual information from each client. If needed, the services of a translator (not a family member) should be used. Because of the vast differences between and within the many cultural groups that rehabilitation professionals serve, it is wise to ask clients about their particular beliefs and practices. Even if one is familiar, for example, with the Lakota Indian health practices, this does not mean that the Navajo will practice precisely the same rituals and observances, although both will value Native American tradition.

African Americans are a group at high-risk for many disabilities and chronic illnesses that warrant rehabilitative care including hypertension, stroke, diabetes, and heart disease. African Americans typically have a close family structure, deep religious affiliations, and share a strong belief against placing older parents in long-term care facilities. They are generally open to rehabilitation programs, and tend to experience disabling conditions at a younger age than their Caucasian counterparts. Career counseling for African Americans with disabilities should take into account the effects of double minority status: disability and racial. Rehabilitation professionals should realize that prejudice, oppression, and stigma are often attached to both these factors, and a multidimensional, multicultural approach to care should be used (Mpofu & Harley, 2006).

Hispanic or Latino Americans enjoy strong family bonds. There is generally good family involvement for clients experiencing rehabilitation. However, severe disability may be seen as a punishment from God for some evil or wrongdoing, and thus may stigmatize a person or family. Hispanics tend to continue to work with a disability, but in some instances may show poorer outcomes, such as adjusting to life after stroke (Cook, Stickley, Ramey, & Knotts, 2005).

Among Asian cultures, there is a diversity of beliefs. However, a respect for healthcare professionals as well as Eastern healers often means that they will seek treatment for rehabilitative conditions. In Chinese and Japanese cultures, there is belief in the need for balance between positive and negative forces, between the hot and cold, between the male and female. These opposing and related forces are referred to as the yin and the yang. When the body is out of harmony, or lacks balance, illness may occur, and emotional problems are linked to a weak character. There may be feelings of guilt and shame in having a disability, as it could indicate punishment for wrong-doing. Work is seen as fundamental to a successful and honorable life, but in Hong Kong, only 2.5% of male Chinese with psychiatric disabilities can seek employment (Yip & Ng, 2002). Asian Americans often seek alternative or complementary medicine, including herbal remedies, in addition to Western medicine and rehabilitation care.

As of the 2000 Census, there were 4.1 million American Indians living in the United States. These groups in general embrace the interrelatedness of the earth with the body and spirit, but tribes often have their own culturally distinct practices. They rely on a relatively private extended community and kinship ties. Most traditional American Indians value folk medicine over Westernized medical treatments and facilities. There is an innate distrust of those outside their community, given their history of oppression. Mortality has been drastically higher for American Indians when compared to the general US population related to the following: alcoholism, 627%; tuberculosis, 533%; diabetes mellitus, 249%; accidents, 204%; suicide, 72%; pneumonia and influenza, 71%; and homicide, 63% [Indian Health Services (IHS), 2001]. Rehabilitation professionals must be aware that today's American Indians may come from a mixed background of tribal customs, and that many will still believe in folk healers.

Several excellent resources are readily available to help develop cultural awareness and sensitivity. A helpful series of monographs online and in booklet form are available to assist rehabilitation professional with cultural information (CIRRIE, 2007). These informative papers provide information on 11 countries of origin for foreign-born groups in the United States including China, Cuba, Dominican Republic, El Salvador, India, Jamaica, Korea, Mexico, Philippines, Vietnam, and Haiti. The Web site is updated regularly at http://cirrie.buffalo.edu/mseries.html. More than a hundred training programs for rehabilitation providers on a variety of issues related to various ethnic groups and disabilities are also available from The National Clearing House of Rehabilitation Training Materials (2007) at www.ncrtm.org/.

Formal and Informal Caregiver Issues

As the population increases and the oldest old become the fastest growing age group, there will be a lack of physicians and nurses prepared to meet the care demand for the number of persons with chronic illness and disability. Currently, there is a lack of qualified physiatrists and nurses in the United States (Verville & DeLisa, 2001; Currie, Atchison, & Fiedler, 2002; Dean-Baar, 2003). The Association of Rehabilitation Nurses (Secrest, 2007) has strongly advocated for certification in rehabilitation; there are nearly 10,000 nurses who hold the Certified Rehabilitation Registered Nurse (CRRN) credential. However, few nursing programs provide rehabilitation education as a separate course or have dedicated content to this specialty area. Getting healthcare professionals such as physicians and nurses interested in the specialty has been difficult because of its limited visibility in traditional educational programs (Neal, 2001; Thompson, Emrich, & Moore, 2003). The European Union has addressed concerns regarding their own shortage of physicians trained in physical medicine and rehabilitation through the Union of European Medical Specialist (UEMS) by beginning to standardize training and education throughout the 28 member countries. Within these countries there are 13,000 specialists and more than 2800 trainees in PRM (physical and rehabilitation medicine) (Ward & Gutenbrunner, 2006), and the specialty is felt to be robust. Still, there is a concerted effort to recruit and educate physicians in PRM in Europe.

With more than 35 million people in America older than 65 years of age, there is an increased need for professionals trained to provide quality care to older adults. Older adults account for almost one fourth of ambulatory care visits, nearly one half of all hospital days, and represent 83% of nursing facility residents (Kovner, Mezey, & Harrington, 2002; Mezey & Fulmer, 2002). Most nursing schools in this country have no full-time faculty certified in geriatric nursing; only a few of the nation's medical schools have a geriatric department, and less than 10% require a course in geriatrics (Remsburg & Carson, 2006). As of 2002, there were 63 master's programs that prepared nurses in geriatrics, but only 4200 certified specialists (Mezey & Fulmer, 2002).

Despite concerted efforts to change it, there continues to be a negative stigma around care of older adults among nursing students. Without education in gerontology, healthcare professionals may not realize the rehabilitation potential of many of these older adults. The common rehabilitative disorders often are seen in the older age

group, and even small improvements in function and independence can allow older adults to age in place and remain at home. Even those making long-term care or retirement communities their home can improve their strength and function with small lifestyle changes and exercise.

There is also a growing number of persons whose caregiving needs go unmet (Kennedy, 2001; LaPlant, Kaye, Kang, & Harrington, 2004). More than 34 million persons are limited in some way from usual activities because of chronic illness. It is estimated that there are 3.8 million adults with disabilities who require assistance with ADLs and 7.8 millions who need help with IADLs (Adams et al., 2007). Persons who need assistance were more likely to be poor, older, and less educated. Persons whose needs are not met with the needed assistance are more likely to experience discomfort, weight loss, dehydration, falls, and burns (LaPlante et al., 2004). Further research is needed to help identify consequences from unmet caregiving needs as well as strategies to address this growing problem.

INTERVENTIONS

The Rehabilitation Process

Rehabilitation is both philosophy and a discipline (Secrest, 2007). Rehabilitation is based on the premise that all individuals have self-worth and are deserving of dignity, respect, and quality health care regardless of their limitations. Many concepts are imbedded in the field of rehabilitation and are reflected through such common sayings as:

- Rehabilitation begins day one
- What you do not use, you lose
- Progress is measured in small gains
- Independence is better than dependence
- Motivation is a key to success
- All care should include rehabilitation principles
- Activity strengthens and inactivity wastes
- If it can be corrected, it probably could have been prevented

Rehabilitation should begin from the first day the person is in the hospital. When healthcare professionals forget the basic principles of rehabilitation, complications such as contractures, pressure sores, and incontinence ensue. Rehabilitation includes nursing, medical, therapies, and social services. It is an interdisciplinary team process focused on maintaining or restoring function, preventing complications, promoting independence and self-care, and enhancing quality of life.

Team Approach

The team approach is most effective when working with clients with complex needs such as those requiring rehabilitative services. Although there are several models used in this approach, the common threads are that the team members work toward goals that are mutually established with the client.

Prevailing models are either multidisciplinary, interdisciplinary, or transdisciplinary. Multidisciplinary teams involve professionals from different disciplines, each treating the client within their various areas; however, they may not coordinate their efforts in the care of a client (Secrest, 2007). The advantage of this type of model is that all professionals bring their education and expertise to promote the best outcomes for the client. However, the major weakness is that communication between and across the disciplines may be lacking.

In the transdisciplinary model, each client has a primary therapist from the team, who may be a nurse, physical therapist, or occupational therapist. One therapist is cross-trained to provide comprehensive care to the client (Secrest, 2007). Although this model may provide for continuity of care, issues surrounding licensure, scope of practice, and accountability abound. In addition, team members are often out of their comfort zone in providing services that they were not specifically trained for. Turf issues often complicate this type of care. Lastly, some organizations that have tried this model have given it up for a different approach because the team was not motivated to embrace it.

TABLE 24-6

Members of the Rehabilitation Team

Physiatrist
Certified rehabilitation registered nurse (CRRN)
Certified nursing assistant
Physical therapist
Physical therapist assistant
Occupational therapist
Certified occupational therapy assistant
Speech therapist/speech–language pathologist
Audiologist
Dietitian/nutritionist
Social worker
Psychologist
Therapeutic recreation specialist
Pastoral counselor
Prosthetist/orthotist
Case manager

The most preferred rehabilitation team model is the interdisciplinary team (see Table 24-6). The interdisciplinary team approach involves each team member communicating on a regular basis with each other and establishing common goals for clients (Secrest, 2007). This is often accomplished through weekly team meetings in which the entire team reviews the progress of each client and mutual goals are discussed and updated. The client and family are an important part of the team as well. Nontraditional team members may be added to the team based on the client's needs. Table 24-6 lists other potential team members in addition to the client and family members.

Evaluation of the Client

An important element in considering rehabilitation as an option for any client is proper evaluation of rehabilitation potential. There are many factors that comprise such an evaluation, but several forces seem to play a major role. These include the severity of the illness, injury, or defect, functional level and cognitive status, willingness to participate, internal or external motivation (Kemp, 1986), social support (Fairfax, 2002), and available resources.

Rehabilitation Potential

For purposes of insurance coverage (i.e., the healthcare payers), clients receiving inpatient rehabilitation need to meet the minimum requirements of being able to tolerate at least three hours of therapy per day. Generally, a professional is assigned to do an evaluation of rehabilitation potential before the client is admitted to a program. This professional may be a social worker, nurse, case manager, clinical nurse specialist, or other clinician with appropriate education and evaluation skills. No one type of client provides a perfect profile of the usual patient. Rather, the evaluator uses his or her assessment skills to consider all the aspects of the person's life that could contribute to success in an intensive therapeutic program such as the likelihood of functional improvement given the person's illness or injury, internal motivation, and available support.

Although there are general criteria followed for admission to a rehabilitation program, the uniqueness of each individual is considered by the evaluator. Over time, healthcare professionals develop an intuition that aids them in the selection of clients who are appropriate rehabilitation candidates. So, there may be occasions when a person with a low functioning level as a result of traumatic brain injury but who is highly motivated and has strong family support has better rehabilitation outcomes than the stroke patient with minimal functional deficits, but whose negative attitude is a deterrent to readiness for intensive therapy. Sometimes clients will be referred to a transitional care unit or post-acute care prior to rehabilitation admission, and then days or weeks later feel the motivation to enter acute rehabilitation.

For each specific disease or condition there are some factors that are associated with either more positive or negative outcomes. For example, history of previous stroke, advanced age, incontinence, and visual–spatial deficits are all associated with poorer outcomes after stroke (Brandstater, 2005). Easton (2001) found that stroke survivors who were older, had more life experience, knew the cause of their stroke, had realistic expectations, good social support, and expressed faith in God seemed to adapt better to their condition after stroke. Outcomes for older stroke survivors have been shown to improve with intensive inpatient rehabilitation (Jett, Warren, & Wirtalla, 2005).

Strengths of the Client, Family, and Environment

Another important factor in the evaluation process is the identification of the client's and family's strengths. Questions to ask during this assessment should include: What can the client do for him/ herself? What does the client see as his or her own strengths and weaknesses? What are the family's strengths and weaknesses? What coping mechanisms does the client typically use, and will they be sufficient for the current crisis? What resources are available to the family and client within the community? What are the client's personal goals? A highly motivated client and supportive family are important to the success of the rehabilitation process.

Functional Assessment

Although functional assessment is important, the evaluator should not forget that a true evaluation of rehabilitation potential must consider all factors, not just physical or function related. Functional assessment includes an evaluation that identifies one's ability to perform self-care and physical activities. The two approaches generally used are asking questions and observation (Guse, 2006).

A number of tools are available to assess function, although these are mainly aimed at screening for disability. Functional assessment tools include: (1) the development of a client problem list, (2) goal setting based on identified strengths and weaknesses of the client, (3) evaluation of the client's

▌CASE STUDY

Mr. Jenkins—Adjustment to Life-Altering Condition

Mr. Jenkins was diagnosed with Parkinson's disease at the age of 55. Previously a hardworking nursing home administrator, the rapid progression of his symptoms led to a forced early retirement. He suffered from bouts of depression and short-term memory loss. The spasticity in his extremities became so severe that at times he was unable to hold papers in his hand or stay seated in a chair. Both his ability to speak and move were exacerbated with stress. His wife was frustrated that her husband had gone from a productive middle-aged man to one with a poor quality of life who still wished to be working and enjoying social functions that were now prevented by his deteriorating condition. A clinical nurse specialist was asked to consult with Mr. Jenkins and his wife about the possibility of deep brain stimulator (DBS) implantation. Mr. Jenkins was found to be an appropriate candidate and underwent surgery to implant a DBS. The results after rehabilitation were significant. Mr. Jenkins was able to ambulate with a near-normal gait and his resting spasticity was dramatically decreased. His quality of life was improved and he reported increased satisfaction with his situation.

Discussion Questions

1. What team members would have been involved in Mr. Jenkins's rehabilitation after deep brain stimulator (DBS) implantation?
2. What goals would be appropriate for Mr. Jenkins before and after surgical intervention?
3. Name two tools or classification systems that would be appropriate in evaluating Mr. Jenkins's functional ability.
4. If you developed a long-term plan of care for Mr. Jenkins, realizing that the DBS is not a cure, and that Parkinson's disease is a chronic disease, what outcomes would be appropriate over a 10-year period?

---

progress and outcomes, (4) measurement of treatment interventions, (5) cost–benefit effectiveness of care, (6) assistance in the rehabilitation program's evaluation and audit, and (7) research (Remsburg & Carson, 2006, p. 601).

Evaluators may use a variety of methods to complete a functional assessment. Generally, a combination of self-report, whether in the form of a questionnaire completed by the person or the interviewer, and observation are used. An example of an easy tool to assess general geriatric health is the Timed Up and Go (TUG) test. The person is asked to rise up from a chair, walk 10 feet, turn around, and sit back down. Increased TUG times have been associated with falls in the elderly (Podsaidlo & Richardson, 1991).

Functional assessment in rehabilitation often focuses primarily on examining the patient's ability to perform ADLs such as dressing, grooming, bathing, eating, and toileting. The Barthel index is a tool based on self-report (see Table 24-7). Respondents are asked to rate themselves on 15 tasks, responding about their level of independence by choosing one of the following options: "can do by myself," "can do with help of someone else," or "cannot do at all." Criticisms of the Barthel index are that it omits some essential information such as scores on comprehension and other cognitive function, so its utility as a single tool for evaluation in rehabilitation is limited. Self-report without observation also introduces the potential for inaccuracies.

The Functional Independence Measure (FIM) (Uniform Data Systems for Medical Rehabilitation, 1997) is the most widely accepted and most used performance-based measure of ADLs (see Figure 24-1). A revised version of the FIM (called the Wee-FIM) is available for pediatric patients. The FIM is an instrument that is completed by a trained evaluator to assess 18 performance items on a 7-level scale. The tool is completed upon admission, at discharge, and often several times in between to monitor progress. The total score of all categories can help to show

improvement over time. The evaluator may be one person, or different team members may complete various parts of the FIM tool based on their expertise. For example, the nurse may complete the sphincter control item and the speech therapist may complete the communication section. Team members base their evaluation on direct observation of the subject. The items assessed include self-care, sphincter control, transfers, locomotion, communication, and social cognition. The evaluator quantifies each category by determining how much assistance is required in each category. A

TABLE 24-7

The Barthel Index

	"Can Do by Myself"	"Can Do with Help of Someone Else"	"Cannot Do at All'"
Self-Care Subscore			
1. Drinking from a cup	4	0	0
2. Eating 6	0	0	
3. Dressing upper body	5	3	0
4. Dressing lower body	7	4	0
5. Putting on brace or artificial limb	0	2	0 (N/A)
6. Grooming	5	0	0
7. Washing or bathing	6	0	0
8. Controlling urination	10	5 (accidents)	0 (incontinent)
9. Controlling bowel movements	10	5 (accidents)	0 (incontinent)
Mobility Subscore			
10. Getting in and out of chair	15	7	0
11. Getting on and off toilet	6	3	0
12. Getting in and out of tub or shower	1	0	0
13. Walking 50 yards on the level	15	10	0
14. Walking up/down one flight of stairs	10	5	0
15. If not walking: Propelling or pushing wheelchair	5	0	0 (N/A)

Barthel total: Best score is 100; worst score is 0

Note: Tasks 1-9, the self-care subscore (including control of bladder and bowel sphincters), have a total possible score of 53. Tasks 10-15, the mobility subscore, have a total possible score of 47. The two groups of tasks combined make up the total Barthel index, with a total possible score of 100.
Source: From Granger, C., & Gresham, G. (1984). *Functional assessment in rehabilitation medicine* (p. 74). Baltimore: Williams & Wilkins. Used with permission.

FIGURE 24-1

FIM Instrument

		NO HELPER
L E V E L S	7 Complete Independence (Timely, Safely) 6 Modified Independence (Device)	**NO HELPER**
	Modified Dependence 5 Supervision (Subject = 100%+) 4 Minimal Assist (Subject = 75%+) 3 Moderate Assist (Subject = 50%+) **Complete Dependence** 2 Maximal Assist (Subject = 25%+) 1 Total Assist (Subject = less than 25%)	**HELPER**

	ADMISSION	DISCHARGE	FOLLOW-UP
Self-Care A. Eating B. Grooming C. Bathing D. Dressing - Upper Body E. Dressing - Lower Body F. Toileting			
Sphincter Control G. Bladder Management H. Bowel Management			
Transfers I. Bed, Chair, Wheelchair J. Toilet K. Tub, shower			
Locomotion L. Walk/Wheelchair M. Stairs	W Walk C Wheelchair B Both	W Walk C Wheelchair B Both	W Walk C Wheelchair B Both
Motor Subtotal Score			
Communication N. Comprehension O. Expression	A Auditory V Visual B Both V Vocal N Nonvocal B Both	A Auditory V Visual B Both V Vocal N Nonvocal B Both	A Auditory V Visual B Both V Vocal N Nonvocal B Both
Social Cognition P. Social Interaction Q. Problem Solving R. Memory			
Cognitive Subtotal Score			
TOTAL FIM Score			

NOTE: Leave no blanks. Enter 1 if patient not testable due to risk.

Source: Copyright © 1997 Uniform Data System for Medical Rehabilitation (UDSmr), a division of UB Foundation Activities, Inc. (UBFA). Reprinted with the permission of UDSmr, University at Buffalo, 232 Parker Hall, 3435 Main Street, Buffalo, NY 14214. All marks associated with IFM and UDSmr are owned by UBFA.

score of 1 means total assistance was needed and the subject provided less than 25% of the effort. A score of 7 signifies complete independence in a timely and safe matter (i.e., the subject was completely independent in that activity).

The usefulness or accuracy of some of these tools has been called into question by some. It is wise to investigate the development of the instrument and which patients groups were used during its development. In addition, the outcomes of a tool are generally somewhat dependent upon the person using it, so it is essential that evaluators are properly educated in the use of the instrument. Many tools have questionable generalizability to older adults and may not take into consideration the normal effects of aging.

Pain Management

Both acute and chronic pain may be present in rehabilitation clients. Acute pain is thought to be of shorter duration and associated with the insult. Chronic pain, more often seen in those clients with chronic illness and disability, is of longer duration, and can result in diminished health, disability, and reduction in quality of life (American Pain Society, 2006; Hertzberg, 2007). Chronic pain has been associated with depression, disability, decreased function, and increased time off of work (Walsh, Dumitru, Schoenfeld, & Ramaurthy, 2005; Harris, 2000; Lipton, Hamelsky, Kolodner, Steiner, & Stewart, 2000). The popularity of pain clinics, whose major purpose is to address chronic, intractable pain, is growing, and referrals are often made to these programs when other interventions fail.

Pain, whether acute and/or chronic, can interfere with rehabilitation goals. Therefore, pain management is a part of most rehabilitation programs. The ARN, in fact, provides specific goals for pain management in their clients, stating that the rehabilitation nurses should seek to "improve the level of functioning and the quality of life for those affected by pain" (ARN, 1994). Pain is a complex problem that requires a comprehensive approach from an interdisciplinary team using a variety of pharmacologic and nonpharmacologic interventions (see Chapter 17).

Rehabilitation Nursing

Rehabilitation is a growing specialty, and nursing is an emerging leader in this field. Specialties such as rehabilitation nursing are often impacted by the wars that create larger numbers of veterans with multiple traumatic injuries that require rehabilitation. Rehabilitation nurses are finding themselves working in a wider variety of settings and subspecialties to meet the growing demand for their services. Several of the settings in which rehabilitation nurses may work are discussed in the following sections.

In 1984, the Association of Rehabilitation Nurses offered the first certification for registered nurses working with rehabilitation clients. This credential, the certified rehabilitation registered nurse (CRRN), is the basic designation for this nursing specialty. In 1997 an advanced practice certification, the certified rehabilitation registered nurse-advanced (CRRN-A) was offered, but because of the smaller number of nurses sitting for the exam and changes in certification methods, it is being phased out in 2009 (Secrest, 2007). The Association of Rehabilitation Nurses (ARN) also supports a variety of specialized practice roles for rehabilitation nurses (ARN, 2007a). Role descriptions that have been developed by the ARN for rehabilitation nurses include the subspecialties of gerontologic rehabilitation, home care, pain management, pediatric rehabilitation, rehabilitation nurse manager, rehabilitation admissions liaison, advanced practice, case manager, staff nurse, nurse educator, and nurse researcher (see Table 24-8).

Rehabilitation Settings

Rehabilitation services are offered in a wide variety of settings. These may include freestanding rehabilitation facilities, acute rehabilitation within hospitals, long-term care facilities, or the home. Regardless of the setting for care, rehabilitation

TABLE 24-8

Rehabilitation Nursing Role Descriptions

Gerontologic Rehabilitation Nurse
Home Care Rehabilitation Nurse
Pain Management Rehabilitation Nurse
Pediatric Rehabilitation Nursing
Rehabilitation Nurse Manager
Rehabilitation Admissions Liaison Nurse
Advanced Practice Rehabilitation Nurse
Rehabilitation Nurse Case Manager
Rehabilitation Nurse Educator
Rehabilitation Staff Nurse
Rehabilitation Nurse Researcher

Source: Association of Rehabilitation Nurses. (2007b). Role description brochures. Retrieved on November 19, 2007 from www.rehabnurse.org/db/members/fs/

services should be provided by an interdisciplinary team of trained professionals. In the past, rehabilitation units, especially those within hospitals, served patients with diverse diagnoses. However, as the specialty has grown and the body of research and evidence-based practice enlarges, it is becoming more common for larger rehabilitation facilities to target services for specific diagnostic groups of clients such as multiple trauma, traumatic brain injury, stroke syndromes, spinal cord injuries, cancer, burns, or HIV, or at least have dedicated units for persons with similar diagnoses.

Hospitals and Freestanding Facilities

Acute rehabilitation is often provided in acute care hospitals or freestanding rehabilitation facilities. A person requiring inpatient rehabilitation is one not just in need of therapy, for if that was the only service required, it could be done on an outpatient basis, as often occurs with such problems as joint replacement surgery. The person needing intensive inpatient rehabilitation is one who also requires 24-hour nursing care to address such problems as medication management, complex comorbidities, nutrition, swallowing disorders, behavior issues, skin care, and bowel and

bladder retraining. Clients in acute rehabilitation may be admitted for a specific diagnosis such as stroke, but also have pre- or coexisting conditions that complicate recovery including hypertension, cancer, diabetes, renal disease, and the like. In addition, the majority of clients treated in acute rehabilitation are older adults. Older adults as a population have unique needs with or without undergoing acute rehabilitation. Generally, to qualify for acute intensive rehabilitation services offered in these facilities, clients must be able to tolerate at least 3 hours of therapy per day, have a goal of discharge to home, and be able to demonstrate progress toward mutually established goals (Easton, 1999). They should also have private insurance or Medicare coverage to cover the high cost of the interdisciplinary services provided by multiple therapies and nursing.

Subacute Care Units

Subacute care units are for patients who require more intensive nursing care than the traditional long-term care facility or nursing home can provide, but less than that provided by the acute care hospital or skilled care unit (Mauk, 2006). These units are sometimes referred to as transitional care units. Clients seen in subacute care are typically those "needing assistance as a result of non-healing wounds, chronic ventilator dependence, renal problems, intravenous therapy, and coma management and those with complex medical and/or rehabilitation needs, including pediatrics, orthopedics, and neurologic. These units are designed to promote optimum outcomes in the least expensive cost setting" (Easton, 1999, p. 15). Clients may stay from days to several weeks. Persons who need rehabilitation services but would be unable to tolerate the intensive therapy of acute rehabilitation may be candidates for this level of care.

Skilled Nursing Facilities

Skilled nursing facilities may also provide rehabilitation and can be housed in acute care hospitals on independent specialty units, or within long-term care facilities. Remsburg cautions that not all skilled nursing facilities provide the same level of rehabilitation services, with services ranging from those who are Commission on Accreditation of Rehabilitation Facilities (CARF)–accredited programs and others that offer some restorative care, so consumers should carefully evaluate options when choosing a facility (Remsburg, Armacost, Radu, & Bennett, 1999; Remsburg, Armacost, Radu, & Bennett, 2001; Resnick & Fleishall, 2002).

Several benefits are seen with SNFs. The pace is generally slower. Often patients will have more continuity of care with nursing staff than in an acute care hospital. Length of stay is generally longer, perhaps weeks or months instead of days. The focus of treatment is on individual outcomes with less regard to speed of progress (Osterweil, 1990).

Long-Term Care Facilities or Retirement Communities

Although long-term care facilities often carry a negative stigma with the general public, rehabilitative services offered in these facilities may be quite appropriate for assisting adults regain independence and function. Long-term care facilities, especially those offering multiple levels of care, may have accredited rehabilitation units housed within them. Persons making a retirement community their home may also avail themselves of therapeutic services offered within a facility. An increasing number of continuous care retirement communities (CCRCs) have physical or other therapists available to assist with rehabilitation after an accident, surgery, or illness in order to help older adults "age in place." In addition, many CCRCs have begun to offer health promotion activities that include state-of-the-art fitness centers with personal trainers to foster primary prevention as well as rehabilitation.

Community-Based Rehabilitation

Community-based rehabilitation may involve a rehabilitation team or involve only nursing.

Community-based nurses may work in outpatient rehabilitation clinics, senior centers, assisted living, home health care, public schools, churches, or function as case managers. According to Parker and Neal-Boylan (2007), community-based rehabilitation is used in a variety of settings including home health care, subacute care, long-term care, and independent living.

Home health care provides services to clients of all ages and emphasizes primary care and case management. It allows individuals and families to remain in the home and still receive services that focus on health restoration and maximizing function. Home care is considered a cost-effective service for those recuperating from an injury or illness, who are not able to completely care for themselves (National Association for Home Care and Hospice, 2007). Unique models may even allow CCRCs to provide home care services covered by Medicare (L. Mullet, personal communication, November 26, 2007).

Subacute care in the community-based model generally provides services to adults through a team-nursing delivery system, with most of the daily care being provided by nursing assistants, with supervision or LPNs and case management by RNs. In the long-term care setting, services are offered mainly to geriatric residents using a team approach, with the RN in the role of case manager. In independent living settings, older adults may receive care from personal care attendants. Here again the RN serves as a care manager and client advocate (Parker & Neal-Boylan, 2007).

Rehabilitation Specialties

Within the discipline of rehabilitation, there are many subspecialties. Although most traditional rehabilitation programs provide care to a mixed-case of clients, there are both population and diagnosis-specific units that cater to the needs of smaller, select groups of patients. These types of specialty programs may be inpatient or outpatient and may include geriatrics, pediatrics, cardiac, pulmonary, cancer, HIV, and Alzheimer's disease.

Geriatric Rehabilitation

By 2030, it is estimated that there will be more than 71 million Americans older than age 65, comprising about 20% of the population (CDC, 2007a). The top chronic illnesses that are considered the greatest health burden to society include arthritis, heart disease and stroke, diabetes, and cancer, and more recently obesity and tobacco (National Centers for Chronic Disease Prevention and Health Promotion, 2007). Of the six leading causes of death in older Americans, five are from chronic illnesses, indicating that rehabilitation in geriatric clients should be a priority.

Geriatric rehabilitation focuses on restoring and maintaining optimal function while considering holistically the unique effects of aging on the person (Clark & Siebens, 2005). Programs specifically designed for older adults may have adjusted expectations such as requiring less intensive rehabilitation and preventing potential complications such as falls, dehydration, pressure sores, immobility, delirium, and polypharmacy that more frequently occur in older adults (Beers & Berkow, 2004; Lin and Armour, 2004; Routasalo, Arve, & Lauri, 2004; Worsowicz, Stewart, Phillips, & Cifu, 2004). Geriatric rehabilitation also focuses on enhancing quality of life through the strengthening of social support systems, family involvement, client education, and connection with community resources.

Mauk and Lehman (2007) suggest that there are two ways in which disability affects older adults: acquired at an advanced age, and aging with an earlier onset disability. Factors that may affect an older adult's rehabilitation potential include: age, frailty, the normal aging process, effects of chronic disease, functional and cognitive status, the use of multiple medications, and the presence of social support (Bagg, Pombo, & Hopman, 2002; Yu, 2005; Bandeen-Roche et al., 2006; Charles & Lehman, 2006; Beaupre et al., 2005). The more common acquired disabilities in older adults include stroke, head injury, and fractures from falls. In addition, the various syndromes (such as delirium, dizziness, incontinence, dehydration, and functional loss) that are seen more often in older adults can negatively impact the rehabilitation process (Mauk & Lehman, 2007). Persons aging with a disability tend to experience a greater degree of complications over time. For example, the person with a lower extremity amputation that occurred in his twenties is much more likely to have arthritis and range of motion problems in his shoulders from overuse of a non–weight-bearing joint than the person who has lost this limb later in life. However, the person with lower extremity amputation as a result of peripheral vascular disease secondary to diabetes is at an increased risk for complications due to advanced age and disease process than a younger person. Therefore, both the disability and the aging process contribute to one's overall rehabilitation potential. Rehabilitation can positively impact older adults by providing services to strengthen both physical and psychosocial functioning.

Pediatric Rehabilitation

Children with functional limitations have different needs and development concerns than adults do. Pediatric rehabilitation involves the collaboration of an interdisciplinary team of professionals to provide a continuum of care for children from the onset of injury or illness until adulthood. The focus of treatment is on adaptation and maximum function to promote independence within the family and society. The Association of Rehabilitation Nurses (ARN, 2007) defines pediatric rehabilitation nursing as "the specialty practice committed to improving the quality of life for children and adolescents with disabilities and their families" (p. 1). Professionals working with children practice family-centered care, must be knowledgeable about normal growth and development, and be able to work with an interdisciplinary team to address interventions that include physical, emotional, cultural, educational, socioeconomic, and spiritual dimensions (Edwards, Hertzberg, & Sapp, 2007).

CASE STUDY

Norma—Technologic Advances

Norma, a 60-year-old woman with severe rheumatoid arthritis, had experienced the effects of this chronic, progressive disease for decades. She kept a positive attitude throughout the course of her chronic illness, and had a supportive husband and adult children. Norma worked with her medical team to manage her pain with a combination of drugs and nonpharmacologic interventions such as aquatic therapy, finding that simple resistive exercises in a warm indoor pool helped to increase her mobility and decrease pain. However, progressive pain and continued loss of function decreased her ability to perform activities of daily living (ADLs). Even simple activities such as dressing herself, shopping, and putting away groceries became impossible over time. Norma underwent replacements of nearly all her major joints over the course of her lifetime including bilateral hips and knees, as well as arthroplasty on both shoulders and wrists. Additional foot surgeries were needed to maintain the ability to walk. The technologic advances in joint replacement therapy, prosthetics, and subsequent rehabilitation allowed Norma to continue to live a productive life despite her degenerative condition. Medical advances and rehabilitation promoted her quality of life well into old age.

Discussion Questions

1. What are some other nonpharmacologic strategies that could be applied to help improve Norma's quality of life?
2. How would the interdisciplinary team assist Norma with developing a long-term plan to cope with the effects of rheumatoid arthritis?
3. What rehabilitation issues and concerns would be involved in Norma's situation?
4. How should the family be involved in the plan of care for Norma?

Some of the common disorders associated with the need for pediatric rehabilitation include: traumatic brain injury, spinal cord injury, burns, cancer, congenital diseases and birth defects, and chronic illness. For example, whether a child sustains a brain injury from an accident or is born with cerebral palsy, the interventions from the interdisciplinary rehabilitation team will be designed to maximize function and help the child attain adulthood as a well adjusted member of society.

Cardiac Rehabilitation

According to the American Heart Association (AHA, 2007a), 79.4 million Americans are affected by cardiovascular disease. Cardiac rehabilitation "enhances recovery, and secondary prevention measures prevent further complications from disease" (Carbone, 2007). Cardiac rehabilitation is appropriate for persons with congenital or acquired heart disease such as those with myocardial infarction, chronic angina, cardiomyopathy, or postsurgical patients. The aims are to improve functional capacity and to reduce related morbidity and mortality (Singh, Schocken, Williams, & Stamey, 2004). Cardiac rehabilitation following a myocardial infarction has four phases: Phase I: Acute phase—during the inpatient stay; Phase II: Convalescent phase—early post-discharge; Phase III: Training phase—structured and supervised exercise program; and Phase IV: Maintenance phase—post-training and lifestyle changes (Shah, 2005; Singh et al., 2004). Measures employed in cardiac rehabilitation include risk factor modification along with medication management and medical interventions. Risk-factor management focuses on smoking cessation, controlling hypertension, decreasing cholesterol, management of diabetes, increasing physical activity, and decreasing stress (AHA, 2007b). Client participation in cardiac rehabilitation is an ongoing problem, with recent research suggesting that the strength of physician recommendation, gender (men participated more than women), and disease severity may be the best predictors of whether clients initiate cardiac rehabilitation (Shanks, Moore, & Zeller, 2007; Ades, Waldmann, McCann, & Weaver, 1992).

Pulmonary Rehabilitation

Chronic obstructive pulmonary disease (COPD), which includes chronic bronchitis and emphysema, is the fourth leading cause of death in America, claiming over 120,000 lives in 2003 [American Lung Association (ALA), 2008]. When asthma and other pulmonary problems are factored in, chronic respiratory problems are a leading cause of functional disability in the United States. The primary risk factor for COPD is smoking, and 80–90% of deaths from COPD are attributed to this cause (ALA, 2008). Because of the large numbers of Americans experiencing pulmonary problems, specific programs have been developed to address these needs. The American Association for Respiratory Care (AARC, 2002) stated that essential components of a pulmonary rehabilitation program include: assessment, patient education, exercise, psychosocial interventions, and follow-up. Smoking cessation programs are a major focus in both the prevention and rehabilitative treatment of respiratory problems.

Cancer Rehabilitation

Deaths from cancer declined about 2.1% per year between 2002 and 2004 (CDC, 2007b). According to the CDC's 2003 data, the top cancer deaths for both males and females across all races include prostate, female breast, lung and colon–rectum (CDC, 2007c). Given these statistics, many cancers detected early are highly treatable and need not

be viewed as a terminal diagnosis with the stigma that cancer historically held. These data suggest that persons with cancer will not only survive, but may require rehabilitation to enhance quality of life and return to optimal functioning after their diagnosis and as part of their treatment." Cancer rehabilitation is the process that assists the person with cancer in obtaining maximum physical, social, psychological, and work-related functioning during and after cancer treatment" (People Living with Cancer, 2006, p. 1). The goals of cancer rehabilitation include maximizing independence in mobility and ADLs, preserving dignity, and promoting quality of life (Beck, 2003; Gillis, Cheville, & Worsowicz, 2001; Vargo & Gerber, 2005), and are individualized to each person, given the stage of their disease. The cancer rehabilitation team includes all of the usual team members of rehabilitation but also includes the oncologist. Quality of life is enhanced through cancer rehabilitation by assistance with ADLs, pain management, improving nutrition, smoking cessation, stress reduction, and improved coping strategies. In one study of women with breast cancer, exercise therapy was found to significantly enhance quality of life (Dale et al., 2007). Rehabilitation can also assist individuals with terminal cancer to live a better quality of life until their end of life.

Dementia or Alzheimer's Programs

Alzheimer's disease is a progressive and fatal brain disease that currently affects more than 5 million Americans. New research from the National Institutes of Health suggests that one in seven Americans older than the age of 71 has some type of dementia (Plassman, 2007). Generally occurring in older adults, there are still believed to be between 220,000 and more than half a million cases of early onset Alzheimer's that affect persons ages in their thirties, forties, and fifties (Alzheimer's Association, 2007). It is the most common type of dementia and has no cure. Although Alzheimer's disease is not generally considered a rehabilitation diagnosis, it certainly fits the profile of chronic illness. Those with early onset Alzheimer's disease would certainly avail themselves of all treatment possible to postpone the inevitable effects of this progressive illness. This would include interventions from the rehabilitation team.

Rehabilitation nurses are often found working in long-term care facilities that serve residents with dementia, and the need is likely to grow. Although the focus of care for older persons with Alzheimer's disease includes rehabilitation goals, realistic outcome planning as the disease progresses will not likely include discharge to home. Persons with Alzheimer's disease may receive services from assisted living, nursing homes, and/or special care units (Alzheimer's Association, 2007). The Alzheimer's unit within the nursing home often becomes the last home that a person with dementia will know. The number of Alzheimer's units within long-term care facilities is increasing owing to the demand for services as the disease progresses, and family caregivers are no longer able to manage persons at home. As their condition deteriorates with advancing dementia, the fundamental principles of rehabilitation still apply to these residents: to assist individuals to remain as independent as possible for as long as possible, to maintain function, and to prevent complications.

HIV/AIDS

Approximately one million Americans are living with HIV or AIDS, with thousands of these unaware of their condition (CDC, 2006a). It is estimated that between 34.6 and 42.3 million people in the world have HIV or AIDS (Monohan et al., 2007) and about 25 million people worldwide have died from AIDS, including about a half million Americans (CDC, 2006b). Although current treatments have dramatically increased the life expectancy for many person with HIV, those developing AIDS experience many associated neurologic, pulmonary, cardiac, and rheumatologic problems. Rehabilitation programs designed to address all levels of prevention along with the associated health problems inherent with HIV/AIDS are becoming more common. Rehabilitation nurses may work with infected patients from before diagnoses through end of life

(Manning & Haldi, 2007). Rehabilitation goals depend on the stage of illness, whether symptomatic, asymptomatic, or terminal, but include interventions such as monitoring client status, careful assessment, addressing psychological needs and responses, balancing energy with rest, medication management, education regarding prevention of transmission, emotional support, and counseling for the person and family.

Ensuring Quality in Rehabilitation Facilities

There are two primary accrediting bodies for rehabilitation providers: The Joint Commission (JC) (formerly Joint Commission on the Accreditation of Healthcare Organizations, JCAHO) and the Rehabilitation Accreditation Commission (CARF). Although JC accreditation is expected for inpatient rehabilitation providers, CARF accreditation is viewed as a mark of distinction that signifies meeting higher standards for rehabilitation.

The Joint Commission

The oldest and best known accrediting body is The Joint Commission (JC), previously known as the Joint Commission on the Accreditation of Healthcare Organizations (JCAHO). The mission of the JC is "to continuously improve the safety and quality of care provided to the public through the provision of health care accreditation and related services that support performance improvement in health care organizations" (JC, 2007, p. 1). The Joint Commission has developed current, professionally based standards for hospitals, long-term care, home health care, and other organizations, and uses a survey process to evaluate the compliance of healthcare organizations with these standards. The Joint Commission has a cooperative agreement with CARF regarding the evaluation of rehabilitation facilities. In 1997, the ORYX initiative allowed the integration of outcomes and standard performance measures into the accreditation process and helped organizations identify care issues that required attention (Black, 2007). The

Joint Commission holds organizations responsible for providing safe care that meets the standards of the industry and protects public safety. Some benefits of JC accreditation and certification include strengthening the trust of the public in the organization, improving risk management, promoting patient safety and comfort, and enhancing staff recruitment into the organization (Black, 2007).

Commission on Accreditation of Rehabilitation Facilities (CARF)

The Commission on Accreditation of Rehabilitation Facilities (CARF) is an independent, not-for-profit organization that accredits rehabilitation programs and services. "CARF reviews and grants accreditation services nationally and internationally on request of a facility or program. Our standards are rigorous, so those services that meet them are among the best available," and CARF accreditation procedures "ensure the highest industry standards possible, providing risk reduction and accountability" (CARF, 2007, p. 1). There are six divisions in CARF's organizational structure: Medical rehabilitation, behavioral health, employment and community services, aging services, child and youth services, and opioid treatment (Black, 2007). The most recent publications for CARF include the Child and Youth Standards Manual, Aging Services Standards Manual, and Stroke Specialty Programs Standards.

OUTCOME MEASUREMENT AND PERFORMANCE IMPROVEMENT

According to Black (2007), outcomes of care are being emphasized as never before. She lists the following benefits of monitoring outcomes (Black, 2007, p. 395):

- Track efficiency and effectiveness
- Identify trends
- Facilitate communication between the patient, family, treatment team, payers, referral source, and other stakeholders

- Assess follow-up measures to determine whether progress is continuing after discharge
- Identify areas for improvement
- Measure access to programs

In rehabilitation, outcomes are key to ensuring that goals are being met. Goal-setting in rehabilitation should be mutual between the client and the healthcare team. Individual goals for clients are reviewed systematically at team conferences. Outcome measurement can be used to look at trends within an organization, be benchmarked against industry standards, and compared with best practices.

There are many ways that outcomes can be measured. Accreditation provides one way to ensure that facilities are meeting the industry standards. A variety of tools can also be used to monitor individual and collective rehabilitation outcomes. One of the most commonly used is the Functional Independence Measure (FIM) instrument (see Figure 24-1). The FIM (Uniform Data Systems for Medical Rehabilitation, 1997) instrument provides a quantitative measure of function on admission, discharge, and follow-up so that data may be compared across time and with other cohorts. This information often provides useful in justifying insurance coverage to demonstrate continued improvement by the client.

There are also many tools and models for performance improvement in health care. Most of these focus on devices to assist team members to improve the quality of care for clients. Diagrams, flow sheets, checklists, charts, and other visuals can enhance performance. Standard setting by national organizations provides an additional means of quality improvement as organizations strive to meet industry aims. Outcomes measurement and documentation of performance improvement is critical as reimbursement under present payment systems require rehabilitation providers to provide evidence of the effectiveness of their programs and services (Johnston, Eastwood, Wilkerson, Anderson, & Alves, 2005).

EVIDENCE-BASED PRACTICE BOX

This study involved secondary analysis of data from 659 women ages 18 to 95 years with a mean age of 47 years. The larger study was a longitudinal survey of health-promoting behaviors and quality of life in persons with multiple sclerosis (MS). Participants responded via e-mail to a survey that included reporting the extent of loneliness for the preceding week. Findings suggested that loneliness in not uncommon for women with MS. It was associated with lower levels of social support, increased functional limitations, lower self-rated health, and greater social demands of illness, and being unmarried. Limitations of the study included a convenience sample, and mainly Caucasian participants, so caution should be used with generalizability of the findings. The researchers concluded that women with MS should be screened for loneliness and social isolation, and that rehabilitation professionals could use this information to identify and implement strategies to help strengthen social support networks for these patients.

Source: Beal, C. C. & Stuifbergen, A. (2007). Loneliness in women with multiple sclerosis. *Rehabilitation Nursing, 32*(4), 165–171.

STUDY QUESTIONS

1. Rehabilitation is both a philosophy and an approach to treatment. Describe the philosophy of rehabilitation and how it relates to treatment from an interdisciplinary team of professionals.
2. Define the following rehabilitation terms in relationship to chronic illness: impairment, functional limitation, disability, and community reintegration.
3. Identify three problems in the provision of rehabilitation services to the chronically ill.
4. Describe the different settings where rehabilitation services can be provided.
5. What specific issues in rehabilitation make doing research difficult?
6. Discuss the advantages and disadvantages of three major functional assessment tools mentioned in this chapter.

INTERNET RESOURCES

Alzheimer's Association: www.alz.org
American Heart Association: www.aha.org
American Stroke Association: www.strokeassociation.org
Association of Rehabilitation Nurses: www.rehabnurse.org
Center for Medicare & Medicaid Services: www.cms.hhs.gov/medicare/
Centers for Disease Control and Prevention: www.cdc.gov/aging/saha.htm
National Institute of Neurological Disorders and Stroke: www.ninds.nih.gov
National Rehabilitation Information Center: www.naric.com
National Rehabilitation Association: www.nationalrehab.org
National Stroke Association: www.nsa.org

REFERENCES

Adams P.F., Dey A.N., & Vickerie J.L. (2007). Summary health statistics for the U.S. population: National Health Interview Survey, 2005. National Center for Health Statistics. Vital Health Statistics, *10*(233). Hyattsville, MD: U.S. Department of Health and Human Services.

Ades, P.A., Waldmann, M.L. McCann, W., & Weaver, S.O. (1992). Predictors of cardiac rehabilitation participation in older coronary patients. *Archives of Internal Medicine, 152*, 1033–1035.

Alzheimer's Association. (2007). Alzheimer's disease. Retrieved on December 1, 2007 from http://www.alz.org/alzheimers_disease_alzheimers_disease.asp

American Association for Respiratory Care (AARC). (2002). AARC clinical practice guideline: Pulmonary rehabilitation. *Respiratory Care, 47*(5), 617–625.

American Cancer Society. (2006). *Cancer facts and figures 2006*. Atlanta: American Cancer Society.

American Heart Association. (2008). Exercise and fitness. Retrieved September 14, 2008 from http://www.americanheart.org/presenter.jhtml?identifier=1200013

American Heart Association. (AHA) (2007b). Heart disease and stroke statistics: 2007 update. Retrieved on May 25, 2007 from americanheart.org/presenter.jhtml?identifier=1543

American Lung Association. (2008). Chronic bronchitis. Retrieved on September 14, 2008 from http://www.lungusa.org/site/c.dvLUK9O0E/b.4061173/apps/s/content.asp?ct=3052285

American Pain Society. (APS). (2006). Pain: Current understanding of assessment, management, and treatments. Retrieved from www.ampainsoc.org/ce/enduring.htm.

Anderson, C., Linto, J., & Stewart-Wynne, E. (1995). A population-based assessment of the impact and burden of caregiving for long-term stroke survivors. *Stroke, 26*, 843–849.

Arbour, K.P., Latimer, A.E., Ginis, K.A. & Jung, M.E. (2007). Moving beyond the stigma: The impression formation benefits of exercise for individuals with a physical disability. *Adapted Physical Activity Quarterly, 24*(2), 144–159.

Association of Rehabilitation Nurses. (2007a). ARN positional statement on the role of the role of the nurse in the rehabilitation team. Retrieved on November 11, 2007 from www.rehabnurse.org/advocacy/roleofnurse.html

Association of Rehabilitation Nurses. (2007b). Role description brochures. Retrieved on November 19, 2007 from www.rehabnurse.org/pubs/role/index.html

Association of Rehabilitation Nurses. (1996). *Scope and standards of advanced clinical practice in rehabilitation nursing*. Glenview, IL: Association of Rehabilitation Nurses.

Association of Rehabilitation Nurses. (2000). *Standards and scope of rehabilitation nursing practice*. Glenview, IL: Association of Rehabilitation Nurses.

Bagg, S., Pombo, A.P., & Hopman, W. (2002). Effect of age on functional outcomes after stroke rehabilitation. *Stroke, 33*, 179–185.

Bandeen-Roche, K., Xue, Q-L., Ferrucci, L., Walston, J., Guralnik, J.M., Chaves, et al. (2006. Pheotype of frailty: Characterization in the women's health and aging studies. *The Journals of Gerontology series A: Biological Sciences and Medical Sciences, 61*, 262–266.

Beck, L.A. (2003). Cancer rehabilitation: Does it make a difference? *Rehabilitation Nursing, 28*(2), 32–37.

Beauchamp, T.L. & Childress, J.F. (2001). *Principles of biomedical ethics*. New York, NY: Oxford University Press.

Beaupre, L.A., Cinats, J.G., Senthilselvan, A., Scharfenberger, A., Johnston, D.W., & Saunders, L.D. (2005). Does standardized rehabilitation and discharge planning improve functional recovery in elderly patients with hip fracture? *Archives of Physical Medicine and Rehabilitation, 86*, 2231–2239.

Beers, M. H., & Berkow, R. (2004). Rehabilitation. The Merck manual of geriatrics. Merck & Co., Medical Services, USMEDA, USHH. Retrieved from www.merck.com/mrkshared/mm_geriatrics/home.jsp

Beam, T.B., & O'Hare, T.P. (2003). *Meeting the Financial Need of Long-term Care*. Bryn Mawr, PA: The American College.

Black, T. (2007). Outcomes measurement and performance improvement. In K.L. Mauk (Ed.). *The specialty practice of rehabilitation nursing: A core curriculum* (pp. 395–411). Glenview, IL: Association of Rehabilitation Nurses.

Brandstater, M.E. (2005). Stroke Rehabilitation. In J. DeLisa and B. Gans (Eds.), *Rehabilitation medicine: Principles and practice* (4th ed.) (pp. 1655–1676). Philadelphia: Lippincott-Raven.

Brandt, E. & Pope, A. (1997). *Enabling America: Assessing the Role of Rehabilitation Science and Engineering.* Committee on Assessing Rehabilitation Science and Engineering. Division of Health Policy. Institute of Medicine. Washington, DC: National Academy Press.

Brouwer, W.B.F., van Exel, N.J.A., van de Berg, B., Dinant, H.J., Koopmanschap, M.A. & van den Bos, G.A. (2004). Burden of caregiving: evidence of objective burden, subjective burden, and quality of life impacts on informal caregivers of patients with rheumatoid arthritis. *Arthritis and Rheumatism, 51*(4), 570–577.

Buchanan, L. (1996). Community-based rehabilitation nursing. In S. Hoeman (Ed.), *Rehabilitation nursing: Process and application* (2nd ed.) (pp.114–129). St. Louis: Mosby.

Bushnik, T., Wright, J., & Burdsall, D. (2007). Personal attendant turnover: Association with level of injury, burden of care, and psychosocial outcome. *Topics in Spinal Cord Injury Rehabilitation, 12*(3), 66–76.

Campinha-Bacote, J. (2001). A model of practice to address cultural competence. *Rehabilitation Nursing, 26*(1), 8–11.

Canam, C., & Acorn, S. (1999). Quality of life for family caregivers of people with chronic health problems. *Rehabilitation Nursing, 24*(5), 192–196.

Carbone, L. (2007). Cardiovascular and pulmonary rehabilitation: Acute and long-term management. In K.L. Mauk (Ed.), *The specialty practice of rehabilitation nursing: A core curriculum*, (pp. 238–259). Glenview, IL: Association of Rehabilitation Nurses.

Center for International Rehabilitation Research Information Exchange (CIRRIE) and the National Institute on Disability and Rehabilitation Research (NIDDR) (2007). The rehabilitation provider's guide to cultures of the foreign-born. Retrieved from cirrie.buffalo.edu/mseries.html

Centers for Disease Control and Prevention. (2007a). The State of Aging and Health in America Report. Retrieved on December 1, 2007 from www.cdc.gov/ aging/saha.htm

Centers for Disease Control and Prevention. (2007b). Report to the nation on the status of cancer. Retrieved on December 1, 2007 from www.cdc.gov/ Features/CancerReport/

Centers for Disease Control and Prevention. (2007c). United States cancer statistics. Retrieved on December 1, 2007 from apps.nccd.cdc.gov/uscs/ Table.aspx?Group=3f&Year=2003&Display=n

Centers for Disease Control and Prevention. (2007d). About minority health. Retrieved on December 8, 2007 from www.cdc.gov/omhd/AMH/AMH.htm

Centers for Disease Control and Prevention. (2006a). Overview. Retrieved on December 2, 2006 from www.cdc.gov/hiv/topics/testing/index.htm

Centers for Disease Control and Prevention. (2006b). Spotlight: Commemorating 25 years of HIV/AIDS. Retrieved December 2, 2006 from http://www.cdc. gov/hiv/spotlight.htm Centers for Medicare and Medicaid Services. (2002). RAI Version 2.0 Manual. Retrieved from www.cms.hhs.gov/quality/ mds20/

Centers for Medicare and Medicaid Services. (2005a). Medicare Information Resource. Retrieved from www.cms.hhs.gov/home/medicare.asp

Centers for Medicare and Medicaid. (2005b). Medicare inpatient rehabilitation facility classification requirements. Retrieved from http://www.cms. hhs.gov/ medicare/

Centers for Medicare and Medicaid. (2005). Medicaid at a Glance 2005. Retrieved from www.cms.hhs. gov/MedicaidGenInfo/Downloads/MedicaidAtA-Glance2005.pdf

Centers for Medicare and Medicaid Services. (2007). Medicare and you 2008. Retrieved from www. medicare.gov/Publications/Pubs/pdf/10050.pdf

Centers for Medicare and Medicaid Services. (2007a). Overview of Inpatient Rehabilitation Facility PPS. Retrieved from www.cms.hhs.gov/InpatientRehabFacPPS/01_Overview.asp#TopOfPage

Charles, C.V. & Lehman, C. (2006). Medications and laboratory values. In K.L. Mauk (Ed.), *Gerontological Nursing: Competencies for Care*, pp. 293–320. Sudbury, MA: Jones & Bartlett.

Clark G. S., & Siebens H. (2005). Geriatric rehabilitation. In J. DeLisa and B. Gans (Eds.). *Physical Medicine and Rehabilitation: Principles and practice* (4th ed.) (pp. 1531–1560). Philadelphia: Lippincott Williams & Wilkins.

Committee on Accreditation of Rehabilitation Facilities. (2007). Payers. Retrieved on November 21, 2007 from www.carf.org/

Cook, C., Stickley, L, Ramey, K., & Knotts, V. J. (2005). Variables associated with occupational and physical therapy stroke rehabilitation utilization and outcomes. *Journal of Allied Health, 34*(1), 3–10.

Council of State Administrators of Vocational Rehabilitation (2004–2005). Investing in America: The gateway to independence public vocational rehabilitation—A program that works. Retrieved from www.rehabnetwork.org/investing_in_america. htm

Currie, D.M., Atchison, J.W., & Fiedler, I.G. (2002). The challenge of teaching rehabilitative care in medical school. *Academic Medicine, 77*(7), 701–708.

Dale, A.J., Crank, H., Saxton, J.M., Mutrie, N., Coleman, R., & Roalfe A. (2007). Randomized trial of exercise therapy in women treated for breast cancer. *Journal of Clinical Oncology, 25*(13), 1713–1721.

D'Andrea, D.C., & Meyer, J.D. (2004). Workers' compensation reform. Clinics in *Occupational & Environmental Medicine, 4*, 259–271.

das Chagas Medeiros, M., Ferraz, M., & Quaresma, M. (2000). The effect of rheumatoid arthritis on the quality of life of primary caregivers. *Journal of Rheumatology, 27*(1), 76–83.

Dean-Baar, S. (2003). Nursing shortages affect all levels of the profession. *Rehabilitation Nursing, 28*(4), 102.

Department of Veterans Affairs. (2007a). Vocational rehabilitation and employment services. Retrieved from www1.va.gov/vetind/

Department of Veterans Affairs. (2007b). Disability compensation benefits. Retrieved from http://www.vba.va.gov/benefit_facts/Service-Connected_Disabilities/English/Compeg_0107.doc

Deutsch, A. & Dean-Baar, S. (2007). Economics and health policy in rehabilitation. In K.L. Mauk (Ed.), *The specialty practice of rehabilitation nursing: A core curriculum*, (pp. 35–53). Glenview, IL: Association of Rehabilitation Nurses.

Doherty, R.B. (2004). Assessing the new medicare prescription drug law. *Annals of Internal Medicine, 141*(5), 391–395.

Draper, B., Bowring, G., Thompson, C., Van Heyst, J., Conroy, P., & Thompson, J. (2007) Stress in caregivers of aphasic stroke patients: A randomized controlled trial. *Clinical Rehabilitation, 21*(2), 122–130.

Easton, K.L. (1999). *Gerontological rehabilitation nursing*. Philadelphia: Saunders.

Easton, K.L. (2001). The post-stroke journey: From agonizing to owning. Doctoral dissertation. Wayne State University, Detroit, MI.

Edwards, P. (2007). Rehabilitation nursing: Past, present and future. In K. Mauk (Ed.), *The specialty practice of rehabilitation nursing: A core curriculum* (5th ed.) (pp. 455–466). Glenview, IL: Association of Rehabilitation Nurses.

Edwards, P., Hertzberg, D., & Sapp, L. (2007). Pediatric rehabilitation nursing. In K. L. Mauk (Ed.), *The specialty practice of rehabilitation nursing: A core curriculum* (pp. 336–358). Glenview, IL: Association of Rehabilitation Nurses.

Edwards, P. (1992). The evolution of rehabilitation facilities for children. *Rehabilitation Nursing, 17*, 191–192.

Ellis, J. R. & Hartley, C.L. (2004). *Nursing in today's world: Trends, issues, and management* (8th ed.). Philadelphia: Lippincott, Williams & Wilkins.

Emmer, S., & Allendorf, L. (2004). The Medicare Prescription Drug, Improvement, and Modernization Act of 2003. *Journal of the American Geriatrics Society, 52*(6), 1013–1015.

Fairfax, J. (2002). Theory of quality of life of stroke survivors. Doctoral dissertation. Wayne State University, Detroit, MI.

Federal Register. (2007). Inpatient Rehabilitation Facility Prospective Payment System for Federal Fiscal Year 2008; Proposed Rule. Department of Health and Human Services, CMS, 72(88), 26230–26479.

Fried, T.R., Bradley, E.H., Williams, C.S., & Tinetti, M.E. (2001). Functional disability and health care expenditures for older persons. *Archives of Internal Medicine, 161*(21), 2602–2607.

Gillis, T.A., Cheville, A.L., & Worsowicz, G.M. (2001). Cardiopulmonary rehabilitation and cancer rehabilitation: Oncologic rehabilitation. *Archives of Physical Medicine and Rehabilitation, 83* (Suppl 1), S47–51.

Grunfeld, E., Coyle, D., Whelan, T., Clinch, J., et al. (2004). Family caregiver burden: results of a longitudinal study of breast cancer patients and their principal caregivers. *Canadian Medical Association Journal, 170*(12), 1795–1801.

Guse, L.W. (2006). Assessment of the older adult. In K.L. Mauk (Ed.), *Gerontological Nursing: Competencies for Care*, (pp. 265–292). Sudbury, MA: Jones & Bartlett.

Halm, M.A., Treat-Jacobson, D., Lindquist, R., & Savik, K. (2007). Caregiver burden and outcomes of caregiving of spouses of patient who undergo coronary artery bypass graft surgery. *Heart & Lung, 36*(3), 170–187.

Harris, J.A. (2000). Understanding acute and chronic pain. In P. Edwards (Ed.), *The specialty practice of rehabilitation nursing* (4th ed.). Glenview, IL: Association of Rehabilitation Nurses.

Hartke, R.J., & King, R.B. (2002). Analysis of problem types and difficulty among older stroke caregivers. *Topics in Stroke Rehabilitation, 9*(1), 16–33.

Havercamp, S.M., Scandlin, D., & Roth, M. (2004). Health disparities among adults with developmental disabilities, adults with other disabilities, and adults not reporting disability in North Carolina. *Public Health Reports, 119*(4), 418–426.

Hertzberg, D. (2007). Understanding acute and chronic pain. In K.L. Mauk (Ed.), *The specialty practice of rehabilitation nursing: A core curriculum*, (pp. 260–274). Glenview, IL: Association of Rehabilitation Nurses.

Hogstel, M.O., Curry, L.C., Walker, C.A., & Burns, P.G. (2004). Ethics committees in long-term care facilities. *Geriatric Nursing, 25*(6), 364–369.

Hughes, J.A. (2004). Ethics in the emergency department. *Academy of Emergency Medicine, 11*(9), 995–996.

Hughes, S., Giobbie-Hurder, A., Weaver, F., Kubal, J., et al. (1999). Relationship between caregiver burden and health-related quality of life. *Gerontologist, 39*(5), 534–545.

Indian Health Service. (2001). *Trends in Indian health.* Retrieved on March 28, 2004 from www.ihs.gov/PublicInfo/Publications/trends98/trends98.asp

Inman, J., McGurk, E., & Chadwick, J. (2007). Is vocational rehabilitation a transition to recovery? *British Journal of Occupational Therapy, 70*(2), 60–66.

Jett, D.U., Warren, R.L., & Wirtalla, C. (2005). The relation between therapy intensity and outcomes of rehabilitation in skilled nursing facilities. *Archives of Physical Medicine and Rehabilitation, 86*(3), 373–379.

Johnson, J.A. (2004). Withdrawal of medically administered nutrition and hydration: the role benefits and burdens, and of parents and ethics committees. *Journal of Clinical Ethics, 15*(3), 307–11.

Johnston, M.V., Eastwood, E., Wilkerson, D.L., Anderson, L., et al. (2005). Systematically assessing and improving the quality and outcomes of medical rehabilitation programs. In J. DeLisa & B.M. Gans (Eds.), *Rehabilitation medicine: Principles and practice* (3rd ed.) (pp. 1163–1192). Philadelphia: Lippincott-Raven.

Joint Commission. (2007). Retrieved on November 21, 2007 from http://www.jointcommission.org/AboutUs/.

Kaiser Commission. (2007). Medicaid and the uninsured. Retrieved on December 14, 2007 from http://www.kff.org/medicaid/upload/7682.pdf.

Kemp, B. (1986). Psychosocial and mental health issues in rehabilitation of older persons. In S. Brody & G. Ruff (Eds.). *Aging and rehabilitation*, (pp. 122–158). New York: Springer.

Kennedy, J. (2001). Unmet and undermet need for activities of daily living and instrumental activities of daily living assistance among adults and disabilities: Estimates from the 1994 and 1005 disability follow-back surveys. *Medical Care, 39*(12), 1305–12.

Kent, B., & Smith, S. (2006). They only see it when the sun shines in my ears: Exploring perceptions of adolescent hearing aid users. *Journal of Deaf Studies & Deaf Education, 11*(4), 461–476.

Kielhofner, G., Braveman, B., Finlayson, M., Paul-Ward A.,Goldbaum, L., & Goldstein, K. (2004). Outcomes of a Vocational Program for Persons with AIDS. *American Journal of Occupational Therapy, 58*(1), 64–72.

King, R.B., Hartke, R.J., & Denby, F. (2007). Problem-solving early intervention: A pilot study of stroke caregivers. *Rehabilitation Nursing, 32*(2), 68–76.

Kirschner, K. L., Stocking, C., Wagner, L. B., Foye, S. J., & Siegler, M. (2001). Ethical issues identified by rehabilitation clinicians. *Archives of Physical Medicine and Rehabilitation, 82* (12 Suppl 2), S2–8.

Kiselica, D., Sibson, B., & McKenzie-Green, J. (2004). Workers' compensation: A historical review and description of a legal and social insurance system. *Clinics in Occupational and Environmental Medicine, 4*, 237–247.

Kolanowski, A.M., Fick, D., Waller, J.L., & Shea, D. (2004). Spouses of persons with dementia: Their healthcare problems, utilization, and costs. *Research in Nursing & Health, 27*, 296–306.

Kosciulek, J.F. (2007). A test of the theory of informed consumer choice in vocational rehabilitation. *Journal of Rehabilitation, 73*(2), 41–49.

Kottke, F., Stillwell, G., & Lehmann, J. (Eds.). (1982). *Krusen's handbook of physical medicine and rehabilitation* (3rd ed.). Philadelphia: Saunders.

Kovner, C.T., Mezey, M., & Harrington, C. (2002). Who cares for older adults? Workforce implications of an aging society. *Health Affairs (Millwood), 21*(5), 78–89.

LaPlante M., Kaye H. S., Kang T., & Harrington C. (2004). Unmet need for personal assistance services: estimating the shortfall in hours of help and adverse consequences. *The Journal of Gerontology, Series B, Psychological Science and Social Science,* 59(2), S98–S108.

Lieberman, M., & Fisher, L. (1995). The impact of chronic illness on the health and well-being of family members. *Gerontologist, 35*(1), 94–102.

Lin, J.L., & Armour, D. (2004). Selected medical management of the older adult rehabilitative patient. *Archives of Physical Medicine and Rehabilitation,* 85(Suppl 3), S76–82.

Lipton, R., Hamelsky, S., Kolodner, K., Steiner, T., & Stewart, W.F.(2000). Migraine, quality of life, and depression: A population-based case-control study. *Neurology, 55*(5), 629–635.

Lloyd, C., & Waghorn, G. (2007). The importance of vocation in recovery for young people with psychiatric disabilities. *British Journal of Occupational Therapy, 70*(2), 50–59.

Lomay, V.T. & Hinkebein, J.H. (2006). Cultural considerations when providing rehabilitation services to American Indiana. *Rehabilitation Psychology,* 51(1), 36–42.

Lutz, B.J., & Bowers, B.J. (2003). Understanding how disability is defined and conceptualized in the literature. *Rehabilitation Nursing, 28*(3), 74–78.

Lysaght, R.M. (2004). Approaches to worker rehabilitation by occupational and physical therapists in the United States: Factors impacting practice. *Work,* 23(2), 139–146.

Manning, K. & Haldi, P. (2007). Specific disease processes requiring rehabilitation interventions. In K.L. Mauk (Ed.). *The specialty practice of rehabilitation nursing: A core curriculum,* (pp. 275–322). Glenview, IL: Association of Rehabilitation Nurses.

Masters-Farrell, P.A. (2007). Ethical, moral, and legal considerations. In K.L. Mauk (Ed.). *The specialty practice of rehabilitation nursing: A core curriculum,* (pp. 27–34). Glenview, IL: Association of Rehabilitation Nurses.

Masters-Farrell, P.A. (2006). Ethical/legal principles and issues. In K.L. Mauk (Ed.). *Gerontological Nursing: Competencies for Care,* (pp. 589–616). Sudbury, MA: Jones & Bartlett.

Mauk, K.L. (2006). Nursing interventions within the Mauk Model of Poststroke Recovery. *Rehabilitation Nursing, 31*(6), 267–263.

Mauk, K.L. & Lehman, C. (2007). Geriatric rehabilitation. In K.L. Mauk (Ed.) *The specialty practice of rehabilitation nursing: A core curriculum,* (pp. 359–383). Glenview, IL: Association of Rehabilitation Nurses.

Mezey, M., & Fulmer, T. (2002). The future history of gerontological nursing. *Journal of Gerontology A Biological Sciences Medical Sciences, 57*(7), M438–441.

Mills, P., Yu, H., Ziegler, M., Patterson, T., & Grant, I. (1999). Vulnerable caregivers of patients with Alzheimer's disease have a deficit in circulating CD62L-T lymphocytes. *Psychosomatic Medicine,* 61(2), 168–174.

Monahan, F.D., Sands, J.K., Neighbors, M., Marek, J.F. & Green, C.J. (2007). *Phipps' medical-surgical nursing: Health and illness perspectives* (8th ed.). St. Louis: Mosby Elsevier.

Morgan, J.E. (2007). Successful outcomes in vocational rehabilitation: The effects of stage of change and relational development. Doctoral dissertation: Brandeis University.

Mpofu, E. & Harley, D.A. (2006). Racial and disability identify: Implications for the career counseling of African Americans with disabilities. *Rehabilitation Counseling Bulletin, 50*(1), 14–23.

Nadash, P., & Feldman, P.H. (2003). The effectiveness of a "restorative" model of care for home care patients. *Home Healthcare Nurse, 21*(6), 421–423.

National Association for Home Care and Hospice (2007). Basic statistics about home care. Retrieved on November 28, 2007 from http://64.233.167.104/search?q=cache:p4PBbH6VpgcJ:www.nahc.org/facts/07HC_Stats. pdf+statistics+on+home+care+visits+2007&hl=en&ct=clnk&cd=1&gl=us

National Cancer Institute. (2007). Rehabilitation. Retrieved on December 8, 2007 from www.cancer.gov/Templates/db_alpha.aspx?CdrID=441257e

National Center for Chronic Disease Prevention and Health Promotion, Centers for Disease Control and Prevention (2007). Quick facts: Economic and health burden of chronic disease. Retrieved on [date] from www.cdc.gov/nccdphp/press/#4.

National Clearing House of Rehabilitation Training Materials (2007). Multicultural catalog. Retrieved on [date] from http://ncrtm.org/.

National Organization on Disability (2004). Executive summary of the 2000 N.O.D./Harris survey of Americans with disabilities. Retrieved on [date] from www.nod.org

Neal, L.J. (2001). Using rehabilitation theory to teach medical-surgical nursing to undergraduate students. *Rehabilitation Nursing, 26*(2), 72–75, 77.

Nelson, W. (2004). Addressing rural ethics issues. The characteristics of rural healthcare settings pose unique ethical challenges. *Healthcare Executive, 19*(4), 36–37.

Niemeier, J.P., Burnett D.M., & Whitaker D.A. (2003). Cultural competence in the multidisciplinary rehabilitation setting: Are we falling short of meeting needs? *Archives of Physical Medicine and Rehabilitation, 84*(8), 1240–1245.

O'Neill, J. H., Zuger, R.R., Fields, A., Fraser, R., & Pruce, T. (2004). The program without walls: Innovative approach to state agency vocational rehabilitation of persons with traumatic brain injury. *Archives of Physical Medicine and Rehabilitation, 85*(4), S68–72.

Ostchega, Y., Harris, T., Hirsch, R., Parsons, V. Kingston, R. & Katzoff, M(2000). The prevalence of functional limitations and disability in older persons in the U.S.: Data from the National Health and Nutrition Examination Survey III. *Journal of the American Geriatrics Society, 48*, 1132–1135.

Osterweil, D. (1990). Geriatric rehabilitation in the long-term care institutional setting. In B. Kemp, K. Brummel-Smith, & J. Ramsdell (Eds.). *Geriatric rehabilitation*, (pp. 347–456). Boston: Little, Brown.

Parker, B. J. & Neal-Boylan, L. (2007). Community and family-centered rehabilitation nursing. In K.L. Mauk (Ed.). *The specialty practice of rehabilitation nursing: A core curriculum*, (pp. 13–26). Glenview, IL: Association of Rehabilitation Nurses.

People Living with Cancer (2006). Rehabilitation. Retrieved on December 1, 2007 from http://www.cancer.net/patient/Survivorship/Rehabilitation/#mainContent.idmainContent

Pierce, L.L., Steiner, V., Hicks, B., & Holzaepfel, A.L. (2006). Problems of new caregivers of persons with stroke. *Rehabilitation Nursing, 31*(4), 166–172.

Pierce, L. Steiner, V., Govoni, A., Hicks, B., Thompson, T. & Friedemann, M. (2004). Caring-Web Internet-based support for rural caregivers of persons with stroke show promise. *Rehabilitation Nursing, 29*(3), 95–99, 103.

Plassman, B. L. et al. (2007). Prevalence of dementia in the United States: The aging, demographics, and memory study. *Neuroepidemiology, 29*, 125–132.

Podsiadlo, D, & Richardson S. (1991). The timed "Up & Go": A test of basic functional mobility for frail elderly persons. *Journal of the American Geriatric Society, 39*, 142–148.

Pryor, J. (2002). Rehabilitative nursing: A core nursing function across all settings. *Collegian, 9*(2), 11–15.

Reichard A., Sacco T.M., & Turnbull H.R. 3rd. (2004). Access to health care for individuals with developmental disabilities from minority backgrounds. *Mental Retardation, 42*(6), 459–470.

Rehabilitation Services Administration. (2007). About RSA. Retreived on December 9, 2007 from www.ed.gov/about/offices/list/osers/rsa/about.html.

Remsburg, R., & Carson, B. (2006). Rehabilitation. In Lubkin, I. & Larsen, P. (Eds.). *Chronic illness: Impact and interventions*, (pp. 579–616). Sudbury, MA: Jones & Bartlett.

Remsburg, R. (2004). Restorative Care Activities. In B. Resnick (Ed.). *Restorative care nursing for older adults: A guide for all care settings* (pp. 74–95). New York: Springer.

Remsburg, R., Armacost, K., Radu, C., & Bennett, R. (1999). Comparison of two models of restorative care in the nursing home. *Geriatric Nursing, 20*(6), 321–326.

Remsburg, R., Armacost, K., Radu, C., & Bennett, R. (2001). Impact of a restorative care program in the nursing home. *Educational Gerontology: An International Journal, 27*, 261–280.

Resnick, B., & Fleishell, A. (2002). Developing a restorative care program: A five-step approach that involves the resident. *American Journal of Nursing, 102*(7), 91–95.

Resnick, B., & Remsburg, R. (2004). Overview of restorative care. In B. Resnick (Ed.). *Restorative care nursing for older adults: A guide for all care settings*, (pp. 1–12). New York: Springer.

Routasalo, P., Arve, S., & Lauri, S. (2004). Geriatric rehabilitation nursing: Developing a model. *International Journal of Nursing Practice, 10*(5), 207–215.

Royal Hospital for Neuro-disability. (2007). Definitions of rehabilitation. Retrieved on December 8, 2007 from www.rhn.org.uk/institute/doc.asp?catid=213&docid=208.

Rusk, H. (1965). Preventive Medicine, curative medicine—The rehabilitation. *New Physician, 59*(4), 156–160.

Santerre, R.E. (2002). The inequity of Medicaid reimbursement in the United States. *Applied Health Economics and Health Policy, 1*(1), 25–32.

Schulz, R., & Beach, S. (1999). Caregiving as a risk factor for mortality: The caregiver health effects study. *Journal of the American Medical Association, 282*(23), 2215–2219.

Secrest, J.A. & Zeller, R. (2007). The relationship of continuity and discontinuity, functional ability, depression, and quality of life over time in stroke survivors. *Rehabilitation Nursing, 32*(4), 158–164.

Secrest, J.A. (2007). Rehabilitation and rehabilitation nursing. In K. Mauk (Ed.). *The specialty practice of rehabilitation nursing: A core curriculum* (5th ed.) (pp. 2–12). Glenview, IL: Association of Rehabilitation Nurses.

Secrest, J. & Thomas, S.P. (1999). Continuity and discontinuity: The quality of life following stroke. *Rehabilitation Nursing, 24*(6), 240–246.

Secrest, J., & Zeller, R. (2003). Measuring continuity and discontinuity following stroke. *Journal of Nursing Scholarship, 35*(3), 243–249.

Shah, S.K. (2005). Cardiac rehabilitation. In J. DeLisa & B.M. Gans (Eds.). *Rehabilitation medicine: Principles and practice* (3rd ed.) (pp. 1811–1842). Philadelphia: Lippincott-Raven.

Shanks, L.C., Moore, S.M., & Zeller, R.A. (2007). Predictors of cardiac rehabilitation initiation. *Rehabilitation Nursing, 32*(4), 152–157.

Shaw, W., Patterson, T., Ziegler, M., Dimsdale, J., et al. (1999). Accelerated risk of hypertensive blood pressure recordings among Alzheimer caregivers. *Journal of Psychosomatic Medicine, 43*(3), 215–227.

Shirey, L., & Summer, L. (2000). *Caregiving: Helping the elderly with activity limitations. Challenges for the 21st century: Chronic and disabling conditions.* National Academy on An Aging Society, Washington, DC.

Singh, V.N., Williams, K., & Stamey, R. (2004). Cardiac rehabilitation. EMedicine. Retrieved on [December 2, 2007] from www.emedicine.com/pmr/topic180.htm

Ski, C. & O'Connell, B. (2007). Stroke: The increasing complexity of carer needs. *Journal of Neuroscience Nursing, 39*(3), 172–179.

Social Security Online (2007). Supplemental Security Income. Retrieved on [date] from www.ssa.gov/pubs/11000.html#part3.

Stuart, H. (2006, September). Mental illness and employment discrimination. *Current Opinion in Psychiatry, 5*, 522–526.

Targett, P., Wehman, P., & Young, C. (2004). Return to work for persons with spinal cord injury: Designing work supports. *Neurorehabilitation. 19* (2), 131–139.

Thompson, T.L, Emrich, K., & Moore, G. (2003). The effect of curriculum on the attitudes of nursing students toward disability. *Rehabilitation Nursing, 28*(1), 27–30.

Uniform Data System for Medical Rehabilitation. (1997). FIM™ Instrument. University at Buffalo, Buffalo, NY, 14214.

Minority Business Development Agency. (1999). Dynamic diversity: Projected changes in U.S. race and ethic composition 1995 to 2050. Retrieved from http://www.mbda.gov/?section_id=6&bucket_id=16&content_id=3195U.S. Census Bureau, Housing and Household Economic Statistics Division. (2004). Health insurance coverage: 2003. Retrieved on [date] from www.census.gov/hhes/www/hlthins/hlthin03.html

U.S. Department of Education (2005). Office of Special Education and Rehabilitation Services. Rehabilitation Services Administration. Retrieved on [date] from http://www.ed.gov/about/offices/list/osers/index.html U.S. Department of Health and Human Services (DHHS) & The Agency for Health Quality and Research (AHRQ). (2003). The National Health Disparities Report. Retrieved on [date] from http://qualitytools.ahrq.gov/disparitiesreport/download_report.aspx

U.S. Equal Opportunity Employment Commission. (2006). Americans with Disabilities Act. Retrieved on [June 1, 2006] from www.eeoc.gov/types/ada.html

Vargo, M.M., & Gerber, L.H. (2005). Rehabilitation for patients with cancer diagnoses. In J. DeLisa and B. Gans (Eds.). *Physical medicine and rehabilitation: Principles and practice* (4th ed.) (pp. 1771–1794). Philadelphia: Lippincott Williams & Wilkins.

Verville, R., & DeLisa, J.A. (2001). The evolution of Medicare financing policy for graduate medical education and implications for PM&R: A commentary. *Archives of Physical Medicine and Rehabilitation, 82*(4), 558–562.

Walsh, N.E., Dumitru, D., Schoenfeld, L.S., & Ramaurthy, S. (2005). Treatment of the patient with chronic pain. In J. DeLisa and B. Gans (Eds.). *Physical medicine and rehabilitation: Principles and practice* (4th ed.) (pp. 493–530). Philadelphia: Lippincott Williams & Wilkins.

Ward, A.B. & Gutenbrunner, C. (2006). Physical and rehabilitation medicine in Europe. *Journal of Rehabilitation Medicine, 38*, 81–86.

Weitzenkamp, D., Gerhart, K., Charlifue, S., Whiteneck, G., & Savic, G. (1997). Spouses of spinal cord injury survivors: The added impact of caregiving. *Archives of Physical Medicine and Rehabilitation, 78*(8), 822–827.

Whyte, J. (1998). Enabling America: A report from the Institute of Medicine on rehabilitation science and engineering. *Archives of Physical Medicine and Rehabilitation, 79*(11), 1477–1480.

World Health Organization. (1980). International classification of impairments, disabilities and handicaps. Geneva: WHO.

World Health Organization. (2002).Towards a common language for functioning, disability and health ICF. Retrieved on January 31, 2002 from: http://www.who.int/classifications/icf/en

World Health Organization. (2007). International Classification of Functioning, Disability, and Health. Classifications. Retrieved on December 5, 2007 from http://www.who.int/classifications/icf/en

Worsowicz, G. M, Stewart, D. G., Phillips, E.M, & Cifu, D.X. (2004) Geriatric Rehabilitation. Social and economic implications of aging. *Archives of Physical Medicine and Rehabilitation, 85*(Suppl 3), S3–6.

Wu, H., Wang, J., Cacioppo, J., Glaser, R., Kiecolt-Glaser, J.K., & Malarkey, W.B.(1999). Chronic stress associated with spousal caregiving of patients with Alzheimer's dementia is associated with down-regulation of B-lymphocyte GH mRNA. *Journal of Gerontology A Biologic Science/Medical Science, 54*(4), M212–215.

Yip, K. & Ng, Y. (2002). Chinese cultural dynamics of unemployability of male adults with psychiatric disabilities in Hong Kong. *Psychiatric Rehabilitation Journal, 26*(2), 197–202.

Yu, F. (2005). Factors affecting outpatient rehabilitation outcomes in elders. *Journal of Nursing Scholarship*. Retrieved on November 1, 2006 from www.blackwellpublishing.com/journals/jns.

Zola, I.K. (1982). *Disincentives to independent living.* Lawrence, KS: Research and Training Center on Independent Living, University of Kansas.